Developments in Psychiatry in India

Savita Malhotra · Subho Chakrabarti
Editors

Developments in Psychiatry in India

Clinical, Research and Policy Perspectives

Springer

Editors
Savita Malhotra
Department of Psychiatry
Postgraduate Institute of Medical Education and Research (PGIMER)
Chandigarh
India

Subho Chakrabarti
Department of Psychiatry
Postgraduate Institute of Medical Education and Research (PGIMER)
Chandigarh
India

ISBN 978-81-322-1673-5 ISBN 978-81-322-1674-2 (eBook)
DOI 10.1007/978-81-322-1674-2

Library of Congress Control Number: 2014958454

Springer New Delhi Heidelberg New York Dordrecht London

Printed on acid-free paper

Springer (India) Pvt. Ltd. is part of Springer Science+Business Media (www.springer.com)

Preface

Developments in psychiatry in India can be referenced to the progress in the field of psychiatry since India's independence, as in the pre-independence era psychiatric services were not only rudimentary, but were also not meant for the treatment and care of the masses. Patients suffering from major mental illnesses, who were too disturbed to be kept within the confines of their homes, needed to be secluded behind the walls of mental hospitals, built outside the city limits. Moreover, there were no training centres for the speciality of psychiatry at that time in India. The first generation of psychiatrists trained abroad, mostly in the UK, established departments of psychiatry in post-independence India, which became the prime centres of psychiatric education. One such department of psychiatry was started in 1963 in the Post Graduate Institute of Medical Education and Research (PGIMER) at Chandigarh, which became a leading centre for postgraduate education in psychiatry, acquiring national and international recognition within a short time, for excellence in the standard of education and research. The alumni of this department are spread over the length and breadth of India and the world, occupying high positions, leading many academic departments and institutes of psychiatry for many years, setting them apart from others by their sheer class and quality. As a group they are a force to reckon with for the quantum and quality of research done by them, and their individual scholarship that is recognized in India and the world. It is these members of the department of psychiatry at PGIMER, Chandigarh, who have come together to author this book, writing perspective papers on subjects to which they have devoted their significant time and energy. Most of them are authorities in their own subjects with seminal contributions to the world literature. The quality of their work, their professional competence and intellectual prowess bear a stamp of the department, in which they were mentored.

The idea of this book emerged during planning for the golden jubilee celebrations of the department in 2013, and was taken up enthusiastically by one and all. There was a large list of possible contributors, out of which only a few could be included due to the constraints of time and the volume size. Therefore, this volume is a tribute to 50 years of research and practice at the department of psychiatry, which has spearheaded most developments in the field in post-independence India.

Psychiatry in India has taken rapid strides since the time of independence. Research has tried to keep pace both with changes in the society, as well as developments in the subject across the world. To encompass all the advances made in the field of clinical, research and policy aspects of psychiatry in India in a single book is a daunting task. It is simply not possible to do justice to the many developments which have taken place in diverse areas of the discipline. Nevertheless, if one were to draw a common thread linking the chapters in this book, it would be the developments in the major subspecialities of psychiatry in India. Therefore, this book has been mainly organized to highlight the developments in general adult psychiatry, child psychiatry, substance use psychiatry, community psychiatry, liaison psychiatry and other subspecialities. In addition developments in related fields, such as psychology and psychodynamics, advances in treatment, and the progress made in legal and educational aspects, have also been emphasized.

Professor Wig's chapter on "The beginnings of psychiatry in India" provides an appropriate anchoring point for viewing these advances and judging how far we have come. The book is also meant to be a bridge between a traditional textbook and one solely on policy and research developments. Thus, all chapters while encapsulating the research data and policy imperatives of a particular area continue to have a decidedly clinical and practical emphasis. We hope that these contributions by stalwarts in their particular field, which are documented in this book, will give us a sense of pride and achievement in what has been achieved. However, the time has not come yet to rest on our laurels. As chapter after chapter in this book demonstrates, there are far too many ills and shortcomings afflicting the practice of psychiatry in India. In this regard, we hope this book will provide some inspiration to those who are dedicating themselves to the cure and care of the mentally ill in India every day of their lives.

We are extremely grateful to all the authors for accepting our request to contribute to this book, and for their painstaking effort in the submission of their chapters. We are also grateful to Springer (India) Private Limited for agreeing to publish this volume within the deadline. It was a great honour and pleasure to work with all the lead authors and our co-alumni. This work would not have been possible without their unquestioning cooperation and commitment.

All the authors in the list of contributors, except for two stalwarts, namely Prof. N.N. Wig and Prof. V.K. Varma, have been the teachers of the other contributors, who have been their students. Prof. Wig and Prof. Varma together built and shaped the department, which has produced generations of students. They occupy a position of highest esteem in the minds of all their ex-students. Graduates from the department have been either taught directly by them, or indirectly by their students.

We consider ourselves highly privileged to have had the opportunity to be trained under the tutelage of Prof. Wig and Prof. Varma. It gives us immense pleasure to dedicate this book to them.

Savita Malhotra
Subho Chakrabarti

Contents

Editors and Contributors

About the Editors

Subho Chakrabarti is Professor of Psychiatry at the Post Graduate Institute of Medical Educational and Research (PGIMER), Chandigarh. He has clinical, teaching and research experience of over 22 years. He has been a Fellow of the Royal College of Psychiatrists, U.K., Fellow of the International Society for Affective Disorders, Fellow of the Indian Psychiatric Society, Fellow of the Indian Association of Social Psychiatry and Member of the National Academy of Medical Sciences, India. Professor Chakrabarti has received 15 national and international awards for best paper or best presentation. He is a member of the editorial board of five national and international journals and member of the Expert Working Group on Mood and Anxiety Disorders for the Revision of ICD-10 Mental and Behavioural Disorders, WHO, Department of Mental Health and Substance Abuse. He has around 170 national and international publications, over 100 of which are indexed in the Index Medicus.

Savita Malhotra is Head of the Child and Adolescent Psychiatry Services at the Department of Psychiatry, Post Graduate Institute of Medical Educational and Research (PGIMER), Chandigarh, India. She is a recipient of the D.L.N. Murthy Rao Oration Award, Bhagwat Award, PPA 1 Award, Bombay Psychiatric Society Silver Jubilee Year Award of the Indian Psychiatric Society; Tilak Venkoba Rao Award of the Indian Council of Medical Research; and WHO Fellowship in Child Mental Health. She has also received the Dr. K.L. Wig Oration Award of the National Academy of Medical Sciences. She is a Life Fellow of the Indian Association for Social Psychiatry and of the Indian Association for Child and Adolescent Mental Health. Professor Malhotra has been actively involved with several national and international societies and organisations: Indian Association for Social Psychiatry (Past President); Indian Association for Child and Adolescent Mental Health (Life President); International Association for Child and Adolescent Psychiatry and Allied Professions (Assistant Secretary

General and Adjunct Secretary); Member and Consultant Education Committee of the World Psychiatric Association; and Temporary Advisor, World Health Organisation, in the past. She is President Elect of the Asian Society for Child and Adolescent Psychiatry and Allied Professions, and Board Member of the Child Psychiatry Section of WPA. She has published over 200 research papers and book chapters and authored/edited several books.

Contributors

A. Avasthi Department of Psychiatry, Postgraduate Institute of Medical Education and Research, Chandigarh, India

S. Balachander Department of Psychiatry, Postgraduate Institute of Medical Education and Research (PGIMER), Chandigarh, India

D. Basu Drug de-Addiction and Treatment Centre, Department of Psychiatry, Postgraduate Institute of Medical Education and Research (PGIMER), Chandigarh, India

R.V. Behere Department of Psychiatry, Kasturba Medical College, Manipal, Karnataka, India

P.B. Behere Department of Psychiatry, Jawaharlal Nehru Medical College, Datta Meghe Institute of Medical Sciences, Wardha, Maharashtra, India

A.P. Behere Department of Child and Adolescent Psychiatry, Mid Coast Mental Health Centre, Rockland, ME, USA; Pen Bay Psychiatry, Belfast, ME, USA

M.C. Bhise Department of Psychiatry, MGM'S Medical College, Aurangabad, Aurangabad, Maharashtra, India

R.K. Chadda Department of Psychiatry, All India Institute of Medical Sciences, New Delhi, India

S.K. Chaturvedi Department of Psychiatry, National Institute of Mental Health and Neurosciences, Bangalore, India

B.S. Chavan Department of Psychiatry, Government Medical College and Hospital, Chandigarh, India

S. Das Department of Psychiatry, Government Medical College and Hospital, Chandigarh, India

K. Deka Department of Psychiatry, Assam Medical College, Dibrugarh, India

Pravin Dullur University of New South Wales, Sydney, NSW, Australia

A. Ghosh Department of Psychiatry, Postgraduate Institute of Medical Education and Research (PGIMER), Chandigarh, India

S.C. Girimaji Department of Child and Adolescent Psychiatry, National Institute of Mental Health and Neurosciences, Bengaluru, India

Sandeep Grover Department of Psychiatry, Postgraduate Institute of Medical Education and Research (PGIMER), Chandigarh, India

R. Gupta Department of Psychiatry, Pt. B.D. Sharma PGIMS, Rohtak, Haryana, India; Pt. B.D Sharma University of Health Sciences, Rohtak, Haryana, India

R.C. Jiloha Department of Psychiatry, Maulana Azad Medical College and G.B. Pant Hospital, New Delhi, India

Natasha Kate Department of Psychiatry, Postgraduate Institute of Medical Education and Research (PGIMER), Chandigarh, India

Sudhir K. Khandelwal Department of Psychiatry, All India Institute of Medical Sciences, New Delhi, India

H. Khurana Department of Psychiatry, Pt. B.D. Sharma PGIMS, Rohtak, Haryana, India; Pt. B.D Sharma University of Health Sciences, Rohtak, Haryana, India

A. Kohli Department of Psychiatry, Postgraduate Institute of Medical Education and Research, Chandigarh, India

Parmanand Kulhara Fortis Healthcare, Chandigarh, India; Department of Psychiatry, Postgraduate Institute of Medical Education and Research (PGIMER), Chandigarh, India

S. Mahajan Clinical Psychology, Postgraduate Institute of Medical Education and Research, Chandigarh, India

Savita Malhotra Department of Psychiatry, Postgraduate Institute of Medical Education and Research, Chandigarh, India

S.K. Mattoo Department of Psychiatry, Postgraduate Institute of Medical Education and Research, Chandigarh, India

M. Mehta Department of Psychiatry, All India Institute of Medical Sciences, New Delhi, India

R.S. Murthy Department of Psychiatry, National Institute of Mental Health and Neurosciences, Bangalore, India; Association for the Mentally Challenged, Bangalore, India

U.S. Naik Department of Psychiatry, Osmania Medical College, Hyderabad, India

R. Nehra Clinical Psychology, Postgraduate Institute of Medical Education and Research, Chandigarh, India

S.K. Padhy Department of Psychiatry, Postgraduate Institute of Medical Education and Research, Chandigarh, India

B. Patra Department of Psychiatry, Postgraduate Institute of Medical Education and Research (PGIMER), Chandigarh, India

Raman Deep Pattanayak Department of Psychiatry, All India Institute of Medical Sciences, New Delhi, India

B.K. Pradhan Assistant Professor of Child, Adolescent and Adult Psychiatry, Cooper University Hospital and Cooper Medical School of Rowan University, Camden, NJ, USA

S.K. Praharaj Department of Psychiatry, Kasturba Medical College, Manipal, Karnataka, India

R. Sagar Department of Psychiatry, All India Institute of Medical Sciences, New Delhi, India

S. Sarkar Department of Psychiatry, Postgraduate Institute of Medical Education and Research, Chandigarh, India

V.K. Sharma International Health Development, University of Chester, Chester, UK; Early Intervention in Psychosis Services, Cheshire and Wirral Partnership NHS Trust, Chester, UK

P.S.V.N. Sharma Department of Psychiatry, Kasturba Medical College, Manipal, Karnataka, India

A. Singh Department of Psychiatry, Postgraduate Institute of Medical Education and Research, Chandigarh, India

P.K. Singh Department of Psychiatry, Patna Medical College, Patna, India

S.M. Singh Department of Psychiatry, Postgraduate Institute of Medical Education and Research, Chandigarh, India

S.P. Singh Mental Health and Wellbeing, Warwick Medical School, University of Warwick, Coventry, UK

B.N. Subodh Drug de-Addiction and Treatment Centre, Department of Psychiatry, Postgraduate Institute of Medical Education and Research (PGIMER), Chandigarh, India

V.K. Varma Department of Psychiatry, Postgraduate Institute of Medical Education and Research, Chandigarh, India

S.K. Verma Clinical Psychology, Department of Psychiatry, Postgraduate Institute of Medical Education and Research, Chandigarh, India

N.N. Wig Department of Psychiatry, Postgraduate Institute of Medical Education and Research, Chandigarh, India

Part I
The History of Psychiatry in India

Chapter 1
The Beginnings of Psychiatry in India

N.N. Wig

1 Introduction

The history of psychiatry in India since independence is essentially the story of how psychiatry has largely come out of mental hospitals and has gradually become a part of mainstream medicine. This is a remarkable change, and in a way, it is a new beginning of psychiatry in India. It is also noteworthy that India has been in the forefront of this movement, at least in the developing world. Hence, in this chapter, my focus will be mainly on how psychiatry has reached this present position. I may have to clarify right at the beginning that history is a continuous process, and divisions of time are only arbitrary lines to understand the whole process better. The mental hospital movement of the colonial period was a very important phase and has given shape and structure to modern psychiatry. However, mental hospital care, which was developed originally in Europe, when applied to Indian conditions, turned out to be a very expensive and a wasteful method of care for the mentally ill requiring large spaces and buildings with large multi-layered staff. Worse still, this system of care further isolated mentally ill away from society without any significant medical benefit. All over the world, services in such isolated mental hospitals gradually tend to deteriorate and become depersonalised and dehumanised. It was much worse in India and other developing countries with very limited financial resources and trained manpower, and a very different cultural background from Europe. The focus of mental hospitals was always on very serious psychiatric conditions such as psychosis or dementia. This further reinforced the stigma against

N.N. Wig, Emeritus Professor

N.N. Wig (✉)
Department of Psychiatry, Postgraduate Institute of Medical Education and Research, Chandigarh, India
e-mail: wignn@yahoo.co.in

S. Malhotra and S. Chakrabarti (eds.), *Developments in Psychiatry in India*,
DOI 10.1007/978-81-322-1674-2_1

mental disorders. Persons with lesser forms of psychotic illness and other common psychiatric disorders, which are so widespread in the community, were generally left out of this system of modern medical care.

Mental hospitals have of course, not totally outlived their utility and usefulness. Many of them are still playing a very useful role in the long-term care of disturbed and chronically mentally ill, especially with criminal and legal background. In Indian settings, some of the hospitals have completely transformed themselves into modern academic institutions such as the National Institute of Mental Health and Neurosciences (NIMHANS), Bangalore, the Central Institute of Psychiatry (CIP), Ranchi, or the Institute of Human Behaviour and Allied Sciences (IHBAS), Delhi, and are playing a very significant role in service, training and research. However, the fact remains that in the second decade of twenty-first century, the bulk of psychiatric patient care in government, private or voluntary sectors is now outside mental hospitals, through general hospital psychiatric units (GHPUs), private clinics, primary care centres and non-governmental organisation (NGO) run services. Similarly, while 50 years ago, training of mental health professionals was confined to few mental hospital-based institutes such as the NIMHANS, Bangalore, and the CIP, Ranchi, now the bulk of training programmes has moved to autonomous medical institutes such as the Postgraduate Institute of Medical Education and Research (PGIMER), Chandigarh, the All India Institute of Medical Sciences (AIIMS), New Delhi, and various major medical colleges in Lucknow, Vellore, Mumbai, Kolkata, Chennai and other big cities. It has changed the whole atmosphere of psychiatric training with proximity to, and interaction with other medical disciplines. Psychiatric research has gained equally by this transformation. While the traditional mental hospitals had very little scope or incentive for research, the newer academic departments in medical institutes and medical colleges are producing much more relevant and valuable research, and also winning recognition in many national and international forums.

2 A Review of Literature on History of Psychiatry in India

I do not plan to go into great details of pre-colonial and colonial periods of history of psychiatry in India, mainly because this subject has been amply covered in many previous articles. Nizamie and Goyal (2010) have written a comprehensive article on the ‘History of psychiatry in India’ in the Indian Journal of Psychiatry. (In fact, I have borrowed the terms, ‘Psychiatry in pre-colonial, colonial and independent India’ from that article, which I acknowledge with thanks). There is an equally good article by Parkar, Dawani and Apte in Journal of Postgraduate Medicine in 2001 (Parkar et al. 2001). A very comprehensive article titled ‘The history of modern psychiatry in India 1857–1947’ by James Mills, a chapter in a book ‘History of Psychiatry’ published by Sage in 2001, is an outstanding piece of research and is worth reading by anyone who is interested in this subject (Mills 2001). While the history of psychiatry in colonial period is well covered in all the above references, my own personal favourite is the article (in two parts) ‘History of psychiatry in India and Pakistan' by Dr. L.P. Varma in the Indian Journal of Psychiatry in 1953, then called Indian Journal of Neurology and Psychiatry (Varma 1953). This is a remarkable article on the history of Indian psychiatry, especially when one keeps in mind that this was being written for the first time by an Indian psychiatrist in an Indian Journal. The article is comprehensive, very well researched (with nearly one hundred references) along with scholarly and insightful comments by late Dr. L.P. Varma who was then First Assistant Superintendent at the Indian Mental Hospital, Kanke, Ranchi and also the Editor of the Journal. The Indian Psychiatric Society from time to time has also covered the subject of history in many of its conferences, souvenirs and journal supplements. One outstanding contribution in recent years has been the issue called 'Icons of Indian psychiatry' brought out by Indian Journal of Psychiatry in 2010 under the leadership of its editor, Rao (2010). It is an excellent volume on history of psychiatry in India, highlighting the contributions by various pioneers from different regions who are no more.

The Directorate General of Health Services, Ministry of Health and Family Welfare, New Delhi has also brought out an excellent book on 'Mental Health—An Indian Perspective 1946–2003' (Agarwal et al. 2003). It contains some very good articles on historical aspects by authors such as D.S. Goel, S.D. Sharma, M. Sarada Menon and others. It has some very interesting appendices, including excerpts from the famous Bhore Committee Report (1946) containing the sections related to mental health. It also has the detailed report by Col. Taylor describing his visits to all the mental hospitals in India at that time, and highly unsatisfactory conditions encountered there (Taylor 1946).

3 Psychiatry During Pre-colonial Period in India

Abnormalities of human behaviour have been known and recognised since the beginning of civilisation all over the world. While it is true that modern science, medicine and psychiatry came to India along with the colonial powers, it does not mean there was no recognition or no methods of treatment and care of the mentally ill in India before that. Both the Ayurveda and Unani systems of medicine, which were widely practiced for hundreds of years in the country, had extensive discourses on signs and symptoms of various types of mental disorders and their management. In the indigenous herbal pharmacopoeia, there were powerful remedies such as opium, cannabis, 'Sarpgandha' and Brahmi, which have been relevant even in modern times. However, at that time, the knowledge of modern anatomy, physiology or pathological changes in brain was rudimentary, and humoral theories such as disturbance of 'Kaph, Pit and Vayu' were the main basis of diagnosis and management. Apart from herbal medicines, religious rituals and faith healing practices were widely prevalent for the treatment of mentally ill. There was, however, one significant difference between pre-colonial and post-colonial periods. While there were no formal asylums or mental hospitals for the care of seriously mentally ill in pre-colonial India, they sprung up with regular frequency during the British colonial period and became the main feature of psychiatry in colonial days. In fact, there was hardly any other psychiatry outside mental hospitals in the European system of medicine for a long time, while the Ayurveda and Unani systems still continued to offer help for various forms of common psychological conditions. Indian medical systems also recognised variations in personality and temperaments. Religious practices such as meditation and yoga were regularly used for psychological treatment, which is gradually being re-incorporated in the modern psychiatry now.

4 Psychiatry During Colonial Period

As is well known, the term 'psychiatry' was coined by Johann Christian Reil in Germany in the year 1808. This is to the credit of Reil that he did not see psychiatry as merely a speciality dealing with 'diagnosis and treatment of mental disorders', but visualised psychiatry as a broad clinical approach utilising psychological knowledge and methods for all medical disorders. Unfortunately, despite Reil's broad vision, the term psychiatry remained limited to diagnosis and management of serious mental disorders such as psychosis, dementia or severe mental retardation. This is particularly true of the development of psychiatry during the colonial period of the eighteenth and nineteenth centuries in British India, when asylums or mental hospitals were the main centres for its practice.

As Dr. L.P. Varma has rightly observed in 1953, 'The history of psychiatry in this country is the history of establishment of mental hospitals and then increasing its accommodation from time to time as the exigencies of the time demanded'. From 1787, when the first regular government asylum was opened in Kolkata for the next one and half century, nothing much was happening in psychiatry, except the opening of mental asylums (as they were then called) in different provinces of the British Raj, such as Bengal, Madras, Bombay, Bihar, U.P. and Punjab. In the beginning, asylums were meant for European patients only. In 1795, for the first time, an asylum was opened in Monghyr, Bihar for Indian sepoys. Gradually, the pressure built up for the use of asylums for civilian population as well.

The story of these asylums is very similar. In the beginning, the space for a 'lunatic asylum' was any old, abandoned building or army barracks. Gradually, new buildings with open spaces and with grounds were provided. Tall boundary wall erected to protect the inmates, or to prevent their escape, was another universal feature. The subsequent history is a sad one. Almost every asylum would open with great hope and expectations, but within a few years, there would be overcrowding, neglect, paucity of staff and resources, combined with almost total indifference of authorities and civil society. Occasionally, there would be some inspection, which would result in scathing reports of neglect and squalor. Some efforts at improvement would follow, followed by another round of neglect and deterioration. In fact, this pattern of neglect, indifference, reforms and again gradual neglect and indifference has continued with regular frequency in most of the mental hospitals in the country till this day, except perhaps, with the exception of some mental hospitals which have turned into academic institutes such as the

NIMHANS, Bangalore, the CIP, Ranchi, or the IHBAS, Delhi, with huge inputs of resources and manpower.

For historical record, it is important to mention some of the landmark events during this period.

(1) After the 1857 Mutiny, the rule of the East India Company ended and direct rule by British Crown was established in India in 1858. The Indian Penal Code drafted earlier by the famous Lord Macaulay was promulgated. One of the provisions in this act was 'authorisation and establishment of asylums for reception and detention of lunatics'.
(2) Till 1905, all lunatic asylums were under the charge of civil surgeons. In 1905, for the first time, some asylums were designated as 'Central Asylums' and placed under the separate charge of an 'Alienist' (this was the name for mental specialists at that time). This was perhaps the first step for the recognition of psychiatry as a separate speciality in this country. There was also an attempt by then Secretary of State in England, John Morley, to establish a separate 'Alienist Department' in India, but this was never realised (Varma 1953).
(3) The year 1912 was a landmark in the history of psychiatry, when the Indian Lunacy Act was passed. Asylums became independent of the general medical administration, and rules for reception and detention were clearly codified.
(4) In the year 1922, the names of all asylums were changed to 'Mental Hospitals'.
(5) Some hospitals remained strictly for the use of Europeans and Anglo-Indians only, e.g. the European Mental Hospital Ranchi, or the Colaba Mental Hospital in Bombay. The Ranchi hospital made a big concession in 1940, when 10 beds were provided for 'Indian paying patients of European habits' (Varma 1953).
(6) Mental Hospital, Bangalore established in 1937 was the first mental hospital in India which avoided high enclosures.

5 Psychiatry After the Independence of India (Till 1960)

Though it is true that the rise of psychiatry as a modern medical speciality largely occurred after the independence of the country in 1947, some of the developments, which significantly influenced this, were already taking place two or three decades before that. One can identify at least three major developments which have given shape to modern psychiatry in independent India. These are as follows:

(1) The rise of psychoanalysis as an intellectual discipline with its impact on psychology, medicine, literature and arts.
(2) Developments in military psychiatry during the World War II, resulting in rapid increase in number of army psychiatrists and treatment facilities outside mental hospitals.
(3) Recommendations of the famous 'Bhore Committee' to provide health services near the people, away from big hospitals. Perhaps out of the three events, the most significant influence on the progress of psychiatry was of the Bhore Committee Report (1946), and we would consider it first.

6 Impact of the Bhore Committee Recommendations

The Bhore Committee Report (1946) was undoubtedly one of the momentous events in the history of the public health movement in India. Even after nearly seventy years of its publication, one continues to marvel at the vision and foresight of its deliberations and recommendations. Much has been written about it over the years. Its emphasis on the importance of primary health care, before developing secondary and tertiary services in the country, has changed the shape of our health services ever since.

Somehow the impact of the Bhore Committee Report on the subsequent developments in psychiatry in India has not received sufficient attention in psychiatric literature. One honourable exception is the chapter 'Mental Health: The pre-independence scenario' by S.D. Sharma in Ministry of Health book 'Mental Health. An Indian Perspective 1946–2003', where he has not only referred to the Bhore Committee Report, but has also included the whole mental health section of the report in the appendix (Sharma 2003).

7 Some of the Important Recommendations of Bhore Committee on Mental Health

The opening sentence of the mental health section sets the tone of the whole report, i.e. *The physical and mental health of an individual are inter-related and no health programme can be considered complete without adequate provision for the treatment of mental ill health and for the promotion of positive mental health.* It is sobering to note that the pioneers of the Bhore Committee in 1946 had already thought that there is no health without mental health, which has become such a popular slogan now in the documents of the Royal College of Psychiatrists and the World Health Organisation (WHO).

Other notable features of the report were:

- Prevention of mental illness and promotion of mental health receive equal emphasis in the report along with the treatment of mental disorders
- The proposals for mental health in the Bhore Committee Report begin by stating *In our view the most important step to be taken, is the formulation of a mental health programme for the country after preliminary investigation of the needs of the individual provinces.* It is sad that it took nearly forty years to develop a National Mental Health Programme (in 1982) in India.
- The Bhore Committee recommended creation of a mental health organisation in the Directorate of Health Services. It finally happened in the shape of National Advisory Committee on Mental Health in the 1980s.
- The Bhore Committee strongly recommended facilities for the training of mental health professionals in India, which resulted in the formation of All India Institute of Mental Health in Bangalore in 1954 (now the NIMHANS).

- It recommended establishment of the AIIMS in New Delhi, where it further recommended undergraduate and postgraduate training in psychiatry and also promotion of research. In a way, this recommendation provided a strong impetus for emergence of GHPUs in all medical colleges in the later years.
- The Bhore Committee was very critical of the existing state of mental hospitals in the country. It strongly recommended their rapid improvement, but felt that mental hospitals alone were grossly inadequate for the total mental health needs of the country.

8 Impact of the Psychoanalysis Movement

Dr. Girindrasekhar Bose would always be remembered for starting the first Indian Psychoanalytical Society in Kolkata in 1922. By that time, psychoanalysis was already making waves in the intellectual life of people in Europe and the USA. Despite strong criticism from some quarters, people were fascinated by its bold theories of the subconscious mind to explain the psychological basis of both normal and abnormal behaviour. The movement soon spread to Bombay where Dr. K.K. Masani was an early pioneer. In Ranchi, Col. Berkley Hill, started the Indian Association of Mental Hygiene and was also closely associated with Psychoanalytical Association in Calcutta. Many universities started courses on psychoanalysis; the popular press and literary magazines were also writing articles on the subject. Hollywood in the USA was also greatly influenced by psychoanalysis movement. A number of movies incorporated the new knowledge of psychoanalytical theories. One memorable film in 1945 was 'Spellbound', a suspense thriller directed by famous director, Alfred Hitchcock. The hero Gregory Peck is a patient with amnesia who is being treated by a lady psychoanalyst, played by Ingrid Bergman. There was a much talked about dream sequence, which had the clue to the hero's amnesia. The sets for this dream sequence were designed by the great surrealist painter of his time, Salvador Dali.

In this liberal atmosphere of the time, many young men and women medical doctors in India were also attracted to psychoanalysis. Psychoanalysis helped to give a new image to psychiatrists. Instead of being a *doctor for the insane,* here was a chance to become a *doctor who understands the mysteries of conscious and subconscious mind.* It was indeed a big shift in the social status of psychiatrists. A number of the top names in Indian psychiatry, who started their career in the 1950s and early 1960s (including the present author), seem to have been inspired by psychoanalysis to take up psychiatry as a career. For example, a pioneer of Indian psychiatry, Dr. Ajita Chakraborty, told me that she had undergone personal analysis in Kolkata, before taking up her distinguished career in psychiatry. Dr. D.N. Nandy was also closely associated with the Psychoanalysis Association in Calcutta. Dr. J.S. Neki, another stalwart of Indian psychiatry, told me that he went to NIMHANS Bangalore in 1956 and joined the Diploma course in Medical Psychology with the hope of learning psychoanalysis. Later, as advised by his teachers he shifted to regular Diploma in Psychological Medicine (DPM) course for medical doctors. The late Doctor Ravi Kapur was also greatly attracted to psychoanalysis and psychotherapy. The list can be easily increased by adding many other names, but the main point, which emerges is that psychoanalysis motivated many early psychiatric pioneers in India.

9 Early Women Psychiatrists of India

In this context, it is also noteworthy that during the 1950s, soon after independence, a number of women doctors came forward to take up psychiatry as their chosen career, which was not common till that time. Even in the first batch of DPM students in Bangalore, there was a woman doctor. All these early women psychiatrists, of course, played a pioneering role in modernising psychiatry in India and have left a powerful impact on it. Some of the well-known names of such early distinguished women psychiatrists are Dr. Ajita Chakraborty, Dr. Sharda Menon, Dr. Roshan Master and Dr. Jaya Nagaraja, who have all made the profession proud by their contributions.

10 Impact of Military Psychiatry

Another area, which deserves a better recognition in the history of Indian psychiatry, is the role of military psychiatry. A large number of early pioneers who have changed the shape of modern psychiatry in India belonged at some time to the Indian Army. Some of these distinguished psychiatrists were Col. M. Taylor, Col. O. Berkley Hill, Major R.B. Davis, Col. Kirpal Singh, Major Vidya Sagar, Major K.C. Dube and many others like them. Recently, Brig. Prabhu has written an excellent article on 'Military psychiatry in India', in which he has provided detailed information, particularly of the period during the World War II (Prabhu 2010). It is a striking fact that at the start of the world war in 1939, these were only four psychiatric specialists in the Indian Military Service. The number rose to 10 in 1942, 31 in 1943 and 86 by end of the war in 1945. How did this phenomenal increase occur and how was this achieved? The need was urgently felt because it was realised that apart from battle wounds, a large number of casualties among the soldiers were psychological in nature, and existing medical services were not adequate to handle it. To rapidly train the medical officers in psychiatry, a short training of 2–4 months was introduced, which was later increased to 9–12 months, after which they were posted as graded specialists. The second important innovation introduced by military psychiatry was that the treatment of psychiatric patients was done not in mental hospitals, but in units resembling GHPUs of the present. A standard psychiatric ward used to have only 25 beds (Prabhu 2010). Looking back it seems that the war time experiences of military psychiatry had a great impact on the civil side after the independence of the country. A large number of senior psychiatrists such as Maj. Davis, Maj. Vidya Sagar, Major K.C. Dube and Capt. Chandorkar had moved to civil side. GHPUs, which flourished during 1960s, used the same Army model of a GHPU of earlier years. The community psychiatry movement of the 1970s also used the military psychiatry model of short training courses for different health professionals.

11 Summary and Conclusions

The rapid growth of psychiatric services after independence of India is a remarkable story of how psychiatry came out of mental hospitals and is now gradually becoming part of mainstream medicine. This paradigm shift took place due to numbers of factors. Most important was perhaps the vision and foresight of the Bhore Committee recommendations of opening of training centres for mental health professionals in the country, and starting of GHPUs in medical colleges and other big general hospitals. This gave a big boost to the development of modern psychiatry. A large number of bright young men and women got attracted to psychiatry as their career. The psychoanalysis movement added to the liberal intellectual attitude towards abnormalities of human behaviour, which further helped the growth of psychiatry as a medical speciality.

In this chapter, I have considered the events up to 1960 or so, but history is a continuous process. Psychiatry took rapid strides in the 1960s and 1970s, moving from mental hospitals to general hospitals and then attempting to provide community psychiatric services through the primary health-care network. This glorious journey must continue till we are able to ensure that the benefits of modern psychiatry are available to all citizens of India, rural or urban, rich or poor, men or women.

References

Agarwal, S. P., Goel, D. S., Ichpujani, R. L., Salhan, R. N., & Shrivastava, S. (2003). *Mental health. An Indian perspective 1946–2003*. New Delhi: Directorate General of Health Services Ministry of Health and Family Welfare.

Bhore Committee. (1946). *Health survey and development committee* (Vol. III). Simla: Government of India Press.

Mills, J. (2001). The history of modern psychiatry in India, 1858–1947. *History of Psychiatry, 12*, 431–458.

National Mental Health Programme for India (1982). New Delhi: Directorate General of Health Services, Ministry of Health and Family Welfare, Government of India.

Nizamie, H. S., & Goyal, N. (2010). History of psychiatry in India. *Indian Journal of Psychiatry, 52*(7), 7–12.

Parkar, S. R., Dawani, V. S., & Apte, J. S. (2001). History of psychiatry in India. *Journal of Postgraduate Medicine, 47*(1), 73–76.

Prabhu, H. R. A. (2010). Military psychiatry in India. *Indian Journal of Psychiatry, 52*(7), 314–316.

Rao, T. S. (2010). Icons of Indian psychiatry. *Indian Journal of Psychiatry, 52*(6), 5–212.

Sharma, S. D. (2003). Mental health: The pre-independence scenario. In S. P. Agarwal, D. S. Goel, R. L. Ichpujani, R. N. Salhan & S. Shrivastava (Eds.), *Mental health. An Indian perspective 1946–2003* (pp. 25–29). New Delhi: Directorate General of Health Services Ministry of Health and Family Welfare.

Taylor, M. (1946). *Report of the health survey and development committee* (Vol. III). Simla: Government of India Press.

Varma, L. P. (1953). History of psychiatry in India and Pakistan. *Indian Journal of Neurology and Psychiatry, 4*(1), 26–53.

Part II
Developments in Psychology and Psychodynamics

Chapter 2
Development of Psychological Testing in India

S.K. Verma

1 Introduction

When I joined the Department of Psychiatry at the Postgraduate Institute of Medical Education and Research (PGIMER), Chandigarh, many of the psychological tests used in most parts of the country suffered from several deficiencies, known and unknown till then. In fact, one cannot work in an area where the tools in use are deficient in many ways. If one has to work honestly in this area, one cannot hide behind these imperfect tools, without doing anything about it. Blaming the tools alone cannot help one for long, particularly, when this happens to be one's chosen field of work and worship. The God is everywhere, seeing everything and forgiving nothing.

But, before I name these deficiencies in tests in use then, I may be allowed to define an ideal test and mention its necessary characteristics. In all fairness, I must accept that no single psychological test can be considered as a perfect test for all types of populations, for all subjects and for all times to come. But, realising our own limitations in knowledge, wisdom and availability of time and resources, a psychological test has to have most of these desirable characteristics, while leaving scope for improvement in the future.

S.K. Verma, Former Additional Professor of Clinical Psychology

---

S.K. Verma (✉)
Clinical Psychology, Department of Psychiatry, Postgraduate Institute of Medical Education and Research, Chandigarh, India
e-mail: savita.pgi@gmail.com

S. Malhotra and S. Chakrabarti (eds.), *Developments in Psychiatry in India*,
DOI 10.1007/978-81-322-1674-2_2

2 Definitions

A psychological test is a standardised method of (a) comparing the behaviour of two or more persons at the same time and/or (b) comparing the behaviour of the same person in different periods of time.

A standard is that in terms of which we measure something, e.g. a gram, a litre, a mile, a rupee or an inch; measurement is attributing a number according to well-defined rules.

Behaviour includes both overt and covert behaviour, observed and expressed verbally and/or measured.

Standardisation is a process of exactly fixing the stimulus variables, the exact situation of administration and of observing the behaviour, in terms of well-defined units of measurement and the exact method of interpretation, in the light of relevant norms, having high reliability and validity.

Objectivity refers to freedom from subjective factors in administration, measurement and interpretation.

Reliability means consistency of scores over a period of time and consistency in administrative methods, administration by self or by others, the method used by scorers as well as the test's internal consistency. It makes one confident that every time a test is used, the same test is used and similar methods are used for administration, scoring and interpretation. Reliability can be of the total score, of various parts of the test or of every individual item. It is mostly measured in terms of coefficients of correlation, but can also be estimated in terms of percentage of agreement or disagreement.

Validity of a test shows whether a test measures what it purports to measure, e.g. a test may measure more than one aspects of behaviour, but one of them may be more specific.

Intelligence tests, for example, must measure intelligence in particular, but may also show the approach in solving a problem, a method of solving problems and how a person reacts to frustrations when difficulties arise while solving a problem. A personality test may also measure one or more aspects of personality, i.e. interest, attitude, preferences and aptitudes. A test is a valid measure of behaviour and may be valid for one aspect of behaviour only. The validities are also of different kinds: face validity, content validity, concurrent validity, construct validity, factorial validity and predictive validity.

Other features of validity of a test are as follows:

- A test is valid for something with which it correlates.
- Validity depends upon the reliability of the test. In fact, validity cannot exceed the under root of its reliability.
- A test may have different validities for different aspects of behaviours.

Norms have to be relevant and meaningful. Local norms have to be used for interpretation. Population, reliabilities and validities are defined by the standardisation process and must be given in the test manuals. Norms have to be specific with regard to location, age, sex, education and all other significant variables likely to influence test scores, reported or not reported so far.

Test manuals should ideally provide all the above information. No test can be culture free and culturally fair unless it is proved, reported and defined. Manuals can also provide cross-validation data, if and when available. That is why a test can be revised and has to be revised after sometime, in order to remain a valid and reliable measure over time.

3 Drawbacks or Deficiencies of Psychological Tests

The following drawbacks were most prominent when I joined the department in 1968:

- Most tests used were in English language only, and on-the-spot translations were being done on the bedside of patients in the general hospital setting. Uniform Hindi translations were needed, with local norms for use with them.
- Patients were illiterate or barely literate and unsophisticated in the use of tests. Some of them were even so frustrated that they were ready to give their thumb impressions, in place of responding to test items.
- Foreign norms were being used while scoring and interpreting the test scores, whereas there was the need to prepare local and relevant norms for use with our patient population.
- The tests used were too time consuming in terms of length of items, e.g. nearly 200 in the General Medical Index Health Questionnaire or the CMI Health Questionnaire (Erdmann Jr. et al. 1952) and 60 in Standard Progressive Matrices (Raven et al. 1998). The language used in Hindi versions of personality tests was complicated, with difficult words, e.g. "*ashrupat*" for tears in the eyes, as in the Hindi Personality Trait Inventory (Verma et al. 1990).
- Tests in simple Hindi were not available, which were constructed using patients' own symptoms with their own expressions, and for which, local norms were available or which could be used at all educational levels.
- A need for modifications of some tests was felt, but no constructive and useful work was done, and at best, only lip service was paid. The problems were noted, but nothing was done to address them. There was a scope for construction of tests in many areas, but much needed work was missing in the absence of a team of clinical psychologists devoted to this work wholeheartedly.
- In a few areas, e.g. Bhatia's battery of performance tests of intelligence in India (Bhatia 1955), where useful, constructive work was done with separate scoring systems for literate and illiterate subjects, there was lack of follow-up work with revision of the scoring system and revision of norms from different parts of the country.
- In addition to the above drawbacks, the attitude of the so-called experts from Indian universities was deplorable, to say the least, because test construction was looked down upon even for a PhD work. In my personal experience, while doing my PhD, the "experts" made one excuse after another for it—such as "It is not sufficient work for PhD" to even saying "One PhD is not sufficient for test construction, or "Test construction in India is not accepted for PhD," or "Only in

North India some universities have accepted a few PhDs in test construction," or "There is nothing original in test construction." Even when evidence to the contrary was available, such excuses continued to be made.

I was lucky enough to have Prof. Wig (who accepted my arguments and allowed me to continue my PhD work) who accepted to be my supervisor and encouraged me to continue my experiments. (That is why I call him my godfather.)

- These "experts", when I approached them for guidance or advice, were of the opinion that we should adopt standardised tests from the West and use them with our population to solve any research problem, a piece of advice, which I could not and did not follow, for obvious reasons. I was too junior a researcher, so I bowed my head in silence, but continued my work, the only way open to me at that time. I do not know what kept me going in those early years, despite the continued opposition by my seniors, colleagues and juniors, both psychiatrists and clinical psychologists, in this Department of Psychiatry (not of Clinical Psychology). But looking back over the years, I can name a few possible "reasons" for it.
- I saw construction of psychological test as writing beautiful poems as a hobby, enjoying the process, as my way of worship to the "God of Measurement", if there is any. (If others can worship other Gods or Goddesses such as *Brahma, Vishnu, Mahesh, Lakshmi or Saraswati*, why cannot I have my own God and worship Him.)
- I had read somewhere the definition of morale (given by a veteran soldier) as "Morale is what keeps your feet going while your head says it can't".
- So I bowed my head and like a good student, started doing my work, as a worship in order to please him (i.e. the God of Measurement), to shower His invisible blessings (no matter if it is seen or appreciated by others or not). To be able to do one's preferred work, is its own reward and can never be replaced by any other award or reward.
- Appeal of my heart—"Do not give up before doing your best, no matter what the consequences". So I did continue my work as worship, on a war footing, if I can call it that.
- My father's advice—"Whenever in difficult circumstances, bow your head in silent prayer and start doing what you think is right, without caring what others say or do". My late father often referred to his own example—when he started his own work as a dentist, people made fun of a dentist as a mere tooth puller, as one who is destined to end up on the road calling people for repairing their broken teeth. But, he never gave up and ended as one of the leading dentists in the city of Varanasi at the time.
- Never-ending faith of my late wife in my ability to overcome my shortcomings, my difficulties and be successful in the end. This moral support proved to be of great help, whenever I happened to be in low spirits and seeing faces of my own children, as if asking me "Water water everywhere nor any drop to drink" (Coleridge in his "Rime of the Ancient Mariner"), as to what messages would my life and efforts leave behind, for them to follow. ("Keep your head above the sea level, in order to survive and win".)

- It is rightly said that "All is well that ends well". At the start of my professional career, opposition to my views was the rule; this was gradually converted into active cooperation by all concerned, from all parts of the country. My prayers were being answered after all and in my life time.
- When there were other PhDs, not only by clinical psychologists but also by psychiatrists of the department, it was more than I could ever expect or imagine or live to see.

In this regard, I must gratefully acknowledge the significant contribution of other fellow clinical psychologists, particularly of Dr. Dwarka Pershad, Ex. Additional Professor of Clinical Psychology, Department of Psychiatry. Indirect encouragement to our efforts was soon available in the form of a few national awards for such tests from professional bodies, including one by the Indian Psychiatric Society, and my own nomination to advisory bodies and editorial boards of various journals in the country. I admit here once again the full and constant support of Professor Wig, without which I would have left this great department long ago. Last but not the least was indirect factors such as constructive criticism by eminent professionals, foremost among them were Prof. N.N. Sen, Prof. G.G. Prabhu and Prof. J.S. Neki, and international authorities on tests such as Prof. H.J. Eysenck, Prof. R.B. Cattell and Prof. Guilford.

4 Our Contributions

Our contribution in this area has to be seen as an insignificant and tiny effort, in the universe of a vast area of research and possibilities. Doing something (however small it might be) is better than doing nothing in the area of construction of psychological tests. I had read somewhere (in a different context though) that:

> A piece of bread is better than nothing.
> Nothing is better than God.
> So, a piece of bread is better than God.

If I may be forgiven, I would like to replace "a piece of bread" by a psychological test in this statement.

Similarly, in another context I have read:

> O God, if there is a God.
> Save my soul, if there is a soul.

If I may be forgiven, I would like to put it as:

> O God of Measurement, if there is a God of Measurement. Accept our small offerings (tests as flowers); if they can be offered and be accepted.

We are not sure (at least I am not sure) that what we have attempted to do in the field of psychological tests would make a difference to the world of measurement and be accepted as such. I have read somewhere—"A difference that makes no difference is no difference".

To put it a little differently, I would like to make the following modified statement as—If a psychological test constructed by us in simple Hindi, for use with our population, majority of which consists of illiterates, barely literates, rural and unsophisticated people is better than a well-standardised Western test for use with their populations when used in India, without doing any modifications, it would make a difference to be called a real difference, in the end. On the other hand, if it does not make any difference, I would most humbly be ready to bow my head to be sacrificed.

5 A Start to Meet the Problems Faced

In order to meet the problems faced by us, we started with assessing the extent of the problems one by one and finding solutions that were available, practical and within our resources.

The first problem I faced was the length of the items in the test, particularly in the CMI Questionnaire (Erdmann Jr. et al. 1952). It was used in English with spot translation in Hindi. It contained nearly 200 items referring to different bodily systems and psychological complaints (A–L for physical section and M–R for psychological symptoms, with A–R referring to total complaints). We attempted to translate it in Hindi, so that the same language could be used with every patient. This took care of uniformity of the items, from tester to tester, and over time.

Another related difficulty arose with regard to the total scores. With the spot translations of English version, perhaps our patients could not relate to their problem correctly and did not endorse many items.

Patients' relative positions with regard to the scores remained the same (as shown by the coefficients of correlation between English and Hindi versions remaining high), but the average score significantly increased with the Hindi version. This justified our attempt at developing a Hindi version, as patients could actually feel that the item really described their own difficulties or problems, versus the exact, literal, on the spot translation as attempted earlier.

Another issue was whether so many items were really required or whether the same results could be achieved by fewer items, which were more reliable and valid. So, item analysis was begun, to find out which items were readily accepted (frequently endorsed) by many patients, as opposed to others, which were rarely (it at all) endorsed by non-patients and patients (patients with both medical and psychiatric problems).

Those items that had zero or nearly zero percentage of endorsement were excluded in order to prepare a shorter version of the scale in simple Hindi.

When literature search for item construction was done, it was found that illiterate or barely literate people related better to items when expressed in first person (I, me, my versus you, your). In the English version, as well as in spot-translated Hindi version, the items were asked in the second person only, e.g. every time the items were "do you have" this or that problem. A need was felt for using first-person expressions in these questions. This shortened and simplified the statements (in place of questions), with the common question at the top asking them to tick the items applicable to them. Thus, the question form was converted into statement form to make it easier, simpler, shorter and quicker, taking less time to complete the test, while it still remained questionnaire (i.e. tick those items that are correct for you).

The "thinking aloud method" was used to make items short, simple and easily comprehensible by our patients. Each item was read aloud, and any difficulties that may be arisen in the patient's mind were addressed to remove all ambiguity, if any, found in expressions. When required, that ambiguity was removed by modifying the item structure, replacing difficult words by its simplest form, without sacrificing the meaning. This critical self-examination was a necessary evil, which proved quite useful in the end.

A cross-cultural examination was done on items with at least 10 % of endorsements, and system-wise comparisons were done.

It was found that our clinic population endorsed more items relating to gastro intestinal problems and of general weakness, as compared to Western cultures, where the systems involved were cardiovascular and respiratory. Keeping this in mind, item selection was done accordingly. All this research was based on different studies, which were published in professional journals.

Thus, the shortened version of the CMI, modified according our own needs, consisting of 38 items was developed. Section A was physical section consisting of 22 items corresponding to A–L section of the CMI, and divided into Sections A and B. Section B was related to M–R section of the CMI and consisted of mental or psychological items. A provision for a total score consisting of all the 38 items was also. This scale was called as PGI Health Questionnaire N-1 (Verma et al. 1985).

This PGI Health Questionnaire N-1 was presented at one of the annual conferences of the Indian Psychiatric Society and won the prestigious Marfatia Award.

This provided much needed confirmation of rightfulness of our efforts and encouraged us to follow the same line in future also.

6 Continuation of the Work

As the next step, we collected the chief complaints of our patients, describing their complaints, in their own words and in Hindi. This was made possible by Prof Wig's foresight and direction to all (staff and students of the Department) to write in verbatim the chief complaints in Hindi, even before translating them. I collected all these complaints for 2 years and put them in proper order and saw to it that all types of patients, male and female, rural and urban, of all age groups, of all educational levels and all types of "neurotic" patients were included in this sample. The next step was to put similar complaints together and select the simplest and most comprehensive expression to represent the group. Fifty items were thus selected in this way. This formed the N-Scale, and we defined "neuroticism as a tendency to develop neurotic symptoms when under stress". Items were numbered 1–50, and the scale was called as PGI HQ N-2. A new scale consisting of 10 lie items was added to this N-2 scale, after a lot of research with "too-good-to-be-true items" selected from the original EPI Lie scale and the PEN scales of H.J. Eysenck, who had taken them from original MMPI scale of Hathway and Mackinley of Minessota (Eysenck and Eysenck 1964; Hathaway and McKinley 1940). These items were translated into simple Hindi and used in number of studies using modified instructions to test for different response biases and selecting tendency to measure social desirability response set (or the "Lie scale"). It was used with the neuroticism scale PGI HQ N-2 (Wig and Verma 1979).

In order to distinguish these "too-good-to-be-true" items from neurotic symptoms, these were kept as separate and numbered 51–60. Thus, the PGI HQ N-2 consisted of 60 items in all. Reliabilities and validity of this new scale were established. It was also cross-validated against samples drawn from psychiatric units, from all parts of India. This scale was constructed and standardised and formed subject matter of my PhD, the first PhD of the department.

The two scales N and L of the PGI HQ. N-2 were found to have low correlation, indicating the freedom from the social desirability response set of this neuroticism scale. These N-scores were found to have positive and significant correlations with other measures of neuroticism existing at the time, when used with English-speaking educated samples (who could take tests in both languages). This confirmed that this N-measure had good validity. N-1 and N-2 showed good correlation as expected. Another quality of these tests (N-1 and N-2) was their low difficulty levels as compared to many other personality tests in Hindi. A research paper published on difficulty levels of some personality tests used in India written by me got a good mention in a Presidential Address in Indian Science Congress (psychology section), and this was sent to Professor Wig. It confirmed that we were on the right track and this was being recognised by senior psychologists of the country. By the way, I would like to mention here that this publication (paper on difficulty levels) was published in Indian Journal of Clinical Psychology. I was elected as editor of this journal in 1974 and was re-elected four times (1974–1983). This was all because of our contribution in this area of psychological testing.

7 Measures of Difficulty Levels in Personality Tests

Here, a mention needs to be made, as to how difficulty levels can be measured and what could be the units of its measurement, so that tests consisting of different length of items could be compared. In test of intelligence, it is done easily by comparing the pass percentage of items, where an easy item is one passed by almost all the subjects, and most difficult item as the one that very few or none could pass. In a personality test (there are no right answers to be called as pass), the difficulty levels can be judged in the following ways:

- The number of words used in a test per 100 items (i.e. in percentages calculated) or the number of letters per 100 items (as unit of measurement). It takes time to read each item, to comprehend each item and to respond thereafter. The assumption being that longer the sentence, it would take relatively longer time and would more difficult. (In fact, we rarely used only one test for each subject e.g. one intelligence test, one questionnaire, one projective test, one memory test and one test for perceptuo-motor function. One had to choose among many tests; hence, one chose short, less difficult tests.)

- The total time taken (greater the time taken, more difficult would be the test).
- The number of difficult words per 100 items. It had to be rated as "difficult" (defined in their own way) by the same group of experts, to be unbiased in rating different tests. This is called the "underlining test", i.e. underlining "difficult" words.
- Instead of each item making a fresh start, if items are gone through in a quick succession, they would be called easy items. The arrangement of items was such that it made it easy to pass through a lot of items in quick succession, e.g. items, starting with "I", could be put together, those with "my" in another group and those with "we" together in a third group.
- Tests could be ranked on each of these criteria, so that the lower the rank number, easier it would be. When ranked in this way, we found our own tests were the least difficult ones, on all these criteria, when comparison was made with other tests.

8 Measurement of Response Biases

Another scale constructed by me was for measuring response biases such as the following:

- Tendency to choose the first response choice, in the list of response choices; for example, in yes/no choice list, it is yes, while in the list of no/yes, it is no more frequently selected. This is independent of the question or statement. Surprisingly, it was found that the same person selects the first response, even when the same question is being asked a second time, but in reverse order, hence indicating the response bias.
- Tendency to choose the extreme responses. This can be seen, where, in a list of choices, extreme ones are selected, e.g. either one is extremely happy or, extremely unhappy, never in between. This shows a response bias.
- Tendency to choose the middle most responses. When people do not agree with extreme responses, when they are not sure whether to agree or disagree, they feel safer by avoiding extreme responses and choosing the middle response instead. This shows a feeling of insecurity.
- Tendency to choose either all positive responses or all negative ones. Those well-adjusted, satisfied persons or maladjusted, dissatisfied persons tend to choose such one-sided responses.

Thus, whenever a particular bias is shown in a test, one is confident that the responses of the person do not correspond to the question or statement. In other words, the responses are independent of the content of the items, hence are untrustworthy and cannot be accepted as true responses.

A scale was prepared where there were no questions or statements—but only responses were given. It is called rightly as "The questionnaire without questions". Here, there were no random answers; otherwise, all response choices would be equally selected as responses by a group of subjects. Deviation from equal chance probability to a significant extent was considered as a "response tendency" for a person or for a group.

The Lie scale used in the PGI HQN-2 was one such a measure, indicating a tendency to give socially desirable responses. A high lie score, thus, indicated the unreliability of N-score in a given situation, by a specific group of subjects.

This was shown to be the case in a number of experimental conditions, where a significant bias was induced by specific directions (e.g. in interviews for jobs or interviews for a decision for compensation).

Matching of normal and neurotic groups:

The "neurotic" group was selected on the basis of case identification in the psychiatric clinics, while the normal group was selected mainly from the relatives or attendants of these patients. The idea behind this was the assumption that both would be from the same or similar socio-economic background and hence would be well matched. In addition, these groups were also matched on relevant socio-economic variables such as age, sex, education and rural or urban residence. This was necessary for meaningful comparison of test scores.

9 The PGI Memory Scale

My esteemed professional colleague, Dr. Dwarka Pershad, wanted to construct a battery of memory scales for use with our clinic population. He started at first with well-known batteries such as the Wechsler Memory Scales and the Boston Memory Scales.

Both were in English and had foreign norms, but were used in our country with spot translations and with varied success, reported and unreported. The limitations were quite apparent, and a need was soon felt for developing our own memory scales in simple Hindi and to develop our own norms, for use with our clinic population, who were mostly illiterate or barely literate, rural and unsophisticated people.

Selecting various areas of measuring memory, he started experimenting with various subjects which included the following:

- General information and personal data for recent memory.
- Areas for recent and remote past.
- Attention span.
- Memory for words and sentences.
- New learning for new unrelated pair of words.
- Recognition of simple designs.
- Retention for old, familiar words.

He, thus, collected material for his battery of memory scales in 10 such areas and formed a battery called PGI Battery of Memory Scale for clinic population (Pershad and Wig 1977; Pershad and Verma 1990).

All those items were in simple Hindi. Experimenting with different time intervals, he finalised standard times for exposure of stimulus material and the time gap before reproduction/recognition of those stimulus materials. Percentile scores were used, and a profile of scores for differentiating between normal and organic cases was generated.

Finding that obtained scores varied significantly with educational levels, and Dr. Pershad decided to develop separate norms for three educational levels:

- 0–5 years of schooling,
- 6–9 years of schooling and
- Above 10 years of schooling.

This was done for the first time in the field of psychological testing in our country and won recognition for Dr. Pershad and for the department, in the field of psychiatry in India. This battery of memory scales was for his PhD work under the guidance of Prof. Wig. This was another major contribution of the department in the field of psychological testing.

10 A Beginning of Teamwork

We (I and Dr. Dwarka Pershad) worked together for the construction of reliable and valid tools for our clinic population, and significant among them were as follows:

- Modified shorter version of Bhatias' battery of performance tests of intelligence (B.B.P.T.). In this pioneering work of Dr. C.M. Bhatia, in the construction of the battery of performance tests, there were many significant contributions such as the following:
  - Separate norms for illiterates—used for the first time in India.
  - Large sample of students, 11–16 years of age, from different areas of Uttar Pradesh.
  - It consisted of 5 subjects—viz. Kohs' Block Design Test, Alexanders Pass—Along Test, Digit Span Test (for literates but alphabets for illiterates), Picture Completion Test and Picture Construction Tests.

We found some good points in it, but also some drawbacks:

- Test norms were more than 15 years old and needed revision.
- Scoring was limited to 1 min or 2 min only, requiring wider range of scoring for greater reliability.
- Extending norms for adult groups also. Means and standard deviations were computed.
- Norms for three educational groups and for different age levels.

When we approached Dr. C.M. Bhatia, he readily agreed for us to carry out the necessary modifications, which we did and published our results in the form of a practice manual. We used deviant IQ directly calculated from the raw scores.

- WAIS-R verbal scales in Hindi. After obtaining the necessary permission from the author and publisher, we selected few verbal scales such as Information, Digit Span, Arithmetic and Comprehension for translation in Hindi and administered them to normal population in different age and education groups. Data were collected from other centres in India such as Agra, Baroda, Bikaner and Ahmadabad with the help of co-investigators there. After calculating means and standard deviations for each education groups, deviant IQs were obtained directly from the raw scores.

This was the deviation from the original method used. This information was given in the manual concerned.

- PGI Battery of Brain Dysfunctions. It consisted of a number of subjects such as the PGI Memory Scale, Bhatias' Short Scale of performance test of intelligence and WAIS-R verbal scales in Hindi. The information about its construction, administration, standardisation reliability, validity and normative data is given in the manual published. Measures of visuo-motor functions were also added after doing research on the BVMG test, the Nahar and Benson scale, and the Hoopers Visual Organization Test (VOT). Dysfunctional Analysis Questionnaire (D.A.Q.) was also prepared to assess the deviation from previous functioning (i.e. before the illness started). Norms for the Standard Progressive Matrices were also established for different age and education groups using deviant IQs (Pershad and Verma 1990).

11 Other Scales or Tests Developed

A number of new psychological tools were prepared and used for research carried out for PhD degrees in the department (including those of other departments where guidance was provided by clinical psychologist of our department).

These include the following:

- A schedule for measuring temperament in children (Savita Malhotra).
- A childhood psychopathology measurement schedule (Savita Malhotra).
- Parental handling questionnaire (Savita Malhotra).
- Psychoticism scale in Hindi (Manju Mehta).
- PGI locus of control scale (D.K. Menon).
- PGI achievement value India (D.K. Menon).
- A shorter way to assess the IQ (Adarsh Kohli).
- Scale for assessment of attitude towards yoga (Poonam Grover).
- Medication attitude scale (Poonam Grover).
- Maternal attitude and maternal adjustment scale (Karobi Das).
- A scale for personality disorders (Pratap Sharan).

- A coping checklist (Ritu Nehra).
- Social support questionnaire (Ritu Nehra).
- Paediatric development screening test (Amita Puri).
- Home based-programme for MR children (Mala Seshadri).

Other psychological tests constructed or used in revised forms for MD thesis, for funded (from WHO, I.C.M.R., I.C.S.S.R. and PGI research schemes) and non-funded departmental projects include the following:

- PGI General Well-Being Scale.
- PGI Quality of Life Scale.
- PGI Job Satisfaction Scale.
- PGI Battery of Assessment of Mental Efficiency in the Elderly.
- Hindi Personality Trait Inventory.
- Bond's Defence Style Questionnaire.
- Learned Helplessness Scale.
- Hope Scale.
- Pleasure Scale.
- Sensation Seeking Scale.
- SPD Scale.
- Sex Knowledge and Attitude Scale.
- Geriatric Depression Scale.
- Eating Attitude Scale.
- Psychiatric Disability scale.
- Relapse Precipitant Inventory.
- Self-efficacy Scale.
- Alienation Scale.
- Cognitive Behaviour Scale.
- Vignettes for Attitudinal Research.
- Hindi MPI Scale.
- Authoritarian Scale.
- Tests for Linguistic Competence.
- Illness Behaviour Questionnaire.
- PGI sentence completion tests—Forms G (General)
  - Form M (Married individuals).
  - Form S (Students).

- Social Burden Scale.
- Family Burden Scale.
- Home Environment Scale.

Projective tests:

A number of projective tests were devised/used, and normative studies conducted on them:

- Draw-a-Person Test—Body Image Concept of Students.
- Body Image Disturbances of Psychiatric Patients.

- Body Image Disturbances of Patients Undergoing Cardiac Surgery.
- Sack's Sentence Completion Test (Hindi).
- Indian Adaptation of T.A.T. (Story-making test).
- Rosenzweig Picture—Frustration Study (Indian adaptation).
  - For adults.
  - For children.
- For studying attitudes of patients:
  - Standard stories were used (vignettes) depicting various illnesses.
  - Standard pictures depicting various psychiatric disorders.

Both these were constructed and used in the department.

- Word Association Test.
- Rorschach Test—(Indian Norms, modified instructions).
- Somatic Inkblot Series.
  - Booklet Form.
  - Card Form.

Indian norms and reliability studies were devised for the following:

- Three Wishes Test.
- Projective Question—(If reborn—what animal you would like to be—and why).
- Draw a Person—Practice Manual and Norms.

12 Manuals

Construction and standardisation of psychological tests is one thing, writing useful and practical manuals, complete in all respects, making it ready for use by other researchers, throughout the country is equally important. This was taken care of by us working in the department. The details are as follows:
Publishers:

A. National Psychological Corporation, Agra.

- Manual for PGI Health Questionnaire N-1 in Hindi (1985).
- Manual for measurement of dysfunction and Dysfunction Analysis Questionnaire (DAQ) in Hindi (1985).
- Abridged manual of CMI Health Questionnaire in Hindi (1983).
- Manual for Bhatia's Battery of Performance Tests of Intelligence (Short Scale) (1988).
- Concept and measurement of Intelligence (1988).
- Manual for Malhotras' Temperament Schedule (1988).
- PGI Battery of Brian Dysfunction (PGIBBD) (1990).
- Manual for PGI Battery for Assessment of Mental Efficiency in the elderly (PGI-AMEE) (1996).

- Draw a Person Tests Manual.
- Manual for ADHD.

B. Ankur Psychological Agency, Agra.

- Manual for PGI General Well-Being scale (Verma and Verma 1989).

C. Rupa Psychological Corporation, Varanasi.

- Manual for Hindi PEN Inventory (1988).
- Manual for PGI Locus of Control Scale (1988).
- Manual for PGI Achievement Value Index (1988).

An ideal test manual is expected to include standard stimulus content, ways to administer the test, way to score objectively, specific, local normative data and standardised method of interpretation, with established reliabilities and validities. All these should be open for inspection and acceptance or rejection. The concept itself has to be well-defined, meaningful and acceptable for critical evaluation by others, if they so desire and when they decide.

As such, things require a great deal of time and effort, and this is difficult for research workers working with limited resources available. This, however, is not an acceptable excuse for poor quality of products and for avoiding criticism. All criticism is healthy and motivates us to do more and better and hence should be welcomed with an open heart.

13 Science and Religion in Measurements

This brings us to look philosophically at the issue of relation between the science and religion and how this can help us in our work. There are many individual facts to be discovered. We cannot limit ourselves to discover facts alone, such as constructing psychological tools to find more and more scientific facts. It is rightly said that "those who refuse to go beyond facts rarely go as far as facts". Facts have to be linked together in a meaningful way and used for a purpose.

Whereas scientific methods help in collection of newer facts and tools to measure something, we have to pursue the search for their meaning and application religiously, like a determined devotee, trying to please the "God of Measurement".

In Hindu Philosophy, there are many Gods such as *Brahma* (for generation/creation), *Vishnu* (for protection), *Mahesh* (for destruction), Vayu Devta (for air), Agni Devta (forfire), Indra Devta (for rain) and *Yamraj* (for death). I may therefore be forgiven for introducing another god, the "God of Measurement", and I am willing to submit myself, all my work on measurement and construction for psychological tests to him. Each test can be visualised as flowers or fruits for offering to get his blessings.

The method is scientific, while the pursuit is religious, i.e. blindly and faithfully, with all our forces and resources applied to get scientific results. Each tool is like another *Brahmastra*, i.e. an instrument or weapon to get "good" results. The weapon should be prepared in a scientific way. The concept has to be clearly and unambiguously defined and religiously followed (with approved *mantras*) to get effective results (to achieve measurement of the concept). We are ready to face others' weapons (criticisms, challenges) with our *Brahmastra* (test scores). Both science and religion are involved. But for the collection of scientific facts, collected religiously, we would still believe that the earth is flat (not round), that sun moves around earth (not earth revolving around the sun), and that an atom is indivisible (not divisible into nucleus and sub-atomic particles).

The same thing is true about newer methods of measurements, and depending upon the newer facts discovered, we modify our tools, e.g. if difficulty levels of language create problems for those not properly educated, we use simpler language and prepare tests that can be used with all education levels, with local norms for different educational groups.

In the West, when Eysenck found the MPI was difficult for lower educational levels, a new test with simpler language, the EPI was constructed (Eysenck and Eysenck 1964), and when Cattell found that 16PF Test Forms A and B were posing problem with education levels, he constructed forms C and D, and even E and F making the language simpler (Cattell 1989).

Surprisingly, our so-called experts (university professors, used to working with highly educated people) denounced any such notion of difficulty levels and still preferred to use English tests as such, advocating their use with our clinic patients as well. We refused to accept the suggestions of "authorities", i.e. senior university professors, as science does not accept any authority, as science starts with doubts and ends with the valid proofs. Religion starts with only beliefs and refuses to accept doubts at any level. We went on using scientific methods religiously, refusing to bow down to the so-called authorities.

While future psychologists working in the department are free to work according to their own faith, in their own selected areas, to realise their own dreams, I would like to again point out my own rebellious attitude, against established authorities, in our more example as another attempt to justify my approach. It is a case of the Seguin Form Board Test. The original norms were devised by Cattell (in the Guide to Mental Testing), based on research done abroad. We were using those norms. A funded research, on large samples (over 500) in each of the three language groups in South India, published in a book form, suggested that children in our country were 20 % less efficient as found in their research. This was taken up as a challenge, and we found many facts that showed poor validity of their claims:

- This test was used by school teachers (not trained clinical psychologists), from school situated on roadsides, with lot of disturbance from continuous traffic (not in a psychology laboratory with no disturbance), and from class rooms, in the presence of other students.
- Standard procedures were not followed. For example, no practice trials were given before starting data collection. Use of preferred hand (right or left) was not strictly followed. Sometimes even both hands were used.
- Age of the children was not reliable (or reported in the book itself by the authors). Many children had the same date of birth filled up by school staff to

enable students get admission without any problem of age. Parents were not sure in most cases about the exact ages.

- Either no stop watch was used and/or the wrist watches were used in wrong manner.
- To "start" spoken aloud was to be taken as actual start of the work and not necessarily when the child actually starts. Most of the children were from rural background, not used to competition and did not realise the importance of doing the work as fast as possible.
- To "stop" was not noted, when the child had actually completed the task, but only when he/she verbally indicated. Many children were not sure when to stop and say I have done the work.

As this is a speed test of intelligence, the above factors had a significant role in influencing the test scores.

It was more a test of somehow compiling the data and not necessarily a test of real intelligence. Role of non-cognitive factors played a part, and results were wrongly interpreted as real slowness of Indian children. All these facts were reported in a paper—"Are Indian children slow?" published in the Child Psychiatry Quarterly (Verma et al. 1980).

This only shows that a common test does not necessarily mean the same test, if not used in a specified (standard) manner, as described in the test manual.

It also shows the importance of publishing test manuals in addition to test construction (to avoid wrong or hasty conclusions). Finally, the importance of religiously following test manuals for deriving or correcting interpretations scientifically was also demonstrated.

14 Concluding Remarks

It is good writing about my first and foremost love—i.e. psychological tests, in the area of measurement. People write their autobiographies to justify their past mistakes and leave it for others to give their judgments. So, writing about our psychological tests in use, I surrender myself before the God of Measurement and give ample opportunity to people who matter and time to give their thoughtful judgments about the quality, reasons and outputs of our department.

I was allowed to work with full devotion to achieve my aims and fulfil my dreams, for which I am indeed very grateful to the God of Measurement, to the Head of the Department, my seniors, colleagues and students of the department. Work is its own reward. There can be no greater reward than the satisfaction of doing ones' work honestly and sincerely, and if any mistakes are made in this process, I take the full responsibility for it.

Let those errors be recognised and corrective measures taken to improve them further. This is my hope and wish.

The journey towards making perfect psychological tests is an endless pilgrimage to reach the vague, undefined, abstract concept of God of Measurement. While the task is difficult, if not impossible, the journey is pleasurable for all the selfless devotees offering their lifetime work to it. So let us all enjoy. The journey continues. The procession is on. Like the normal probability curve, this curve approaches the baseline, but never touches the baseline. There is always a scope for hope, for better endings, by better or smarter people. After all, "God is in the Heaven; everything is right with the world, with the department and with the movement of psychological tests".

References

Bhatia, C. M. (1955). *Performance intelligence test battery*. Bombay: Oxford University Press.

Cattell, H. B. (1989). *The 16PF: Personality in depth*. Champaign, IL: Institute for Personality and Ability Testing Inc.

Erdmann, A. J, Jr, Brodman, K., Lorge, I., & Wolff, H. G. (1952). Cornell Medical Index-Health Questionnaire: v. Outpatient admitting department of a general hospital. *Journal of the American Medical Association, 149*(6), 550–551.

Eysenck, S. B. G., & Eysenck, H. J. (1964). An improved short questionnaire for the measurement of extraversion and neuroticism. *Life Sciences, 305*, 1103–1109.

Hathaway, S. R., & McKinley, J. C. (1940). A multiphasic personality schedule (Minnesota): I. Construction of the schedule. *Journal of Psychology, 10*, 249–254.

Pershad, D., & Wig, N. N. (1977). *The construction and standardization of clinical test of memory in simple Hindi*. Agra: National Psychological Corporation.

Pershad, D., & Verma, S. K. (1990). *Handbook of PGI battery of brain dysfunction*. Agra: National Psychological Corporation.

Raven, J. C., Court, J. H., & Raven, J. (1998). *Manual for Raven's standard progressive matrices*. Oxford, England: Oxford Psychologists Press.

Verma, S. K., Pershad, D., & Randhawa, A. (1980). Are Indian children slow? Report on enquiry with a speed measure of intelligence. *Child Psychiatry Quarterly, 13*(1), 67–71.

Verma, S. K., Wig, N. N., & Pershad, D. (1985). *Manual for PGI Health Questionnaire, N-1, a simple neuroticism scale in India*. Agra: National Psychological Corporation.

Verma, S. K., & Verma, A. (1989). *Manual for PGI general well-being measure*. Lucknow: Ankur Psychological Agency.

Verma, S. K., Pershad, D., & Mahajan, A. (1990). Hindi translation of Personality Trait Inventory. *The Creative Psychologist, 2*(1), 23–26.

Wig, N. N., & Verma, S. K. (1979). *Construction and standardization of PGI Health Questionnaire N2*. Agra: Agra Psychological Research Cell.

Chapter 3
Psychometry as an Adjunct to Psychiatry: An Indian Perspective

R. Nehra, S. Sarkar and S. Mahajan

1 Introduction

Like other branches of medicine, psychiatric practice is benefitted by diagnostic tests to supplement the clinical examination and case formulation (Rapaport 1950). Diagnostic assessment in psychiatry is the process of appraising the patient's condition, and psychometry can serve as a vital adjunct to the process of diagnostic assessment and management (Venkatesan 2010). Psychometry involves research related to the construction of instruments and procedures for measurement, and the development and refinement of theoretical approaches to mental measurements. It includes measurement of knowledge, skills, abilities, aptitudes, attitudes, intelligence, memory, creativity, adjustment and personality. The field uses measuring instruments like questionnaires, schedules, inventories, checklists and objective performance tests to make inferences.

More recently, psychometry is also being applied to measure beliefs, interests, motivation, academic achievement and health-related issues. A related concept clinimetrics refers to the application of psychometric tests to psychiatric practice. Psychodiagnostics is another related phrase that refers to the process of psychological evaluation (Verma and Nehra 1997) and has two components: psychological evaluation and diagnosis.

The process of psychodiagnostics includes both qualitative and quantitative assessment and has diagnostic, prognostic and therapeutic implications.

Psychometric testing is not synonymous with psychological assessment as the latter is a broader, more encompassing term. Psychometric testing refers to a process

R. Nehra, Additional Professor of Clinical Psychology; S. Sarkar, Senior Resident; S. Mahajan, Senior Resident

R. Nehra (✉) · S. Sarkar · S. Mahajan
Clinical Psychology, Postgraduate Institute of Medical Education and Research, Chandigarh, India
e-mail: ritu_nehra@rediffmail.com

S. Malhotra and S. Chakrabarti (eds.), *Developments in Psychiatry in India*,
DOI 10.1007/978-81-322-1674-2_3

wherein a particular scale is administered to obtain a specific score, and a descriptive meaning is applied to the score on the basis of normative, nomothetic findings. In contrast, psychological assessment is concerned with the clinician taking the test scores in the context of the history, referral information and behavioural observations to understand the patient as a whole and to relevantly answer the referral question.

It is a difficult task to classify psychometric tests, because there are a great variety of such tests, each with differences in domains looked into, the assessment protocol, requirements of instruments, scoring procedures and interpretation of results. For the sake of simplicity, we have classified the psychometric tests into tests of intelligence, neuropsychological tests and tests of personality characteristics. The representative tests are depicted in Table 1.

Table 1 Some representative psychometric tests

Intelligence tests
Verbal Adult Intelligence Scale (VAIS)
Bhatia Battery of Performance Tests of Intelligence (BBPT)
Malin's Intelligence Scale for Indian Children (MISIC)
Vineland social maturity scale (VSMS)
Gessell's Drawing Test (GDT)
Stanford-Binet Test (SFBT)
Raven's Coloured Progressive Matrices (CPM)
Neuropsychological assessments
PGI memory scale
PGI battery of brain dysfunction
AIIMS comprehensive neuropsychological battery in Hindi
NIMHANS neuropsychological battery
Bender Visual-Motor Gestalt Test
Block Design Test
Trail Making Test
Digit Span Test
Digit Symbol Substitution Test
Wisconsin Card Sorting Test (WCST)
Personality tests
Minnesota Multiphasic Personality Inventory
Multiphasic Personality Questionnaire
Eyesenck Personality Questionnaire
PEN Inventory
Rorschach Inkblot Test
Thematic Apperception Test
PGI Sentence Completion Test
Draw a person test
Others
PGI-Health Questionnaire (N_2)
Temperament Measurement Schedule
Social Support Questionnaire
Coping Checklist

A lot of work has been done from India, at many centres on these tests. Institutions like the All India Institute of Medical Sciences, New Delhi (AIIMS), National Institute of Mental Health and Neurosciences, Bangalore (NIMHANS), and Central Institute of Psychiatry, Ranchi (CIP), have all been quite involved in development and validation of psychometric tests. The tests that have been developed notably include the AIIMS Battery and the NIMHANS Battery for neuropsychological testing (Gupta et al. 2000; Rao et al. 2004). However, the Division of Psychology of Department of Psychiatry at the Postgraduate Institute of Medical Education and Research, Chandigarh (PGIMER), has been the forerunner in the field of psychometry. A number of tests have been developed or adapted for Indian settings, both for clinical use and research. Keeping in mind the cultural variations and the different populace, norms have been created for local use. Clinical use of psychometrics has been expanded and consolidated as a consequence of research into the psychological testing. Psychologists are being increasingly involved in psychometric testing for clinical diagnosis and making management decisions. This chapter takes a look at the different psychometric tests available in India, especially those from the Department of Psychiatry in PGIMER, Chandigarh. This chapter also provides an overview of the challenges faced by the psychometric testing worldwide and answers the queries raised about relevance and importance of these tests.

2 The Need for Psychometric Testing

Psychological and psychometric tests are required for a variety of reasons. All mental health professionals rely on interviews and observations as the key sources of information to make a diagnosis. Although generic interviews are efficient and effective ways to obtain data, they have their own limitations. The patients may give poor histories and/or present biased information. For example, neurologically impaired patients frequently lack awareness of their deficits or personality changes, which can be brought into light by psychometric testing. Also, response styles, such as defensiveness or exaggeration, affect the way patients are viewed by clinical interviewers or observers. Taking assistance of psychometric tests would help patients being less misunderstood, mischaracterised or misdiagnosed, and hence less than optimally treated (Meyer et al. 2001).

Psychological testing is often done to confirm, refute or modify the impressions about the diagnosis and assists in the overall management of the patient. Testing aids in describing current functioning of the patients, including cognitive abilities, severity of disturbance and capacity for independent living. Psychometric tests can also monitor treatment over time to evaluate the success of interventions and identify new issues, which may require attention as original concerns are resolved. These tests can help in managing risks and in providing skilled and empathic feedback, which may work as a therapeutic intervention (Meyer et al. 2001).

3 Intelligence Tests

Intelligence tests are the most widely used psychometric tests in the clinical practice. A variety of intelligence tests have been used in a variety of clinical situations. Since there are different theoretical conceptualisations of what intelligence is, and each measure of intelligence looks at non-overlapping areas of functioning, 'intelligence' is at times subsumed as 'what the intelligence test measures'. Some of the intelligence tests that have been validated in India are the Verbal Adult Intelligence Scale (VAIS) (Pershad and Verma 1988), the Malin's Intelligence Scale For Children (MISIC) (Malin 1969), the Bhatia Battery of Performance Tests (BBPT) (Murthy 1966), the Wechsler Adult Performance Intelligence Scale (WAPIS) (Ramalingaswamy 1974) and others like the Draw a Person test for Indian children (Pathak 1966).

The VAIS (Pershad and Verma 1988) has been developed as an Indian adaptation of the Wechsler Adult Intelligence Scale, and it has only four subscales, i.e. Information, Digit span, Arithmetic and Comprehension. The test yields separate quotients for the four subscales, and a verbal quotient can be obtained from the mean of all subscales. Norms have been developed for age, gender and different educational achievement backgrounds. The Bhatia battery (BBPT) (Murthy 1966) comprises of 5 subtests which include the Koh's Block Design, the Alexander Pass Along test, the Pattern Drawing Test, the Immediate Memory for sounds and the Picture Construction Test. All these tests are time tested, and age correction is applied to the norms to obtain the performance quotient.

The MISIC (Malin 1969) is an Indian adaptation of Wechsler Intelligence Test for Children and comprises of 6 verbal and 5 performance scales. Norms are available for 6–15 years of age, and yield verbal and performance quotients, the mean of which is the intelligence quotient. The WAPIS (Ramalingaswamy 1974) comprises of 5 performance subtests, i.e. Picture Completion, Digit Symbol, Block Design, Picture Arrangement and Object Assembly. The reliability coefficients of these tests have been found to be good, and Indian norms are available. The Seguin Form Board Test (Verma et al. 1980) is a performance test, which can be used for children as young as 3½ years of age to 11 years of age. The performance can be converted into the mental age of the child.

Intelligence tests have many applications. Formal diagnosis of mental retardation is still based on the intelligence quotient (IQ). The overall IQ is a good measure of intellectual functioning, but the indices and subtest scores are perhaps of even more practical help. For example, high scores on the Verbal Comprehension Index indicate good verbal abilities and suggest that the person could benefit from formal education. In contrast, a slower processing speed suggests that the person would have difficulty in processing information quickly, and difficulties are likely to be encountered when training such individuals. IQ scores have implications in predicting future academic and occupational achievement. They also provide standardised procedures for assessing a person's performance in various areas, which can be compared with that of age-related peers. The IQ score can aid the clinician in assessing improvement in different functions with time, or with treatment.

The tests of intelligence have certain limitations too. The usefulness of these tests is quite limited in predicting non-test or non-academic skills like creativity, motivational level, problem-solving abilities, social acumen and success in dealing with people. IQ Scores are not measures of an innate and fixed ability, and the performance on these tests may change with time. Their use in classifying minority groups has been questioned, as these are based on norms based on majority population. These tests lay emphasis on understanding the end product of cognitive functioning and show a relative neglect in appreciating underlying cognitive processes. Irrespective of the above limitations, IQ tests are a robust measure of overall cognitive functioning.

4 Personality Assessment

Personality assessment attempts to understand the personality of an individual, i.e. the deeply ingrained and enduring behaviour patterns, manifesting themselves as inflexible responses to a broad range of personal and social situations. Assessment of personality can be carried out using tests, which can be objective and subjective in the way interpretations are made. In objective personality tests, patients are asked specific and standard questions in a structured format. Each patient is typically asked the same questions, and data obtained from a given patient is compared to that of a normative group. The degree to which the patient deviates from the norm is noted and is used for interpretation. Patients' responses are scored according to certain agreed-upon criteria.

The Minnesota Multiphasic Personality Inventory (MMPI; Hathaway and McKinley 1940) and the Multiphasic Personality Questionnaire (MPQ; Murthy 1970) are some of the well-known objective personality tests. Subjective tests often give ambiguous or open-ended stimuli to the individual, and responses are subjectively graded. These tests are based on the phenomenon of projection, i.e. the unconscious tendency of ascribing repressed mental processes to the external world. These tests provide ambiguous stimuli and require the subject to respond with his own constructions and responses in accordance with his basic personality traits. The test takers are unaware of the type of interpretation that will be made of their responses, and trying to feign the test is difficult as the test bypasses the conscious defences of the respondents. The Rorschach Inkblot Test and the Thematic Apperception Test (TAT) are commonly used subjective tests.

Various objective tests of personality assessment are also available. Of these, the MMPI is the most well-known objective psychometric test (Hathaway and McKinley 1940). The test had been designed originally as an aid to psychiatric diagnosis. The test has 10 clinical scales and 4 validity scales and is useful both in psychiatric assessment and the description of normal personality. The MPQ (Murthy 1970) had been derived from the MMPI and contains 100 true-or-false-type questions. It measures personality profile for anxiety, depression, mania, paranoia, schizophrenia, hysteria and psychopathic deviation and has indicators for lie scale and repressor sensitizer. The Personality Trait Inventory is based on the MMPI and has been adapted by in Indian settings (Sen 1966).

It has 90 dichotomous items. It measures 8 general personality traits activity, cyclothymia, superego, dominance, paranoid tendency, depressive tendency, emotional instability, introversion and social desirability. The Eysenck Personality Questionnaire (EPQ) measures major dimensions of personality, i.e. psychoticism, extraversion and neuroticism. The PEN Inventory (Menon and Verma 1988) is the Indian adaptation of the EPQ and is available in Hindi. The inventory has four dimensions of psychoticism, neuroticism, extraversion and lie scale.

Projective tests are those that are based upon the phenomenon of projection, i.e. ascribing one's own ideas and feelings onto another object. They can be of many types based on the response required. These tests use association with inkblots or words, e.g. the Rorschach Inkblot Test and the Sentence Completion Test. They can be based upon construction of stories or sequences, e.g. the TAT or the Childhood Apperception Test. It can be based upon completion of sentences or stories, e.g. Sentence Completion Test and Picture frustration study. They can alternatively be based upon arrangement or selection of pictures or verbal choices (e.g. the Szondi test), or on expression with drawings or play, e.g. the Draw a Person Test, or the House–Tree–Person Test.

The Rorschach Inkblot Test is the most widely utilised projective test and was developed by Hermann Rorschach in 1910. It consists of 10 inkblots (bilaterally symmetrical), each printed on a separate card. The patient is handed the cards one at a time and asked what each blot resembles.

The examiner writes down verbatim what the patient says during the above 'free association' or 'response proper' phase. After the patient has given responses to all ten cards, an enquiry phase of administration begins. Different scoring systems are available and include those of Beck, Klopfer, Pitrowski, Hertz, Rapaport and Exner. There are some pathognomonic signs of schizophrenia and organicity (Pitrowsky signs), and indices for schizophrenia, depression, hypomania, hysteria, anxiety and obsessions can be calculated. Applications of the Rorschach test include diagnosis, clarifying treatment targets, identifying potential obstacles to progress, and providing a basis for evaluating treatment change and outcome (Weiner 1994). Indian norms have been developed for this test (Asthana 1971), and a manual has been developed from the PGIMER (Pershad and Parekh 2010).

Certain controversies have also emerged with respect to the use of the Rorschach test. Doubts have been raised about accuracy and cultural generalisability of the norms. There is little research on differential validity across different racial or cultural groups. The adequacy of norms has been doubted as they are outdated and are based on small samples. The discrepancies in the norms tend to overpathologise normal individuals. The use of the test itself has been suggested to harm clients and be contrary to the ethical principles (Wood and Lilienfeld 1999). The reliability of this test has been questioned as only about half of the variables attain acceptable threshold of reliability criteria (Acklin et al. 2000). The field reliability as well as test–retest reliability remains questionable, and the validity has been low (Hunsley and Michael 1999; Wood et al. 1996).

The TAT is another test to assess reactions to ambiguous interpersonal stimuli. The term 'apperception' denotes that respondents actively interpret the TAT stimuli in accordance with their personality traits and life experiences. The Indian Adaptation was developed by Chawdhury (1967). It is useful, primarily for hypothesising the subjects' personality dynamics, and for contributing to treatment planning. However, scoring systems are rarely used for TAT, and the test suffers from lack of stimulus standardisation. The test may not differentiate between a person's present attribute and fantasy. Other potential issues with the test are lack of norms, questionable test–retest reliability, untested field reliability and the effect of cultural bias in responses (Groth-Marnat 2009). The Children's Apperception Test and the Seniors' Apperception Test are also available for use in the Indian population (Chowdhury 1960a, b).

The PGI Sentence Completion Test (Verma et al. 1985) is an indirect, disguised and relatively understudied method for finding out subjective realities, i.e. attitudes, fears, aspirations, conflicts and frustrations. It is based on the Rotter's Incomplete Sentence Blanks. Three forms of the test are available, the G form (general form, 35 items), the M form (married form, 25 items) and the S form (student form, 20 items). The test can be used effectively with children to diagnose intellectual difficulties, attention deficit disorder and stress, depression, anxiety, thought disturbance, and defensiveness. However, the test does not have a standard scoring procedure, interpretation is subjective, responses can be fabricated, and there is a lack of reliability and validity studies.

5 Neuropsychological Tests

Neuropsychology is concerned with understanding the relationship between brain structure and human function. The aim of a neuropsychologist is to diagnose brain damage by quantifying the cognitive status and interpreting these changes in terms of the models of brain function (Hallett 1994). Two approaches have been used in the field of neuropsychology to diagnose brain damage: the unitary approach and multifactorial approach. The unitary approach is based on the assumption of functional unity of the brain as a whole and is assessed by tests of unitary functions, e.g. tests for memory, intelligence and perceptuo-motor functions. The Bender Visual-Motor Gestalt Test and the Trail Making Tests are among the commonly used tests for assessing unitary functions. The multifactorial approach is based on assumption that different parts of brain have adaptability, equipotentiality, and compensatory function and that they are governed by mass action rather than localisation. The multifactorial approach is assessed by comprehensive batteries of tests such as the Halsted-Reitan Neuropsychological Battery and the Luria Nebraska Neuropsychological Battery.

The PGI Bhatia Battery of Brain Dysfunction (Pershad and Verma 1990) is a comprehensive assessment tool for measuring a range of neuropsychological dysfunctions. It comprises of the PGI Memory Scale, the Revised Bhatia Short Scale of Intelligence, the Verbal Adult Intelligence Scale, the Nahor Benson test and the Bender Visual-Motor Gestalt Test.

The test is fully validated and well acclaimed. Norms are available for age group 20–50 years with respect to age, education and gender. The PGI Memory Scale (Pershad and Wig 1977) measures memory function comprehensively and has 10 subtests: remote memory, recent memory, mental balance, attention and concentration, delayed recall, immediate recall, retention for similar pairs, retention for dissimilar pairs, visual retention and recognition. The scale assesses various aspects of memory and can be used with ease in an illiterate population. The Bender Visual-Motor Gestalt test measures visuo-constructive ability and is a screening instrument for assessing brain damage. The test involves 3 broad stages, i.e. sensory reception, interpretation and organisation, and motor performance of the figure. In general, patients with lesions in their right hemispheres tend to approach visuo-constructive tasks in a fragmented, piecemeal fashion in which they often lose the overall gestalt of the design. In contrast, patients with left hemisphere lesion are likely to duplicate the overall gestalt of the design, but often omit important details of the drawing. Many studies have demonstrated the test's ability to discriminate brain damaged from non-brain-damaged populations with fair diagnostic accuracy (Piotrowski 1995). The Wisconsin Card Sorting Test has also been validated in the Indian setting (Kohli and Kaur 2006).

Batteries for neuropsychological evaluation have also been developed at the AIIMS and the NIMHANS (Gupta et al. 2000; Rao et al. 2004). The AIIMS battery has 160 items and 10 subscales. It is useful for both diagnosis and rehabilitation and can help in detection, and lateralisation and localisation of discrete brain lesions in patients.

The NIMHANS battery has 19 subtests, which measure different neuropsychological deficits. The test has been validated in the age range of 16–65 years, and factorial and criterion-related validity of the battery is well established.

Neuropsychological tests have many uses. One of the most important uses of neuropsychological testing is for differential diagnosis. Many neurological and psychiatric disorders have similar clusters of symptoms. For example, impaired attention and concentration are commonly found among patients who present with a history of psychiatric disorders (e.g. depression, posttraumatic stress disorder or anxiety), or any of several types of neurological disorders that are associated with subcortical involvement (e.g. Parkinson's disease, multiple sclerosis or HIV-related cognitive decline). These tests can be used to identify pseudodementia, which may mimic presentation of dementia. Neuropsychological testing gives an objective measure of different aspects of attention and memory and can help in differentiating normalcy, minimal cognitive impairment and dementia. These tests can help in detecting early dementia, so that prompt treatment can be instituted, and rapid deterioration is avoided to the extent possible. Neuropsychological testing can help in diagnosing certain disorders like specific learning disabilities. Neuropsychological testing can also be of use in documenting cognitive deterioration and provide an objective means of monitoring treatment efficacy. When used appropriately in skilled hands, this is an invaluable tool for diagnostic, prognostic and therapeutic decision-making.

Follow-up assessments can help to objectively examine improvement or worsening of cognitive sequelae and any deviation from the expected trajectory. Such testing is also useful for evaluation of decision-making capacity and judgment, when assessments are made for financial and legal matters, health care and medical treatment, and the ability to work or practice in a given profession (e.g. air traffic controllers, surgeons or financial advisors). Neuropsychologists may also be called in for forensic evaluation to evaluate deficits and opine about possibility of malingering.

There are certain advantages of the psychometric approach to neuropsychological assessment. Neuropsychological tests lay emphasis on standardisation and normative data and thus rely less on clinical intuition. These tests offer objectivity and focus on individual strengths and weaknesses. These aid to correct diagnosis and offer amenability for statistical analysis and are attractive tools for comparative research (Hallett 1994). The psychometric approach to neuropsychological assessment has some disadvantages too. Findings from these tests may not correlate exactly with brain lesions or pathology. It takes quite a long time to administer these tests, and patient's adequate cooperation is required for the results to be dependable (Hallett 1994). It fosters the idea that a poor score on a certain test is invariably related to specific damage, which may not be the case. Complex cognitive processing in the brain reflecting networked interactions between separate cortical and subcortical areas of the brain means that interpretations should be made with caution.

6 Other Relevant Psychological Scales of Clinical Use

Many other tests have been developed in India for psychological assessment. It is difficult to succinctly enumerate all such tests; hence, the focus is upon tests that have been developed or adapted at the PGIMER for assessment of psychological functioning.

The PGI Well-Being Scale is an instrument to measure the subjective well-being of individuals (Verma et al. 1983). It is a 20-item scale with good inter-rater reliability and is applicable to all educational levels. The PGI Quality of Life Scale-Revised is a 26-item scale rated on 5-point Likert scale that measures quality of life (Moudgil et al. 1983).

The PRIME-MD Patient Health Questionnaire is an instrument to diagnose common mental disorders in the primary health care. The Indian adaptation (Avasthi et al. 2008) includes 8 diagnostic categories, and there is a high degree of correlation with the psychiatrists' diagnoses. The disorders covered include major depressive disorder, panic disorder, other anxiety disorder, bulimia nervosa and other subthreshold disorders such as other depressive disorder, probable alcohol dependence, somatoform and binge eating disorder. A 26-item scale has also been developed to assess eating attitudes (Nehra et al. 2001) and has good reliability and validity. Similarly, a scale has been developed to assess the attitude, cognition and reaction towards body shape, which has 34 items and is available in Hindi (Nehra et al. 2006).

To assess the sexual knowledge and attitudes, the Sexual Knowledge and Attitudes Questionnaire (SKAQ) has been developed (Avasthi et al. 1992).

The questionnaire has 35 items in the knowledge part and 20 items assessing the attitude. It is a simple test and shows a high degree of reliability. A scale for assessing the knowledge and attitudes towards use of condoms has been also developed which consists of 62 items, and tested in the clinical setting (Avasthi et al. 1998).

A coping checklist in Hindi has been adapted from the scale of Scazufca and Kuipers (1999) for use in the Indian population (Nehra et al. 2002). The scale has 14 items divided into 5 domains: problem focused, seeking social support, avoidance, collusion and coercion. Significant correlation has been found between the English and the Hindi versions.

The Social Support Questionnaire has been developed as a measure for social support (Nehra et al. 1998). It is an 18-item questionnaire which has both positively and negatively worded items. The scale is a short, simple and easy to score instrument that can be used in variety of clinical population. The total score ranges from 18 to 72 with higher scores reflecting a greater social support. The test retest reliability of the modified version is found to be high.

The temperament measurement schedule is a 15-item scale that measures the temperament of the children (Malhotra et al. 1983). The scale is applicable with patients as well with healthy population. The test shows a good test–retest validity and inter-rater reliability. Factorial and construct validity are found to be satisfactory.

Instruments have also been made available for assessing patients with substance use disorders. The Sensation Seeking Scale (Basu et al. 1993) is self-administered scale with 40 items, which evaluates the inclination to seek new sensations and the willingness to take risk for the same. The Motivation for Addiction Treatment is an 18-item self-rated Likert-type scale in Hindi for assessing motivation for treatment of substance use disorders (Mattoo et al. 2002). The Hindi adaptation of the Relapse Precipitant Inventory has been developed at PGIMER and has shown robust psychometric properties (Mattoo and Malhotra 2000). The Attitudes Towards Drinking and Alcoholism scale is a 29-item scale that assesses attitudes towards alcohol use. Satisfactory results have been obtained regarding stability of attitudes, and the test takes around 15 min to complete (Basu et al. 1998). A similar scale has been developed about attitudes to drug-taking behaviour (Basu et al. 1997). Thus, many tests have been developed at PGIMER with wide variety of applicability and clinical utility as adjuncts to usual clinical practice.

7 Usefulness of Psychometric Tests in Psychiatry

The 1990s saw a declining trend of use of psychometric tests in the United States as they were considered time-consuming, and their validity and utility in clinical health care setting was increasingly challenged. It was also difficult to obtain authorisation and reimbursement for psychological assessments from third-party payers (Meyer et al. 2001). In response, a Psychological Assessment Work Group

(PAWG) was established in 1996 and commissioned to evaluate contemporary threats to psychological and neuropsychological assessment services.

The Work Group reviewed the evidence about validity and utility of psychological assessment in clinical practice.

Several clinical and health care applications of psychometric tests were judged to be best supported by evidence gathered by the PAWG. These included description of clinical symptomatology and differential diagnosis; description and prediction of functional behaviour; prediction of psychotherapy, forensic and mental health outcomes; and identification of patient characteristics that affect treatment.

Psychometric tests have been evaluated for their ability to identify, describe and quantify important patient characteristics and have been shown to be useful for differential diagnosis (Kubiszyn et al. 2000). In a meta-analysis of 77 studies, neuropsychological tests were found to be effective in differentiating the normal elderly from patients with mild, moderate or severe dementia (Christensen et al. 1991). Meta-analytic and narrative reviews have also shown that neuropsychologists make reliable and accurate judgments when they use a battery of test data to make inferences about cognitive impairment due to brain damage (Garb and Schramke 1996; Russell 1995), which cannot be obtained simply through interviews or informal observation (Roca et al. 1982; Schwartz and Wiedel 1981). Among the personality tests, the MMPI was found to have strong validity as a descriptor of personality in meta-analyses (Atkinson 1986; Parker et al. 1988).

The MMPI and MMPI-2 helped with differential diagnosis between neurotic and psychotic disorders, depression and anxiety disorders, schizophrenia and affective disorders, and between non-patients and patients with psychiatric disorders (Ben-Porath et al. 1991; Zalewski and Gottesman 1991). In diagnosing depression, the MMPI had been found to have good positive and negative predictive power (Ganellen 1996). The test also differentiates various conditions on Axis I (clinical disorders) or Axis II (personality disorders) of the DSM-IV.

Among the projective tests, the Rorschach test and the TAT seem to be the best studied. Several meta-analytic reviews have demonstrated the utility of the Rorschach test in describing symptomatology (Atkinson 1986; Parker et al. 1988). Rorschach produces fairly large validity coefficients when used in research conducted with a sound rationale. The utility of the Rorschach test or the TAT for descriptive and diagnostic purposes is also reported to be fair (Exner 1986; Gartner et al. 1989). A strong relationship was found between ego deficits as measured by the Rorschach test and general impairment in social and occupational functioning (Perry et al. 1995). Personality test scores from this test predict behaviours such as absenteeism from work, success on the job, problem-solving ability, creativity, disciplinary problems, irresponsible behaviour, and initiative in both non-clinical settings and medical or psychiatric settings (Robertson and Kinder 1993).

Psychometric tests can be used for prediction of psychotherapy outcomes. A meta-analysis showed that the Rorschach test had a powerful ability to predict psychotherapy outcomes at 1 year after baseline testing (Meyer and Handler 1997). In adults, Rorschach test scores have predicted ratings of the ability to engage in short-term dynamic therapy as well as its outcome (Alpher et al. 1990). The

Rorschach test also measures ego strength and could predict response to antidepressant and outcome (Perry et al. 1995).

Psychometric tests also have a role in prediction of mental health outcomes. In children, baseline self-reports of negative emotionality predicted behaviour problems and subsequent clinical outcomes (Mattison et al. 1990). In adults, baseline self-reported neuroticism is a better predictor of long-term clinical outcome in depression (Hirschfeld et al. 1986). In general, elevated baseline neuroticism scores predispose people to negative outcomes in individual and marital therapy (Luborsky et al. 1993). Baseline neuropsychological testing can usefully predict the subsequent onset of dementia in otherwise asymptomatic patients, or patients who had age-associated memory impairment on initial evaluation (Crystal et al. 1996).

Psychometric tests have a role in prediction of forensic outcomes. The Hare Psychopathy Checklist (PCL) is used to predict outcomes in a criminal context (Salekin et al. 1997). The instrument is able to predict subsequent violent behaviour, recidivism and sexual sadism or deviant sexual arousal.

In addition, the PCL has proved to be a better predictor of these outcomes than virtually all other variables or procedures, including criminal history, psychiatric history, age, substance use or a diagnosis of antisocial personality disorder (Bonta et al. 1998; Hanson and Bussiere 1998).

Psychological testing probably has the greatest predictive value for individual or group psychotherapy for identifying the best match between patient characteristics and therapist–treatment characteristics (Garfield 1994; Piper et al. 1998). Patients with externalising symptoms (e.g. acting out, projecting, avoidant defences) do better in treatment that is more structured or therapist directed. Patients with internalising symptoms (e.g. self-punishment, anxiousness, worry) do better in treatments where they set the pace and determine the structure (Blatt 1992).

It is interesting to draw comparisons of psychological tests to medical tests. Both psychological and medical tests have varying degrees of validity ranging from tests that are essentially uninformative for a given criterion, to tests that are strongly predictive of appropriate criteria. Validity coefficients for many psychological tests are indistinguishable from those observed for many medical tests; for example, the ability to detect dementia is at least as good with neuropsychological tests ($r = 0.68$) as it is with magnetic resonance imaging ($r = 0.57$) (Meyer et al. 2001). However, it should be mentioned that results from the medical tests (e.g. X-Ray or biochemical tests) do not depend on certain individual factors like motivation or rapport, unlike psychological assessments.

8 Current Perspective and Future Directions

A wide variety of psychometric tests and instruments are in use. Some of these tests are validated across strict criteria, while some are not. Further references to the individual tests are available from other sources (Nehra and Kulhara 2011; Venkatesan 2010).

There are some limitations in clinical utility of psychometric tests in the Indian population. Most of these assessments have been developed in Western countries and have been subsequently adapted for the Indian population. Their applicability to a culturally distant and different setting is a matter of concern and consideration. Biases inherent in the test due to cultural factors need to be eliminated, or controlled for. Testers continue to use antiquated norms, which would hardly be applicable for the present generation The wide variability of language across India, even with usage of different forms of Hindi, limits the applicability of these tests across the country. Many of these tests do not have adaptable norms for the mentally ill, for those with special needs and for minority groups; this, thus, restricts the inferences made from these tests. Non-availability of well-trained and experienced professional also limits the use of these tests, as they are best delivered in experienced hands. Moreover, due to the cost and time spent on testing, and the shortage of trained clinical psychologists in the country, these may not be feasible or appear as an exciting proposition in the busy Indian clinical settings.

Nonetheless, it should be emphasised that psychometric tests function as an important part of the therapeutic armamentarium in clinical practice.

However, interpretations from these tests should be made with a few caveats in mind. Clinicians should take decisions after taking into consideration the case history, clinical observation, mental status examination and inputs from family members. They should not base their decisions solely on psychometric test conducted only once in the course of the illness. It is important to judge the expected benefits of psychometric assessments relative to the costs incurred. The latest available and culturally appropriate norms should be used for making interpretations of the test findings. Psychometric assessment is likely to yield the greatest yield when treating clinician or patient has salient questions. Thereafter, relevant testing procedures can be utilised, and a hypothesis can be made, which can be put to test subsequently (Finn and Tonsager 1997).

In the future, there is a need for shift in the research focus from microlevel testing (testing psychometric reliability and validity of tests) to a macrolevel testing (practical value of these tests to clinician). There is a need for periodic revalidation of psychometric tests. Norms need to be periodically revised for different subgroups of population, so that they give valid and clinically useful results. Research of relationship of these tests in concurrence with neuroimaging may help develop better prognostic markers. The search for a brief and concise test with high sensitivity and specificity still continues. Developing an instrument, which reduces the time required for administration without compromising on range and depth of information gleaned, may be of a greater assistance to clinicians. There is a need for proper training of professionals for applying the psychometric tests correctly.

Professionals need to update their knowledge, especially when using the newer versions or revisions of the older tests.

An extensive research base exists by now, which supports the validity and utility of psychological assessment instruments for a range of applications in psychometric testing. But, it needs to be understood that they are only tools analogous to medical tests like the X-ray or the MRI. Thus, they can only act as aids to the diagnosis, and they are not substitutes for clinical interviews. Tests do not think for themselves, nor do they directly communicate with patients. Their worth cannot be separated from the sophistication of the clinician who draws inferences from them, and then communicates with patients and other professionals. The application of the tests requires critical appraisal of the method of the test, the way findings are obtained and the meaning of the results.

References

Acklin, M. W., McDowell, C. J, I. I., Verschell, M. S., & Chan, D. (2000). Interobserver agreement, intraobserver reliability, and the Rorschach Comprehensive System. *Journal of Personality Assessment, 74*, 15–47.

Alpher, V. S., Perfetto, G. A., Henry, W. P., & Strupp, H. H. (1990). The relationship between the Rorschach and assessment of the capacity to engage in short-term dynamic psychotherapy. *Psychotherapy: Theory, Research, Practice, Training, 27*, 224–229.

Asthana, H. S. (1971). *Normative data on Rorschach Inkblot for Indian sample*. Saugar: Department of Psychology, Saugar University.

Atkinson, L. (1986). The comparative validities of the Rorschach and MMPI: A meta-analysis. *Canadian Psychology, 27*, 238–247.

Avasthi, A., Nehra, R., Kumar, B., & Pershad, D. (1998). Quantification of knowledge and attitude towards use of condom. *Indian Journal of Clinical Psychology, 25*, 159–164.

Avasthi, A., Varma, S. C., Kulhara, P., et al. (2008). Diagnosis of common mental disorders using PRIME-MD Patient Health Questionnaire. *The Indian Journal of Medical Research, 127*, 159–164.

Avasthi, A., Varma, V. K., Nehra, R., & Das, K. (1992). Construction and standardization of a sex knowledge and attitude questionnaire (SKAQ) in simple Hindi for Northern Indian population. *Indian Journal of Psychiatry, 34*, 24–27.

Basu, D., Malhotra, A., Varma, V. K., & Khanna, R. (1997). Attitude towards drug taking behavior: A factor analytic study. *Journal of Indian Academy Applied Psychology, 23*, 31–35.

Basu, D., Malhotra, A., Varma, V. K., & Khanna, R. (1998). Development of a scale to assess attitude towards drinking and alcoholism. *Indian Journal of Psychiatry, 40*, 158–164.

Basu, D., Verma, V. K., Malhotra, S., & Malhotra, A. (1993). Sensation seeking scale: Indian adaptation. *Indian Journal of Psychiatry, 35*, 155–158.

Ben-Porath, Y. S., Butcher, J. N., & Graham, J. R. (1991). Contribution of the MMPI-2 content scales to the differential diagnosis of schizophrenia and major depression. *Psychological Assessment: A Journal of Consulting and Clinical Psychology, 3*, 634–640.

Blatt, S. (1992). The differential effect of psychotherapy and psychoanalysis with anaclitic and introjective patients: The Menninger Psychotherapy Research Project revisited. *Journal of the American Psychoanalytic Association, 40*, 691–724.

Bonta, J., Law, M., & Hanson, K. (1998). The prediction of criminal and violent recidivism among mentally disordered offenders: A meta-analysis. *Psychological Bulletin, 123*, 123–142.

Chowdhury, U. (1960a). *An Indian modification of the children's apperception test*. New Delhi: Manasayan.

Chowdhury, U. (1960b). An Indian modification of the thematic apperception test. *Journal of American Social Psychology, 51*, 245–263.

Chowdhury, U. (1967). *An Indian modification of thematic apperception test*. Calcutta: Bookland Publishers Private Limited.

Christensen, H., Hadzi-Pavlovic, D., & Jacomb, P. (1991). The psychometric differentiation of dementia from normal aging: A meta-analysis. *Psychological Assessment: A Journal of Consulting and Clinical Psychology, 3*, 147–155.

Crystal, H. A., Dickson, D., Sliwinski, M., et al. (1996). Associations of status and change measures of neuropsychological function with pathologic changes in elderly, originally nondemented subjects. *Archives of Neurology, 53*, 82–87.

Exner, J. E. (1986). Some Rorschach data comparing schizophrenics with borderline and schizotypal personality disorders. *Journal of Personality Assessment, 50*, 455–471.

Finn, S. E., & Tonsager, M. E. (1997). Information-gathering and therapeutic models of assessment: Complementary paradigms. *Psychological Assessment, 9*, 374–385.

Ganellen, R. J. (1996). Comparing the diagnostic efficiency of the MMPI, MCMI II, and Rorschach: A review. *Journal of Personality Assessment, 67*, 219–243.

Garb, H. N., & Schramke, C. J. (1996). Judgment research and neuropsychological assessment: A narrative review and meta-analyses. *Psychological Bulletin, 120*, 140–153.

Garfield, S.L. (1994) Research on client variables in psychotherapy. Wiley, New York.

Gartner, J., Hurt, S. W., & Gartner, A. (1989). Psychological test signs of borderline personality disorder: a review of the empirical literature. *Journal of Personality Assessment, 53*, 423–441.

Groth-Marnat, G. (2009) *Handbook of psychological assessment*. New York: Wiley

Gupta, S., Khandelwal, S. K., Tandon, P. N., et al. (2000). The development and standardization of a comprehensive neuropsychological battery in Hindi (adult form). *Journal of Personality and Clinical Studies, 16*, 75–109.

Hallett, S. (1994). Neuropsychology and psychometry. In D. Tantam & M. Birchwood (Eds.), *Seminars in psychology and the social sciences* (pp. 107–135). London: Gaskell.

Hanson, R. K., & Bussiere, M. T. (1998). Predicting relapse: A meta-analysis of sexual offender recidivism studies. *Journal of Consulting and Clinical Psychology, 66*, 348–362.

Hathaway, S. R., & McKinley, J. C. (1940). A multiphasic personality schedule (Minnesota): I. Construction of the schedule. *Journal of Psychology, 10*, 249–254.

Hirschfeld, R. M., Klerman, G. L., Andreasen, N. C., et al. (1986). Psycho-social predictors of chronicity in depressed patients. *British Journal of Psychiatry, 148*, 648–654.

Hunsley, J., & Michael, J. (1999). The clinical utility of the Rorschach: Unfulfilled promises and an uncertain future. *Psychological Assessment, 11*, 266–277.

Kohli, A., & Kaur, M. (2006). Wisconsin card sorting test: Normative data and experience. *Indian Journal of Psychiatry, 48*, 181–184.

Kubiszyn, T. W., Meyer, G. J., Finn, S. E., et al. (2000). Empirical support for psychological assessment in clinical health care settings. *Professional Psychology: Research and Practice, 31*, 119–130.

Luborsky, L., Diguer, L., Luborsky, E., et al. (1993). Psychological health-sickness (PHS) as a predictor of outcomes in dynamic and other psychotherapies. *Journal of Consulting and Clinical Psychology, 61*, 542.

Malhotra, S., Malhotra, A., & Randhawa, A. (1983). Children's temperament: Factorial validity. *Indian Journal of Clinical Psychology, 10*, 309–406.

Malin, A.J. (1969) Manual for Malin's intelligence scale for Indian children. Nagpur Child Guidance Centre, Nagpur.

Mattison, R. E., Handford, H. A., Kales, H. C., et al. (1990). Four-year predictive value of the children's depression inventory. *Psychological Assessment: A Journal of Consulting and Clinical Psychology, 2*, 169–174.

Mattoo, S. K., Basu, D., Malhotra, A., & Malhotra, R. (2002). Motivation for addiction treatment (Hindi) scale: development and factor structure. *Indian Journal of Psychiatry, 44*, 131–137.

Mattoo, S. K., & Malhotra, R. (2000). Relapse precipitant inventory: Hindi adaptation and factor structure. *Indian Journal of Clinical Psychology, 27*, 278–285.

Menon, D. K., & Verma, S. K. (1988). *Manual for Hindi pen inventory*. Varanasi: Rupa Psychological Centre.

Meyer, G. J., Finn, S. E., Eyde, L. D., et al. (2001). Psychological testing and psychological assessment. A review of evidence and issues. *American Psychologist, 56*, 128–165.

Meyer, G. J., & Handler, L. (1997). The ability of the Rorschach to predict subsequent outcome: A meta-analysis of the Rorschach prognostic rating scale. *Journal of Personality Assessment, 69*, 1–38.

Moudgil, A. C., Verma, S. K., & Kaur, K. (1983). PGI quality of life scale—revised form. *Indian Journal of Clinical Psychology, 13*, 175–184.
Murthy, H. N. (1966). A short scale of Bhatia's performance tests. *Indian Psychological Review, 2*, 133–134.
Murthy, H. N. (1970). *Multiphasic personality questionnaire*. Bangalore: All India Institute of Mental Health.
Nehra, R., Kulhara, P., & Verma, S.K. (1998). Adaptation of social support quetionnaire in Hindi. *Indian Journal of Clinical Psychology, 23*, 33–39.
Nehra, N., Mohanty, M., Sharan, P., et al. (2001). Assessment of the psychometric properties of the Eating Attitudes Test (EAT-26) in a targeted population. *Indian Journal of Clinical Psychology, 28*, 241–245.
Nehra, N., Mohanty, M., Sharan, P., et al. (2006). Assessment of the body shape questionnaire in a targeted population. *Indian Journal of Clinical Psychology, 33*, 122–126.
Nehra, R., Chakrabarti, S., Sharma, R., & Kaur, R. (2002). Psychometric properties of the Hindi version of the coping checklist of Scazufca and Kuipers. *Indian Journal of Clinical Psychology, 29*, 79–84.
Nehra, R., & Kulhara, P. (2011). *Psychometric assessment tools*. Chandigarh: Indian Psychiatric Society.
Parker, K. P., Hanson, R. K., & Hunsley, J. (1988). MMPI, Rorschach, and WAIS: A meta-analytic comparison of reliability, stability, and validity. *Psychological Bulletin, 103*, 367–373.
Pathak, P. (1966). *Draw a man test for Indian children*. Pune: Anand Agencies.
Perry, W., McDougall, A., & Viglione, D, Jr. (1995). A five-year follow-up on the temporal stability of the Ego Impairment Index. *Journal of Personality Assessment, 64*, 112–118.
Pershad, D., & Verma, S. K. (1988). Translation and adaptation of WAIS-R verbal scale in Hindi. In D. Pershad & S. K. Verma (Eds.), *The concept and assessment of intelligence* (pp. 71–89). Agra: Indian Perspect. National Psychological Corporation.
Pershad, D., & Verma, S. K. (1990). *Handbook of PGI battery of brain dysfunction (PGI-BBD)*. Agra: National Psychological Corporation.
Pershad, D., & Parekh, S. C. (2010). *The Rorschach test: A practical manual*. Agra: H.P. Bhargava Book House.
Pershad, D., & Wig, N. N. (1977). *PGI memory scale*. Agra: National Psychological Corporation.
Piotrowski, C. (1995). A review of the clinical and research use of the Bender-Gestalt Test. *Percept Motor Skills, 81*, 1272–1274.
Piper, W. E., Joyce, A. S., McCallum, M., & Azim, H. F. (1998). Interpretive and supportive forms of psychotherapy and patient personality variables. *Journal of Consulting and Clinical Psychology, 66*, 558–567.
Ramalingaswamy, P. (1974). *Manual for the Wechsler adult performance intelligence scale, form PR*. Delhi: Manasayan Psychological Corporation.
Rao, S. L., Subbakrishna, D. K., & Gopukumar, K. (2004). *NIMHANS neuropsychology battery-2004, manual*. Bangalore: National Institute of Mental Health and Neurosciences.
Rapaport, D. (1950). Diagnostic testing in psychiatric practice. *Bulletin of the New York Academy of Medicine, 26*, 115–125.
Robertson, I. T., & Kinder, A. (1993). Personality and job competencies: The criterion-related validity of some personality variables. *Journal of Occupational and Organizational Psychology, 66*, 225–244.
Roca, R. P., Klein, L. E., & Vogelsang, G. (1982). Inaccuracy in diagnosing dementia in medical inpatients. *Clinical Research, 30*, 305A.
Russell, E. W. (1995). The accuracy of automated and clinical detection of brain damage and lateralization in neuropsychology. *Neuropsychology Review, 5*, 1–68.
Salekin, R. T., Rogers, R., & Sewell, K. W. (1997). Construct validity of psychopathy in a female offender sample: A multitrait–multimethod evaluation. *Journal of Abnormal Psychology, 106*, 576.
Scazufca, M., & Kupiers, E. (1999). Coping strategies in relatives of people with schizophrenia before and after psychiatric admission. *British Journal of Psychiatry, 174*, 154–158.

Schwartz, S., & Wiedel, T. C. (1981). Incremental validity of the MMPI in neurological decision-making. *Journal of Personality Assessment, 45*, 424–426.

Sen, N. N. (1966). *Personality trait inventory*. New Delhi: NCERT.

Venkatesan, S. (2010). Indian scales and inventories. *Indian Journal of Psychiatry, 52*, S378–S385.

Verma, S., & Nehra, A. (1997). Psychodiagnostics. *Psychiatry Today, 2*, 81–84.

Verma, S. K., Dubey, B. L., & Gupta, D. (1983). PGI general well being scale: Some correlates. *Indian Journal of Clinical Psychology, 10*, 299–304.

Verma, S. K., Khanna, B. C., & Wig, N. (1985). Construction of PGI sentence completion tests (in Hindi). *Mind, 11*, 7–14.

Verma, S. K., Pershad, D., & Randhawa, A. (1980). Are Indian children slow? Report on enquiry with a speed measure of intelligence. *Child Psychiatry Quarterly, 13*, 67–71.

Weiner, I. B. (1994). The Rorschach Inkblot Method (RIM) is not a test: Implications for theory and practice. *Journal of Personality Assessment, 62*, 498–504.

Wood, J. M., & Lilienfeld, S. O. (1999). The Rorschach Inkblot Test: A case of overstatement? *Assessment, 6*, 341–352.

Wood, J. M., Nezworski, T., & Stejskal, W. J. (1996). The comprehensive system for the Rorschach: A critical examination. *Psychological Science, 7*, 3–10.

Zalewski, C. E., & Gottesman, I. I. (1991). (Hu)man versus mean revisited: MMPI group data and psychiatric diagnosis. *Journal of Abnormal Psychology, 100*, 562–568.

Chapter 4
Cultural Psychodynamics and the Indian Personality

V.K. Varma

1 Introduction: No One Was Moving Around on Foot

This was my first dispatch home on landing in the U.S. in the last days of 1960 from my home in India. I had just landed in the medium-sized city of Canton in the State of Ohio in the United States. Compared to the crowded city of my hometown, Patna, in Bihar, as I stepped out in Canton, everything seemed to be quite sparse. In my first letter home, I remarked how very few people one saw on the city streets. Almost all the people were going around in cars. One could find barely few people moving around or going on the streets on foot.

People have a natural curiosity for other places, other people and other cultures. They like to compare it with their own as the frame of reference. Places differ from one another in material culture; buildings, cars, bridges; in people, racially and otherwise; and in social relationships. In the same way, they differ in the overall, or the average or modal personality.

Kluckhohn (1962), the well-known cultural anthropologist, famously stated that every man is in certain aspects, (a) like all other men, (b) like some other men and (c) like no other man. The three ways of looking at men can be said to translate into the biological, the sociocultural and the individual, respectively. The first point is that we human beings are all similar as we are members of the same human race, of the species *Homo sapiens,* and share the same biology. The second point is that we all are similar to people of our cultural and social group. The final point is that, in the final analysis, we are all unique. Each one of us has one's own

V.K. Varma, Former Professor and Head

V.K. Varma (✉)
Department of Psychiatry, Postgraduate Institute of Medical Education and Research, Chandigarh, India
e-mail: vijoyv@frontier.com

S. Malhotra and S. Chakrabarti (eds.), *Developments in Psychiatry in India*,
DOI 10.1007/978-81-322-1674-2_4

biology, own DNA and own inheritance. Not only that each one of us has our own unique early life experience, nurture, which has shaped our personality.

The present paper deals mostly with the second variable of us as people. Some 10 years ago, there was a survey reported in Reader's Digest, which listed (then) Bombay as the rudest city in the world. The rudeness was measured by such things as not saying 'thank you', and/or not picking up a piece of paper if someone accidently dropped it; not holding a door for someone. I circulated a commentary on this to our own group of Indian psychiatrists, which was deeply and hotly discussed. Most Indians rejected the Reader's Digest conclusion. However, with my considerable travel experience, I have no doubt that 'not lending a hand' remains the hallmark of the Indian personality.

Dubois (1944), in her landmark study of the people of Alor, gave the concept of the modal personality, as the personality that is 'modal' among the adult members of a particular culture. Although apparently useful, this concept has been widely criticised. The opponents of this concept discredit it as it obscures variations within a particular culture, may lead to stereotypes and breed prejudice.

There are many ways of looking at trans-cultural or cross-cultural psychiatry. We all have a frame of reference in almost everything we deal with. If places can differ in material culture such as buildings and roads, parks, cities and people can differ in race, religion and belief system, why not in the personality?

As I have elaborated in Varma (2009a, b), a rather simple method of understanding the culture and personality issue could be as follows: many things differ across places, societies and cultures. There are geographic and social and cultural differences. To illustrate, when I travel from India to the United States and back, on my return, people ask me what America is like. 'On my return, I tell them of the skyscrapers in New York City. I tell them that the people look different from us Indians. Most people are White or Caucasian, although a significant proportion of them are black. I tell them of the climate, how it differs from India, and varies across the U.S. I also tell them of the differences in certain social customs. For example, in the U.S., you do not just walk into someone's house without a prior appointment, like you do in India' (Varma 2009b).

However, none of these differences are absolute. 'There are tall buildings in India also, as are tenements in America. There are the '*pucca sahibs*' in India who ape the norms taught to us by the English. There are groups of affluent people in India whose lifestyle could approach that of Americans. There are people in India who copy the social lifestyle of the English and the Europeans. One of the first things I learnt about the English was not to use a loud voice when calling someone. Follow the appointment and the queue system. Any number of things' (Varma 2009b).

One way that the differences can be explained is statistical. We can follow the statistical technique called the analysis of variance. This compares differences **within** a group with that **across** groups, if differences across groups are only just as much as within groups, or they are more than what is observed within groups. As per this method, in comparing groups, in so far as the differences across groups significantly exceed those within groups, the groups can be said to differ significantly from each other.

2 Culture and Personality

'The study of culture and personality seeks to understand the growth and development personal and social identity as it relates to the surrounding social environment' (Barnouw 1963). Through the examination of individual personalities, broader correlation and generalisations can be made about specific culture of its members. This has led to an examination of national characters, modal personality types and configurations of the personality.

> The field of culture and personality draws on psychology and anthropology. Born out of Freud's psychoanalysis, anthropologists began searching for common aspects that would characterise differing peoples by their cultures. In an attempt to avoid racist, hierarchical culture models, a new breed of anthropologists sought to describe cultures based on the individuals within a society and the similarities that they shared (McGhee-Snow and Lawrence, www.as.ua.edu/ant/Faculty/murphy/cult&per.htm).

The culture and personality approach has to assume that there is an **average** personality in a culture. Within a culture, people will vary from one another, but there is a mean or average; what people are **generally** like. There are various ways of denoting the mean, from the 'modal personality' of Cora Dubois, to the 'national character' of Inkeles and Levinson (1969), to the 'ethnic personality' of Devereaux (Varma 2009a, b).

In spite of its critics, the concept of an average personality in a culture has deep roots, going back to Hippocrates (460–377 BC). As I have mentioned elsewhere (Varma and Gupta 2008), 'C.P. Snow, the famous British intellectual, talking about a culturally determined personality pattern, put it simply as 'without thinking about it, they respond alike. That is what culture means (Murphy and Leighton 1965)'.

A general question can be raised: Why would the personality differ from culture to culture, society to society and country to country? The culture and personality approach initially linked it to the differences in child rearing practices and produced a lot of research on it.

One way of looking at it could be that the personality develops in its attempt to deal with the attempts of the individual to deal with the demands of the environment so as to survive in a most optimal fashion. Societies and cultures differ in the material culture, demanding different coping mechanisms. There may be scarcity of something and abundance of another. Material things may be abundant and sex scarce.

A more seminal point may be that a culture may require differential quanta of autonomy versus dependence/inter-dependence at the level of the individual. To illustrate, in an agrarian society, people need to toil together to produce. On the other hand, in an industrial society, each person works at an assigned place in the assembly line. A society may be more or less dependent on the nature and may require different adaptive mechanisms; to deal with it, or even to explain it.

To start with, we humans were hunters and gatherers. We hunted and gathered and saved our food. The first major change occurred with the advent of agriculture. This gave us rootedness; to a piece of land. It also attuned us to seasons and a timetable, to the necessity to save the produce so as to last through all seasons. Many agricultural processes required people to work together in a team.

Generally speaking, the development of agriculture itself is taken to herald the beginning of human civilisation. The agricultural society continued for several millennia, till it was replaced, as recently as 300–400 years ago, by an industrial society. The industrial society capitalised on the industrial revolution, which harnessed energy and put it to use, in things such as manufacturing and innovation. The assembly line became the prototype of 'work'. Every worker became 'a cog in the wheel'. He became responsible only for his little piece of work. He was not responsible for the work of others in the line. It thus led to more of autonomy and less of dependence.

In reading historical novels, I am struck how they differentially depict dependence/inter-dependence in some societies and autonomy and fierce individualism in others. Although works of fiction and written centuries after the story depicted, perhaps there is something carried over from the epoch and locale that the story is about.

> Whatever may be the reasons and explanations, the resultant personality, as it develops, differs across cultures. This is the whole idea of culture and personality (Varma and Gupta 2008).

3 Sociocultural Variables of Personality

The variables affecting the personality can be genetic and environmental—the nature versus nurture controversy. The environment can be viewed influencing the individual, varying across persons, or it can be viewed differing across societies and cultures. The latter can be called 'sociocultural'. One such variable I have called the continuum of 'dependence/autonomy,' ranging across cultures.

3.1 Dependence Versus Autonomy

As opposed to other animals, including other mammals, the human being is born immature. Man is an altricial animal. I have explained it as follows (Varma 2009a, b):

'On account of the disparity between the size of the birth canal and the projected size of the head, the human infant must be born immature, not fully developed, 'partly baked' so to say, and much of the development must occur after birth' (Varma 1985a, 1986). To perform all the human functions, the brain must be of a particular size and must be housed in a cranium of sufficient dimensions. Such a cranium cannot be born through the dimensions of a birth canal. Accordingly, the human infant is born relatively immature.

> This leads in humans a protracted period of dependence. This early dependence permeates and influences all inter-personal relationships throughout life. Cultures differ from each other in the quantity of dependence and autonomy (Varma 2009a).

Although born immature, the further development of the human infant progresses according to the genetic programme. The epigenetic theory explains that the development is already programmed in the genes; further development proceeds like the blossoming of a flower in a timely fashion.

Even compared with other mammals, the human infant is born less complete, less capable of looking after himself. Look at cows; soon after birth, the calf can stand up and can move around. In the human, all milestones are more protracted. We make a thorough analysis of developmental milestones in the human, standing unsupported, walking, saying words and talking a three-word sentence. The entire industry of infant and baby clothes and shoes, not to mention toys, depends on the developmental prerogatives.

In the beginning, the human infant is totally dependent on others for most functions. Some instincts help in the survival process. For example, the process by which he sucks milk from mother. One wonders what would have happened if the infant lacked this ability.

Although dependence can be called a universal hallmark of the human infant; for some reasons, it varies from society to society.

If we dichotomise the world into the technologically advanced societies of the West and the traditional, developing countries of the West, and compare them with one another, it has been pointed out that a greater amount of dependence develops in the East (Neki 1976a, b; Varma 1985a, b, 1988). Hoch (1990) has submitted that the Indian personality attaches importance to the development of a unique, distinctive personality and to individual 'self-realisation'. Marriott (1976, 1979, The open Hindu person and humane sciences. Unpublished paper) has pointed out that in contrast to the generally closed, homogeneous and enduring mental integrations attributable to the adult persons in the West, Hindu adults are posited as persons 'who are open, composed of exogenous elements, substantially fluid… and thus necessarily changing and inter-changing in their nature. …Given the vulnerability of open Hindu persons to a cosmos of inter-personal flow, persons as wholes cannot be thought of enduring or bounded 'egos' in any western sense'.

Comparing the industrialised societies of the West with the developing, traditional East, I have surmised as follows (Varma 2009a):

> Traditional, developing, Eastern cultures can be said to exemplify dependence, and developed, industrialised societies of West, autonomy. In dependence-prone societies there is greater dependence, chronologically in that order, on parents, peer groups, spouse, and finally on one's children. This leads to a beautiful system of inter-relationships, with everybody leaning on everybody else.
>
> Why does this occur? It may be hypothesised that in traditional Eastern societies, there is less clear compartmentalisation of roles and responsibilities. In both personal and professional lives, a person is generally expected to be able to switch/modify his roles as per need of the situation. Another point could be that in traditional societies (like India), a

> child grows up in a family where co-existence and co-dependence of functioning (especially at personal levels) with other members is expected and probably the norm than otherwise. Hence, even on achieving cognitive maturity or adult functioning, the person is not able to fully demarcate his 'self' from others leading to possible lack of clear demarcation (and consequent blurring) of ego boundaries.
>
> To illustrate, Indian patients have been observed to feel freer in terms of being dependent. Most patients will approach the doctor (therapist) with the expectation of getting advice and guidance from him and would expect it to be very similar to that which would be available from their parents and family elders (Roland 1995). It has been further mentioned that Indian patients are brought up with an attitude of being receptive to such advice and guidance as they expect a caring, concerned, and nurturing attitude that goes along with the advice in their familial hierarchical relationships (Varma 2009a).

After having mastered the nutritional needs, the human infant addresses to toilet training, requiring control over the sphincters. Control over the sphincters becomes the prototype of control over oneself—of autonomy. Compared the East with the West, I have commented as follows (Varma 2009a):

'On the other hand, the control over one's sphincters becomes the prototype of control over oneself—of autonomy'. 'The social inter-relationship in the technological advanced countries of the West is more characterised by individual autonomy'. 'This is me and this is my body bounded by my epidermis. Everything within the layer of epidermis is me; and I have, or I should have, complete control over it, over its needs, wishes and desires. I should assume full responsibility over my desires, emotions and actions. Just like I take full responsibility over myself, everybody should take full responsibility for himself or herself.' An autonomous man is more cognisant of his rights and prerogatives, responsibilities and actions. 'Both dependence and autonomy generate its own unique character traits in the members of a society' (Varma 2009a).

As such, the Western man develops with a keener sense of his individuality; his rights, prerogatives and responsibilities. As he or she is responsible for himself or herself, he or she expects and demands others also to be so for themselves. These can be considered to include the following (Varma 2009a):

Traits of a dependence-prone society:

1. An on-going active social inter-relationship between the individual and the society.
2. Pre-occupation with giving and receiving, in day-to-day behaviour, as also in language, idioms and folklore.
3. Lesser idea of individuality: of individual rights, prerogatives and responsibilities.
4. Piety, sacrifice, submission and gratitude as character traits.
5. Development of an 'oral' personality.
6. Strong sense of identity with the primary, filial group.
7. Greater differentiation between 'us' and 'them', with clearly different codes of conduct in dealing with these.
8. Lack of an impersonal 'fairness' and sense of justice.

Attributes of autonomy-prone personality:

1. Clearly demarcated ego-boundaries.
2. Control over one's body—over one's actions, thoughts and emotions. Concern with lack of control over one's body.
3. Greater self-reliance.
4. An acute sense of one's rights and prerogatives.
5. An acute sense of one's duties and responsibilities.
6. Righteous indignation, punitive superego.
7. Self-reliance for one's bodily needs.

The autonomous personality develops in the pursuit of independence and negation of dependence. In an autonomy-prone society, there is a pejorative connotation of dependence. You should be self-reliant and independent, and should not depend on others. In pursuit of asserting oneself, the autonomous person becomes competitive and acquisitive. He is more cognisant of his rights and prerogatives, including the right to keep secrets. He makes clearer distinction between him and others. He judges others, including elders, and does not follow blindly. As he is pursuing his goals, he is also more keenly aware of his own limitations and failings; this gives rise to guilt-proneness. He does not explain things on fate. As he judges himself, he also judges others and pins blame and responsibility. No job is completed till blame is fixed, people punished, and heads roll.

The autonomous individual also has limitations in dealing with members of the immediate family. Marriage, for example, requires ceding one's rights to the spouse. Limitations in ceding such rights can lead to marital problems. The autonomous person is also hampered in accepting limitations arising out of age and disability. As such, as a child, he is in a hurry to grow up to adulthood, as an old person, he is reluctant to seek help from younger family members.

> Doi and Neki (cited in Neki 1976a, b) have developed the concepts of dependence in the cross-cultural context.

> However, it is obvious that neither total dependence nor total autonomy is possible in any society. These are always relative. A total dependence relegating a person to just a mass of protoplasm will not be tolerated. A complete autonomy is also not possible—negating that man has social needs. No man can be an island unto himself (Varma 2009a).

Further:

> The western ethos lauds self-reliance. One should look after himself. It abhors dependence and its manifestations in all forms. The ability to assert himself and to hold to one's own is considered worthy of praise and applause. However, it is the manifestations of man's dependence on each other that brings out the moist eye!

> The dependence-prone individual, on the other hand, lives in a continuous, ongoing relationship with his social milieu. Not only the milieu is taken for granted, the individual becomes an inextricable part of it. The goals and objectives of the group become his goals and objectives. In such a situation, there is no room for exchange of gratitude.

In a dependence-oriented society, friendship is very important. Friendship is always eulogised. 'My friend, right or wrong!' The western society, however, revolves around fair play and egalitarianism. Let the best man win. Egalitarianism holds that all human beings are equal and should be treated as such. There should be no favourites. All friendships are only relative.

In the Western society, the pressure to achieve autonomy is so great that biological limitations to have it are ignored. Children strive for it from a very young age. You are not complete unless you are self-sufficient. From a very young age, children try for economic self-sufficiency. They take up a paper route, do babysitting, wash cars and mow lawns. They are eager to 'grow up,' be like adults. In the process, they deprive themselves of the sheer joy and bliss of a carefree childhood. In the same way, the elderly try their best to continue to be self-reliant as long as possible, even when biological imperatives make it difficult to impossible. However, it has been observed that although age-related de-compensation starts late in the West, once it starts, it is more precipitous and complete, in contrast to the slow-onset relative de-compensation of traditional societies (Varma 2009a).

One other manifestation of the blind pursuit for autonomy and personal rights is the breakdown of conjugal relationships. Marriage revolves around give and take. If both partners insist on total personal rights, it is likely to break down. With the breakdown of the family structure and support, the Western man and woman finally take refuge in the institution of marriage; looks on the spouse to fulfil all the needs for emotional support. All the expectations are pinned on that one person. The spouse is expected to be firm like a father, conciliatory like a grandmother, deferential like a favourite nephew and a friend like a brother. How can one person fulfil all these varied expectations? No wonder, marriage is doomed from the start.

The blind quest for autonomy leads to the development of a judgmental society. The autonomous self-reliant person is solely responsible for his actions. He expects others also to be responsible for themselves. This is opposed to the dependence-prone societies where responsibilities are often viewed as common and communal rather than individual and specific. Each person is constantly evaluated—good versus bad, competent versus incompetent, easy or hard to get along with, pious or sinful. This goes on forever; you have to continuously prove yourself. I have noticed that, in America, in a particular job situation, it takes at least a year or two to get fully accepted. A judgmental society is also quick to assign responsibilities and lay blame for any mishaps. Just like he assigns blame to other, he also does it to self, leading to guilt-proneness.

Although a sense of autonomy can be said to contribute to the individuation process, it can bring about a chasm between men. There is no unquestioning acceptance of people as they are. They are constantly being evaluated. The human relationships become ephemeral and superficial. Open and confiding relationships are compromised, between friends or even spouses.

The autonomous individual is keenly aware of his rights and prerogatives. He jealously guards his privacy and resists any intrusion from others into it. 'Mind your own business,' and 'it is none of your business' are often-heard retorts to such encroachments.

I have pointed out that man's dependence and his capacity for empathy are perhaps the two key (and inter-related) aspects of his social interactions. Neki (1976a, b) has pointed out that "man being an altricial organism, dependence is the fate of every human infant".

Doi (cited in Neki 1975, 1976a, b) has given a well-respected exposition of dependence in the Japanese culture. He has introduced, to the English readers, terms such as amae and amaeru. Amae refers to the feeling that all normal infants at the breast harbour towards the mother. It is dependence, the desire to be loved; the unwillingness to be separated. Amaeru is such a child desiring dependence, whereas amai is the mother allowing the child to behave self-indulgently. (More than the calf wanting to suck, the mother wants to suckle!) These terms are not translatable to other languages; as such concepts may not occur universally. However, I recall a word, larhiyana, meaning acting like a highly dependent, demanding child, the amaeru of Doi, which occurs in my colloquial dialect of Hindi, though not in proper Hindi (Varma 2009a)

As I have pointed out elsewhere (Varma 2002):

- The relentless pursuit of autonomy in Western countries has had undesirable consequences which are now being increasingly recognised. The heightened sense of self-reliance does not permit dependence even in situations where it is a biological imperative; in children, in the aged, in the infirm and disabled. This has given rise to what can be termed "death of childhood" and "death of old age."
- This has led to an intense righteous indignation, assigning responsibility to specific individual to every lapse and mishap. Nothing happens by chance, everything is caused by individuals, and responsibility must be fixed. It leads to finger-pointing, a particularly American trait, and litigiousness. It ignores the fact that the cause-effect relationship between events is neither straightforward nor linear. Many mishaps such as traffic accidents are just that – accidents, in which chance plays a large role and imponderables determine its occurrence. In America, no job is finished until (the paper work is done and) responsibility (for it) is fixed, until heads roll.
- On the other hand, the Eastern dependence admits that we all live in a social system, in an on-going relationship with our environment, and the variables are multiple and often intangible. It teaches us greater understanding in judging our fellow human beings. Short of a stand of intellectual nihilism, we can all use a great deal more humility in judging others!

As Hsu (1972) has put it, 'however, it is obvious that no individual can be self-reliant. In fact, the very foundation of the human way of life is man's dependence upon his fellow human beings'.

Although we have for the sake of simplicity and better understanding, clearly demarcated autonomy and dependence, it must be appreciated that autonomy dependence is a continuum. Furthermore, it needs to be recognised that a society is constantly changing. In a country such as India, autonomy-proneness is probably a more understandable concept in urban population, whereas dependency-proneness is probably more relevant in the rural population. Hence, one may find that the dynamics (or concepts) related to autonomy and dependence may present in a more mixed than a purist approach.

3.2 *The Indian Personality*

There are many ways of understanding the Indian personality. I have summarised it as follows (Varma 2009b):

1. The Indian personality is a 'dependence-prone' personality. The traits of dependence as mentioned in this chapter are manifest to a large degree.
2. The Indian personality is a traditional personality. It is shaped around the primary group, the family. It makes a clear differentiation between the primary group, the family, the in-group and those outside. Responsibilities, commitments and fidelities are all different between the in-group and the out-group.

3. The Indian personality is a religious personality. It has an absolute belief in God, the ultimate creator, and reserves absolute duties to Him or Her. The person will go to any extent to show the commitment and obeisance to our Creator.
4. The Indian society is a technologically developing society. Compared to the West, it is struggling to develop the material resources for life.
5. The Indian personality follows certain beliefs and cognitive styles of its own. This includes a theory of science and of causality. The cognitive style is synthetic.

Putting together the above influences, I have identified the following as the key attributes of the Indian personality (Varma 1985a, b, 1986, 2009a, b):

1. Dependence: Dependence as a key attribute of the Indian personality has already been discussed. Indians are more dependent on each other than is the case in West. As children, we are dependent on our parents. As we grow older, there is dependence on the peer group and the spouse. When we grow old, the tables are turned and we become, in turn, dependent on our children. The ego boundaries around people are loose and people take each other more readily for granted. The Western politeness as evidenced by the use of phrases such as ‘please’, ‘thank you’ and ‘excuse me’ are infrequently used, as they consider all individuals as parts of their own social system. If you touch a hot object and then withdraw your finger, the finger does not say ‘thank you’ to the CNS for conveying and reacting to a noxious stimulus. In the same way, components of a society need not express gratitude to each other.
2. Lack of obsessionality: One thing that may strike a Westerner about India is a relative lack of obsessionality; thoroughness in work. The caution that Lord Chesterton is credited with saying, ‘if anything is worth doing at all, it is worth doing it well’, is relatively lacking. The approach seems to be, what would be the least that one can get by. To give a mundane example, if you attaching a wire to a plug, the person with the minimum approach would stop when the attachment would hold at all, the one who believes in being thorough, would pull at the wire with a considerable force to ensure that it will not lose the connection. There is a relative lack of pride in doing a job well.
3. Identification: As a traditional society, the identification in India is mainly with the primary group, such as the family. Family is more important than friends. Many of the apparent oddities in Indian values are due to the fact that the codes of conduct are different as it applies to those within the primary group and those outside; ‘inside–outside’. Although hospitality is highly extolled as a virtue, it applies largely to the in-group. Indians can be quite rude and callous to an outsider. The Western egalitarian value of due respect and consideration to someone simply because he or she is a member of the human race—simply because he walks on two legs rather than four—seems to be relatively lacking. The differentiation is also manifest in differential generosity to the in-group versus the out-group, and the tendency to draw people, one wants, to the in-group.

4. Selfishness: The typical Indian approach seems to be personal rather than communal. It has been pointed out by cultural anthropologists such as Hsu (1961), that as compared to the Chinese 'situation-centredness', the basic Hindu personality has a supernatural-centredness. The Chinese society has 'mutual dependence' as opposed to the 'unilateral dependence' in India. The Indian person is keenly concerned about his personal mores, such as personal cleanliness, bathing and washing frequently; but he is least concerned about the communal cleanliness, he does not care where the polluted water goes. The selfishness is most manifest in religion, in one's relationship with his or her God. Almost no obstacle is too great to fulfil one's religious duties; for the holy dip at the Ganga (particularly at the holy Kumbh mela), one does not mind if he has to trample over 10 women and 20 children.
5. Codes of conduct: As compared to many societies, the code of conduct in India is largely personalised. The ultimate arbiter to conduct is to empathise, to see how one would feel if he were at the receiving end. *Atmavat sarv bhootanam*. Do not do unto others what you would not have done to you. The code can be summed up by three simple things: consider all women as mother, consider others' belonging as lumps of clay, and consider everybody as yourself. This simplicity stands in sharp contrast to the elaborate rules that have characterised some religions and societies, particularly the Jewish.
6. Fairness: The Western concept of fairness just does not exist. It is not enough that a decision is taken simply because it is 'fair'. Decisions and actions are interpreted depending on whether it is favourable or unfavourable to the members of the primary group.
7. Omnipotence: Just in any culture, a certain amount of omnipotence pervades the Indian personality. Man cannot reconcile himself to the fact that he is just a speck in the universe. He is just one of over six billion people in the world, which itself is just a speck in the known universe. One must develop a certain amount of importance to feel good about himself in such a universe. Such omnipotence reflects itself in mythology and epics in which the person identifies himself with its characters.
8. In-built contradictions: Just as in other cultures, there are in-built contradictions in the Indian values. These are evidenced by the contradiction between free will and determinism, fate and own action. You must submit yourself totally to God but, at the same time, you must do your best. Although your social position, your fate and even your wisdom are determined by karma relating to previous births, you must do your best to improve.
9. Preoccupation with peace: One is struck with the preoccupation with peace, especially at religious functions, where everything begins and ends with incantations of peace (Om shanti). This may indicate a violent past. There is a preoccupation with peace, with a fear of aggression.
10. Traditionalism: The Indian mind can be seen as highly tradition-oriented. This has made change slow and more difficult.
11. Negative values: Certain Western values seem to be lacking, at least relatively. For example, there is not as much of concern over a loss of control

over oneself, and does not evoke the same amount of anxiety and guilt. The Western abhorrence of dependence is less apparent. The punitive superego and the righteous indignation of the Western man; that someone must be punished even if it serves no useful functions, which is also difficult for an Indian to understand. Man is not created in sin.

12. High tradition orientation: Tradition orientation can be viewed as a mechanism to ensure safety and security. It takes away a certain amount of uncertainty in what to do and what not to do.
13. Argumentativeness, challenging and 'sparring': To an outsider, it may appear that we Indians are always quarrelling and arguing. It seems to be much more than in a Western setting. However, it must be seen that much of this is just dialectics, just an exercise, actual violence seldom erupts or long-term animosity takes place.

3.2.1 Interpretation of the Indian Personality

Very loose ego boundaries within the primary group with very sharp distinction between 'we' and 'they'. Low level of compulsivity and high primary narcissism are present. Person is unbounded, exogenous. Preoccupation with peace and high tradition orientation betray a decadent rather than developing society. It can be characterised as passive-dependent personality with evidence of oral aggression.

Lately, the Nobel laureate economist, Sen (2005), wrote 'The Argumentative Indian'. My own views are somewhat similar. We Indians seem to be more argumentative in social situations. Or, seem to be. However, much of the time, the arguments are merely dialectical. It seems to me, though, that people in the eastern parts of India can be more argumentative. However, when it comes to actually being assertive, they may not be so. A common Bengali saying goes like this: 'He beat me; that is OK, but why did he call me names?'

4 Conclusion

- Just as mental health and illness are dependent on individual biological and psychological variables, they are also correlated with sociocultural factors, which must be taken into account for their full understanding. Cross-cultural psychiatric and anthropological research has drawn attention to the considerable differences across cultures in the incidence, typology, manifestations and outcome of mental illness, as in the personality configuration.
- Needs of societies are similar to needs of individuals. Like individuals, society develops by trying to master the basic human needs, biological, social, existential, cognitive and communicative. Societies can be characterised by more or less of dependence, inter-dependence and autonomy. There can be varying

levels of 'oral' and 'anal' traits in various cultures, with reference to food, self-control and obsessionality. The relationship between individuals and the society is complex.

- People differ both within and across societies. As members of *H. sapiens*, we are alike in many ways. However, where the differences across cultures significantly exceed those within it, it can be said that the culture plays a significant role in the shaping of the personality.
- In so far differences across cultures in these exceed those within a cultural group, culture can be said to play a significant role. As such, a macro-level analysis is essential to their understanding.
- In understanding illness as also health, it is not adequate to limit oneself to individual differences. Social and cultural factors are just as important.

References

Barnouw, V. (1963). *Culture and personality*. Homewood, Illinois: Dorsey Press.

DuBois, C. (1944). *The people of Alor*. New York: Harper Row.

Hoch, E. M. (1990). Experiences with psychotherapy in India. *Psychotherapy and Psychosomatics, 53*, 14–20.

Hsu, F. L. K. (1961). *Psychological anthropology*. Homewood, Illinois: Dorsey Press.

Hsu, F. L. K. (1972). *Psychological anthropology*. Cambridge: Schenkman Publishing Co.

Inkeles, A., & Levinson, D. J. (1969/1954). The handbook of social psychology (Rev. ed.). Addison-Wesley, Reading, MA.

Kluckhohn, C. (1962). *Culture and behavior*. Oxford, England: Free Press Glencoe.

Marriott, M. (1976). Interpreting Indian society: A monistic alternative to Dumont's dualism. *Journal of Asian Studies, 36*(1), 189–195.

Murphy, J. M., & Leighton, A. H. (1965). *Approaches to cross-cultural psychiatry*. Ithaca: Cornell University Press.

Neki, J. S. (1975) Psychotherapy in India: past, present, and future. *American Journal of Psychotherapy, 29*(1), 92–100.

Neki, J. S. (1976a). An examination of the cultural relativism of dependence as a dynamic of social and therapeutic relationship. I. Socio-developmental. *British Journal of Medical Psychology, 49*, 1–10.

Neki, J. S. (1976b). An examination of the cultural relativism of dependence as a dynamic of social and therapeutic relationship. II. Therapeutic. *British Journal of Medical Psychology, 49*, 11–22.

Roland, A. (1995). Value issues involving western psychoanalysis with Asian patients. *Journal of the American Academy of Psychoanalysis, 23*, 283–292.

Sen, A. (2005). *The argumentative Indian*. New York: Farrar, Straus and Giroux.

Varma, V. K. (1985a). Psychosocial and cultural variables relevant to psychotherapy in the developing countries. In P. Pichot, et al. (Eds.), *Psychiatry: The state of the art* (Vol. 4, pp. 159–165)., Psychotherapy, psychosomatic medicine Vienna: Plenum Press.

Varma, V. K. (1985b). The Indian mind and psychopathology. *Integrative Psychiatry, 3*, 290–296.

Varma, V. K. (1986). Cultural psychodynamics in health and illness. *Indian Journal of Psychiatry, 28*, 13–34.

Varma, V. K. (1988). Culture, personality and psychotherapy. *International Journal of Social Psychiatry, 34*, 142–149.

Varma, V. K. (2002). Reflections on human existence: A social psychiatric perspective. *Indian Journal of Social Psychiatry, 18*(1–4), 5–12.

Varma, V. K., & Gupta, N. (2008). *Psychotherapy in a traditional society: Context, concept and practice*. New Delhi: Jaypee Brothers Medical Publishers (P) Ltd.

Varma, V. K. (2009a). Culture and the Indian personality. In V. K. Varma, A. K. Kala, & N. Gupta (Eds.), *Culture, personality and mental illness* (pp. 177–187). New Delhi: Jaypee Brothers Medical Publishers (P) Ltd.

Varma, V. K. (2009b). Epidemiology, manifestations and outcome of schizophrenia: East and west. In V. K. Varma, A. K. Kala, & N. Gupta (Eds.), *Culture, personality and mental illness* (pp. 258–274). New Delhi: Jaypee Brothers Medical Publishers (P) Ltd.

Selected Bibliography on Culture and Personality

Barnard, A., & Spencer, J. (1996). *"Culture" encyclopedia of social and cultural anthropology*. London: Routledge.

Benedict, R. (1934). *Patterns of culture*. New York: Mentor.

Benedict, R. (1946). *The chrysanthemum and the sword*. Boston: Houghton Mifflin.

Bock, P. (1980). *Rethinking psychological anthropology*. New York: W. H. Freeman and Co.

Bohannan, P., & Mark, G. (1988). *High points in anthropology*. New York: Alfred A. Knopf.

DuBois, Cora. (1961). *The people of Alor*. New York: Harper Row.

Freud, S. (1950). *Totem and taboo*. New York: Norton.

Goodenough, W. H. (1996). *"Culture" encyclopedia of cultural anthropology*. New York: Henry Holt.

Honigman, J. J. (1954). *Culture and personality*. New York: Harper and Brothers.

Hsu, F. L. K. (1954). *Aspects of culture and personality*. New York: Abelard Schuman.

Mead, Margaret. (1949). *Coming of age in Samoa*. New York: Mentor.

Singer, M. (1964). A survey of culture and personality theory and research. In Studying personality cross-culturally. New York: Elmsford.

Toren, Christina. (1996). *"Culture and personality" encyclopedia of social and cultural anthropology*. London: Routledge.

Varma, V. K., Kala, A. K., & Gupta, N. (2009). *Culture Personality and Mental Illness* (pp. 258–274). New Delhi: Jaypee Brothers Medical Publishers (P) Ltd.

Wallace, A. (1970). *Culture and personality*. New York: Random House.

Part III
Developments in General Adult Psychiatry

Chapter 5
Psychiatric Nosology, Its Philosophy and Science

P.K. Singh

1 Introduction

Psychiatric nosology is currently under intense international scrutiny, both by the public and the professionals. Everybody is a stakeholder and everyone is speaking out, because it is a matter of their personal lives, more particularly of their private mental life. Everybody is also a stakeholder, because everybody has a mind and potentially everyone is a psychiatric patient. The right to liberty, right to expression and right to life empower them to assert their views. It is being questioned as to whether the recently published DSM-5 is a nosology of disorders, or just a list of labels of doubtful validity. Against this backdrop, the status of the psychiatric nosology needs to be examined dispassionately and objectively. Its limits, its strengths and weaknesses should be acknowledged explicitly to obviate undue criticism. A more fundamental analysis of the possible sources of this perpetual ambiguity in terms of the validity and applicability of the principles employed in formation of such nosologies is a matter of urgent concern.

Nosology has been defined as a branch of medicine that deals with classification of diseases.[1] Disease again is a medical concept, which signifies departure from health or the converse of health (Pearce 2011). As the concept of a particular disease evolves to 'mature' form, its symptoms get reliably defined and described.

An erratum of this chapter can be found under DOI 10.1007/978-81-322-1674-2_33

P.K. Singh, Junior Resident

[1] Nosology—Wikipedia, the free encyclopaedia

P.K. Singh (✉)
Department of Psychiatry, Patna Medical College, Patna, India
e-mail: pkspostline@yahoo.com

S. Malhotra and S. Chakrabarti (eds.), *Developments in Psychiatry in India*,
DOI 10.1007/978-81-322-1674-2_5

This is followed by delineation of its pathogenesis in terms of disruption of structure and function and, still later, its aetiology is determined. One of the first indicators of departure from health, at least to the primitive man, must have been the pain and suffering associated with the activities of daily life.

Sufferings of purely mental nature must also be equally old, because it is the mental dimension that truly defines the essence and uniqueness of man. Recorded medical history does bear testimony to this. Man is primarily and pre-eminently a mental organism. Evolution has allowed a massive quantum jump in his mental faculties. It is a paradox though that despite this massive enhancement of his cognitive abilities, he still appears condemned to remain a mystery unto himself. Actually, he is existentially structured to be so. This is so because mental dimension of man is not accessible to objective observation and analysis in the same way as his physical dimension is. It is not surprising, therefore, that the human race had to wait for several millennia, till the arrival of the 'information age', for such massive attention to get focused on the sufferings involving his mental dimension. Yet it appears to be just a prelude to the beginning. This is testified by the sudden emergence of many fierce and some pessimistic reactions to the just published DSM-5, with some calling it 'a snap-shot of a field in flux,' (Jabr 2012) while the National Institute of Mental Health (NIMH), USA, calling it at best a dictionary.[2]

2 The Dilemmas

Psychiatric nosology is to psychiatry what the soul is to individual human beings. Like the soul, nosology also continues to remain at the existential centre of psychiatry, but all the same continue to remain elusive and indefinable. The most fundamental issue surrounding psychiatric nosology is the issue of validity of its diagnostic categories.

Even though reliability has certainly improved tremendously through intensive international efforts, no progress has been made in the area of establishing validity. The search for validity is important, because that alone will separate real entities from pseudo-entities. Only real entities will be definite, definable and stable. Only real entities will permit predictability and be amenable to control. In fact, the validity issue has become further murky in modern times, because of the accumulation of an enormous amount of data from population and general hospital-based observations and studies. There is near universal applicability of 'spectrum phenomena' to almost all categories, a very high occurrence of co-existing or co-morbid diagnoses, and increasing necessity for use of not otherwise specified or not elsewhere classified categories (NOS/NEC) (Goldgerg 2010). Uncertainty about validity gets further highlighted by the frequent observation of diagnostic instability over time at the individual level, as well as by substantial changes made in the nature of categories and criteria, even by the international bodies in the subsequent editions of their classificatory systems. 'Zone of rarity' as a paradigm of separating different entities and defining their boundaries has not been supported by the observational data. The above mentioned observations are possibly because of

[2] NIMH Blog, http://www.nimh.nih.gov/about/director/2013/transforming-diagnosis.shtml

extremely large number of factors operating simultaneously leading to enormous variability at the level of mental or behavioural phenomena. Very large number of factors lead to generation of innumerable, mostly unique 'disposition-profiles' of both normal and abnormal states, which defy classification as categories. Since it is not repetitive, it will not form a class and thereby would not permit classification. This raises a more fundamental question.

How valid and applicable is the notion that validity of psychiatric conditions can be established on the same parameters as that for other medical conditions? This notion is intrinsically flawed.

The intrinsic flaw is that we overlook the boundary between the physical and the mental when it comes to the issue of examining the validity of disorders in these two domains. We treat them both with the same yardstick. It would be a matter of common sense to presume that medical disorders would have features of physical domain, whereas psychiatric disorders would have features of mental domain. Physical and mental domains are qualitatively different. The physical domain is constituted of matter, whereas the constituents of mental domain are unknown. Properties of matter would apply to physical domain, but would not apply to mental domain. Therefore, the concept of validity as applicable to material domain would not be the same as that applicable to mental domain.

Inherent in the search for validity is the premise that the real has to be separated from the artefacts. The real is the one that exists 'on its own' in nature, whereas artefacts would be the subjective creations of human mind. It is something like the relationship between the waking experience and the dream experience. The physical or the material domain exists purely in the objective realm, whereas the mental domain exists exclusively in the subjective realm. It is not accessible to 'objective' observation. We cannot observe somebody else's mind in the same way as we can observe his body and its different parts. As regards the mind, only subjective individual introspection is possible. Its existence beyond the immediate conscious experience remains unknown.

But, introspection is not considered a valid scientific method of observation, because it cannot be consensually validated through its agencies of observation. All the same, the validity of introspective truths cannot be denied; we have to focus our creative energies to devise paradigms for convergence of introspective and observational truths. Till the time we are able to do that, we have to make do with limited 'validity' for the psychiatric entities, commensurate with the primary dimension to which it refers to, that is the mind. In fact, international efforts should focus more on unravelling and establishing the nature of mind rather than its neurophysiologic correlates.

Modern age is dominated by doctrines of science. Science is dominating, because it has empowered people in their struggle against nature and has also transformed their lives. Science is a product of the human mind, but, unfortunately scientific methods are not applicable to the study of mental phenomena. Even most advanced neurophysiologic studies should not be equated with the study of mental phenomenon per se. At best, it can be a specific or a non-specific substrate for the other. The two cannot be considered interchangeably. Forcing a universal 'brain' explanation for all mental phenomena is like forcing a square into a circle. This is one of the reasons why such limited progress has been made in this area of brain–behaviour relationships, despite so much investment of resources of time, talent and treasure. Since psychiatry is a relatively recent offshoot of modern scientific medicine, it is still nurturing fond and nascent hopes, and aspirations of being similar to its brethren from the world of physical medicine. This natural-looking, seemingly acceptable goal appears completely oblivious of the fact that the physical and mental dimensions of man are completely and qualitatively different from each other. Even though they are seamlessly one and mutually interdependent, they are not on the same plane. They complement and supplement each other into emergence of a 'supra-ordinary' being, with some limited autonomy to impose certain rules of its own on itself and the milieu.

3 The Differences

Some of the qualitative differences between the physical and mental domain has already been mentioned above. Further, it appears that even the concept of aetiology may not be uniformly applicable to both the mental and physical dimensions. Mental events and its manifestations are quite often dictated and guided by the goals or the end points to be achieved, which becomes obvious when we analyse our speech and behaviour. All our speech and behaviour is always guided by a goal. On the other hand, physical events are guided and dictated by the antecedent or the initiating influence. One is guided by the past, whereas the other seemingly is guided by the future as set from beforehand. This is a mystery as well as a paradox that both kinds of operating paradigms should not only co-exist within the same organism, but also should work seamlessly in consonance with each other. In fact, this should be considered as one of the most important attainments of the evolutionary process. Evolution is not simply about movement from amoeba to homo sapiens; it is as well a movement from antecedent driven causality to consequence driven causality, from 'command' driven causality to 'demand' or 'goal' driven causality. It is a very fundamental difference; therefore, different yardsticks become obligatory to be used for these two domains. In fact, it may be conceptualised that emergence of consciousness was necessitated to provide a transcendent plane where goals and directions could be preset for emergent behaviours to be expressed by organism. This would also make the behaviour of the organism predictable, and thus, setting the stage for collective living to form societies, civilizations and cultures.

There are a few other ways in which aetiology for psychiatric disorders would be different from aetiology for physical disorders. Because of a higher order multi-factoriality of psychiatric disorders, the possibility that several factors may be equally contributing to the causation of disordered states is very high as against solitary factors, which are often sufficient to cause specific disorders on the physical plane. In this context, it will be more prudent to talk of 'aetiology-spectrum' for psychiatric disorders as against mostly single aetiological factor for physical disorders. This appears to be an interesting combination of 'spectrum clinical phenomena' linked to 'aetiology-spectrum' of causes. Another very important difference is that mental plane is in dynamic equilibrium with not only itself, but also with social, spiritual as well as physical planes. Therefore, a causal influence may be located in any of these planes. Accordingly, causation of mental phenomena would be 'trans-dimensional,' as against predominantly 'iso-dimensional' causation for physical phenomena, where cause and effect take place on the same plane, that is the material plane.

Another unique feature about mental phenomena is that they operate at different levels of consciousness, which is the primary quality of this domain. Events and influences get stratified into conscious, subconscious and unconscious compartments, which keep interacting. There is no such arrangement in the physical dimension. There is nothing like the sub-material plane. On the top of all these differences, there is the confounding variable of 'autonomy' available on the mental plane. Autonomy implies personal control over self, of whatever limited magnitude it may be. In instances of disorder, the surface manifestation of the disorder at the mental plane may get modified by the exercise of this faculty of autonomy, which may be used either to react or adapt or compensate. So the final picture of psychopathology that emerges in any particular instance would be the net result of the sum total of all the commands and demands of all the dimensions as modified by the autonomy-based responses of the individual. This would be very different from the generally linear iso-dimensional cause and effect relationship seen on the dimension of physical plane. The identity of a disorder on the physical plane is at the aetiology level, whereas the identity of a disorder at the mental plane should ideally and desirably be at the manifest level, that is the consequence or the product level. The aetiology in such situations are generally multiple, diverse and scattered along different co-variate dimensions.

4 The Difficulties

There is absolute lack of clarity about the nature of the mind. There is further lack of clarity about the nature of relationship between the mind and the body. In the absence of any reasonable answer or even hypothesis about these two questions, we, the mental health professionals, are in complete darkness. However, most of us seem blissfully unaware of it. We keep exploring and experimenting about mental disorders as if we are under full noon sun. The often discussed neural-circuitry or a chemical imbalance can be a substrate for a particular emotion or an idea, but it cannot be a substitute for them. A neural-circuitry or a neurotransmitter is not the same as any emotional or cognitive experience. Any mental phenomenon can best be described only in terms of mental attributes and not in terms of neurophysiology or neurochemistry. It is absolutely improbable that there ever shall be a neurophysiologic dictionary of different mental states. While it is commendable that we should direct research efforts to discover the physiological substrates for different mental states in health and disease, we should also keep ourselves cognisant of its severe limitations. We have several examples today wherein the same drug molecule is equally effective against widely diverse type of symptomatology. The classic drug haloperidol is effective not only against thought disorders, but also against motor and mood symptoms of great diversity.

Another difficulty relates to the cut-off line that requires to be drawn between normal and abnormal, between order and disorder. For physical, bio-medical sciences it is much simpler. A cut-off value, inclusive of a range, is determined on the basis of population-based sample studies. But the value remains stable and static. The same does not hold true for mental dimension. Here, the cut-off line has to be dynamic and different not only for different individuals, but also sometimes within the same individual. The cut-off line, most often, cannot be defined in absolute terms. It can be meaningfully defined only in terms that are relative to the concerned individual. Every individual provides his own measure of comparison in terms of the baseline of his functional state. Now, this baseline is not a static entity. It is a dynamic entity and changes with the changing socio-economic and cultural context of the individual (Rosenberg 2006). Human capacity to adapt and change is tremendous and this would lead to changing parameters of judgment for states of disorder, because with every adaptation the baseline changes. A simple example from the physical world will make the statement more explicit. Human capacity to see visually ranges from pitch darkness to extremely bright sunlight, which would represent a difference of several thousand times in terms of brightness, requiring very specialised modes of adaptation for the visual apparatus. Similar adaptation, multiplied manifold, is also seen at the level of mental plane.

5 The Realities

The reality is that we have a huge burden of mental sufferings and dysfunctions at the population level. The pattern of suffering also exhibits bewilderingly diverse variety of presentations. Mental ‘pain’ quite often is more excruciating than any kind of physical pain. One mentally sick person in the family has a distressing and disruptive impact on the whole family. Therefore, there is an urgent and immediate need for reducing the nosologic complexity to make it comprehensible and manageable by average human cognitive abilities. We need to simplify our system of classification to be able to deliver the services to alleviate sufferings of people. Individual life and its sufferings cannot wait till the issue of validity is resolved. What we need to pragmatically do is to modify our expectations from the massive international efforts being put in preparation of psychiatric nosologies. There appears to be some merit in the comment that it is just a dictionary, but the reality is that compilation of a dictionary of this nature and magnitude is definitely a step forward, and therefore an achievement. All the same, there is general international consensus that our categories do not have established validity. It is also true that we have not been able to comprehensively and effectively define psychiatric disorders and also that our disorders do not meet the set medical criteria of disease.

Till the time we are able to address the above mentioned issues adequately, we should stop calling our compendium of sufferings as a nosology, but continue at the same time to evolve strategies to remedy the mental maladies. We should try not to match our discipline with the profile of physical sciences. Many distortions which creep into psychiatric nosology are because of our anxiety and compulsion to match with the ‘hard sciences’. Methods of science are aptly applicable only for the material sciences. As mental health professionals, we should accept this difference and evolve a different set of concepts and principles to deal with the immaterial phenomenon of inaccessible mind and its expressions through body which are amenable to observation. In that sense, it is half science and half beyond-science. We should acknowledge our ignorance about this 'beyond-science' component, and let it be reflected in our system of classifications internationally. All knowledge does not and need not fall within the jurisdiction of science alone. We should not feel compelled to be called a science to acquire validity. Validity will originate from valid and stable human experiences of qualitatively different nature. Knowledge of those dimensions which are beyond the realm of sensory observation can only be gained through internal revelations, which were the method and practice of our ancient sages.

Even in the field of material sciences, there has been a trend to move towards paraphysics, (Shamasundar 2008) to explain some of the unpredictable behaviours of subatomic particles by invoking an element of consciousness. On the other hand, we, the trustees of consciousness, tend to look backwards and try to wear the mask of definitive material sciences to assume validity and acquire respectability. This is an unrealistic aspiration and endeavour and, therefore, is likely to fail. In the final analysis, even the most valid truth shall remain a relative truth, relative to the existential human predicament. None of our truths can be truer than the truth quotient that can be assigned to our existence in this cosmos. Therefore, we should accept the 'surface' manifestations of disordered psychiatric states as valid and true. Nothing that may be discovered in the name of putative aetiology of the disorder can be truer than the surface psychopathology. At best, it can be equally true. If someone were to ask for the validity of my perception of an object and its colour, it cannot come from any source other than me. No one else can validate my perception. The only ways available at present for such validation is the demonstration of stability over time and collective concordance of experience.

6 Indian Contributions

India has generally been at the forefront of discourses relating to mind, intellect and soul. It may be considered one of the world leaders. However, its contribution to the field of psychiatric nosology in the recent past has been very limited. This may be a reflection of very small size of psychiatric professionals in our country. Apart from some bold proposals and suggestions from Wig (1967), Varma (1971), Teja (1971), Singh (1980) and Rao (1971) in the initial part of last half-century, no significant effort to comprehensively address this fundamental issue has been made. One notable contribution has been the description of a culture-specific syndrome, the 'Dhat Syndrome' by Dr. N.N. Wig and its subsequent international acceptance (WHO 1992). These attempts have been beautifully reviewed by Khandelwal (2000) and Jacob (2010).

In the latter part of last half of the century, some robust contributions have been made by Indian psychiatrists to classification of mental disorders, but it has been restricted to acute and transient psychosis, possession states and post-traumatic stress disorder.[3] Malhotra (2007) has extensively contributed to and reviewed the area of acute and transient psychosis, and Dalal (2009) has examined in depth the challenges facing psychiatric classification. The contributions made by earlier indigenous system of medicine, which is known by the abbreviation AYUSH, have been comprehensively reviewed and documented by Murthy (2001). AYUSH includes all those systems of medicine, which either originated in India or flourished significantly on the Indian soil. It also includes yoga because yogic practices are intimately linked to maintenance and restoration of health. Ayurveda, Unani, Siddha and Homoeopathy systems have their own vocabulary and nomenclature for the mental afflictions, but none of them have gone beyond the surface to make any great revelations. In that sense, psychiatric nosology has not made any progress till date, because the present so-called modern psychiatric nosologies are also stuck at the same level. There has been no further evolution.

Avasthi (2011) has made a strong case for the need for Indianizing psychiatry and not globalising it. This is based on the uniqueness of the Indian psyche, Indian culture and value system, Indian family and social support system, spiritual orientation of Indian masses and to some extent ethno-genetic differences. Despite these differences, he acknowledges that evidence for substantive India-specific syndromes or symptom complexes is yet to come. There was no evidence for this in the International Pilot Study of Schizophrenia (IPSS); however, it may be seen in other categories which have not been studied so far. Part of the reason for this may be the fact that all the tools for study used by us have been validated in the West.

7 Conclusions

Human mind, if at all it exists, is very different from human body. They are qualitatively different even though they function seamlessly as an integrated whole. In case it does not exist, still it is a vital, crucial and practical construct of the indomitable and dominant dimension of man, which does seem to operate independently as well as in conjunction with the body. Deviations and disruptions within this dimension can best be described and understood only in terms of the language of the variables of mind. If we truly want to make progress in the area of psychiatric disorders, we must address some of the most fundamental issues on a priority basis relating to mind. It is most paradoxical as well as surprising that we do not know what mind is, but continue to discuss mental disorders. The simplest corollary of this is that if we don't know what mind is, we cannot know what mental disorders are. Another corollary would be that we can know only as much about mental disorders as much we know about the mind. Under the circumstances, the

[3] Report of the Indian Psychiatric Society's Task Force on the Diagnostic and Statistical Manual-5 (2012).

most scientific and rational approach would be that if we do not understand what mental disorders are, we should acknowledge it and not force them to fit into the scheme of physical disorders. Once we are able to develop a scheme for mental disorders, it should have the provision for accommodating the uniqueness of man as well as uniqueness of his suffering.

A combination of categorical and dimensional approach appears to be the most viable alternative. The categorical approach will take care of the similarities at the more basic level, whereas the dimensional approach will take care of the differences at the higher individual level. This will take care of both the basic and unique aspects of individual's suffering. However, since almost none of our diagnostic categories meet the criteria of a medical disease, it will be a misrepresentation at the moment, if we present them as nosology to the public, because it gives an impression of knowledge, wherein we are actually ignorant. If we agree to replace the word nosology with a word that would mean being a precursor to the nosology, that would take care of the matter, and silence many of the current criticisms. That will also be a bold and de facto statement of the present predicament. Psychiatric nosology of today can at best be an album of the spectrum of psychiatric conditions, which require professional attention and intervention.

Therefore, we should urgently coordinate to focus international attention on unravelling the nature of mind and its relationship with somatic, social and spiritual dimensions of man. Let us first try to understand what the mind is. We will automatically understand better what mental disorders are.

References

Avasthi, A. (2011). Indianizing psychiatry—Is there a case enough. *Indian Journal of Psychiatry, 53*(2), 111–120.

Dalal, P. K., & Sivakumar, T. (2009). Moving towards ICD-11 and DSM-V: Concept and evolution of psychiatric classification. *Indian Journal of Psychiatry, 51*, 310–319.

Goldgerg, D. (2010). Should our major classifications of mental disorders be revised? *The British Journal of Psychiatry, 196*, 255–256.

Jabr, F. (2012). Psychiatry's diagnostic guidebook gets its first major update in 30 years. *Scientific American*, May 7, 2012, 6.

Jacob, K. S. (2010). Indian psychiatry and classification of psychiatric disorders. *Indian Journal of Psychiatry, 52*, 104–109.

Khandelwal, S. K. (2000). Classification of mental disorders : Need for a common language. In R. Srinivasamurthy (Ed.), *Mental Health in India: Essays in Honour of Professor N.N. Wig*. Bangalore: People's Action for Mental Health.

Malhotra, S. (2007). Acute and transient psychosis: A paradigmatic approach. *Indian Journal of Psychiatry, 49*, 233–243.

Murthy, R. S., & Wig, N. N. (2001). Psychiatric diagnosis and classification in developing Countries. *WPA Book-Psychiatric Classification.*

Pearce, J. M. S. (2011). Naming diseases. *Hektoen International A Journal of Medical Humanities*, *3*(4), (internet article).

Rao, A. V. (1971). Classification of depression. *Indian Journal of Psychiatry, 13*, 21–26.

Rosenberg, C. (2006). Contested boundaries: Psychiatry, disease, and diagnosis. *Perspectives in Biology and Medicine, 49*(3), 407–424.

Shamasundar, C. (2008). Relevance of ancient Indian wisdom to modern mental health—A few examples. *Indian Journal of Psychiatry, 50*(2), 138–143.

Singh, G., & Tewari, S. K. (1980). Morbid grief—its clinical manifestation and proposed classification. *Indian Journal of Psychiatry, 22*, 74–80.

Teja, J. S. (1971). Proposed classification of "other psychoses" for use in India. *Indian Journal of Psychiatry, 13*, 7–13.

Varma, V. K. (1971). Classification of psychiatric disorders for use in India (neuroses). *Indian Journal of Psychiatry, 13*, 1–6.

Wig, N. N., & Singh, G. (1967). A proposed classification of psychiatric disorders for use in India. *Indian Journal of Psychiatry, 8*, 157–171.

World Health Organization (1992). International classification of disease 10. Clinical descriptions and diagnostic guidelines. Geneva: WHO.

Chapter 6
Common Mental Disorders in India

R.K. Chadda

1 Introduction

Conventionally, the discipline of psychiatry is often identified with severe mental illnesses like schizophrenia and other psychotic disorders. The movement of psychiatry from inside the walls of the mental hospitals to the community, accompanied by the growth of the general hospital psychiatric units, led to a focus on non-psychotic psychiatric illnesses like depression, anxiety and other neurotic disorders, which also occur more commonly in the community. Goldberg and Huxley (1992), recognising the public health implications and disability associated with these illnesses, introduced the term common mental disorders (CMDs) in the literature. CMDs included anxiety disorders, depression and related neurotic disorders. Though these illnesses exist as separate categories in the classification systems, they often occur as comorbid conditions, and their treatment also tends to be along similar principles. These associations made the term popular, since it was convenient to group these illnesses under this umbrella term. The CMD group would also include somatoform disorders, which commonly present in primary care and general medical settings, and tend to have associated anxiety and depressive symptoms. CMDs are especially important for their public health implications, since these often remain unrecognised in the primary care and medical settings, and are responsible for increased health-care burden and costs (World Health Organisation 2001). Effective treatments exist for the CMDs, and thus, an early diagnosis and management might reduce this huge drain on resources.

R.K. Chadda, Professor

R.K. Chadda (✉)
Department of Psychiatry, All India Institute of Medical Sciences, New Delhi, India
e-mail: drrakeshchadda@gmail.com

S. Malhotra and S. Chakrabarti (eds.), *Developments in Psychiatry in India*,
DOI 10.1007/978-81-322-1674-2_6

This paper discusses epidemiology, nosology, clinical presentation, public health aspects and management of the CMDs with a special focus on the Indian research on the subject.

2 Epidemiology

Epidemiological studies have shown that the CMDs may have an annual prevalence of about 10–12 % with lifetime prevalence going up to 20–25 % (World Health Organisation 2001). Patients with CMDs constitute about 7.3–52.5 % of the clinic populations of primary care settings (Goldberg and Lecrubier 1995). Prevalence of CMDs in primary care settings has varied from about 11–34.6 % in different Indian studies (Nambi et al. 2002). Reasons for this wide variation in prevalence could be due to differences in the inclusion criteria (Nambi et al. 2002). A recent study from India reported a prevalence of 42 % in patients attending a medical outpatient clinic in a tertiary care hospital (Avasthi et al. 2008). About 10 % of the patients presenting in general practice settings have been reported to suffer from depression (Ormel et al. 1993). Prevalence of generalised anxiety disorder in primary care settings is reported to be in range of 5–16 % (Wittchen 2002) and that of panic disorder as 1.5–13 % (Craske et al. 2002).

CMDs are more common in women and in persons belonging to lower socio-economic strata and the marginalised populations (Patel and Kleinman 2003; Patel et al. 2006a).

CMDs can cause significant patient suffering and disability and lead to substantial health-care costs (Smith et al. 1986). Patients with CMDs are more often seen in primary care and general medical settings, rather than in psychiatric services (Manderscheid et al. 1993). Most people with anxiety or depression visit their general practitioner, whether or not they complain of their psychological symptoms (Goldberg and Huxley 1992). Primary care physicians fail to diagnose and treat nearly 50–75 % of patients suffering from CMDs, presenting in their clinical practice (Ormel et al. 1991; Borus et al. 1988).

3 Risk Factors for CMDs

As is the case with most psychiatric disorders, aetiology of CMDs is multi-factorial, with the socio-economic stressors probably triggering a biological process in vulnerable individuals leading to development of the illness.

Poverty, economic deprivation, low educational status and unemployment have been identified as common risk factors for the development of CMDs (Fryers et al. 2003; Pothen et al. 2003; Shankar et al. 2006). Poverty, being married, tobacco use, history of abnormal vaginal discharge, history of chronic physical illnesses like cardiovascular diseases, diabetes and spinal or back disorders and physical disability are associated with increased risk of developing CMDs in the developing countries (Patel and Kleinman 2003).

Gender disadvantage, exposure to intimate partner violence, sexual and reproductive complaints (e.g., excessive vaginal discharge) and tobacco use have been found to predispose to development of CMDs in women (Prasad et al. 2003; Patel et al. 2006b). Higher prevalence in women is not apparently due to hormonal or other biological mechanisms, but the gender disadvantage especially in form of intimate partner violence and low levels of autonomy in decision making could be the key risk factors for higher prevalence of CMDs in women (Patel et al. 2006b).

4 Clinical Presentation

Patients with CMDs often present with physical complaints, frequently in primary care settings. Clinical presentation is no different in secondary or tertiary care settings.

The patients commonly present with complaints of subjective weakness, headache, vague somatic sensations, pain in extremities, palpitations, giddiness or dizziness, bodily tremors, numbness or tingling sensations (Chadda et al. 1991; Srinivasan et al. 1986). The Indian patient frequently comes out with a symptom of vague somatic sensations, which is described in words like *bharipan* (heaviness of parts of the body), *halkapan* (lightness of the body parts), heat or cold or pin-pricking sensation, *houl* (restlessness) or gas in body. The person may use different colloquial words to describe the symptoms. An unpleasant sensation may be described as travelling from one body part to other and finally leaving from the head or the feet, defying all anatomical boundaries. Some of the symptoms like difficulty breathing, chest pain, pounding heart or gaseous abdomen are a part of sympathetic overactivity or psychogenic autonomic dysfunction (Chadda 2011).

On screening for psychological symptoms, it is often possible to elicit the specific symptoms of the primary psychiatric illnesses (Chadda 2000, 2010a, b). There may be an admixture of anxiety and depressive symptoms. On the standard classificatory systems, patients with CMDs may receive a diagnosis of depressive episode, generalised anxiety disorder, mixed anxiety depression, panic disorder, undifferentiated somatoform disorder, dysthymia or other anxiety or somatoform disorders (Chadda and Bhatia 1990). Many of them may not fulfil the criteria for a specific disorder and receive a diagnosis of anxiety disorder, unspecified type or depression, unspecified type (Chadda et al. 1991).

Explanatory model interviews have shown that a significant proportion of patients with CMDs, presenting with unexplained physical symptoms in the primary care settings, hold a combination of medical and non-medical views about their condition (Nambi et al. 2002; Shankar et al. 2006). Many of these patients consider that they are having a specific medical disease and attribute their symptoms to a variety of causes. They perceive their illness as serious, and also fear death and major disability. Only a minority of patients presenting in primary care attribute their problems to psychological causes, though many would admit having emotional problems secondary to the physical symptoms (Nambi et al. 2002; Shankar et al. 2006).

Patients, who present with CMDs in psychiatry outpatient settings on being referred from other specialties, may deny having a psychiatric illness. They, however, would accept the treatment offered by the psychiatrist and are also willing to come for follow-up. A belief in somatic model of illness and stigma of being identified as mentally ill could be the reason for the phenomenon.

5 Assessment

Recognition of the CMDs is poor in primary care, with less than one-third of clinically significant morbidity detected (Ustun and von Korff 1995). Patients presenting with non-specific somatic symptoms with no apparent physical cause are often prescribed various symptomatic medications, such as vitamins, iron supplements or pain killers, since the primary care physician may not be able to diagnose the underlying CMD. Many such patients are also subjected to unnecessary investigations. A multi-centric study conducted by WHO on mental health problems in general health care reported that nearly 10 % of primary care attendees with CMDs in the Indian study centre were prescribed psychotropic drugs (Linden et al. 1999). The majority of prescriptions were for tranquilisers (benzodiazepines), rather than antidepressant drugs.

In a busy primary care clinic in India and neighbouring countries, the physicians have a very limited time available to screen for CMDs. More so, the primary care physicians have received a limited exposure to psychiatry during their undergraduate training, though some of them might have attended the orientation programmes on mental health conducted under the National Mental Health Programme. Thus, the primary care physicians have an inadequate knowledge of the CMDs and are often unable to reach a correct diagnosis in such patients, since they are not familiar with the appropriate questions to be asked. Undetected psychiatric morbidity in primary care commonly leads to unnecessary investigations, medications and continued suffering of the patient. This inevitably leads to impaired family, occupational and social functioning, thus making it crucial for primary care and general practice physicians to be equipped with the necessary skills and measures for detecting CMDs in their patients and providing the necessary treatment.

In the last two decades, a number of structured screening instruments have been developed for screening the patients presenting with CMDs in primary care settings. Though originally developed for the Western populations, most of these have also been standardised in the Indian population. Some of these are also available in Indian vernacular languages. These include the General Health Questionnaire-12 (GHQ-12) (Gautam et al. 1987; Jacob et al. 1997), the Self-Report Questionnaire (SRQ) (Harding et al. 1980), and the Primary Care Evaluation of Mental Disorders (PRIME-MD)—Patient Health Questionnaire (PHQ) (Avasthi et al. 2008). All of these can be easily administered in 5–10 min. The PRIME-MD-PHQ also provides a psychiatric diagnosis.

Another brief instrument, the Mental Health Inventory (MHI), a 5-item subscale of the Short Form Health Survey (SF-36), can also be used to screen for CMDs in primary care settings. The MHI has 5 basic questions, which can be easily incorporated in clinical assessment. This does not take more than 2–3 min to administer. The five questions are as follows: in the past 4 weeks: (a) Have you been very nervous? (b) Have you felt so down in the dumps that nothing could cheer you up? (c) Have you felt calm and peaceful? (d) Have you felt downhearted and depressed? and (e) Have you been happy? (Fone et al. 2007). The items are rated from 1 to 5. The response scores are converted to scoring on 0–100, where 100 is indicative of best mental health.

Once a patient screens positive on a screening instrument, a formal psychiatric assessment to screen for the specific CMD can be undertaken. This would include screening for depression and anxiety disorders.

6 Public Health Aspects

CMDs are associated with substantial disease burden and disease-related disability. As per the Global Burden of Disease (GBD) study, mental and neurological disorders were responsible for 10.5 % of the total disability-adjusted life years (DALYs) in 1990 (Murray and Lopez 1996). This was the first time that mental disorders were identified as responsible for a high burden as a result of years lost due to all diseases and injuries. The figure increased to 12.3 % in 2000 (World Health Organisation 2001). Depression has been identified as a fourth leading cause of the DALYs in the 15–44 year age group. In the recently published GBD estimates for the year 2010 (Murray et al. 2012), mental and behavioural disorders were responsible for 7.4 % of all the DALYs. This included major depressive disorder (2.5 %), anxiety disorders (1.1 %), drug use disorders (0.8 %), alcohol use disorders (0.7 %), schizophrenia (0.6 %) and others. In the GBD 2010 report, there was a global shift in the burden of disease from communicable, maternal, neonatal and nutritional disorders to non-communicable diseases and injuries. There was an increase in DALYs from 54,010 to 74,264 (37.6 % increase) due to depression and from 19,664 to 26,826 (36.4 % increase) due to anxiety disorders during the period 1990–2010. On adjusting for the increase in the world population during this period, the increase in DALYs due to depression and anxiety disorders comes out to be 5.8 and 5.0 %, respectively. Mean rank of depression has risen from 15 to 11 in the diseases listed in order of causing DALYs (Murray et al. 2012). Thus, the GBD 2010 report further emphasises the significance of CMDs in relation to disease-related disability and burden associated with this group.

There have also been a number of studies in India which have assessed disability and psychosocial dysfunction due to CMDs. In one of the earliest studies, patients presenting with somatic symptoms with a depressive diagnosis were found to suffer more severe psychosocial dysfunction than those who received a somatoform diagnosis (Chadda et al. 1993). Dysfunction was especially seen in personal, social, familial and vocational functioning and was minimal in cognitive areas. This is understandable, since the CMDs are not expected to affect the higher mental functions. CMDs have been reported to be associated with impaired functioning in family situations, social relations and work performance (Nambi et al. 2002). In the study by Nambi et al., 69 % of the subjects reported their work being affected by the illness, and around 40 % felt that the illness affected their family and social life.

CMDs as well as their subthreshold symptoms pose a substantial risk of functional disability and absence from work (Rai et al. 2010). The disability rises in increments with increasing psychiatric symptom load, not just for depression but for the entire spectrum of CMDs. Disorders like mixed anxiety depression, which are generally considered mild, are also significantly disabling. Similarly, a higher number of medically unexplained physical symptoms are associated with more disability. In a study by our group, nearly three-fourths of the patients with somatisation disorder suffered moderate-to-severe disability (Kushwaha et al. (2013) A study of disability and its correlates in somatization disorder (Kushwaha et al 2014). Disability showed a positive correlation with duration of illness, number of somatisation symptoms, number of prior consultations and anxiety and depression scores. In another study on caregiver burden and disability in somatization disorder (Krishnan et al. 2013), disability suffered by the patients with somatisation disorder was comparable to that seen in patients with chronic depression and schizophrenia. The study had, however, included clinically stable patients with schizophrenia. But even then, it highlights the public health significance of the CMDs. The patients with depression as well as somatisation disorder were found to lead to similar levels of burden in their caregivers, as those of schizophrenia. These two studies had used the ICD 10 definition of somatisation disorder, which is much broader than the earlier narrower definitions of the illness. Such patients also form a significant proportion of the CMDs presenting in various medical care settings.

7 Public Health Initiatives in India

One of the objectives of the National Mental Health Programme of India was integration of mental health in general health care. The basic purpose underlying the objective was that the treating physician should be able to diagnose and manage the psychiatric morbidity presenting in general medical and primary care settings. The programme has been in existence since 1982 (Murthy 2011). Under its flagship programme, the District Mental Health Programme and orientation programmes in mental health have been undertaken for the primary care doctors. There has not been much follow-up of such training programmes. Most of such training programmes have focused on lectures and case demonstrations.

In a modification of the orientation programmes, Chadda et al. (2009a, b) used a problem-based learning approach for sensitising primary care doctors with the CMDs. A series of one-day workshops were organised, with each workshop being attended by about 40 doctors. The participants were divided into groups of 6–8 each. The workshops were conducted by 3 psychiatrists. Each workshop was divided into 3 sessions, one each on anxiety disorders, depression and somatoform disorders. Each session comprised of a group task with a case vignette, presentation of the management plan by one of the group members and a brief discussion. Each group was given a case vignette along with 5 questions about the case like further information required to make a diagnosis, provisional diagnosis, differential diagnosis and treatment. Each group made a presentation about their case, key issues and its management. Each session included an interactive lecture by a psychiatrist followed by discussion. The programme was well received by the participants.

In the recent past, the National Mental Health Programme has taken a number of more initiatives by covering more districts in the country, as well as in manpower development in psychiatry, clinical psychology, psychiatric social work and psychiatric nursing. A large number of the tertiary care centres in the country have also developed community outreach programmes at the respective centres (Murthy 2011). All these efforts would be helpful in improving management of CMDs in primary care and in reducing the associated burden and disability.

8 Management

The most important component of the management of CMDs is the early recognition. Since the patients present mostly in the primary care settings, the primary care physicians need to be sensitised about early recognition and management of the patients with CMDs in their clinical practice. Once diagnosed, the CMDs are not difficult to manage. A number of brief self-administered screening questionnaires have been developed in the recent past, as discussed in one of the previous sections. Any one of these can be used to screen the primary care attendees, which would help in early recognition of the patients with CMDs.

Most of the patients with CMDs can be easily managed at the primary care level itself. The management includes psychotherapeutic interventions and medications. Psychotherapeutic interventions have a crucial role in management. In addition, antidepressant and antianxiety medications often need to be used. Selective serotonin uptake inhibitors have efficacy against both anxiety as well as depressive symptoms and also relieve the associated somatic symptoms. Other antidepressants like venlafaxine and tricyclic antidepressants also have efficacy against both anxiety as well as depressive symptoms, but these are more often the second-line medications. Venlafaxine and tricyclic antidepressants can be used in patients who do not respond or are unable to tolerate SSRIs (Chadda 2010, 2011).

Cognitive behaviour therapy (CBT)-based interventions have specifically been used in management of CMDs. Efficacy of psychotherapeutic interventions in CMDs has been demonstrated in a few Indian studies (Patel et al. 2003, 2010; Kushwaha et al. 2013). The interventions include psychoeducation, relaxation exercises (simple breathing exercises or progressive muscular relaxation), defocusing from physical symptoms, activity scheduling, distraction and problem solving. The therapy sessions may be given as individual sessions or in group settings. Since the patients often have a focus on physical symptoms, ABC charting (antecedent of symptom or its worsening, contingent behaviour and the consequence) for the symptoms may be used to identify the antecedents to the appearance or worsening of symptoms, which can be discussed in the subsequent sessions. Focus in the later sessions needs to be on cognitive restructuring by defocusing from the physical symptoms, distraction and engagement on pleasurable activities and activity scheduling. Patients should be advised to practise the techniques at home (Kushwaha et al. 2013). In an 8-week intervention study in patients with somatisation disorder, CBT-based psychotherapeutic intervention in combination with fluoxetine brought about significantly more improvement in neuroticism, anxiety, depression and disability, compared to the control group which had received supportive therapy along with fluoxetine. The control group had also shown improvement on various parameters.

Vikram Patel and coworkers have done extensive work in the area in community settings in Goa, India. In an earlier study, Patel et al. (2003) found fluoxetine to be superior to placebo and psychological treatment at 2 months. The difference in improvement was not sustained in the long term, though the treatment was cost effective both at short term as well as long term. The study continued for 12 months. Psychological treatment in the study included explanation about the treatment and reassurance, breathing exercises for relaxation, treatment for specific symptoms like activity scheduling for tiredness or establishing sleep patterns for sleep disturbance and problem solving. The course of therapy lasted for 3 months. Reasons for lack of response to psychological treatments, as discussed by Patel et al., included absence of adequate structure in therapy, the patients' expectations for medications for their symptoms, or the nature of life circumstances and problems faced by the patients.

In a later study, the same research group (Patel et al. 2010) found that a trained lay counsellor-led psychotherapeutic intervention can lead to an improvement in patients with CMDs attending public primary care facilities. A stepped-care approach involving a trained lay counsellor or a primary care physician and a visiting psychiatrist was used. Interventions included psychoeducation by the lay counsellor and antidepressants, or 6 sessions of interpersonal psychotherapy for patients with moderate or severe CMDs. Psychoeducation was given to all the patients with CMDs and included educating patients about association of their symptoms and illness with interpersonal difficulties, teaching them need to share the emotional symptoms with their doctor and share the personal difficulties with the family members. The patients were also taught breathing exercises for anxiety symptoms and scheduling activities for depressive symptoms. The need to adhere to treatment was also emphasised.

Thus, antidepressants and a psychological intervention tailored to the needs of an individual patient remain the mainstay of management of CMDs. In the primary care settings in India and other developing countries, feasibility of instituting a structured psychological treatment remains difficult. However, antidepressants like fluoxetine, which is also included in the national essential drugs list of India and many other countries, could be more freely used. The National Mental Health Programme of India includes short orientation programmes for doctors and paramedical workers including nursing professionals. The primary care physicians need to be encouraged to use the principles of psychological methods in their clinical practice and also include the nursing professionals and other health workers in management of CMDS, especially in psychological interventions. Nurses and other health workers can be trained to administer some of the psychotherapeutic interventions like psychoeducation, teaching relaxation techniques and activity scheduling.

9 Conclusion

Patients with CMDs have often been ignored both by the physicians and the mental health professionals. The focus of physicians has been on the physical illnesses and that of psychiatrists on severe mental illnesses like schizophrenia, bipolar disorders and severe depression. CMDs, besides being common, are associated with substantial distress to the patients and disability. CMDs are a major public health issue, and it is high time that the mental health professionals as well the health policy makers pay due attention to the CMDs.

References

Avasthi, A., Varma, S. C., Kulhara, P., Nehra, R., Grover, S., & Sharma, S. (2008). Diagnosis of common mental disorders by using PRIME-MD Patient Health Questionnaire. *Indian Journal of Medical Research, 127*, 159–164.

Borus, J. F., Howes, M. J., Devins, N. P., Rosnberg, R., & Livingston, W. W. (1988). Primary health care providers' recognition and diagnosis of mental disorders in their patients. *General Hospital Psychiatry, 10*, 317–321.

Chadda, R. K. (2000). Presentation of affective disorders in Indian clinics. In: P. Kulhara, A. Avasthi & P. Sharan (Eds.), *Affective disorders—Indian scene department of psychiatry, Postgraduate Institute of Medical Education & Research*, Chandigarh.

Chadda, R. K. (2010a). Anxiety disorders. *Current Medical Journal of India, 16*, 7–14.

Chadda, R. K. (2010b). Prevention in psychiatry. *Journal of Mental Health and Human Behaviour, 15*, 69–76.

Chadda, R. K. (2011). Medically unexplained physical symptoms. *Current Medical Journal of India, 17*, 11–20.

Chadda, R. K., & Bhatia, M. S. (1990). A clinical study of somatising patients attending psychiatric outpatient clinic. *Indian Journal of Psychiatry, 32*, 39–43.

Chadda, R. K., Bhatia, M. S., & Shome, S. (1991). Physical symptoms in psychiatry—diagnostic uncertainties and clinical characteristics. *Indian Journal of Psychiatry, 33*, 200–205.

Chadda, R. K., Bhatia, M. S., Shome, S., & Thakur, K. N. (1993). Psychosocial dysfunction in somatising patients. *British Journal of Psychiatry, 163*, 510–513.

Chadda, R. K., Sood, M., & Kumar, N. (2009a). Sensitising primary care physicians to common mental disorders using a problem-based learning approach. *International Psychiatry, 6*, 25.

Chadda, R. K., Sood, M., & Kumar, N. (2009b). Experiences of a sensitization programme on common mental disorders for primary care physicians using a problem-based learning approach. *Indian Journal of Psychiatry, 51*, 289–291.

Craske, M. G., Roy-Byrne, P., Stein, M. B., Donald-Sherbourne, C., Bystritsky, A., Katon, W., et al. (2002). Treating panic disorder in primary care: A collaborative care intervention. *General Hospital Psychiatry, 24*, 148–155.

Fone, D. L., Dunstan, F., John, A., & Lloyd, K. (2007). Associations between common mental disorders and the mental illness needs index in community settings. Multilevel analysis. *British Journal of Psychiatry, 191*, 158–163.

Fryers, T., Melzer, D., & Jenkins, R. (2003). Social inequalities and the common mental disorders: A systematic review of the evidence. *Social Psychiatry and Psychiatric Epidemiology, 38*(5), 229–237.

Gautam, S., Nijhawan, M., & Kamal, P. (1987). Standardisation of the Hindi version of Goldberg's General Health Questionnaire. *Indian Journal of Psychiatry, 29*, 63–66.

Goldberg, D., & Huxley, P. (1992). *Common mental disorders: A biosocial model*. London: Tavistock/Routledge.

Goldberg, D. P., & Lecrubier, Y. (1995). Form and frequency of mental disorders across centres. In T. B. Üstün & N. Sartorius (Eds.), *Mental illness in general health care: An international study* (pp. 323–334). Chichester: Wiley.

Harding, T. W., De Arango, M. V., Baltazar, J., Climent, C. E., Ibrahim, H. H. A., Ladrigo-Ignacio, L., et al. (1980). Mental disorders in primary health care: A study of their frequency and diagnosis in four developing countries. *Psychological Medicine, 10*, 231–241.

Jacob, K. S., Bhugra, D., & Mann, A. H. (1997). The validation of the 12 item General Health Questionnaire among ethnic Indians living in UK. *Psychological Medicine, 27*, 1215–1217.

Krishnan, V., Sood, M., Chadda, R. K. (2013). Caregiver burden and disability in somatization disorder. *Journal of Psychosomatic Research, 75*, 376−380.

Kushwaha, V., Chadda, R. K., & Mehta, M. (2013). Psychotherapeutic intervention in somatisation disorder: Results of a controlled study from India. *Psychology, Health & Medicine, 18*, 445–450.

Kushwaha, V., Sinha Deb, K., Chadda, R. K., & Mehta, M. (2014). A study of disability and its correlates in somatization disorder. *Asian Journal of Psychiatry, 8*, 56–58

Linden, M., Lecrubier, Y., Bellantuono, C., Benkert, O., Kisely, S., & Simon, G. (1999). The prescribing of psychotropic drugs by primary care physicians: An international collaborative study. *Journal of Clinical Psychopharmacology, 19*, 132–140.

Manderscheid, R. W., Rae, D. S., Narrow, W. E., Locke, B. Z., & Regier, D. A. (1993). Congruence of service utilization estimates from epidemiologic catchment area project and other sources. *Archives of General Psychiatry, 50*, 108–114.

Murray, C. J. L., Lopez, A. D. (Eds.) (1996). *The global burden of disease: A comprehensive assessment of mortality and disability from diseases, injuries and risk factors in 1990 and projected to 2020*. Cambridge, MA, Harvard School of Public Health on behalf of the World Health Organization and the World Bank (Global Burden of Disease and Injury Series, Vol. I).

Murray, C. J., Vos, T., Lozano, R., Naghavi, M., Flaxman, A. D., Michaud, C., et al. (2012). Disability-adjusted life years (DALYs) for 291 diseases and injuries in 21 regions, 1990–2010: a systematic analysis for the Global Burden of Disease Study 2010. *Lancet, 380*(9859), 2197–2223.

Murthy, R. S. (2011). Mental health initiatives in India (1947–2010). *National Medical Journal of India, 24*, 98–107.

Nambi, S. K., Prasad, J., Singh, D., Abraham, V., Kuruvilla, A., & Jacob, K. S. (2002). Explanatory models and common mental disorders among patients with unexplained somatic symptoms attending a primary care facility in Tamil Nadu. *National Medical Journal of India, 15*(6), 331–335.

Ormel, J., Koeter, M. W., van den Brink, W., & van de Willige, G. (1991). Recognition, management and course of anxiety and depression in general practice. *Archives of General Psychiatry, 548*, 700–706.

Ormel, J., Oldehinkel, T., Brilman, E., vanden Brink, W. (1993). Outcome of depression and anxiety in primary care. A three-wave 3 1/2-year study of psychopathology and disability. *Archives of General Psychiatry, 50*, 759–766.

Patel, V., Kirkwood, B. R., Pednekar, S., Weiss, H., & Mabey, D. (2006a). Risk factors for common mental disorders in women: Population-based longitudinal study. *British Journal of Psychiatry, 189*, 547–555.

Patel, V., Kirkwood, B. R., Pednekar, S., Pereira, B., Barros, P., Fernandes, J., et al. (2006b). Gender disadvantage and reproductive health risk factors for common mental disorders in women: a community survey in India. *Archives of General Psychiatry, 63*, 404–413.

Patel, V., & Kleinman, A. (2003). Poverty and common mental disorders in developing countries. *Bulletin of the World Health Organization, 81*, 609–615.

Patel, V., Chisholm, D., Rabe-Hesketh, S., Dias-Saxena, F., Andrew, G., & Mann, A. (2003). Efficacy and cost-effectiveness of drug and psychological treatments for common mental disorders in general health care in Goa, India: a randomised, controlled trial. *Lancet, 361*(9351), 33–39.

Patel, V., Weiss, H. A., Chowdhary, N., Naik, S., Pednekar, S., Chatterjee, S., et al. (2010). Effectiveness of an intervention led by lay health counsellors for depressive and anxiety disorders in primary care in Goa, India (MANAS): A cluster randomised controlled trial. *Lancet, 376*(9758), 2086–2095.

Pothen, M., Kuruvilla, A., Philip, K., Joseph, A., & Jacob, K. S. (2003). Common mental disorders among primary care attenders in Vellore, South India: nature, prevalence and risk factors. *International Journal of Social Psychiatry, 49*, 119–125.

Prasad, J., Abraham, S., Akila, B., Joseph, A., & Jacob, K. S. (2003). Symptoms related to the reproductive tract and mental health among women in rural southern India. *National Medical Journal of India, 16*, 303–308.

Rai, D., Skapinakis, P., Wiles, N., Lewis, G., & Araya, R. (2010). Common mental disorders, subthreshold symptoms and disability: Longitudinal study. *British Journal of Psychiatry, 197*, 411–412.

Shankar, B. R., Saravanan, B., & Jacob, K. S. (2006). Explanatory models of common mental disorders among traditional healers and their patients in rural south India. *International Journal of Social Psychiatry, 52*, 221–233.

Smith Jr., G. R., Monson, R. A., & Ray, D. C. (1986). Patients with multiple unexplained symptoms: their characteristics, functional health, and health care utilization. *Archives of Internal. Medicine, 146*, 69–72

Srinivasan, K., Murthy, R. S., & Janakiramaiah, N. (1986). Anosological study of patients presenting with physical complaints. *Acta Psychiatrica Scandinavica, 173*, 1–5.

Ustun, T. B., & Von Korff, M. (1995). Primary mental health services: Access and provision of care. In T. B. Ustun & N. Sartorius (Eds.), *Mental illness in general health care: An international study* (pp. 323–334). Chichester: Wiley.

Wittchen, H. U. (2002). Generalized anxiety disorder: Prevalence, burden, and cost to society. *Depression and Anxiety, 16*, 162–171.

World Health Organization. (2001). *The World Health Report 2001: Mental health: New understanding*. New Hope. Geneva: World Health Organisation.

Chapter 7
Early Intervention in the Indian Context

S.P. Singh

1 Introduction

Psychotic disorders such as schizophrenia afflict the young, are highly disabling, rob patients of their most productive years, cause huge suffering and place enormous burden on families and carers. India, with a population of 1.2 billion, a national median age of less than 25 years, and only 3,500 psychiatrists, has a large pool of undetected and untreated patients with psychotic disorders (between 7 and 8 million) living mainly in remote rural areas (Saxena and Sharan 2004). Evidence-based packages of care for these disorders have been developed and piloted for such settings. However, the actual delivery of treatments remains a significant challenge and is a global mental health priority (Lamers et al. 2006; Sullivan and Ghushchyan 2006; Chisholm et al. 2007; Patel et al. 2008; Saxena et al. 2011). The greatest hope for reducing the burden of schizophrenia in India comes from identifying and treating psychotic patients early and offering evidence-based interventions. Such cohorts also offer unique opportunities to explore the sociocultural and neurobiological influences on outcome of schizophrenia.

S.P. Singh, Professor and Head of Division

S.P. Singh (✉)
Mental Health and Wellbeing, Warwick Medical School, University of Warwick, Coventry, UK
e-mail: S.P.Singh@warwick.ac.uk

S. Malhotra and S. Chakrabarti (eds.), *Developments in Psychiatry in India*,
DOI 10.1007/978-81-322-1674-2_7

2 Rationale for Early Intervention

The concept of intervening early in psychosis is neither new nor revolutionary; in 1938, Cameron observed that "the therapeutic results to be obtained [in schizophrenia] are considerably better in patients in whom there is little progression towards chronicity" and advocated a public health approach to early detection of cases in the community (Cameron 1938). The mid-twentieth century witnessed the major service reform of deinstitutionalisation, driven by clinical, sociopolitical and financial imperatives. Antipsychotics had engendered therapeutic optimism in schizophrenia, the anti-psychiatry movement had revealed a disturbing violation of the rights of the incarcerated mentally ill, and funding restraints necessitated the development of community-based alternatives, thought to be both cheaper and more humane. The focus of these changes was where and how care was delivered, rather than the quality and effectiveness of that care (Geller 2000).

Studies in the 1980s (Johnstone et al. 1986; Rabiner et al. 1986) and Wyatt's seminal papers (Wyatt 1991) confirmed the prognostic influence of length of untreated psychosis on outcome. In the 1990s, three emerging and interwoven strands of evidence supported the case for specialised early intervention (EI) services. First, the existence of an early window of opportunity, "the critical period", was postulated on the basis of strong evidence that early trajectory and disability were strongly predictive of long-term course and outcome (Wiersma et al. 1998; Harrison et al. 2001), and the greatest impact on the illness might be made during this period of neuronal and psychosocial plasticity (Birchwood et al. 1998). Second, the association between longer periods of untreated psychosis and poorer outcomes became firmly established (Marshall et al. 2005; Perkins et al. 2005). Third, it became clear that even well-resourced community services were not meeting the needs of young people in their first psychotic episode and had not improved their outcomes (Singh et al. 2000, 2003). Politically, an important lever for change was pressure from service users and their carers determined to tackle the "scandal of delays in care" for young people with emerging psychosis (Rethink 2002).

This chapter reviews the rationale for early intervention, describes the range of early interventions, summarises their evidence base and considers clinical and policy implications of implementing early intervention strategies in an Indian context.

3 Duration of Untreated Psychosis (DUP) and Outcome

DUP refers to the time period between the emergence of psychotic symptoms and the commencement of adequate treatment. Since frank psychotic symptoms are usually preceded by non-psychotic symptoms and behavioural changes, DUP is distinguished from duration of untreated illness (DUI), which is the period between the start of the "prodrome" and the commencement of treatment. The conceptual, clinical and methodological problems in ascertaining DUP and DUI have been well documented (McGorry 2000; Norman et al. 2001; Singh et al.

2005; Malla et al. 2011). Several structured instruments and methods have been proposed for measuring DUP and are routinely used in clinical and research settings (Hafner et al. 1992; Singh et al. 2005; Singh 2007; Large et al. 2008).

Two systematic reviews have explored the relationship between DUP and outcomes in psychosis. Marshall et al. (2005) reviewed 26 first-episode studies to find that while baseline presentation in first-episode studies was not poorer in those with longer DUP, there was a significant correlation between DUP and outcome at 6 months (for all symptoms and overall functioning), 12 months (for symptoms, functioning and quality of life) and 24 months (for positive symptoms, functioning and quality of life). The association between DUP and positive symptoms at follow-up was significant even after controlling for pre-morbid functioning. In a review of 43 studies, Perkins et al. (2005) found an association between shorter DUP and better antipsychotic treatment response as measured on psychopathology, positive and negative symptom severity, and global functioning. Both reviews concluded that there was convincing evidence of an association between DUP and outcome following treatment. However, several questions remain. The relationship between DUP and outcome is not linear (longer the DUP, poorer the outcome), but is there a critical cut-off beyond which longer DUP predicts poorer outcome? Is DUP confounded by pre-morbid and illness-related variables? Is DUP neurotoxic? Is reducing DUP at a population level a worthwhile public mental health strategy? (Verdoux et al. 2001; Friis et al. 2004; Killackey et al. 2007; Singh 2007; Malla et al. 2011).

4 DUP in the Resource-Poor Settings

Early intervention services (EISs) exist mainly in the developed world and are the source of the bulk of DUP data (Chiliza et al. 2012). A review of 11 studies from eight low- and middle-income (LAMI) countries including India, Mexico, Poland, China, Turkey, Brazil, South Africa and Indonesia found that longer DUP was associated with lower treatment response in these settings (Farooq et al. 2009a, b). Given the paucity of mental health services in LAMI, it is reasonable to anticipate that those coming into psychiatric care will have long DUP. Average mean DUP is indeed longer in countries with lower gross domestic product in the LAMI. DUP is reduced by 6 weeks for each US$1,000 GDP purchasing power increase (Large et al. 2008). However, this relationship between DUP reduction and rising GDP does not hold true for high-income countries. A study of untreated patients from Chennai, South India (Tirupati et al. 2004), found that treatment response is evident even in cases with DUP longer than 15 years. In this study, a DUP of less than 5 years predicted good clinical but not occupational outcome.

Recent studies from LAMI suggest that the relationship between DUP, service availability, economic development and outcomes is complex. In Pakistan, Naqvi et al. (2009) reported a mean DUP of 64 weeks in a cohort of patients with schizophrenia. Most patients had a psychiatric contact as their first help-seeking encounter, highlighting the scarcity of primary care or community-based services in the study area. Since this was not an epidemiologically ascertained cohort, it is difficult to draw conclusions about undetected and untreated patients in the base population. In Sao Paulo Brazil, Oliveira et al. recruited an epidemiological cohort of first-episode psychosis (FEP) ($n = 200$) and found a very short DUP (median 4.1 weeks), with longer DUP length associated with patients living alone. A South African study of first hospitalisation patients found an association between longer DUP and spiritual/traditional attributions for psychosis causation and help-seeking through traditional healers (Burns et al. 2011).

5 The Range of Early Interventions

Some of the controversy surrounding early intervention is generated by the different ways in which the term "early intervention" is used. It can mean improving outcomes in established cases of psychosis by facilitating and consolidating recovery, detecting hidden morbidity in the community by identifying untreated cases or preventing the emergence of psychosis through pre-psychotic interventions. These are different aims, requiring different service models and strategies, and have differing levels of supporting evidence.

6 Prodromal Interventions

Preventing psychosis by intervening in the prodrome remains ethically contentious and clinically challenging, given the non-specificity of prodromal symptoms and their low predictive power in identifying cases that will make a transition to psychosis. Table 1 summarises the potential benefits and pitfalls of pre-psychotic and prodromal interventions, as articulated by proponents from both sides of the debate (McGorry 1998; Yung et al. 1998; Warner 2002, 2005; McGorry et al. 2003). In the absence of markers of true prodrome, it is unclear whether the risks of mislabelling and inappropriately treating the "false positives" outweigh the potential benefits of preventing the illness in the "true positives". McGlashan et al. (2001) considers our knowledge in the area to be in "equipoise", i.e. genuine uncertainty, justifying clinical intervention but demanding greater research in the efficacy of such interventions.

Table 1 Pros and cons of prodromal interventions

Against intervention	For intervention
No good screening tests	Help-seeking, symptomatic population with dysfunction and disability
No effective preventive strategy	Targeted rather than universal screening/treatment
Unnecessary treatment of acute and transient psychoses and "false positives"	Safe and efficacious treatments available
Unnecessary stigmatisation	Challenging stigma is part of the solution, not the problem
Research samples are highly selected	Help-seeking groups with prodromal presentation come to clinical services

Correll et al. (2010) reviewed seven randomised trials (a total of 603 "at-risk" individuals), three of which were placebo controlled. Many interventions were used including antipsychotics alone, antipsychotics with CBT, CBT alone and omega 3 fatty acids. Of these, five showed reduced transition rates with CBT (Bechdolf et al. 2004; Morrison et al. 2004); amisulpride (Ruhrmann et al. 2008); ethyl EPA (Berger et al. 2008); and risperidone plus CBT (McGorry et al. 2002). One negative study had a very high dropout, but trend favouring olanzapine (McGlashan et al. 2006). A second negative study had very low transition rates in both groups (Yung et al. 2008). Lower rates of transition ion the active treatment group last only as long as patient receive active treatment; on stopping active treatment, intervention arm patients catch up with control arm in transition rates, with the exception of one study of omega 3 fatty acids (Ethyl EPA). However, this last finding has as yet not been replicated. Another review and meta-analysis of "at-risk" studies concluded that while the benefits for any specific intervention have not been robustly proven, there is tentative evidence that it might be possible to delay or prevent transition to psychosis (Stafford et al. 2013).

Correll et al. (2010) also reviewed specific risk markers such as neuroanatomical abnormalities and cognitive dysfunction predating the emergence of frank psychotic symptoms and concluded that currently valid markers of true psychosis remain unknown. It is unclear whether the risks of mislabelling and inappropriately treating the "false positives" outweigh the potential benefits of preventing the illness in the "true positives". McGlashan et al. (2001) consider our knowledge of the value of treating the prodrome to be in a state of equipoise or genuine uncertainty, justifying needs-based clinical intervention but demanding greater research in the efficacy of such interventions.

7 Early Detection in the Community

In mental health, the routes of access to care are diverse and varied. Patients with FEP access care through a number of agencies, including social services and the criminal justice systems (Singh and Grange 2006). There have been some attempts at developing and evaluating early detection strategies for FEP with mixed results. The first comprehensive trial was the Scandinavian TIPS study which ran over 4 years in four health sectors in Norway and Denmark (Friis et al. 2005; Johannessen et al. 2005; Melle et al. 2005). Both the intervention and control area had similar specialised EISs. In addition, in the intervention arm, GPs and other health professionals were trained face-to-face, schools visited for providing information on psychosis to students, teachers and counsellors, and general public educated about psychosis and help-seeking through information leaflets and a media campaign. TIPS also conducted a historical comparison with DUP data prior to the development of early detection services. Despite a short median DUP in the control area, the TIPS trial found significant further reduction in DUP in the intervention arm. Patients from early detection sectors presented with less severe psychotic symptoms and milder functional deficits prior to treatment initiation. Early detected cases had significantly less suicidal ideation and suicidal attempts at baseline. TIPS is the first large and comprehensive study to show that a community's median DUP can be significantly reduced with clinical advantages both at intake and at follow-up.

Lloyd-Evans et al. (2011) conducted a systematic review of 11 studies which used eight early detection initiatives. They found that general practitioner education campaigns and dedicated EISs do not reduce DUP or increase the number of patients seeking help for psychotic disorders. Multi-focus initiatives such as a mixture of public education campaigns combined with ease of access to care had better, but still mixed results. The authors concluded that the most promising evidence was for identifying hidden cases in the community via intensive public awareness campaigns.

Facilitating recovery in first-episode psychosis: There is now considerable evidence from EISs around the world that effective and assertive intervention in first-episode psychosis improves short- and medium-term outcomes. Besides several naturalistic studies, there have been 12 trials comparing specialised EISs with standard care from Denmark, Spain, Australia, UK, Holland, USA and China. Of these, the OPUS study from Denmark (Nordentoft et al. 2006; Bertelsen et al. 2007, 2008) is the largest (sample size 547), and also the one of two with a 5-year follow-up, the other being the LEO trial (Craig et al. 2004). In the OPUS study, participants received integrated care consisting of high-fidelity assertive community treatment supplemented by behavioural family therapy and social skills training. Standard care consisted of care at a community mental health centre. At 2 years, participants receiving specialist EIS care had better clinical outcomes, including better symptom control and functioning and reduced hospitalisation. After 2 years of specialist input, all patients in the trial received standard care and were followed up for further 3 years. At the five-year follow-up, there were no differences between the two groups on clinical outcomes although the EIS-treated group were more likely to be living independently. Similarly, the LEO trial in the UK showed that specialised EIS was better than a generic community team in improving short-term outcomes in FEP (Craig et al. 2004).

Specialised teams also appear to be cost-effective. McCrone and Knapp (2007) conducted Markov modelling to compare costs between specialist and generic team care for FEP and found that specialist teams incurred lower costs, primarily due to lower hospitalisation and readmission rates. Similar cost savings have been demonstrated from Danish, Swedish and Italian studies (Valmaggia et al. 2009).

Overall, trials confirm that FEP patients treated under specialist EIS teams have better outcomes than standard care. However, the effect of specialist care lasts only as long as the early intervention approach is maintained. Like the OPUS 5-year results, findings from longer follow-up of LEO sample also showed loss of early intervention gains when patients were discharged back to standard care (Gafoor et al. 2010). It appears therefore that once the EI "grip is relaxed", clinical gains are lost; interventions are therefore effective only as long as actively implemented. This suggests that the heterogeneous trajectories of early psychosis require differentiation, with EI provision being tailor-made for longer periods for those with poorer early outcomes. EIS is a complex intervention with several interacting components, and we are yet to determine the active "therapeutic ingredients" within EIS and how these are exerting their effect (Singh 2010).

8 Early Intervention in the Indian Context

Many patients with emerging psychosis in India receive little or no treatment, with major barriers to access and availability of care and the economic impediments especially for the remote and rural population groups. It is hard to justify setting up prodromal services in such a context, given the limited evidence for such interventions and the clinical, resource and policy imperative of prioritising care for those already ill over those who may become ill in the future. Detection of all, not just first-episode, untreated cases in the community is, however, a public mental health priority. Treating these cases effectively in the first episode and preventing relapse must be another key priority demanding urgent action. In countries such as India, schizophrenia is the sixth leading cause of years lost due to disability (DALYs), higher than iron deficiency anaemia, and only slightly less than cataract. The goal of an integrated approach to meeting the challenge of untreated psychosis should combine a public awareness programme particularly dealing with stigma and lack of awareness of treatment options, training primary care workers and general practitioners identifying cases and using the emerging power of the Internet and the voluntary sector in India.

Farooq et al. (2009a, b), Farooq (2013) have argued for a public health approach to psychosis similar to those being applied for infectious and non-communicable diseases. This would require public education campaigns with particular focus on traditional healers and care provision through a network of primary care workers and social welfare organisations. Such an approach is being used by non-profit organisation such as Schizophrenia Research Foundation (SCARF) in Chennai, which is providing early intervention programmes with emerging evidence of success (Rangaswamy et al. 2012). Telepsychiatry is another promising innovation which can allow clinician access to remote areas overcoming the obstacles of time and travel and using mobile connectedness of rural India to considerable advantage (Thara et al. 2008; Thara 2012; Malhotra et al. 2013; Thara and Sujit 2013). Widespread adoption of these innovative models will depend upon policy makers prioritising mental health care and integrating mental health provision into general health care delivery especially in rural and remote areas. In the West, user voice was eventually heard after a sustained campaign by carers, voluntary organisations and concerned clinicians. The emerging economic power of India should not leave behind among the most vulnerable of its citizens, the untreated psychotic patients languishing in the community.

References

Bechdolf, A., Knost, B., et al. (2004). A randomized comparison of group cognitive-behavioural therapy and group psychoeducation in patients with schizophrenia. *Acta Psychiatrica Scandinavica, 110*(1), 21–28.

Berger, G. E., Wood, S. J., et al. (2008). Ethyl-eicosapentaenoic acid in first-episode psychosis. A 1H-MRS study. *Neuropsychopharmacology, 33*(10), 2467–2473.

Bertelsen, M., Jeppesen, P., et al. (2007). Suicidal behaviour and mortality in first-episode psychosis: The OPUS trial. *British Journal of Psychiatry, 51*(Suppl), s140–s146.

Bertelsen, M., Jeppesen, P., et al. (2008). Five-year follow-up of a randomized multicenter trial of intensive early intervention vs standard treatment for patients with a first episode of psychotic illness: The OPUS trial. *Archives of General Psychiatry, 65*(7), 762–771.

Birchwood, M., Todd, P., et al. (1998). Early intervention in psychosis. The critical period hypothesis. *British Journal of Psychiatry, 172*(Suppl 33), 53–59.

Burns, J. K., Jhazbhay, K., et al. (2011). Causal attributions, pathway to care and clinical features of first-episode psychosis: A South African perspective. *International Journal of Social Psychiatry, 57*(5), 538–545.

Cameron, D. E. (1938). Early schizophrenia. *American Journal of Psychiatry, 95*(3), 567–582.

Chiliza, B., Asmal, L., et al. (2012). Early intervention in schizophrenia in developing countries: Focus on duration of untreated psychosis and remission as a treatment goal. *International Review of Psychiatry, 24*(5), 483–488.

Chisholm, D., Flisher, A. J., et al. (2007). Scale up services for mental disorders: A call for action. *Lancet, 370*(9594), 1241–1252.

Correll, C. U., Hauser, M., et al. (2010). Research in people with psychosis risk syndrome: A review of the current evidence and future directions. *Journal of Child Psychology and Psychiatry, 51*(4), 390–431.

Craig, T. K., Garety, P., et al. (2004). The Lambeth Early Onset (LEO) Team: Randomised controlled trial of the effectiveness of specialised care for early psychosis. *BMJ, 329*(7474), 1067.

Farooq, S. (2013). Early intervention for psychosis in low-and middle-income countries needs a public health approach. *British Journal of Psychiatry, 202*(3), 168–169.

Farooq, S., Large, M., et al. (2009a). Early intervention in psychosis in developing countries: Evidence and action. *World Psychiatry, 8*(2), 123.

Farooq, S., Large, M., et al. (2009b). The relationship between the duration of untreated psychosis and outcome in low-and-middle income countries: A systematic review and meta analysis. *Schizophrenia Research, 109*(1–3), 15–23.

Friis, S., Melle, I., et al. (2004). Does duration of untreated psychosis bias study samples of first-episode psychosis? *Acta Psychiatrica Scandinavica, 110*(4), 286–291.

Friis, S., Vaglum, P., et al. (2005). Effect of an early detection programme on duration of untreated psychosis: Part of the Scandinavian TIPS study. *British Journal of Psychiatry, 48*(Suppl), s29–s32.

Gafoor, R., Nitsch, D., et al. (2010). Effect of early intervention on 5-year outcome in non-affective psychosis. *British Journal of Psychiatry, 196*(5), 372–376.

Geller, J. L. (2000). The last half-century of psychiatric services as reflected in psychiatric services. *Psychiatric Services, 51*(1), 41–67.

Hafner, H., Riecher-Rossler, A., et al. (1992). IRAOS: An instrument for the assessment of onset and early course of schizophrenia. *Schizophrenia Research, 6*(3), 209–223.

Harrison, G., Hopper, K., et al. (2001). Recovery from psychotic illness: A 15-and 25-year international follow-up study. *British Journal of Psychiatry, 178*, 506–517.

Johannessen, J. O., Larsen, T. K., et al. (2005). Pathways to care for first-episode psychosis in an early detection healthcare sector: Part of the Scandinavian TIPS study. *British Journal of Psychiatry, 187*(Suppl 48), s24–s28.

Johnstone, E. C., Crow, T. J., et al. (1986). The Northwick park study of first episodes of schizophrenia. I. Presentation of the illness and problems relating to admission. *British Journal of Psychiatry, 148*, 115–120.

Killackey, E., Yung, A. R., et al. (2007). Early psychosis: Where we've been, where we still have to go. *Epidemiologia Psichiatria Sociale, 16*(2), 102–108.

Lamers, L. M., McDonnell, J., et al. (2006). The Dutch tariff: Results and arguments for an effective design for national EQ-5D valuation studies. *Health Economics, 15*(10), 1121–1132.

Large, M., Farooq, S., et al. (2008a). Relationship between gross domestic product and duration of untreated psychosis in low-and middle-income countries. *British Journal of Psychiatry, 193*(4), 272–278.

Large, M., Nielssen, O., et al. (2008b). Measurement and reporting of the duration of untreated psychosis. *Early Intervention Psychiatry, 2*(4), 201–211.

Lloyd-Evans, B., Crosby, M., et al. (2011). Initiatives to shorten duration of untreated psychosis: Systematic review. *British Journal of Psychiatry, 198*(4), 256–263.

Malhotra, S., Chakrabarti, S., et al. (2013). Telepsychiatry: Promise, potential, and challenges. *Indian Journal of Psychiatry, 55*(1), 3–11.

Malla, A. K., Bodnar, M., et al. (2011). Duration of untreated psychosis is associated with orbital-frontal grey matter volume reductions in first episode psychosis. *Schizophrenia Research, 125*(1), 13–20.

Marshall, M., Lewis, S., et al. (2005). Association between duration of untreated psychosis and outcome in cohorts of first-episode patients: A systematic review. *Archives of General Psychiatry, 62*(9), 975–983.

McCrone, P., & Knapp, M. (2007). Economic evaluation of early intervention services. *British Journal of Psychiatry, 191*(51), s19–s22.

McGlashan, T. H., Miller, T. J., et al. (2001). Pre-onset detection and intervention research in schizophrenia psychoses: Current estimates of benefit and risk. *Schizophrenia Bulletin, 27*(4), 563–570.

McGlashan, T. H., Zipursky, R. B., et al. (2006). Randomized, double-blind trial of olanzapine versus placebo in patients prodromally symptomatic for psychosis. *American Journal of Psychiatry, 163*(5), 790–799.

McGorry, P. D. (1998). "A stitch in time" … the scope for preventive strategies in early psychosis. *European Archives of Psychiatry and Clinical Neuroscience, 248*(1), 22–31.

McGorry, P. D. (2000). Evaluating the importance of reducing the duration of untreated psychosis. *Australian New Zealand Journal of Psychiatry, 34*(s2), S145–S149.

McGorry, P. D., Yung, A. R., et al. (2002). Randomized controlled trial of interventions designed to reduce the risk of progression to first-episode psychosis in a clinical sample with subthreshold symptoms. *Archives of General Psychiatry, 59*(10), 921–928.

McGorry, P. D., Yung, A. R., et al. (2003). The "close-in" or ultra high-risk model: A safe and effective strategy for research and clinical intervention in prepsychotic mental disorder. *Schizophrenia Bulletin, 29*(4), 771–790.

Melle, I., Haahr, U., et al. (2005). Reducing the duration of untreated first-episode psychosis—effects on baseline social functioning and quality of life. *Acta Psychiatrica Scandinavica, 112*(6), 469–473.

Morrison, A. P., French, P., et al. (2004). Cognitive therapy for the prevention of psychosis in people at ultra-high risk: Randomised controlled trial. *British Journal of Psychiatry, 185*, 291–297.

Naqvi, H. A., Hussain, S., et al. (2009). Pathways to care: Duration of untreated psychosis from Karachi, Pakistan. *PLoS ONE, 4*(10), e7409.

Nordentoft, M., Petersen, L., et al. (2006). OPUS: A randomised multicenter trial of integrated versus standard treatment for patients with a first-episode psychosis--secondary publication. *Ugeskrift for Laeger, 168*(4), 381–384.

Norman, R. M., Townsend, L., et al. (2001). Duration of untreated psychosis and cognitive functioning in first-episode patients. *British Journal of Psychiatry, 179*, 340–345.

Patel, V., Garrison, P., et al. (2008). The Lancet's series on global mental health: 1 year on. *Lancet, 372*(9646), 1354–1357.

Perkins, D. O., Gu, H., et al. (2005). Relationship between duration of untreated psychosis and outcome in first-episode schizophrenia: A critical review and meta-analysis. *American Journal of Psychiatry, 162*(10), 1785–1804.

Rabiner, C. J., Wegner, J. T., et al. (1986). Outcome study of first-episode psychosis. I: Relapse rates after 1 year. *American Journal of Psychiatry, 143*(9), 1155–1158.

Rangaswamy, T., Mangala, R., et al. (2012). Early intervention for first-episode psychosis in India. *East Asian Archives Psychiatry, 22*(3), 94–99.

Rethink (2002). *Reaching people early*. London: Rethink.

Ruhrmann, S., Paruch, J., et al. (2008). Reduced subjective quality of life in persons at risk for psychosis. *Acta Psychiatrica Scandinavica, 117*(5), 357–368.

Saxena, S., Lora, A., et al. (2011). Mental health services in 42 low-and middle-income countries: A WHO-AIMS cross-national analysis. *Psychiatric Services, 62*(2), 123–125.

Saxena, S., & Sharan, P. (2004). Supporting mental health research publications from low-and middle-income countries. *Revista Brasileria Psiquiatria, 26*(2), 73–74.

Singh, S. P. (2007). Outcome measures in early psychosis; Relevance of duration of untreated psychosis. *British Journal of Psychiatry, 191*(50), s58–s63.

Singh, S. P. (2010). Early intervention in psychosis. *British Journal of Psychiatry, 196*(5), 343–345.

Singh, S. P., Cooper, J. E., et al. (2005). Determining the chronology and components of psychosis onset: The Nottingham Onset Schedule (NOS). *Schizophrenia Research, 80*(1), 117–130.

Singh, S. P., Croudace, T., et al. (2000). Three-year outcome of first-episode psychoses in an established community psychiatric service. *British Journal of Psychiatry, 176*, 210–216.

Singh, S. P., Wright, C., et al. (2003). Developing early intervention services in the NHS: A survey to guide workforce and training needs. *Psychiatric Bulletin, 27*(7), 254–258.

Stafford, M. R., Jackson, H., et al. (2013). Early interventions to prevent psychosis: Systematic review and meta-analysis. *BMJ, 346*, f185.

Sullivan, P. W., & Ghushchyan, V. (2006). Mapping the EQ-5D index from the SF-12: US general population preferences in a nationally representative sample. *Medical Decision Making, 26*(4), 401–409.

Singh, S. P., & Grange, T. (2006). Measuring pathways to care in first-episode psychosis: a systematic review. *Schizophrenia Research, 81*(1):75–82.

Thara, R. (2012). Using mobile telepsychiatry to close the mental health gap. *Current Psychiatry Reports, 14*(3), 167–168.

Thara, R., John, S., et al. (2008). Telepsychiatry in Chennai, India: The SCARF experience. *Behavioral Sciences and the Law, 26*(3), 315–322.

Thara, R., & Sujit, J. (2013). Mobile telepsychiatry in India. *World Psychiatry, 12*(1), 84.

Tirupati, N. S., Rangaswamy, T., et al. (2004). Duration of untreated psychosis and treatment outcome in schizophrenia patients untreated for many years. *Australian and New Zealand Journal of Psychiatry, 38*(5), 339–343.

Valmaggia, L. R., McCrone, P., et al. (2009). Economic impact of early intervention in people at high risk of psychosis. *Psychological Medicine, 39*(10), 1617–1626.

Verdoux, H., Liraud, F., et al. (2001). Is the association between duration of untreated psychosis and outcome confounded? A two year follow-up study of first-admitted patients. *Schizophrenia Research, 49*(3), 231–241.

Warner, R. (2002). Early intervention in schizophrenia: A critique. *Epidemiologia Psichiatria Sociale, 11*(4), 248–255.

Warner, R. (2005). Problems with early and very early intervention in psychosis. *British Journal of Psychiatry, 187*(Suppl 48), s104–s107.

Wiersma, D., Nienhuis, F. J., et al. (1998). Natural course of schizophrenic disorders: A 15-year followup of a Dutch incidence cohort. *Schizophrenia Bulletin, 24*(1), 75–85.

Wyatt, R. J. (1991). Neuroleptics and the natural course of schizophrenia. *Schizophrenia Bulletin, 17*(2), 325–351.

Yung, A. R., Nelson, B., et al. (2008). Validation of "prodromal" criteria to detect individuals at ultra high risk of psychosis: 2 year follow-up. *Schizophrenia Research, 105*(1–3), 10–17.

Yung, A. R., Phillips, L. J., et al. (1998). Prediction of psychosis. A step towards indicated prevention of schizophrenia. *British Journal of Psychiatry, 172*(33), 14–20.

Chapter 8
Acute and Transient Psychosis: An Overview

S. Malhotra and A. Singh

1 Introduction

The acute and brief psychotic states present with florid psychotic symptoms of a sudden or acute onset. However, once the acute episode has remitted, the premorbid level of functioning is reached again, and the personality reappears basically intact. Thus, these disorders seem to contradict the traditional notion of severe mental disorder as a systematically progressive disease that frequently ends in the weakening or destruction of mental faculties (Ackerknecht 1968). This apparent paradox has made brief and acute psychoses a controversial, but highly stimulating area in the study of functional psychoses for more than 150 years.

The International Classification of Mental and Behavioural Disorders, tenth revision (ICD-10) in 1992, has brought together several clinical concepts such as the bouffée délirante, cycloid psychosis, the reactive psychosis and schizophreniform psychoses under the broad rubric of acute and transient psychosis (F23).

However, the ICD-10 (World Health Organisation 1992) states that '*The limited data and clinical traditions... do not give rise to concepts that can be clearly defined and separated from each other.... The nomenclature of these acute disorders is as uncertain as their nosological status*'.

S. Malhotra, Professor and Head; A. Singh, Junior Resident

S. Malhotra (✉) · A. Singh
Department of Psychiatry, Postgraduate Institute of Medical Education and Research, Chandigarh, India
e-mail: savita.pgi@gmail.com

S. Malhotra and S. Chakrabarti (eds.), *Developments in Psychiatry in India*,
DOI 10.1007/978-81-322-1674-2_8

2 Evolution of Concept

In the present diagnostic systems, acute psychotic states are allocated to acute and transient psychotic disorders (ATPD, F23) in ICD-10 (World Health Organisation 1992) and to brief psychotic disorder (BPD) in the Diagnostic and Statistical Manual of Mental disorders, fourth edition (DSM-IV; APA, 1994). Although the operational criteria are new, the descriptions involved show the traces of a long and divergent history of the concept of brief and acute psychoses. In fact, different psychiatric schools, often of a regional or national character, have provided concepts for transient psychotic states.

Descriptions of acute psychosis as a condition characterised by short duration, often having an intensive or even dramatic symptomatology, but with full remission, can be traced back to middle of the nineteenth century.

Researchers of all periods have been faced by three major issues with regard to the concept and definition of ATPD:

(1) ATPD has to be accommodated in the respective nosological system
(2) Diagnostic criteria have to be assigned to delineate these from other psychotic disorders
(3) Need for aetiological explanation for the coexistence of severe disturbance and good prognosis

3 Concepts of Acute and Polymorphous Psychoses—Past and Present

3.1 From Kahlbaum to Kraepelin

Numerous authors have described psychotic states of a transient or periodic nature during the history of psychiatry, even if they did not allocate them to a specific diagnostic category as manifestations of an ongoing disease process passing through several stages (Berrios and Porter 1995). Ludwig Kahlbaum (1828–1899) in his influential work *Die GruppirungpsychischerKrankheiten* (1863) conceived psychotic disorders in their typical forms ('vesania typica'). Although a number of varieties of 'vesania typica' were possible, they had in common the postulated disease process of a progressive nature. There were also disorders, however, in which a psychotic syndrome appeared—often in a severe form—but then remitted without showing the typical sequence of disease states and without leaving a lasting alteration.

Kahlbaum used the term '*dysphrenia*' to denote these disorders, which he believed were not the direct expressions of a typical progressive disease process. Rather, he presumed that some different process, e.g. of epileptic, sexual or rheumatic nature, must have elicited the expression of the syndrome. Thus, the provoking process would stimulate the immediate pathological process 'without leaving a lasting alteration in the elements that serve its expression' (Kahlbaum 1863). It is noteworthy that Kahlbaum's concept of *dysphrenia* connected three elements that were to be found again in later concepts of brief and acute psychoses: an atypical (non-progressive) course, a mixed or impure symptomatic picture and the supposition of some provoking aetiological principle, e.g. an epileptic, sexual or rheumatic process.

During the same time in around 1878, German psychiatrist, Karl Westphal, described *paranoia acuta*—an acute form of paranoia with an outburst of perceptual hallucinations, consisting mostly of hallucinatory voices and delusions, with clouding of consciousness. In 1890, Meynert repeated the clinical description but named the condition *amentia*.

While Kahlbaum's classification of mental disorders did not succeed and concept of Westphal and Meynert did not have an impact on the world either, it was the approach of Emil Kraepelin (1856–1926) that dominated psychiatry in the twentieth century. This fact was of crucial significance for later concepts of brief and acute psychoses, since Kraepelin's notion of dementia praecox with its emphasis on a deleterious outcome cannot readily be reconciled with the existence of acute psychoses of good prognosis. The early editions of his textbook already contain the vivid description of a severe psychotic state, developing in 2–3 days, characterised by vivid hallucinations, delusions and changing mood, and remitting after a number of weeks or months. These difficulties persisted despite the fact that Kraepelin himself, in his later years, was somewhat less dogmatic about psychiatric classification. In 1899, Kraepelin included all the endogenous and functional psychosis under *dementia praecox* and all manic and melancholic periodic disorders in a single-group *manic–depressive insanity* with no place between these two diagnostic categories.

However, if we think on this dichotomy currently, we may argue that nature does not take leaps; there are always overlaps, bridges or something else in between. But why should the psyche take leaps?

In 1920, Kraepelin, in his paper 'The manifestations of types of insanity', wrote:

> *No experienced psychiatrist will deny that there are an alarmingly large number of cases in which, despite the most careful observation, it seems impossible to arrive at a reliable diagnosis. We therefore will have to get used to the fact that the symptoms we have used so far are not sufficient to always reliably distinguish between manic–depressive insanity and dementia praecox, but that there are overlaps based on the origin of these symptoms from given preconditions*

However, he still adhered to the notion of two separate disease processes, one of these destructive (schizophrenic) and another one completely balanced (manic–depressive). Thus, although Kraepelin did not abandon his concept of two opposing disease processes, he admitted the existence of phenomenological pictures that could not be grouped unambiguously with either disease.

In 1911, Bleuler replaced the single disease dementia praecox by the concept of a *group of schizophrenias* of various clinical forms. He noticed that schizophrenia often began with an acute excitatory episode lasting from a few hours to a few years. He described a wide variation of outcome of acute forms of psychosis, but he separated acute schizophrenias from simple schizophrenia as he believed that acute forms did not necessarily end in deterioration. However, the problem of brief, good prognosis psychosis was not solved.

However, in several countries around the world, such as in Germany, France, Scandinavia and Japan, forms of psychoses were described that defied Emil Kraepelin's dichotomic system, as well as Eugen Bleuler's conception of schizophrenia. These were the concepts of bouffeė délirante (Valentin 1886); motility psychosis (Wernicke 1894); *cycloid disorder* (Kleist 1929); *reactive psychosis* (Jaspers 1963); *psychogenic psychoses* (Wimmer 1816; Langfeldt 1937); *acute schizoaffective psychosis* (Kasanin 1933); *Schizophreniform psychosis* (Langfeldt 1937); *hysterical psychosis* (Hollender and Hirsch 1964); and *atypical psychoses* (Mitsuda 1965). *There were also concepts of remitting schizophrenia; good prognosis schizophrenia; acute psychotic reaction*; *acute primitive psychosis; acute paranoid psychosis; transient psychosis; acute psychotic reaction*; *acute psychosis of uncertain origin; hysterical psychosis; acute psychosis without antecedent;* and *acute schizophrenic episode*. These descriptions led to the possibility of a 'third psychosis' apart from schizophrenia and manic–depressive psychosis. A brief account of some of these descriptive forms can help clarify the basic elements of such disorders.

4 Historical Roots of ATPD

(a) Bouffée délirante

For more than 100 years, 'bouffée délirante' has been one of the most eminent and influential diagnostic concepts in French psychiatry. It was created by Valentin (Valentin 1886) Magnan (1835–1916), the eminence grise of French psychiatry (Shorter 1997) and one of the most important French nosologists in the pre-Kraepelinian era. Magnan worked at the Paris mental hospital Sainte-Anne. He devoted much of his professional interest to the study and propagation of the idea of 'degeneration', introduced by Bénédict-Augustin Morel in 1857. The concept of degeneration combined three assumptions that (1) a number of psychiatric disorders and deficits originate from a common disposition or diathesis (the degenerate state) which is partly hereditary in nature, (2) this disposition can be recognised by somatic and psychological abnormalities (the degenerate 'stigmata'), and (3) the related conditions progressively deteriorate as the degenerate diathesis is passed from generation to generation.

Core features of 'bouffée délirante' include a sudden onset of delusional ideas and the rapid evolution of an intense symptomatology, conferring different and often changing contents, for example megalomania, persecution and hypochondriasis (Magnan 1893). Complete remission usually followed after a short time (Pichot 1986).

According to Magnan, in the 'degenerates', psychosis manifested itself through the imbalance of constitutionally labile nervous centres, some irritated and some weakened. In this theoretical framework, bouffée délirante, among other acute psychoses, displays a level of destructuration, intermediate to manic–depressive illness and schizophrenia, hallmarks of which are oneroid phenomena. It is this intermediate level of disturbance that explains the benign prognosis of the bouffée délirante. Bouffée délirante has its firm place in French psychiatry, documented by its inclusion in the national classification system INSERM (1969) and the formulation of operational criteria by Pull and colleagues (Pull et al. 1984, 1987).

(b) Cycloid psychoses

The concept of cycloid psychosis is closely connected to the 'Wernicke–Kleist–Leonhard school of psychiatry'. Carl Wernicke (Wernicke 1894) (1848–1905) gave vivid clinical descriptions of 'anxiety psychosis' and 'motility psychosis' which he conceived as transient psychotic disorders of generally good prognosis (Wernicke 1900). Anxiety psychosis is dominated by anxious affect, leading to other symptoms including psychotic—often paranoid—phenomena. Motility psychosis shows all kinds of motor symptoms and was divided into hyperkinetic, akinetic and mixed ('complete') forms. Wernicke's main concern was to base his classification of mental disorders on pathogenetic hypotheses formulated in terms of the dysfunction of specific brain systems, not on prognosis or aetiology. Wernicke's pupil, Karl Kleist, later coined the term 'cycloid psychoses' (Kleist 1924, 1929), which in its original formulation comprised motility psychosis and confusional psychosis.

Cycloid psychoses 'manifest themselves in multiple phases during life, come and go in an autochthonous way, often show antagonistic syndromes—confusion and stupor, hyperkinesis and akinesis—and do not lead to mental defects' (Kleist 1928).

(c) Reactive psychoses

At the beginning of the twentieth century, several authors described acute psychotic states arising in severely stressful situations such as imprisonment or combat (Kleist 1918; Siefert 1907; Wilmanns 1908). In his Allgemeine Psychopathologie, Jaspers (1963, 1965) determined three conditions, under which a psychopathological state can be recognised as 'reactive':

(1) an adequate precipitating event in close temporal relationship with the reactive state
(2) a comprehensible connection between the content of the event and that of the abnormal reaction
(3) resolution of the abnormality with the course of time or, especially, with the cessation of the primary cause

The concept of reactive/psychogenic psychoses proved particularly popular in Scandinavian countries. Wimmer (1916) professor of psychiatry at the University of Copenhagen, in his work, 'psychogenic forms of mental disorders', attempted to draw together under a single entity to a variety of psychotic disorders in which psychogenic factors or emotional stress played an important role. Wimmer gave concept of psychogenic psychosis. He emphasised the fact that it is not only that psychosis develops in association with an emotional trauma, but also the course and symptomatology reflect the trauma. Wimmer (1816) published a monograph on psychogenic psychoses in 1916. He wrote:

> *As psychogenic psychoses we designate . . . the various, clinically independent psychoses, the main features of which is that they – usually on a (definite) predisposed foundation – are caused by mental agents ('mental traumata'), and in such a way that these pathemata determine the point in time of the start of the psychosis, the fluctuations (remissions, intermissions, exacerbations) of the disease, very often also its cessation. Likewise the form and the content of the psychosis are, more or less directly and completely ('comprehensibly'), determined by the precipitating mental factors. To these criteria can, finally, be added the predominant tendency of these disorders to recovery and, more specifically, that they never end in deterioration.*

Later, the term 'reactive' was used interchangeably with 'psychogenic', and finally, 'reactive' was preferred because it conveyed fewer theoretical assumptions. The phenomenology of reactive psychoses, as the diagnosis is applied, covers a broad spectrum ranging from psychogenic twilight states to depressive symptoms to chronic delusional development.

Kasanin (1933) described this group to be suffering from *schizoaffective psychosis*, which are characterised by sudden onset, generally preceded by severe mental stress in the setting of marked emotional turmoil, followed by good recovery. Patients originally diagnosed by Wimmer as having psychogenic psychosis were followed up by Faergeman (1946, 1963) 15–25 years after their index admission. He reported that 50 % of patients could be considered confirmed cases of psychogenic psychosis and pointed towards the need for recognising these as separate groups of disorders, which were quite different from schizophrenia and affective psychosis.

The findings of Faergeman partly concurred with those of the Langfeldt (1937), who tried to differentiate 'true schizophrenia' from 'schizophreniform states' (Langfeldt 1939). He did not assume the schizophreniform psychoses to be a distinct diagnostic entity, but rather an aetiologically heterogeneous group. Langfeldt (1937) coined the term 'schizophreniform' psychosis to define a group of psychosis disorders in which symptoms subsided spontaneously and had a good prognosis.

(d) Schizophreniform disorder (SFD)

The concept of SFD was given by Langfeldt in 1937.

The characteristics of this group were as follows:

- Sudden onset
- Associated mood symptoms
- Clouding of consciousness
- Benign course

Forty years later, this disorder was officially included in DSM-III under psychosis NOS and was maintained with little change in DSM-IV-TR.

Kendler (1980) suggested that SFD belongs within the 'schizophrenia spectrum'. Changes from *DSM-III* to *DSM-III-R* regarding the schizophreniform category include the stipulations that the clinical picture must not meet the criteria for brief reactive psychosis and that there is no evidence that an organic factor initiated and maintained the illness.

DSM-III-R includes a subcategory of good prognostic features, which includes at least two of the following:

(1) Onset of prominent psychotic symptoms within 4 weeks of first noticeable change in usual behaviour or functioning
(2) Confusion, disorientation or perplexity at the height of the psychotic episode
(3) Good premorbid social and occupational functioning
(4) Absence of blunted or flat affect

The centrality of symptom duration as a change from *DSM-III* to *DSM-III-R* regarding the schizophreniform category includes the stipulations that the clinical picture must not meet the criteria for brief reactive psychosis and that there is no evidence that an organic factor initiated and maintained the illness.

(e) Hysterical psychosis

Hollander and Hirsch (1964) described hysterical psychosis as an illness, which begins suddenly and dramatically, temporally related to stressful event and recedes as suddenly and as dramatically as it had begun. They also emphasised the importance of patients with histrionic personality premorbidly would usually tend to develop this illness.

The features of hysterical psychosis are as under:

- Sudden onset
- Onset related to an event which is profoundly upsetting
- Manifestations in form of delusions, hallucinations, depersonalisation or grossly unnatural behaviour
- Affectivity not usually altered; it is usually in direction of volatility and not flattening
- Disorder is generally circumscribed and transient
- Acute episode, seldom lasts longer than 1–3 weeks
- Psychosis recedes as dramatically as it began, leaving practically no residue
- Second and third episodes may occur
- Common in those with hysterical personality and in women
- Hysterical psychosis is the end point on a continuum beginning from hysterical character

Langness (1967) found that hysterical psychosis occurs in males and females related to culturally defined stressful events and is transient. He also found that behaviour during the attack is stereotyped and is shaped and directed by the particular event. On similar note, Martin (1971) considered that hysterical psychosis was a type of coping mechanism used when all other mechanisms fail.

Mallett and Gold (1964) described a similar clinical entity as pseudo-schizophrenic hysterical syndrome, which primarily involved woman with history of superficial object relations, multiple somatic complaints, moderate to severe depression associated with loneliness, emptiness and moderate to severe social and sexual dysfunction.

(f) Atypical psychoses
The term 'atypical psychoses' has been used by many authors to characterise various conditions not fitting the classical Kraepelinian dichotomy. In DSM-III and DSM-III-R, 'atypical psychoses' were employed as a synonym for the residual category of psychotic disorders not otherwise specified, including, for example, post-partum psychoses not fulfilling the criteria of any other psychotic or organic disorder, psychoses failing to meet the duration criteria of a specific disorder and psychoses with unclear or unusual clinical symptoms that could not be classified elsewhere. However, 'atypical psychosis' has most consistently been used as a diagnostic entity in Japanese psychiatry. Its founder was Hisatoshi Mitsuda, who first published on the topic in 1941. According to Mitsuda (1965), the clinical picture is characterised by a kaleidoscopic appearance and rapid fluctuation. At the initial stage, emotional disturbances are frequent, followed by confusional or oneroid states, hallucinations and delusions. Some impairment or clouding of consciousness is often found. The clinical course of 'atypical' psychosis is, in most cases, episodic or periodic, and the prognosis is presumed to be usually favourable. Complete remission is not obligatory, however, and the development of a defect syndrome has been found in a proportion of patients (Hatotani 1996; Kimura et al. 1980). Still, the differentiation of atypical psychosis from schizophrenia has been a major concern for most authors involved.

It was apparent that the historical concepts of acute psychotic states often contain aetiological assumptions, each of a very specific nature but with quite different implications. These assumptions reflect the preferences of their times as well as the underlying ideas of the respective psychiatric schools. A psychogenic or (later the preferred term) reactive aetiology of psychotic states can be traced back to the writings of Jaspers, but appeared most convincing to psychiatrists in northern Europe. From there, the notion of reactive psychoses influenced American psychiatry, including DSM-III. A related tradition stressed the aetiological significance of an emotionally vulnerable personality in conjunction with specific triggering experiences. In apparent contrast, a number of authors have always postulated a close connection between brief and acute psychoses and organic abnormalities such as epilepsy or metabolic disturbances. The coexistence of reactive and organic hypotheses can be observed, even in recent publications: both fever and acute stress have been suggested as aetiological factors in acute brief psychoses in India (Malhotra et al. 1998).

Thus, to summarise, it may be concluded that Kahlbaum and Kraepelin set the stage on which brief and acute psychoses appeared 'atypical'. The concept of 'bouffée délirante', cycloid psychoses, reactive (psychogenic) psychoses and atypical psychoses has provided diverging, but interrelated ways to delineate brief and acute psychoses and to determine their nosological status.

When all these entities were evaluated, it was found that they had following common features:

1. Acute or sudden onset
2. Variable and unstable symptomatology
3. Associated anxiety
4. Affective symptoms, most commonly fear
5. Clear relation with a stressor
6. Good premorbid adjustment
7. Rapid and complete recovery

There was further evidence emerging from the WHO multi-centre collaborative studies such as International Pilot study of Schizophrenia (IPSS), determinants of outcome of severe mental health disorders (DOSMeD) and cross-cultural study of acute psychosis (CAP), which supported the notion of non-affective, non schizophrenic, acute psychotic states occurring in significant proportion of cases of functional psychosis.

5 International Pilot Study of Schizophrenia (IPSS 1968–1970)

This international multi-centric study was initiated in 1965. This was a nine-country study on schizophrenia funded by World Health Organisation (1973). It was a prospective follow-up study, in which cases were selected through a series of screening procedures and examined with standard instruments. Nine field research centres selected were Aarhus (Denmark), Agra (India), Cali (Columbia), Ibadan (Nigeria), London (UK), Moscow (USSR), Taipei (Taiwan), Washington (USA) and Prague (Czechoslovakia). In this study, patients between 15 and 44 years of age with history of defined symptoms indicative of mental disorder with duration less than 5 years were included.

The aims of study were as follows:

1. Whether schizophrenia existed in different parts of world?
2. What were common/differing clinical presentations?
3. What was course and outcome among different cultures?

In this study, 1,202 patients were recruited and followed up at 1 year, 2 years and 5 years.

The major conclusions of the study were as follows:

- The study demonstrated that it was possible to carry out a large-scale international psychiatric study involving the psychiatrists and mental health workers from different cultures and socio-economic background.
- Similar groups of patients with schizophrenia were identified from all the countries involved in study.

- It was also noted that there was a great variability in the course and outcome of schizophrenia.
- More than half of the patients were in best outcome group.
- Twenty-six percentage of subjects with schizophrenia had good outcome and had only one episode.
- Developing countries had better course and outcome than developed countries. Best course was seen in patients from Ibadan, followed by patients from Agra. However, Aarhus patients had worst course and outcome.
- From different centres, it was found that insidious onset; marital status of widowhood, divorced or separated; social isolation; long duration of episode; and past history of psychiatric treatment were predictors of poor outcome.
- It was hypothesised that culture has an important effect on course and outcome of schizophrenia and that social variables have a greater predictive importance in terms of prognosis than symptomatic variables.

  The results obtained from IPSS study paved the way for further studies on schizophrenia.

6 Determinants of Outcome of Severe Mental Health Disorders (DOSMeD; 1978–1980)

This study (Sartorius et al. 1986) was designed in late 1970s to further investigate some of the findings of the IPSS. It was planned that a more representative sample of patients with schizophrenia at the initial stages of illness would be studied. In this, new cases of schizophrenia occurring over a specified time period were included. Twelve centres in ten countries were included in the study, and they were Aarhus (Denmark); Agra and Chandigarh (India); Cali (Columbia); Dublin (Ireland); Honolulu and Rochester (USA); Ibadan (Nigeria); Moscow (USSR); Nagasaki (Japan); Nottingham (UK); and Prague (Czechoslovakia). Some of these centres had earlier also participated in the IPSS study. The main aim of the study was to assess the incidence of schizophrenia in different cultures and to provide definite evidence about course and outcome of schizophrenia in the different parts of world. In this study, all cases of first-onset psychosis within a specified catchment area and specified age range were taken.

The main findings of the study were as follows:

1. Incidence of schizophrenia: Incidence differed from 'broadly defined' schizophrenia (including reactive and unspecified psychosis, as per ICD-9)(1.5–4.2/lac/year) and 'narrowly defined' schizophrenia (CATEGO S + SFRS)(0.7/lac/year). Broadly defined schizophrenia included a group of acute onset reactive and unspecified psychosis.
2. It was also found that the peak of incidence of broadly defined schizophrenic conditions in males was at 24 years in majority of centres. The peak age of incidence in males was at 20–24 years, but in females, it shifted towards onset at older age.

3. Morbid risk of schizophrenia was found around 0.53 % in Honolulu, about 1.74 % in rural Chandigarh for broad diagnosis of schizophrenia.
4. There was a group of patients who had non-affective psychosis, which remitted completely. They were called non-affective, acute, remitting psychosis (NARP). The incidence of such NARP cases was 10 times higher in developing countries.
5. These patients from developing countries exhibited a benign course at 2 years follow-up.
6. Fifty percentage of patients had single psychotic episode followed by complete or incomplete remission and 16 % had unremitted, continuous illness.

In both the IPSS and the DOSMeD, predictors of good outcome were mainly the following:

- Acute onset
- Developing country setting

Following these results, the WHO conducted another study on acute psychotic states. It was called the **CAP (Cross-cultural Study of Acute Psychosis, 1980–1982).**

This study (Cooper et al. 1990) was an off-shoot of DOSMeD study done in 14 centres and 7 countries. The main objectives of the study were to know the following:

1. Whether there are acute psychotic states that can be defined, which are descriptively different from schizophrenia and MDP?
2. How is acute psychosis related to psychological and physical stress?

One thousand and four patients meeting the criteria of acute onset psychotic symptoms were included in the study. The main findings of the study were as follows:

- Forty-two percentage had stress at onset of symptoms
- Higher prevalence in lower socio-economic status
- Two-thirds of patients had no relapse at 1 year
- Forty-one percentage had schizophrenic symptoms
- Twenty percentage had affective symptoms
- Thirty-five percentage had other symptoms of psychosis
- Outcome of patients with acute psychosis with schizophrenic symptoms was similar to those with only affective symptoms

Taken together, the findings of these three major WHO studies provided strong evidence in favour of occurrence of acute onset psychotic disorders, which were different from both schizophrenia and MDP, and formed the basis for recognition of these entities as one disorder by WHO in 1992 by including it in ICD-10 as ***ATP (acute and transient psychosis)***.

Similarly, the concept of reactive (psychogenic) psychosis was never fully accepted. A category of 'brief reactive psychosis' was introduced in DSM-III (APA 1980). However, the 'brief reactive psychosis' of DSM-III differs from the Scandinavian concept by virtue of the restrictive criteria for trigger, symptomatology and duration. In DSM-IV, it was replaced by '**brief psychotic disorder**'. For this diagnosis, a triggering event is no longer necessary. Thus, the modern classifications, namely the ATPD of ICD-10 and the BPD of DSM-IV, reflect the varied history of the concept.

7 Post-ICD-10 ATP Validation Studies

1. Analysis of the DOSMeD data:
   This study was done by Susser and Wanderling in 1994. It was aimed to study first-onset psychosis cases and acute psychosis cases, identified as non-affective, acute remitting psychosis (NARP). It was also found that these cases were more prevalent in developing countries and among females. The incidence of NARP in men was about one half the incidence in women, and the incidence in the developing country setting was reported about tenfold the incidence in the industrialised country setting. These associations with sex and with setting were different from schizophrenia. It was also reported that the duration of episode among NARP had a bimodal distribution with point of rarity between the clusters of symptoms with 80 % patients had duration less than 28 weeks and 20 % had duration of more than 1 year. Acute remitting psychosis was found to have a modal distribution of 2–4 months, which was greater than 1–3 months period given by the ICD-10. These findings suggested that the typical duration of the episodes of ATPD was about 28 weeks, and it was longer than the time period recognised by the ICD-10.
2. Chandigarh ATP course and outcome study:
   It was 5-year follow-up study of ICD-10 ATP cases by Rozario et al. (1999), Acute and transient psychotic disorders: A follow-up study. Unpublished MD thesis: PGIMER, Chandigarh in 1999. In this study, it was found that 75 % had good outcome in the form of complete recovery, and there were no residual symptoms. Various good outcome predictors were identified such as female gender, presence of stress at onset and absence of schizophrenic symptoms. It was also reported that in their study group, about 65 % patients had single episode psychosis, and only 35 % of cases had recurrence. Besides this, it was found that 77 % of patients had good adjustment in their social functioning. About 84 % of patients were completely asymptomatic at time of follow-up, of which significantly greater number had stress present.
   There was another 20 years follow-up study by Malhotra et al. 2000, Twenty-year follow-up of WHO CAP study cohort, Unpublished in 2000. It was the study of the WHO CAP study cohort. In this long-term study, it was found that 82 % patients had excellent outcome with no relapse and no residual symptoms.
3. Study on Recurrent ATPD by Malhotra et al. (2005):
   The study was done in 2005 (Malhotra et al. 2005) and was aimed at determining different correlates of recurrent ATPD. The correlates were also compared with non-recurrent forms. It was found that while the two groups of recurrent and

non-recurrent ATP were comparable with respect to sex, occupation, education, income, religion, family type and locality, there was significant difference when compared on marital status. Recurrent ATPD was found more likely in married than the unmarried individuals. Among the clinical correlates, it was reported that acute onset of illness was more common with non-recurrent ATPD. However, response to treatment was better in recurrent ATP than non-recurrent ATP. It was also found that recurrence was fairly common in ATPD (47 %). The psychopathology as well as the diagnostic stability of ATPD was retained over episodes. However, there appeared to be no major predictors of recurrence in ATPD.

4. The Halle Study on Brief and Acute Psychoses:
   The 'Halle study on brief and acute psychoses' (HASBAP) (Marneros and Pillman 2002) was the most comprehensive study carried out in Germany. In this study, a prospective approach was adopted. A consecutively recruited inpatient sample with a diagnosis of 'acute and transient psychotic disorder' or 'BPD' was included. A cohort of 42 patients with ATPD was followed up for a mean of 4.7 years after the index episode or 10.6 years after the first episode. The findings in the study were as follows:

- Incidence rate of ATPD was around 8.5 %, and the frequency of ATPD was found to be higher countries of the third world
- Socio-biographic features: more common in female 78.6 % versus 21.4 % males
- Most frequently between the thirtieth and forty-fifth years of age
- Acute stress played a major role
- Duration of psychotic episode: average around 13 days
- Psychopathology of the acute episode: schizophrenic first-rank symptoms were found in more than 70 % of patients with ATPD, i.e. though insertion, thought broadcasting, delusions of being influenced
- Disturbances of affectivity were also found in all patients, with depressed mood, euphoria and anxiety, all being present in most of the patients at some point in time; a 'polymorphic picture: rapidly changing mood, rapidly changing symptoms and bipolarity of symptoms'. In this, not only the quickly changing mood seems to be characteristic of an ATPD episode, but also quickly changing topics of delusions, which were very unstable. Bipolarity (i.e. change between hyperthymic and depressed mood) was found in 29 % of patients within the same episode, often even within one day. This rapid changing of affect especially in the polymorphic group shows the similarity of some such states with the cycloid psychoses or the bouffée délirante
- Because of the short duration of the episode, the effectiveness of the pharmacological treatments has repeatedly been questioned. It has been supposed that the psychotic episode could as well remit without psychopathological picture, which is dramatic and acute as a rule, and is often accompanied by suicidal tendency.

Till now, if we summarise the understanding of acute and transient psychosis, then we may conceptualise the knowledge in form of following questions:

Q. What is their significance in psychiatry?
According to Marneros (2006), from the clinical point of view, the majority of people with ATPD occupy a special position different from that of people with schizophrenia or schizoaffective or affective disorders. Their educational and occupational status and level of functioning are not significantly different from those of the mentally healthy population. They also have an average level of social interaction and activities, as well as the same frequency of stable heterosexual partnerships as mentally healthy people. Their illnesses have symptoms, course and outcome, which distinguish them from other psychotic disorders.

The theoretical point of view is that the ATPD demonstrates the importance of differential diagnosis and of exact final diagnosis in creating a homogeneous group for research. Clinical features, course and outcome of ATPD exclude this kind of psychotic disorder from other psychotic groups such as schizophrenia and from affective or schizoaffective disorders. Patients can also develop affective, schizoaffective and schizophrenic episodes during the long-term course of ATPD, perhaps providing a strong argument in favour of a psychotic continuum or a set of bridge to classical mental disorders such as schizophrenia and melancholic depression.

8 Diagnostic Validity of Acute Psychosis

According to Robin and Guze (1970) in psychiatric illness for any valid diagnosis to exist, it must have a specific clinical description which could be supported by laboratory studies, which could be separated from other entities, and on follow-up must be stable and there must be familial aggregation. However, over the years, the scheme has been modified due to the limited and disparate evidence the research findings are presented according to Kendler (1980) three main classes of potential 'validators':

(1) Antecedent factors: demographic factors, premorbid personality, precipitating factors and familial aggregation
(2) Concurrent validators: biological and psychological factors, symptom measures
(3) Prognostic validators: diagnostic stability, response to treatment, course and outcome

9 Antecedent Validators

1. Demographic factors

   Incidence of ATPD:
   Two studies reported on incidence of ATPD. Singh et al. in 2004 estimated an annual rate of 3.9 per 100,000 population in Nottingham (UK), with a male/female ratio of 1.87.
   In another study by Castagnini et al. in 2008, the incidence of ATPD based on data from the Danish National Register was estimated to be 9.6 per 100,000,

though it was also recorded that about 60 % of cases tended to change diagnosis on subsequent admissions. In Germany, Jäger et al. in 2003 found a frequency of 7.9 % in first admissions for non-affective psychoses, similar to that reported by Albus et al. in 1990 and Marneros et al. in 2004. A comparative study of the ICD-10 diagnoses used in German and Danish psychiatric hospitals by Lange et al. in 2002 pointed to higher rates of ATPD in the latter. Researchers have repeatedly noted the higher incidence of non-affective acute psychoses in developing compared with industrialised countries (Jørgensen et al. 1997; Susser et al. 1996; Das et al. 1999).

Developing countries:

In a study by Susser and Wanderling in 1994, it was found that for non-affective acute remitting psychosis, the incidence in the developing country setting was about tenfold higher than the incidence in the industrialised country setting.

Sex distribution:

Female preponderance has been found in different studies. In a study by Malhotra et al. in 1998, ATP was reported as being more common in females and in patients with a rural background. In another study in 1999, Das et al. (1999) reported that ATPD was more common in females with a mean age in the early middle adulthood. Similarly, in the 'Halle study on brief and acute psychosis (HASBAP) (Marneros and Pillman 2002) at Germany in 2003, it was found that majority of patients diagnosed as having ATPD were females and the female/male ratio was about 3.7:1. Susser and Wanderling (1994) reported male/female ratios of NARP of 0.96 in the developing countries and 0.44 in industrialised settings. The incidence of cycloid psychosis in Sweden (Lindvall et al. 1993) was also reported to be higher in women (0.05 per 1,000) than in men (0.036 per 1,000). In a study by Castagnini et al. in 2008, it was found that among ATPD subgroups, despite the relatively small number of cases, those with schizophrenic features (F23.1 and F23.2) showed a reverse gender distribution, being prevalent in males, indicating a close kinship with schizophrenia. Similar evidence was found in the Danish registry sample, where incidence rates were found only slightly higher in females (9.8 vs. 9.4 per 100,000).

Age:

Age at onset of non-affective psychoses varies considerably across studies. In the DOSMeD, the mean age at onset of NARP was 22.4 years for both sexes in developing countries and 25.5 years for men and 24.9 years for women in industrialised countries (Susser and Wanderling 1994). Similar results have been reported from studies in Iran (Alaghband-Rad et al. 2006a); however, the mean age at onset of NARP was reported around mid-1930s in an incidence cohort from New York (Mojtabai et al. 2003) and Germany (Marneros et al. 2003). In Denmark (Castagnini et al. 2008), the age at onset of ATPD was also higher and differed between men and women (46.2 years females vs. 37.8 years for males).

In a community study in northern Norway (Kørner et al. 2009), the 5-year (1940–1944) prevalence of constitutional (reactive) psychoses in the population over 60 years was found to be 2.2 %. In the study by Jørgensen et al. in 1997, it was found that patients suffering from late first-contact acute and transient psychosis were at a 10 times higher risk of subsequently getting a dementia diagnosis compared to patients with osteoarthritis and at eight times higher risk compared to the general population.

Overall, the similarities among these epidemiologic studies of non-affective acute psychoses were that these conditions appear to be more common in females than males, distinguishing this syndrome from schizophrenia. Second, the non-affective acute psychoses appear to be more common in developing country settings than in industrialised settings. Finally, the average age at onset was higher than the age at onset of schizophrenia.

Socio-biographical data:

In study by Malhotra et al. in 1998, it was found that lower socio-economic status and rural population have more prevalence of ATP. In the HASBAP study, it was reported by Marneros et al. in 2003 that a broken home situation was found significantly in ATPD than in healthy controls. A broken home situation was defined as a disruption in the continuity of caregiving in the patient's family before the age of 15 years (when one of the following criteria was met: death of one or both parents, divorce or separation of parents, caregivers other than parents, severe addiction of one/both parents).

2. Premorbid personality:

   In study conducted by Kuruvilla, it was found that hysterical psychosis was more common in hysterical personalities. Similarly, Tasman et al. reported that ATPD was seen more commonly in personality disorders such as histrionic, paranoid, schizotypal, narcissistic and borderline. Pillmann et al. (2003) carried out a comparison between ATPD patients and control groups with schizophrenia, schizoaffective disorder and healthy subjects using the 5-NEO Factor Inventory (neuroticism, extraversion, openness to experience, agreeableness and conscientiousness). They reported no relevant difference between ATPD and healthy controls; however, it was found that patients with schizoaffective disorder and particularly those with schizophrenia showed markedly higher neuroticism, and lower extroversion and conscientiousness. The latter also had fewer premorbid social relation functions and difficulty in entertaining stable relationships. In a study done by Jørgensen et al. (1996) in 1995, it was observed that almost two-thirds of the patients with ATPD in their study group qualified for a concomitant diagnosis of personality disorder; however, this rate dropped significantly 1 year later. In this study, a high rate (63 %) of personality disorders was observed among an inpatient sample of ATPD patients shortly after recovery from symptoms. However, this rate decreased at 1-year follow-up to 46 % using ICD-10 criteria and 29 % using DSM-IV criteria. It was concluded that personality disorder could be a transient consequence of psychotic decompensation or an effect of pharmacological treatment because most patients were taking neuroleptic drugs on hospital discharge. These findings were consistent with studies of Singh et al. in 2004 and Suda et al. in 2005, who also reported that cases with ATPD did not have significant premorbid dysfunctions.

3. Precipitating factors

   Stress:

> ICD-10 defines ‘acute stress’ as events that would be regarded as stressful for most people in similar circumstances (bereavement, unexpected loss of partner or job), occurring within 2 weeks before onset of psychotic symptoms. Also, acute stress within 2 weeks of onset of psychosis is noted as defining criteria for ATPD. However, as reported by Das et al. in 2001, only 10–69 % patients in their study group experienced acute stress in this time frame. They also reported that patients with family history of psychiatric illness in their first-degree relatives require significantly less amount of stress prior to onset of acute psychotic illness. Stress in this study was construed as a major event that either had a negative impact or involved a significant increase in the responsibilities of the patient. Thus, they emphasised that it was moderate to severe form of stress that preceded the onset of psychosis.

Similarly, in the study by Sajith et al. in 2002, life events were involved in two-thirds of cases, and most often the symptoms had an abrupt onset (less 48 h). These findings were similar to study by Okasha et al. in 1993, in which it was found that 74 % of their Egyptian patients with acute psychosis experienced some stressful event. In a study by Malhotra and Malhotra in 2001, it was reported that stress preceding the onset of symptoms was present in about 60 % of ATPD patients. This study supported the results of earlier studies that stress was more common in female subjects and additionally found that it was associated with better outcome.

In a study from India in 2001 Das et al. (2001) to study the stress-vulnerability hypothesis, it was reported that 32.5 % of patients experienced stress within two weeks before the onset of symptoms. The main finding of this study was that ATPD patients with a positive family history of psychiatric disorder in their first-degree relatives reported significantly less amount of stress prior to the onset of their acute psychotic illness. It was also hypothesised that the positive family history confers a certain degree of vulnerability on the probands, and thereby, these patients need a lesser amount of stress for the occurrence of ATPD in them.

A study from India by Collins et al. (1996) in 1996 reported that recent life events (characterised as job distress for men and leaving or returning to parental village for women) were more common among the brief psychotic cases with acute onset than among those with non-acute onset.

Similarly in a Danish sample Jørgensen et al. (1996), psychosocial stressors were reported within the two weeks prior to the onset of first psychotic symptoms for 53 % of patients and those with preceding stressors were more likely to experience an abrupt onset. On the other hand, ATPD tends to have an abrupt onset in European countries, and ‘acute stress’ was recorded only in a small number of cases (Singh et al. 2004; Marneros and Pillmann 2004; Jørgensen et al. 1997).

Apart from variations between industrialised and developing countries, (Das et al. 2001; Susser et al. 1995) where social and cultural factors are usually associated with acute psychoses, these studies have disproved the hypothesis that stress factors trigger ATPD.

Different researchers have tried to identify different correlates of stress. It was found that the role of stress may vary by gender and frequency of episodes. In a study by Malhotra et al. in 1998, it was reported that stress is more common in female as compared to male patients. In this study group, stress was present in over 50 % of the female subjects and in 26 % of the male subjects. It was also postulated that the female subjects are more vulnerable to the development of psychosis under conditions of stress than males, and that could perhaps partly explain the female preponderance of this disorder. In a similar study by Rozario et al. in 1999, it was found that in patients in whom stress precipitated the illness, in 60 % of them, stress was reflected in their symptomatology.

It was found that many cases of psychosis in the post-partum period can be characterised as cases of non-affective acute psychoses. The post-partum period may be an especially stressful period for women both physically and psychologically. In a study sample by Pfuhlmann et al. in 1998, of consecutively admitted women with post-partum psychosis, it was reported that 21 % of the patients met the diagnostic criteria for acute and transient polymorphous psychotic disorders, and 54 % met the criteria for cycloid psychosis.

There is also some evidence of increased rates of non-affective acute psychosis in immigrants. In a Portuguese sample (Alexandre et al. in 2010, it was found that black immigrants were more likely than non-immigrant white patients to receive a diagnosis of schizophrenia or ATPD. In a similar study in 2009, of foreign domestic workers admitted to a psychiatric hospital in Hong Kong, (Lau et al. 2009) 63 % received a diagnosis of ATPD. Similarly, West African and Caribbean immigrants (Littlewood and Lipsedge 1981) living in Britain have been reported to experience an increased frequency of acute psychotic reactions, although increased rates of schizophrenia also have been reported in this patient population.

4. Family genetic studies:

   Family history of psychotic illness increases the risk of ATP, and presence of family history is hypothesised as a constitutional vulnerability. In a study by Das et al. in 1999, it was found that (a) ATPD was three times more frequent in first-degree relatives of patients with ATPD than family members of schizophrenics; (b) the risk of schizophrenia was significantly increased in first-degree relatives of schizophrenic patients; (c) the risk of affective disorders did not exceed that expected in the general population. It was also found that first-degree relatives of patients with schizophrenia-like symptoms were more likely to develop schizophrenia than ATPD. In this study, it was reported that there is a genetic overlap between ATPD, schizophrenic symptoms and schizophrenia. ATPD is a genetically heterogeneous category including a subgroup that overlaps with schizophrenia or at the interface between the two disorders, whereas there is no relationship to affective psychoses. ATPD subtypes with schizophrenic symptomatology (ICD-10 codes F23.1 and F 23.2) had more family history of schizophrenia than the rest of the ATP subtypes. A later study by Das et al. in 2001 reported that ATPD patients with a family history of mental disorders experienced fewer life events and scored less cumulative stress before illness onset than those without familial psychiatric morbidity. They also hypothesised that these findings lend support to the view that cases with ATPD may be regarded as having an altered sensitivity on the basis of a familial predisposition that render them susceptible to stress effects. In the same study, it was also found that family history of mental illness in first-degree relatives was present in 20.3 % in ATPD patients and 3.6 % for healthy controls. Similarly, the proportion of first-degree relatives with psychotic disorders was 3.4 % for the ATPD group and 0.7 % for controls without mental disorder.

The findings in this study were supported by another study from India in 1988 by Chavan and Kulhara (1988). They reported more family history of psychiatric illness in patients of reactive psychosis. However, there were also some studies that have not replicated such results. Marneros and Pillmann in 2004 reported a higher rate of mental disorders in family members of patients with ATPD than the relatives of healthy controls, but found that there was no significantly raised risk of psychotic disorders.

Increased risk of cycloid psychoses in family members of patients with cycloid psychoses (Perris 1974) also has been noted. However, a twin study of patients with cycloid psychosis found little evidence supporting heritability (Franzek and Beckmann 1998). Also, first-degree relatives of schizophrenic probands had significantly higher prevalence of schizophrenia than those of ATP probands. ATP subtypes with schizophrenic symptomatology (ICD-10 codes F23.1 and F 23.2) had more family history of schizophrenia than the rest of the ATP subtypes.

10 Concurrent Validators

Infections

Acute psychosis has also been described in patients with specific infections such as the viral infection, (Klein et al. 1984; Jarvis et al. 1990) meningoencephalitis (Wise et al. 1977; Frasca et al. 1993) and neurocysticercosis (Shriqui and Mileltte 1992). Viral infections such as influenza, Epstein-Barr virus infection and the herpes simplex virus have been associated with psychotic symptoms. These studies have also found a relationship between the course of psychotic symptoms and changes in serum and CSF viral antibodies (Srikanth et al. 1994). It was proposed by Lycke and Ziegler in 1983 that the stress of recent illness and fever may lead to reactivation of the latent virus, resulting in an acute and short-lived manifestation of psychotic symptoms. It could also be possible that the acute infection and fever initiate an auto-immune response, predisposing to the development of psychosis in the weeks after the fever itself subsides.

Fever

The association with fever assumes importance in view of common occurrence of acute brief psychotic states (Castagnini et al. 2008; Collins et al. 1996, 1999) as well as fever in developing countries with greater prevalence of infectious diseases. It is also proposed that this may be reason for higher incidence of these disorders in developing countries. It was proposed that fever could act as a physiological stressor, leading to hormonal and biochemical changes in the brain resulting in psychosis (Malhotra et al. 1998). It is also possible that acute infection and fever initiate an auto-antibody response that predisposes to the development of psychotic symptoms in the weeks after the fever itself subsides (Collins et al. 1999). The association with fever and ATPD was significant because both fever and acute brief psychoses are common in developing countries. In the same study, Collins et al. found a strong association (odds ratio = 6.2) between antecedent fever and acute brief psychosis and proposed that antecedent fever might be a biological correlate of acute brief psychosis.

According to Malhotra et al. (1998), the association of fever within 4 weeks prior to the onset of psychosis in the DOSMed and CAPS samples (the presence of fever was an exclusion criterion in the FAT PD group) were compared. A significantly higher number of patients were found to have fever in the study group (16.8 % vs. 4.9 %, odds ratio 3.95, 95 % confidence limits 0.81, 26.22). In about 16.8 % of patients in the study group, fever occurred within 4 weeks preceding the onset of psychosis, which was significantly in excess of that in the control group. It was non-specific fever of a moderate to high degree (not necessarily as measured by a thermometer), without associated impairment of consciousness or any possibility of brain involvement. Fever was self-remitting or remitted by non-specific treatment given locally within 2–7 days without any residual systemic effects. Patients in this study group often reported that psychotic symptoms occurred after a variable period of about 1–2 days to 1–2 weeks following the onset of fever. However, the clinical examination and routine laboratory investigations of acute psychosis patients with fever revealed no positive evidence to characterise the pathology.

Hypothalamic—pituitary axis abnormalities

In 1998, a case–control study was done by Malhotra et al. (1998). In this study, the comparative samples of patients with acute non-affective remitting psychoses and of non-affective, non-remitting psychoses or schizophrenias were drawn from the three major study cohorts generated by different teams of investigators at different points in time during the period 1978–1995 (Collins et al. 1996; Varma et al. 1992). In this study, it was found that as compared to the control group, significantly higher proportion of married females (21.7 %) reported childbirth within 3 months prior to the onset of psychosis, (4.5 %; odds ratio 5.83, 95 % confidence limits 0.72, 264.9). Another significant finding of this study was the higher incidence of childbirth in the study sample (10 of 77 cases; 13 %) compared to the controls (1 of 32 cases; 3 %). Of the married female subjects, about 21.7 % of cases involved childbirth in acute psychosis patients, compared to 4.5 % in the controls (an excess of nearly fivefold). Thus, childbirth appears to be a significant factor associated with acute psychosis among female patients.

In this study, it was hypothesised that childbirth acts as a psychophysiological stressor with major hormonal changes which could trigger a psychotic illness. Since acute psychoses occur more often among women, predominantly in the reproductive age group, childbirth may make an important contribution to the aetiology of these disorders. In the study done by Kumar (1994) on post-partum psychosis in different cultures, it was reported that the relative risk of psychosis among women after childbirth was 16- to 20-fold higher, and it was higher for primipara, i.e. 35-fold higher than for the equivalent time prior to conception (Kendell et al. 1981). However, Wieck et al. (1991) proposed that the aetiology of post-partum psychosisis is a specific physiological cerebral dysfunction, rather than psychosocial in nature.

Seasonal pattern
Malhotra et al. in 1998 observed that there was a summer peak (May–September) in acute psychotic states. They reported that the number of patients with onset between May and September in the study group was significantly higher (58.5 %). Since there are no data on the month of onset of acute psychotic states available in the literature, this finding remained incomparable. The reasons for acute psychoses with onset in the peak summer months when temperatures range between 30 and 45 °C maximum are not known. They, however, proposed that the developing countries often have hot and temperate climates, and rural patients may not have enough resources to protect themselves from the direct effects of heat. They further added that exposure to heat may act as a physiological stressor, triggering neuroendocrine changes that are responsible for psychosis. These changes might be rapidly reversed by the alteration of environmental conditions and amelioration of stress, or by treatment, leading to rapid and complete recovery from psychosis.

Neurophysiological basis

A. Role of amino acids: Pepplinkhuizen et al., Fekkes and Pepplinkhuizen in 1997 and 2003 argued that metabolic changes in amino acid (serine) pathways are responsible for acute polymorphic psychotic disorders by doing an analogy with the clinical phenomena induced by psychedelic drugs. In this study, it was reported that many patients with acute polymorphic psychotic disorders also suffer from psychosensory phenomena (APP+) in form of congruent and fleeting delusions and hallucinations, distorted sensory perceptions and intense emotional states. It was found that most of these patients were exhibiting a low plasma serine concentration and a high TSM ratio (taurine–serine–methionine ratio), indicating a disturbed serine metabolism. It was proposed that these biochemical markers might be a useful diagnostic tool in discriminating APP+. In this study, after an oral challenge with serine in the remitted APP+ patients, it was found that the characteristic dysperceptions and psychedelic symptoms were induced. Besides that, the plasma concentrations of serine and methionine were decreased, and the concentration of taurine was increased. Fibroblast experiments also suggested that the activities of the serine metabolizing enzymes serine hydroxymethyltransferase and cystathionine fi-synthase were increased in these patients. However, no other studies have been published on the occurrence of amino acid abnormalities in transient acute polymorphic psychosis and due to limited data available, the proposed metabolic changes in amino acid (serine) pathways as a cause of acute polymorphic psychotic disorders cannot be compared and verified.

B. P300: Roth and McClelland (1979) in 2005 examined EEG recordings of patients with ATPD, but did not found an increased pattern of cerebral activity. This was clearly distinct from EEG recordings of residual schizophrenia and all other psychiatric disorders investigated. From the neurophysiological point of view, this study suggested that cycloid psychosis should be considered separately from schizophrenic disorders. It was also proposed that the P300 might contribute useful information for the prognostic evaluation of the course of the disorder after remission of an acute psychotic episode. Low amplitudes and right-sided peaks appear to be the domain of core schizophrenia with chronic or subchronic course and incomplete remissions, while high amplitudes and normal P300 topography indicated the presence of schizophrenia-like cycloid psychosis with a good prognosis. Duncan et al. (Strik et al. 1994) in 1987 described an increase in P300 amplitudes after successful treatment in the patients with ATPD, and no correlation between P300 amplitudes and neuroleptic dosages was found. The finding of higher-than-normal amplitudes in cycloid psychosis was consistent in different studies (Strik et al. 1994, 1997; Pfefferbaum et al. 1989; Duncan et al. 1987), and this group typically had an excellent prognosis in form of full recovery and complete restitution of social competence. As the P300 amplitudes correlate with attentional performance and with higher levels of norepinephrine metabolite in CSF, it was proposed that higher-than-normal amplitudes might be an indication of higher levels of arousal in the cycloid psychosis group (Strik et al. 1997).

C. Cerebral blood flow: In 1992, Warketin et al. (1992) studied the relation between cycloid psychosis and regional cerebral blood flow. They reported that patients with cycloid psychosis have a significantly elevated level of cortical blood flow when they are in an acute state of their illness, presenting overt and florid symptoms. They also found that the flow normalises again with neuroleptic treatment and clinical remission. In other words, the findings indicate that during an acute exacerbation of symptoms, the cortex was highly aroused in these patients. These flow variations seen during a cycloid episode were different from those usually seen in normal subjects. This was particularly evident in the great variability of hemispheric flow, which in some patients was as large as 25–30 % during the psychotic episode. They also found that hemispheric blood flow levels seen at admission were significantly related to the clinical state of the patients. The higher was the cortical blood flow, the more the patient was behaviourally disturbed. This was particularly evident in relation to the negative symptoms, such as impoverished emotional expression, reactivity and feelings.
D. 5-HT2A receptors: In a study of first-episode psychosis by Arranz et al. in 2009, it was found that then, NARP patients had significantly fewer 5-HT2A receptors compared with patients with paranoid schizophrenia and with healthy controls. They reported that this pattern was quiet distinct from affective disorders. These results supported the results of previous studies that NARP was distinct from affective psychosis and schizophrenia.
E. Ventricular abnormalities: An imaging study (Franzek et al. 1996) from Germany was done by Franz et al. in 1996. It was aimed at comparing the diagnoses of psychiatric patients with ventricular abnormalities and patients without such abnormalities. They found that a higher prevalence of cycloid psychosis was associated with ventricular abnormalities in the form of ventricular enlargement and/or asymmetry.

F. Antibodies: In the study by Karlsson et al. in 2012, it was found that the offspring who were exposed to high levels of antibodies directed at gliadin in the intrauterine life were at an elevated risk of developing non-affective psychoses in the later life. Antibodies of the IgG class were detected in the neonatal blood samples and were predominantly derived from the maternal circulation and transferred across the placenta during pregnancy. These antibodies were therefore likely to represent maternal reactivity to gliadin and thus suggest that mothers who produce high levels of these antibodies during pregnancy give birth to children who have an elevated risk of developing a non-affective psychosis later in life. This is the first study to show an association between high levels of maternal antibodies directed at gliadin and the later development of non-affective psychoses in offspring.

11 Prognostic Validators

The parameters used by different researchers for the assessment of course and outcome of ATPD are the stability of diagnosis, recovery, relapses, readmissions and socio-occupational functioning. Most of the existing studies, on course and outcome of acute psychoses, point towards an excellent prognosis and distinctness of the group from other functional psychoses. Various studies have reported a favourable prognosis of ATPD (Chavan and Kulhara 1988; Susser et al. 1998; Varma et al. 1996).

12 Diagnostic Stability, Course and Outcome

In developing countries, ATPD has a relatively high diagnostic stability (54–73 %) and low rates of relapse (Thangadurai et al. 2006; Amini et al. 2005; Alaghband-Rad et al. 2006b). A long-term follow-up study in a developing country setting has compared the course of acute brief psychosis with that of other remitting psychoses at 5, 7 and 12 years after onset (Susser et al. 1998). In the study, the long-term prognosis of acute brief psychosis was found to be excellent and remarkably homogenous, with only one out of seventeen subjects developing a chronic psychotic illness at 12-year follow-up. On the contrary, the long-term prognosis of other remitting psychoses was often poor, with frequent relapses and one half of cases being ill at 12-year follow-up, possibly schizophrenia.

In another follow-up study of unspecified non-organic psychosis, Chaturvedi and Sahu (1986) reported change in diagnosis in 46 % (21 % affective, 16 % reactive psychosis, 9 % schizophrenia) cases.

In 2000, Gupta and Bhardwaj (2000) studied the outcome of ATPD after 10 years. In this study, patients recruited in ICMR study in 1982 were assessed after the completion of 10 years. It was found that 25 % of patients were having continuous illness with first-rank symptoms, 56 % patients never had any psychotic illness during the course of follow-up, 9 % had multiple episodes in the interval period and were diagnosed to have bipolar disorder, whereas 11 % had been diagnosed with schizophrenia.

A small study of first-episode psychotic patients in Iran found that 100 % of those diagnosed with ICD-10 ATPD and DSM-IV BPD maintained the same diagnosis over 12 months of follow-up (Amini et al. 2005). Another study of 60 patients with a first episode of psychosis from Iran (Alaghband-Rad et al. 2006b) reported that 10 cases with ATPD had their diagnosis confirmed 1 year later. Likewise, from different studies, it was concluded that the acute remitting psychoses have high stability particularly in developing countries, where the disorder also shows a favourable prognosis (Amini et al. 2005; Alaghband-Rad et al. 2006b; Susser et al. 1998; Mojtabai et al. 2000).

On the other hand, in European countries, the diagnostic stability of ATPD was found significantly different from developing countries. Apart from an early follow-up study of Jørgensen (1995), which reported a fairly high diagnostic stability, in Europe, it was found that more than 50 % of cases with ATPD changed diagnosis into another category of 'schizophrenia and related disorders' or affective disorders (Castagnini et al. 2008; Jäger et al. 2003). Even the frequency of recurrences was increased compared with rates observed in developing countries. Marneros and Pillmann in 2004 reported that three-quarters of their cases with ATPD had a recurrent affective or psychotic episode, 30 % developed affective disorders, and a relatively small number converted into either schizoaffective disorder or schizophrenia.

In a study by Pillmann and Marneros in 2005, it was found that only one-third of the patients enjoyed a stable remission and discontinued medication after 7 years. The outcome of ATPD proved to be more favourable than in schizophrenic patients by follow ups from the Nottingham first-episode psychosis study, though two-thirds of cases changed diagnosis over 3 years. However, a Munich study covering 15 years of registry data found a 39 % stability rate of ATPD, with 60 % of the total ATPD sample developing another psychiatric disorder by their third admission (Möller et al. 2010). Similarly, diagnostic stability over 5 years in a first-episode psychotic sample in China was 35 % for those diagnosed with ATPD, and it was found that 29 % of ATPD patients transitioned to schizophrenia. In this study, it was also found that group of ATPD patients who later developed schizophrenia had a 'non-polymorphic' subtype at baseline, whereas patients with a 'polymorphic' subtype at baseline were rediagnosed with bipolar disorder (Chang et al. 2009). In 2008, Castagnini et al. (2008) conducted a six-year analysis of readmission patterns of all subjects listed in the Danish psychiatric central register. They included all patients who were admitted to hospital or treated in outpatient services for the first time with a diagnosis of ATPD from 1 January to 31 December 1996. They reported that more than 80 % of patients diagnosed with ATPD in their study were readmitted on at least one further occasion during the study period. They also reported that during their last admission, 60 % patients changed diagnosis; half were shifted to another F2 category; and 11 % were shifted to affective disorders. The overall stability rate for ATPD was about

39 %. Due to this poor diagnostic stability, authors also argued against attempts to separate ATPD from schizophrenia and other related disorders.

There was, however, one study that reported the stability of NARP in an industrialised country setting; 6 % of the NARP patients from a New York sample changed to a schizophrenia or schizoaffective diagnosis by the 2-year follow-up period, whereas the majority (77 %) of individuals with other remitting psychoses at baseline transitioned to a schizophrenia or schizoaffective diagnosis (Sajith et al. 2002).

Comparing schizophrenia-like and non-schizophrenic subgroups of ATPD, Singh et al. (2004) also found stability rates were markedly lower for 'polymorphic psychotic disorder' and 'predominantly delusional disorder'. They also suggested that female gender and good premorbid adjustment predicted favourable outcome. In another study, it was also found that stress reactivity is mediated through an emotional-driven pathway leading to florid psychotic disorders with good prognosis, whereas cognitive impairment involved in insidious-onset psychoses associated with negative symptoms and poorer outcome (Myin-Germeys et al. 2001).

It was reported by different researchers that ATPD has an episodic course with longer remissions than cases that later develop schizophrenia (Marneros and Pillmann 2004; Jäger et al. 2007). It was also found that patients with ATPD have a favourable response to drug treatment, but are usually prescribed antipsychotic medications for long periods to prevent recurrences (Marneros and Pillmann 2004). Abrupt or acute onset, female gender and good premorbid functioning predicted diagnostic stability and favourable outcome in ATPD (Singh et al. 2004; Das et al. 2001). Marneros and Pillmann in 2004 reported from the follow-up studies that more than half of those affected with ATPD changed to another F2 category 'schizophrenia and related disorders' or mood disorders. The frequency of recurrent affective and psychotic episodes has been interpreted as indicating that ATPD bridges schizophrenia to affective psychoses, from the point of view of psychotic spectrum.

Coryell and Tsuang (1982) reported that outcome of acute psychosis is best if the duration of admission is shorter, i.e. between 2 weeks to a month. On the basis of duration of psychosis, Susser et al. (1995) also showed that the duration of psychotic illness episode in non-affective acute psychoses have a bimodal pattern of distribution, with a point of rarity between two symptom score clusters. In 80 % of the cases, the duration was less than 28 weeks, and in the rest of the 20 % cases, it was more than a year. In a study from Germany in 2010, after 15 years of follow-up, it was reported that 30 % of ATPD patients experienced a single episode, 50 % had an episodic-remitting course, and 20 % had a chronic course (Möller et al. 2010). Perris (1974) reported that patients with cycloid psychosis have on average about five episodes throughout their lifetime. Throughout 2 years of follow-up, 48 % of patients with NARP remained in full remission, compared with 14 % of patients with other types of remitting psychoses (e.g. schizophrenia, delusional disorder). The course of non-affective acute psychoses may be even more benign in developing countries. In the Chandigarh site of the DOSMeD study, only one (6 %) of 17 patients followed up to 12 years had remaining symptoms of illness at the follow-up (Susser et al. 1998).

Different researchers have reported different recurrence rate for ATPD. In study conducted by Malhotra et al. in 2005 in India, a recurrence rate of 46.6 % was found over an 8-year follow-up. In the same study, different correlates of recurrence were found. They reported that recurrence was more common in females (59 %) and in the patients who were married (about 71 %). No catatonic features were present in recurrent group, and they also responded better to treatment (96 %).The different recurrence rate reported in various studies ranged from 11 to 35 %. In 1995, Susser et al. (1995) reported a recurrence rate of 22 % in a 5-year follow-up study and in 1998 reported recurrence rate of 12 % in a 12-year follow-up study. Similarly, Rozario et al. (1999), Acute and transient psychotic disorders: A follow-up study, Unpublished MD thesis: PGIMER, Chandigarh in 1999, reported a 35 % recurrence rate in a 5-year follow-up study.

Different studies were done on the social impairment in ATPD. In 1999, Vázquez-Barquero et al. (1999) examined 76 patients with schizophrenia 3 years after their first episode. They found that 42 % of this sample had a poor social adjustment at follow-up. However, in study done by Jäger et al. in 2003, it was found that 78 % of the patients had good functioning with respect to personal care, 48 % with respect to occupation, 51 % with respect to family and household and 49 % with respect to the broader social context. Only a few patients had developed a severe social impairment as 1 % had poor functioning with regard to personal care, 11 % with regard to occupation, 4 % with regard to family and household and 10 % with regard to the broader social context. Overall, 12 % had a poor social adjustment in at least one of the four domains. As expected, patients with relapse had a more unfavourable social functioning. However, only a minority of these showed severe social impairment: 2 % with respect to personal care, 19 % with respect to occupation, 7 % with respect to family and household and 17 % with respect to the broader social context. Otherwise, patients without relapse showed excellent social functioning in the year prior to the follow-up examination. It was concluded that overall, the patients in the study could be divided into three groups: who experienced no relapse (42 %), those with relapse, but without marked deficits in the social adjustment (46 %) and patients with relapse as well as a severe social impairment (12 %). It was also hypothesised that from a longitudinal point of view, the subgroup with severe social impairment is not compatible with the concept of a 'transient' psychotic disorder, but rather with the concept of schizophrenia in terms of a chronic disorder.

It was also hypothesised that persisting 'negative' and/or 'depressive' symptoms in patients with ATPD might predict an unfavourable outcome in terms of a chronic schizophrenic disorder. Predictors of diagnostic stability and favourable outcome were identified as sudden onset, female sex, duration less than 1 month and good premorbid functioning. Examining a small group of individuals with ATPD, 40 % of whom later developed schizophrenia, and Suda et al. (2005) found no significant differences in severity or duration of psychotic symptoms during the initial hospitalisation. They reported that acute insomnia was predictive of a single episode of ATPD. Confusion and perplexity were listed among the good prognostic indicators of SFD in the DSM-IV (American Psychiatric Association 2000); however, few recent empiric data are available on the predictive validity of this feature. In a review of 13 follow-up studies of ATPD, Castagnini et al. (2008) noted that studies in developing settings tend to show higher diagnostic stability and lower rates of relapse than in Western settings.

From the various studies, the indicators of good prognosis in ATPD can be summarised as good premorbid adjustment, few premorbid schizoid traits, severe precipitating stressors, sudden onset of symptoms, confusion and perplexity during psychosis, little affective blunting, short duration of symptoms and absence of family history of schizophrenia.

It has been suggested by some of the researchers (Susser et al. 1996; Mojtabai et al. 2000) that diagnostic stability of ATPD might be improved by excluding affective features (emotional turmoil) and extending duration up to 6 months.

13 Relationship of ATPD with Schizophrenia and Affective Disorders

There were lots of attempts by various researchers in post-ICD-10 era to identify relationship between ATP, schizophrenia and affective disorders. It was seen that risk of affective disorders among the first-degree relatives of patients with schizophrenia was 6–8 % and the risk of schizophrenia among relatives of affective disorders was 0.5–3.5 %, and both of these risks were more than the risk of either disorder in general population. Clinical research in last 50 years and genetic research have sufficiently shown that there is no gap between schizophrenia and affective disorder, but there are bridges and overlaps. This lead to the concept of 'continuum hypotheses' for schizophrenia and affective disorders. Winokur, Crow and Maier suggested that there was schizophrenia-affective disorder continuum.

13.1 Where Does ATP Stand in This Continuum?

As previously discussed, in the family genetic studies of ATPD, it was found that family history of ATPD was three times greater and that of schizophrenia was four times lower in first-degree relatives of patients with ATPD, as compared to first-degree relatives of patients with schizophrenia. The findings also suggest that ATPD is genetically distinct from MDP and there is genetic overlap between ATPD and schizophrenia and schizophrenic symptoms. The question still remains whether ATPD and schizophrenia are manifestations of same entity though of different severity? And whether we can club them together as one psychotic group? Some of the researchers argued that the unstable longitudinal course of ATPD, showing a frequent change from ATPD episodes into affective, schizoaffective and schizophrenic disorders, is strong evidence against the nosological independence of ATPD and supports the assumption of a psychotic continuum between schizophrenia and affective disorders (Valentin 1886).

14 Can We Predict Who All Can Develop F20 in Future if They Have ATPD?

Different researchers have compared ATPD and its related disorders with schizophrenia. It was reported that ATPD is associated with better premorbid social adaptation, (Marneros et al. 2003) more precipitating stress, less non-schizoid premorbid personality, more acute onset, less psychological impairment and better global functioning in the follow-up period (Stephens et al. 1982). However, different studies also reported that considerable proportion of the ATPD patients would develop schizophrenia and other mental disorders in the course of their illness. So, it became a topic of interest that whether we can predict who all patients of ATPD will develop chizophrenia in future.

Dahl in 1994, in a review of the studies on ATPD prognosis, reported that the question whether there is a real diagnostic shift in the way that ATPD develops into schizophrenia or whether the disorder has been schizophrenia all along with a debut phase more influenced by life events remains unanswered.

In 2005, Suda et al. (2005) found that ATPD leading to onset of schizophrenia had a greater tendency to recur with a shorter inter-psychotic episode period, which was distinct from those with the ATPD-only course. Similarly, difference was found in symptom manifestation in early stages of the episode. Acute occurrence of insomnia before admission was seen significantly more often among patients who had an ATPD-only course than among patients who later developed schizophrenia. It was also reported that schizophrenia-developing patients had significantly poorer premorbid heterosexual relations. In another study by Stephens et al. (1982), it was reported that patients with ATPD had less premorbid schizoid personality features than those with schizophrenia. The differences found in these studies suggested that the ATPD occurring in those patients who would later develop schizophrenia should be seen as a prodromal process and is different from the ATPD occurring in those patients who will remain in an ATPD-only course. Suda et al. (2005) therefore proposed that the former ATPD episodes might be aborted schizophrenic episodes that failed to develop to their full form, possibly on account of the protecting effect of the patient's favourable concurrent adaptations (Robins and Guze 1970).

15 Psychopathology

Marneros and Pillmann (2004) in 2005 reported that the most important differences regarding phenomenology between ATPD and the other psychotic disorders were the 'rapidly changing delusional topics', 'rapidly changing mood' and anxiety. They also found that in ATPD, delusional topics were found to be widespread including delusions of reference, persecution, religious and grandiose delusions, delusions of guilt and delusional misidentifications. They found that more than one half of the patients with ATPD in their study group change form and topic of delusion very rapidly within some minutes. Although hallucinations did not change in the same rapid frequency as delusional topics, the richness of the hallucinations was found to be very impressive. They reported that the most characteristic psychopathological feature of ATPD episodes was the rapid changing mood between anxiety/agitation and normal state or ecstatic. Two other characteristics of the symptoms of ATPD episodes reported were their acute onset and the short duration of the psychotic period. The polymorphic features, in particular the quickly changing state of mood, confirm the relationship of ATPD to cycloid disorders (Leonhard 1961). It was also reported that the polymorphic and dramatic symptomatology of ATPD has an acute or even an abrupt onset and a short duration with or without an antipsychotic treatment (Marneros and Pillmann 2004).

16 Psychodynamics of ATPD

Psychodynamically, ATPDs indicate deficient ego strength where under the face of acute and severe stress, there is breakdown of ego functions. In reactive psychoses, it has been shown that the psychotic symptoms reflect the stress and the psychotic breakdown is used as a defence serving as a wish fulfilment or escape from reality. Psychosis appears to be environmentally induced in a person who is vulnerable by virtue of deficient socio-emotional coping or deficient ability to handle intense emotions.

17 Diagnostic Criteria

ICD-10

The ICD-10 category of ATPD is rather broad and provides criteria for several subtypes. The structure of ATPD as described by ICD-10 reflects that WHO tried to integrate the various schools of thought and regional concepts of acute psychosis. These concepts include the bouffeed elirante of French psychiatry and cycloid psychoses, both stressing a 'polymorphous' symptom picture; the reactive psychoses of Scandinavian psychiatry with an emphasis on psychogenic triggers; and acute brief psychoses believed to be prevalent in developing countries. The category 'acute polymorphic psychotic disorder' (F23.0) includes schizophrenic symptoms (F23.1). Taking the concepts of bouffe´e de´lirante and Leonhard's cycloid psychoses, the clinical picture in ICD-10 is characterised by onset within 2 weeks of varied delusions, hallucinations, perceptual disturbances, perplexity and emotional turmoil shifting from day to day or even from hour to hour. The other categories listed under ATPD have acute onset and early remission as common features. F23.2—acute schizophrenia-like psychotic disorder—incorporates the concept of schizophreniform psychosis and replaced the ICD-9 category 'acute schizophrenic episode'; F23.3—acute predominantly delusional disorder—involves relatively stable delusions and hallucinations that do not fulfil requirements for ‘polymorphic psychotic disorder’ or schizophrenia; F23.8 other ATPD’ and F23.9 ‘acute and transient psychotic disorder unspecified’ are residual classes for cases that cannot be accommodated otherwise. Apart from ‘acute schizophrenia-like psychotic disorder’, the field trials of ICD-10 (Varma et al. 1996) reported that the other categories failed to achieve ‘good’ reliability with kappa values of 0.42–0.54.

Current diagnostic criteria and categories are as follows:

1. An acute onset [within 2 weeks]
2. Presence of typical syndromes—

- Rapidly changing variable [polymorphic] state
- Typical schizophrenic symptoms

3. Presence of associated acute stress

Recovery in most cases occurs within 2–3 months

Along with these, there are diagnostic guidelines which include the following:

1. That should not meet criteria for manic or depressive episodes although affective symptoms may be present
2. Absence of organic causation although perplexity, confusion and inattention may be present
3. Absence of obvious intoxication by drugs or alcohol

Types of ATP according to ICD-10

F 23.0—acute polymorphic disorder without symptoms of schizophrenia
F 23.1—acute polymorphic psychotic disorders with symptoms of Schizophrenia
F 23.2—acute schizophrenia-like psychotic disorder
F 23.3—acute predominantly delusional psychotic disorders

Brief Psychotic disorder (DSM-IV)

DSM-IV provides the category of BPD. In contrast to DSM-III-R, in brief reactive psychosis, a severe antecedent stressor is no longer mandatory. In DSM-IV, some psychotic disorders of brief duration may be coded as SFD if they fulfilled DSM-IV criteria for schizophrenia for 1 month (or less, if successfully treated) but remit before the time of 6 months. Some cases can be classified as delusional disorder (in DSM-IV, the time criterion for delusional disorder requires a duration of more than 1 month, compared with more than 3 months in ICD-10) or as psychotic disorder not otherwise classified.

By comparing ICD-10 and DSM-IV, it can be seen that while in ICD-10, acuteness of onset is considered to be the defining characteristic, in DSM-IV, duration of psychosis of less than 6 months is the distinguishing feature.

Diagnostic criteria

A. Presence of one (or more) of the following symptoms:

1. Delusions
2. Hallucinations

3. Disorganised speech (e.g. frequent derailment or incoherence)
4. Grossly disorganised or catatonic behaviour

Note: Do not include a symptom if it is a culturally sanctioned response

B. Duration of an episode of the disturbance is at least 1 day but less than 1 month, with eventual full return to premorbid level of functioning.
C. The disturbance is not attributable to depressive or bipolar disorder with psychotic features, schizoaffective disorder or schizophrenia and is not associated with the direct physiological effects of a substance (e.g. a drug of abuse, a medication) or another medical condition.

Specify if With Marked Stressor(s) (brief reactive psychosis): if symptoms occur in response to stressful events
Without Marked Stressor(s): if psychotic symptoms do not occur in response to stressful events
With Post-partum Onset: if onset is within 4 weeks post-partum

18 Concordance Between the ICD-10 Diagnosis of ATPD and the DSM-IV Diagnosis of Brief Psychotic Disorder–Cross-System Comparisons

As there were differences in the criteria for diagnosing ATPD and BPDs, it was important to understand how the two diagnoses relate to each other. Few studies were done to explore the concordance between the ICD-10 diagnosis of ATPD and the DSM-IV diagnosis of BPD.

In a Scandinavian study by Jørgensen et al. in 1997, it was found that ATPD does not conform to any specific category in DSM-IV: only one-third of cases in the study group fulfilled the criteria for BPD, 41 % those for SFD and 25 % unspecified psychotic disorder. Among ATPD subcategories, it was found that 'polymorphic psychotic disorder without schizophrenic symptoms' only partially overlaps with BPD, while 'schizophrenia-like psychotic disorder' has closer similarities to SFD. These findings were similar to the one reported by Heijden et al. in 2004. They reported that in their study group, less than half of patients with 'polymorphic psychotic disorder' met the criteria for BPD. However, a previous study by Pitta and Blay in 1997 reported an unusually high number of cases with a positive diagnosis for both disorders.

In a prospective and longitudinal study by Pillman et al. in 2002, a group of 42 patients fulfilling ICD-10 criteria of ATPD were selected. It was found that out of these, 61 $\pm$ 9 % fulfilled the DSM-IV criteria of BPD; 31 $\pm$ 0 % of SFD; 2 $\pm$ 4 % of delusional disorder; and 4 $\pm$ 8 % of psychotic disorder not otherwise specified. BPD showed significant concordance with the polymorphic subtype of ATPD, and DSM-IV SFD showed significant concordance with the schizophreniform subtype of ATPD. It was found that BPD patients had a significantly shorter duration of episode and more acute onset compared with those ATPD patients who did not meet the criteria of BPD (non-BPD). However, it was found that the BPD group and the non-BPD group of ATPD were remarkably similar in terms of socio-demographical factors (especially female preponderance), course and outcome, which was rather favourable for both groups. BPD showed considerable overlap with ATPD. In this study, it was also found that psychosocial stress was not the characteristic feature of BPD, thus supported the abandonment of the DSM-III-R concept of brief reactive psychosis in DSM-IV. It was concluded that DSM-IV BPD was a psychotic disorder with broad concordance with ATPD as defined by ICD-10 and the DSM-IV time criteria for BPD might be too narrow. It was found that there was a significant, but only moderate concordance between BPD and the polymorphic subtype of ATPD (F23.0) and between DSM-IV SFD and the schizophrenia-like subtype of ATPD (F23.2). The group of acute psychotic disorders with good prognosis extends beyond the borders of BPD and includes a subgroup of DSM-IV SFD.

19 Treatment

The patients of ATPD may require short-term hospitalisations for a comprehensive evaluation and safety.

Pharmacological treatment
In the short term, antipsychotic drugs are often most useful along with benzodiazepines.

Long-term use of medication is often not necessary and should be avoided. If maintenance medications are necessary, the diagnosis may need to be revised. Clearly, the newer antipsychotic agents have a better neurological side effect profile and would be preferred over the typical agents (Tasman et al. Tasman III edition).

In 2005, Ehlis et al. (2005) studied the beneficial effect of atypical antipsychotics on prefrontal brain function in acute psychotic disorders. They found that there were mild deficits in prefrontal response in the patients of acute psychosis. It was also reported that there was a highly significant positive correlation between the amount of atypical neuroleptic medication and the NoGo-anteriorization (NGA) during performance of the CPT (Continuous Performance Test, Rosvold et al. 1956), which was used as a measure of prefrontal brain function in this study. Since the NGA is assumed to be a neurophysiological correlate of prefrontal response control, this finding supported the notion of a beneficial influence of atypical neuroleptic drugs on prefrontal brain function.

In another study by Jabs et al. (Ehlis et al. 2005) in 2002, involving the preliminary functional imaging, an 'acute hyperfrontality' was found in some cases of cycloid psychoses. It was reported that acute hyperfrontality returned to normal in the course of the treatment.

Non-pharmacological treatment
Psychotherapy is necessary to help the person reintegrate the experience of psychosis and possibly the precipitating trauma. Individual, family and group

therapies are found to be useful in acute and transient psychosis. Gonzalez de Chavez in 2007 described that acute and transient psychoses could be considered as identity breakdowns with fragmentation of its structure, paranoid mechanism and cognitive regression. He emphasised that psychotherapies favour evolution of psychotic identity through disorder awareness and knowledge of aspects of patients that make them more vulnerable to psychotic experiences.

There are few data available regarding the treatment of acute and transient psychosis as a distinct entity. In the Marneros and Pillmann (2004) study of brief and acute psychoses, 95 % of patients received an antipsychotic, 21 % an antidepressant and 7 % lithium during the initial episode. Compared with patients with schizophrenia or bipolar schizoaffective disorder, a smaller proportion of ATPD patients were still taking psychotropic medications over the follow-up period, and the authors reported good levels of functioning in all patients who were no longer taking medication. NARP patients in a first-episode study from Iran (Alaghband-Rad et al. 2006b) were found to have received fewer months of antipsychotic medication than patients with other non-affective psychotic disorders, which likely reflect faster remission of these psychoses compared with other first-admission psychotic disorders. Similarly, a study by Perris (1974) found that patients with cycloid psychosis on continuous lithium treatment experienced fewer repeat episodes. General treatment recommendations for patients presenting with their first episode of psychosis, including psychotic disorders with acute onset, include a comprehensive assessment to evaluate comorbidities and rule out organic and substance-induced causes (Thomas et al. 2009). A typical antipsychotics, often at low initial doses, are recommended as the first line of medication treatment, with continuation of treatment for 1 year (Jabs et al. 2002). It is also recommended that there should be coordination between treating team, the patient's family and/or friends to help ensure treatment adherence and to educate them about the disorder (Thomas et al. 2009). There is also need for international treatment guidelines for acute episode of ATPD. Guidelines were given by Gaebel et al. (2005) but more research is required in this field. It is also important to have separate guidelines for recurrent category.

20 Mortality in ATPD

Little is known about mortality associated with acute transient psychoses. There are few reports on the increased mortality associated with conditions such as reactive psychosis currently incorporated under ATPD (Jørgensen and Mortensen 1990). In a Danish study by Castagnini and Bertelsen in 2011, it was found that the most unnatural deaths associated with ATPD were from suicide and most of them were within the first 2 years after the initial admission. The standardised mortality ratio for suicide/from unnatural causes was higher and varied by gender (11.1 for males vs. 9.1 for females). Besides this, it was 30.9 times than that expected, with an overall standardised mortality ratio of 2.9 for ATPD patients compared with the general population. There was also an increased risk of suicide/unnatural death in males with ageless than 40 years. It was also found that the standardised mortality ratio for and was particularly high for suicide (30.9). However, there are few studies with which to make meaningful comparisons. A similar trend was previously reported from earlier studies (Thomas et al. 2009) on mortality of reactive psychoses. It was reported that there was a significantly raised mortality risk in reactive psychosis, and suicide was the largest cause of premature death. From these studies, it can be concluded that ATPD is associated with excess mortality from both natural and unnatural causes, particularly from suicide in younger subjects.

However, there were few studies that did not support this result. Contradictory evidence was found in a study by Pillmann et al. in 2003. No suicide was reported in a series of patients with ATPD 5 years after the index episode, as opposed 2 cases with schizophrenia and 3 with bipolar schizoaffective disorder had died of suicide. In this study, it was also found that suicidal behaviour was linked to acute symptomatology, which is characterised typically by varied delusions, hallucinations, agitation and emotional turmoil shifting from day to day or even from hour to hour in otherwise well-adjusted subjects. It was also found that the rate of suicidal behaviour during the course of ATPD was 35.7 % and was comparable to the rate found in schizophrenia (40.5 %).

21 Conclusion

ICD-10 and DSM-IV incorporate the rich history of the concepts involved, but still leave many questions open to further research. Having two different diagnostic systems which classify these conditions very differently also hampers the research and limits the generalisation of the results. Therefore, there is need to harmonise these two diagnostic systems. To conclude, acute and transient psychoses remain a challenge for nosological considerations in the area of psychotic disorders. It brings into question the nosological boundaries within endogenous psychoses and the concept of psychotic continuum.

References

Ackerknecht, E.H. (1968). *A short history of psychiatry* (2nd rev. ed.). New York: Hafner.

Alaghband-Rad, J., Boroumand, M., Amini, H., et al. (2006a). Non-affective acute remitting psychosis: A preliminary report from Iran. *Acta Psychiatr Scandinavica, 113*(2), 96–101.

Alaghband-Rad, J., Boroumand, M., Amini, H., et al. (2006b). Non-affective acute remitting psychosis: A preliminary report from Iran. *Acta Psychiatrica Scandinavica, 113*, 96–101.

Albus, M., Strauss, A., & Stieglitz, R. D. (1990). Schizophrenia, schizotypal and delusional disorders (section F2): Results of the ICD-10 field trial. *Pharmacopsychiatry, 23*, 155–159.

Alexandre, J., Ribeiro, R., & Cardoso, G. (2010). Ethnic and clinical characteristics of a Portuguese psychiatric inpatient population. *Transcult Psychiatry, 47*(2), 314.

American Psychiatric Association. (2000). *Diagnostic and statistical manual of mental disorders* (Rev. 4th ed.). Washington, DC: American Psychiatric Association.

Amini, H., Alaghband-rad, J., Omid, A., et al. (2005). Diagnostic stability in patients with first episode psychosis. *Australasian Psychiatry, 13*, 388–392.

Arranz, B., San, L., Ramírez, N., et al. (2009). Clinical and serotonergic predictors of non-affective acute remitting psychosis in patients with a first-episode psychosis. *Acta Psychiatrica Scandinavica, 119*(1), 71–77.

Berrios, G. E., & Porter, R. (eds.) (1995). *A history of clinical psychiatry*. New York: New York University Press.

Castagnini, A. C., & Bertelsen, A. (2011). Mortality and causes of death of acute and transient psychotic disorders. *Social Psychiatry and Psychiatric Epidemiology, 46*, 1013–1017.

Castagnini, A., Bertelsen, A., & Berrios, G. E. (2008). Incidence and diagnostic stability of ICD-10 acute and transient psychotic disorders. *Comprehensive Psychiatry, 49*(3), 255–261.

Chang, W. C., Pang, S. L. K., Chung, D. W. S., et al. (2009). Five-year stability of ICD-10 diagnoses among Chinese patients presented with first-episode psychosis in Hong Kong. *Schizophrenia Research, 115*(23), 351–357.

Chaturvedi, S. K., & Sahu, R. N. (1986). Clinical and follow-up study of unspecified non-organic psychosis. *Indian Journal of Psychiatry, 28*, 73–77.

Chavan, B. S., & Kulhara, P. (1988). A clinical study of reactive psychosis. *Acta Psychiatrica Scandinavica, 78*, 712–715.

Collins, P. Y., Wig, N. N., Day, R., et al. (1996). Psychosocial and biological aspects of acute brief psychoses in three developing country sites. *Psychiatric Quarterly, 67*(3), 177–193.

Collins, P. Y., Varma, V. K., Wig, N. N., et al. (1999). Fever and acute brief psychosis in urban and rural settings in north India. *British Journal of Psychiatry, 174*(6), 520.

Cooper, J. E., Jablensky, A., Sartorius, N. (1990) WHO collaborative studies on acute psychosesusing the SCAAP schedule. In C. N. Stefanis, A. D. Rabavilas & C. R. Saldatos (Eds.), *Psychiatry: A world perspective* (pp. 185–192), vol. 1. Pub Elsevier.

Coryell, W., & Tsuang, M. T. (1982). DSM-III schizohreniform disorder: Comparison with schizophrenia and affective disorder. *Archives of General Psychiatry, 39*, 66–69.

Dahl, A. A. (1994). The validity of the Scandinavian concept of reactive psychoses. *Seishin Shinkeigaku Zasshi, 96*, 660–675.

Das, S. K., Malhotra, S., & Basu, D. (1999). Family study of acute and transient psychotic disorders: comparison with schizophrenia psychotic disorders: Precursors, epidemiology, course and outcome. *British Journal of Psychiatry, 185*, 452–459.

Das, S. K., Malhotra, S., Basu, D., et al. (2001). Testing the stress—vulnerability hypothesis in ICD–10–diagnosed acute and transient psychotic disorders. *Acta Psychiatr Scandinavica, 104*(1), 56–58.

Duncan, C. C., Morihisa, J. M., Fawcer, W. T., et al. (1987). P300 in schizophrenia: State or trait marker? *Psychopharmacology Bulletin, 23*, 497–501.

Ehlis, A. C., Zielasek, J., Martin, J., et al. (2005). Beneficial effect of atypical antipsychotics on prefrontal brain function in acute psychotic disorders. *European Archives of Psychiatry and Clinical Neurosciences, 255*, 299–307.

Faergeman, P. (1963). *Psychogenic psychoses: A description and follow-up of psychoses following psychological stress*. London: Butterworth.

Fekkes, D., & Pepplinkhuizen, L. (1997). Amino acid studies in transient acute polymorphic psychosis. *Amino Acids, 12*, 107–117.

Franzek, E., & Beckmann, H. (1998). Different genetic background of schizophrenia spectrum psychoses: A twin study. *American Journal of Psychiatry, 155*(1), 76.

Franzek, E., Becker, T., Hofmann, E., et al. (1996). Is computerized tomography ventricular abnormality related to cycloid psychosis? *Biological Psychiatry, 40*(12), 1255–1266.

Frasca, J., Kilpatrick, T. J., & Burns, R. J. (1993). Protracted form of encephalitis with good outcome. *Medical Journal of Australia, 158*, 629–630.

Gaebel, W., Weinmann, S., Sartorius, N., et al. (2005). Schizophrenia practice guidelines: International survey and comparison. *British Journal of Psychiatry, 187*(3), 248.

Gonzalez de Chavez, M. (2007). Psychotherapies in acute and transient psychoses. *Psilogos, 4*(1), 32–40.

Gupta, L. N., & Bhardwaj, P. (2000). Acute non-organic psychosis: Outcome after 10 yrs. *Indian J Psychiatry, 42*(4), 356–363.

Hatotani, N. (1996). The concept of 'atypical psychoses': Special reference to its development in Japan. *Psychiatry and Clinical Neurosciences, 50*, 1–10.

Heijden, F. M. M. A. V., Tuinier, S., Kahn, R. S., et al. (2004). Nonschizophrenic psychotic disorders: The case of cycloid psychoses. *Psychopathology, 37*, 161–167.

Hollender, M. H., & Hirsch, S. J. (1964). Hysterical psychosis. *American Journal of Psychiatry, 120*, 1066–1077.

Jabs, B. E., Pfuhlmann, B., Bartsch, A. J., et al. (2002). Cycloid psychoses—from clinical concepts to biological foundations. *Journal of Neural Transmission, 109*, 907–919.

Jäger, M. D. M., Hintermayr, M., Bottlender, R., et al. (2003). Course and outcome of first-admitted patients with acute and transient psychotic disorders (ICD-10: F23): Focus on relapses and social adjustment. *European Archives Psychiatry and Clinical Neuroscience, 253*, 209–215.

Jäger, M. D. M., Riedel, M., & Möller, H. J. (2007). Akute vorübergehende psychotische Störungen (ICD-10: F23). Empirische Befunde und Implikationen für die Therapie. *Nervenarzt, 78*, 749–752.

Jarvis, W. R., Wasserman, A. L., & Fodd, R. D. (1990). Acute psychosis in a patient with Epstein-Barr virus infection. *Journal of American Academy of Child and Adolescent Psychiatry, 29*, 468–469.

Jaspers, K. (1963). General psychopathology. In J. Hhoenig & M. W. Hamilton (Eds.), *Manchester University Press*. UK: Manchester.

Jaspers, K. (1965). *Allgemeine psychopathologie. Achte unveränderte auflage*. Berlin: Springer.

Jørgensen, P. (1995). Comparative outcome of first admission patients with delusional beliefs. *European Psychiatry, 10*, 276–281.

Jørgensen, P., & Mortensen, P. B. (1990). Reactive psychosis and mortality. *Acta Psychiatrica and Scandinavica, 81*, 277–279.

Jørgensen, P., Bennedsen, B., Christensen, J., et al. (1996). Acute and transient psychotic disorder: comorbidity with personality disorder. *Acta Psychiatr Scandinavica, 94*(6), 460–464.

Jørgensen, P., Bennedsen, B., Christensen, J., et al. (1997). Acute and transient psychotic disorder: A 1-year follow-up study. *Acta PsychiatrScandinavica, 96*(2), 150–154.

Kahlbaum, L. (1863). Die Gruppirung psychischer Krankheiten. Danzig.

Karlsson, H., Blomström, A., Wicks, S., et al. (2012). Maternal antibodies to dietary antigens and risk for nonaffective psychosis in offspring. *American Journal of Psychiatry, 169*, 625–632.

Kasanin, J. (1933). The acute schizoaffective psychoses. *American Journal of Psychiatry, 13*, 97–126.

Kendell, R.E., Rennie, D., Clarke, J.A., et al. (1981). The social and obstetric correlates of psychiatric admissions in puerperium. *Psychological Medicine, 11*, 341–350.

Kendler, K. S. (1980). The nosologic validity of paranoia (simple delusional disorder). *Archives of General Psychiatry, 37*, 699–706.

Kimura, S., Fujito, T. and Wakabayashi, T. (1980). A contribution to the course and prognosis of the atypical psychosis. *Folia Psychiatrica et Neurologica Japonica, 34*, 419–432.

Klein, R. F., Betts, R., Hom, R., et al. (1984). Acute psyshosis in a 45-year old man with bipolar disorder and primary Epstein-Barr virus infection: A case report. *General Hospital Psychiatry, 6*, 13–15.

Kleist, K. (1918). Schreckpsychosen. *Allgemeine Zeitschrift für Psychiatrie, 74*, 432–510.

Kleist, K. (1924). Über die gegenwärtigen Strömungen in der klinischen Psychiatrie. *Allgemeine Zeitschrift für Psychiatrie, 81*, 389–393.

Kleist, K. (1928). Über cycloide, paranoide und epileptoide Psychosen und über die Frage der Degenerationspsychosen. *Schweizer Archiv für Neurologie, Neurochirurgie und Psychiatrie, 23*, 3–37.

Kleist, K. (1929). Liber cykloide, paranoid and epileptoidepsychosen and iiber the question of Degeneratiouspsychosen Switzerland. *Arch NeurolPsychiatr, 23*, 3–37.

Kørner, A., Lopez, A. G., & Lauritzen, L. (2009). Acute and transient psychosis in old age and the subsequent risk of dementia: A nationwide register-based study. *Geriatrics and Gerontology International, 9*, 62–68.
Kumar, R. (1994). Postnatal mental illness. A transcultural perspective. *Social Psychiatry Psychiatric Epidemiology, 29*, 250–264.
Lange, W., Munk-Jørgensen, P., Bertelsen, A., et al. (2002). Comparison of psychiatric ICD-10 diagnoses in Denmark and Germany. *Psychopathology, 35*, 36–47.
Langfeldt, G. (1937). The diagnosis in schizophrenia and the factors influencing the course of disease. *ActaPsychiatrNeurol(s), 13*.
Langfeldt, G. (1939). *The schizophreniform states*. Kopenhagen: Munksgaard.
Langfeldt, G. (1969). Schizophrenia: Diagnosis and prognosis. *Behavioural Science, 14*, 173–182.
Langness, L. (1967). Hysterical psychoses: the cross-cultural evidence. *American Journal of Psychiatry, 124*, 143–152.
Lau, P. W. L., Cheng, J. G. Y., Chow, D. L. Y., et al. (2009). Acute psychiatric disorders in foreign domestic workers in Hong Kong: A pilot study. *International Journal of Social Psychiatry, 55*(6), 569.
Leonhard, K. (1961). Cycloid psychoses—endogenous psychoses which are neither schizophrenic nor manic-depressive. *Journal of Mental Sciences, 107*, 633–648.
Lindvall, M., Axelsson, R., & Ohman, R. (1993). Incidence of cycloid psychosis. A clinical study of first-admission psychotic patients. *European Archives Psychiatry Clinical and Neurosciences, 242*(4), 197–202.
Littlewood, R., & Lipsedge, M. (1981). Acute psychotic reactions in Caribbean-born patients. *Psychological Medicine, 11*(02), 303–318.
Magnan, V. (1893). *Leçons cliniques sur les maladies mentales* (2nd ed.). Paris: Battaille.
Malhotra, S., & Malhotra, S. (2001). Acute and transient psychosis: Conceptual understanding and current status. In R. S. Murthy (Ed.), *Mental Health in India 1950–2000* (pp. 17–41). Bangalore: PAMH.
Malhotra, S., Varma, V. K., Misra, A. K., et al. (1998). Onset of acute psychotic states in India: a study of sociodemographic, seasonal and biological factors. *Acta Psychiatr Scandinavica, 97*(2), 125–131.
Malhotra, S., Gupta, N., & Gill, S. (2005). *Recurrence in acute and transient psychoses: 13th world congress of psychiatry, September 2005*. pp. 10–15. Cairo: Egypt.
Mallett, B. L., & Gold, S. (1964). A pseudo-schizophrenic hysterical syndrome. *British Journal of Medical Psychology. 37*, 59–70.
Marneros, A., & Pillman, F. (2002). Acute and transient psychotic disorders. *Psychiatry, 13*, 276–286.
Marneros, A., & Pillmann, F. (2004). *Acute and transient psychoses*. Cambridge: Cambridge University Press.
Marneros, A., Pillmann, F., Haring, A., et al. (2003a). Features of acute and transient psychotic disorders. *European Archives Psychiatry Clinical and Neurosciences, 253*(4), 167–174.
Marneros, A., Pillmann, F., Haring, A., Balzuweit, S., & Bloink, R. (2003b). What is schizophrenic in acute and transient psychotic disorder? *Schizophrenia Bulletin, 29*, 311–323.
Marneros, A. (2006). Beyond the Kraepelinian dichotomy: Acute and transient psychotic disorders and the necessity for clinical differentiation. *British Journal of Psychiatry, 189*, 1– 2.
Martin, P. A. (1971). Dynamic considerations in the hysterical psychosis. *American Journal of Psychiatry, 128*, 101–104.
Mitsuda, H. (1965). The concept of atypical psychoses from aspects of clinical genetics. *Acta Psychiatr Scandinavica, 41*, 372.
Mojtabai, R., Varma, V. K., & Susser, E. (2000). Duration of remitting psychoses with acute onset: Implications for ICD-10. *British Journal of Psychiatry, 176*, 576–580.
Mojtabai, R., Susser, E. S., & Bromet, E. J. (2003). Clinical characteristics, 4-year course, and DSM-IV classification of patients with nonaffective acute remitting psychosis. *American Journal of Psychiatry, 160*(12), 2108–2115.

Möller, H. J., Jäger, M., Riedel, M., et al. (2010). The Munich 15-year follow-up study (MUFUSSAD) on first hospitalized patients with schizophrenic or affective disorders: Comparison of psychopathological and psychosocial course and outcome and prediction of chronicity. *European Archives of Psychiatry and Clinical Neurosciences, 260*, 367–384.

Myin-Germeys, I., van Os, J., & Schwartz, J. E. (2001). Emotional reactivity to daily life stress in psychosis. *Archives of General Psychiatry, 58*, 1137–1144.

Okasha, A., Dawla, A. S., Khalil, A. H., et al. (1993). Presentation of acute psychosis in an Egyptian sample: A transcultural comparison. *Comprehensive Psychiatry, 34*, 4–9.

Pepplinkhuizen, L., van der Heijden, F. M. M. A., Tuinier, S., et al. (2003). The acute transient polymorphic psychosis: A biochemical subtype of the cycloid psychosis. *Acta Neuropsychiatrica, 15*, 38–43.

Perris, C. (1974). A study of cycloid psychoses. *Acta Psychiatr Scandinavica, 50*(s253), 7–79.

Pfefferbaum, A., Ford, J. M., White, P. M., et al. (1989). P300 in schizophrenia is affected by stimulus modality, response requirements, medication status and negative symptoms. *Archives of General Psychiatry, 46*, 1035–1044.

Pfuhlmann, B., Stöber, G., Franzek, E., et al. (1998). Cycloid psychoses predominate in severe postpartum psychiatric disorders. *Journal of Affective Disorders, 50*(2–3), 125–134.

Pichot, P. (1986). The concept of 'bouffée délirante' with special reference to the scandinavian concept of reactive psychosis. *Psychopathology, 19*, 35–43.

Pillmann, F., & Marneros, A. (2005). Longitudinal follow-up in acute and transient psychotic disorders and schizophrenia. *British Journal of Psychiatry, 187*, 286–287.

Pillmann, F., Haring, A., Balzuweit, S., et al. (2002). The concordance of ICD-10 acute and transient psychosisand DSM-IV brief psychotic disorder. *Psychological Medicine, 32*(3), 525–533.

Pillmann, F., Balzuweit, S., Haring, A., et al. (2003). Suicidal behavior in acute and transient psychotic disorders. *Psychiatry Research, 117*, 199–209.

Pitta, J. C., & Blay, S. L. (1997). Psychogenic (reactive) and hysterical psychoses: A cross-system reliability study. *Acta Psychiatrica Scandinavica, 95*, 112–118.

Pull, C. B., Pull, M. C., & Pichot, P. (1984). Des critères empiriques français pour les psychoses. I. Position du problème et méthodologie. *Encéphale, 10*, 119–123.

Pull, C. B., Pull, M. C., & Pichot, P. (1987). Des critères empiriques français pour les psychoses. II. Consensus des psychiatres français et définitions provisoires. *Encéphale, 13*, 53–57.

Robins, E., & Guze, S. B. (1970). Establishment of diagnostic validity in psychiatric illness: Its application to schizophrenia. *American Journal of Psychiatry, 126*, 107–111.

Rosvold, H., Mirsky, A., Sarason, I., et al. (1956). A continuous-performance test of brain damage continuous-performance test of brain damage. *Journal of Consulting Psychology, 20*, 343–352.

Roth, M., & McClelland, H. (1979). The relationship of 'nuclear' and 'atypical' psychoses: Some proposals for a classification of disorders in the borderlands of schizophrenia. *Psychiatria Clinical, 12*, 23–54.

Rozario, A. (1999). Acute & Transient psychosis: A follow-up study. Unpublished MD Thesis submitted to Postgraduate Institute of Medical Education and Research, Chandigarh, India

Sajith, S. G., Chandrasekaran, R., Sadanandan Unni, K. E., et al. (2002). Acute polymorphic psychotic disorder: Diagnostic stability over 3 years. *Acta Psychiatr Scandinavica, 105*, 104–109.

Sartorius, N., Jablensky, A., Korten, A., et al. (1986). Early manifestations and first contact incidence of incidence of Schizophrenia in different cultures. A preliminary report on the initial evaluation phase of the WHO collaborative study on determinants of outcome of severe mental disorders. *Psychological Medicine, 16*, 909–928.

Shorter, E. (1997). *A history of psychiatry: From the era of the asylum to the age of Prozac*. New York: Wiley.

Shriqui, C. L., & Mileltte, P. C. (1992). You drive me carzy: A case report of acute psychosis and neurocysticerosis. *Canadian Journal of Psychiatry, 37*, 121–124.

Siefert, E. (1907). *Über die geistesstörungen der strafhaft*. Halle: Marhold.

Singh, S. P., Burns, T., Amin, S., et al. (2004). Acute and transient psychotic disorders: Precursors, epidemiology, course and outcome. *British Journal of Psychiatry, 185*, 452–459.

Srikanth, S., Ravi, V., Poornima, K., et al. (1994). Viral antibodies in recent onset, non-organic psychoses, correspondence with sympathetic severity. *Biological Psychiatry, 36*, 512–517.

Stephens, J. H., Shaffer, J. W., & Carpenter, W. T, Jr. (1982). Reactive psychoses. *Journal of Nervous and Mental Disease, 170*, 657–663.

Strik, W. K., Dierkst, Franzck E., et al. (1994). P300 asymmetries in schizophrenia revisited with reference-independent methods. *Psychiatry Research: Neuroimaging, 55*, 153–166.

Strik, W. K., Fallgatter, A. J., Stoeber, G., et al. (1997). Specific P300 features in patients with cycloid psychosis. *Acta Psychiatrica Scandinavica, 95*, 67–72.

Suda, K., Hayashi, N., & Hiraga, M. (2005). Predicting features of later development of schizophrenia among patients with acute and transient psychotic disorder. *Psychiatry and Clinical Neurosciences, 59*(2), 146–150.

Susser, E., & Wanderling, J. (1994). Epidemiology of nonaffective acute remitting psychosis vs schizophrenia: Sex and sociocultural setting. *Archives of General Psychiatry, 51*(4), 294–301.

Susser, E., Fennig, S., Jandorf, L., et al. (1995a). Epidemiology, diagnosis, and course of brief psychoses. *American Journal of Psychiatry, 152*, 1743–1748.

Susser, E., Varma, V. K., Malhotra, S., et al. (1995b). Delineation of acute and transient psychotic disorders in a developing country setting. *British Journal of Psychiatry, 167*, 216–219.

Susser, E., Finnerty, M. T., & Sohler, N. (1996). Acute psychoses: A proposed diagnosis for ICD-11 and DSM-V. *Psychiatric Quarterly, 67*(3), 165–176.

Susser, E., Varma, V. K., Mattoo, S. K., et al. (1998). Long-term course of acute brief psychosis in a developing country setting. *British Journal of Psychiatry, 173*, 226–230.

Thangadurai, P., Gopalakrishnan, R., Kurian, S., et al. (2006). Diagnostic stability and status of acute and transient psychotic disorders. *British Journal Psychiatry, 188*, 293.

Thomas, P., Alptekin, K., Gheorghe, M., et al. (2009). Management of patients presenting with acutepsychotic episodes of schizophrenia. *CNS Drugs, 23*(3), 193–212.

Valentin M, Ck Ey H, Bernard P, Brisset C (1886) Manuel *de Psychiatrie* (2nd ed.) (p. 245). Masson: Paris; 1963.

Varma, V. K., Malhotra, S., & Jiloha, R. C. (1992). Acute non-organic psychotic states in India: Symptomatology. *Indian Journal of Psychiatry, 34*, 89–101.

Varma, V. K., Malhotra, S., Yoo, E. S., et al. (1996). Course and outcome of acute non-organic psychotic states in India. *Psychiatric Quarterly, 67*, 195–207.

Vázquez-Barquero, J. L., Cuesta, M. J., Herrera Castanedo, S., et al. (1999). Cantabria first-episode schizophrenia study. *British Journal of Psychiatry, 174*, 141–149.

Warketin, S., Nilsson, A., Karlson, S., et al. (1992). Cycloid psychosis: Regional cerebral blood flow correlates of a psychotic episode. *Acta Psychiatrica Scandinavica, 85*, 23–29.

Wernicke, C. (1894). *Floor plan of psychiatry in clinical lectures*. Leipzig: Thieme.

Wernicke, C. (1900). *Grundriss der Psychiatrie in klinischen Vorlesungen*. Leipzig: Thieme.

Wieck, A., Kumar, R., Hirsta, D., et al. (1991). Increased sensitivity of dopamine receptorsand recurrence of affective psychoses after childbirth. *British Medical Journal, 303*, 613–616.

Wilmanns, K. (1908). *Über gefängnispsychosen*. Halle: Marhold.

Wimmer A. (1916). Psykogenesindssygdomsformer (Psychogenic form of mental disorders). In *St. Hans Hospital, 1816–1916* (pp. 82–216). Jubilee Publication: Gad, Copenhagen.

Wise, T. N., Lebuffe, F. P., & Granger, S. T. (1977). Meningo-encephalitis presenting as an acute paranoid psychosis. *International Journal of Psychiatry, 8*, 405–414.

World Health Organisation. (1973). *Report of the international pilot study of schizophrenia*. Geneva: WHO.

World Health Organisation. (1992). *The ICD-10 classification of mental and behavioural disorders*. Geneva: World Health Organisation.

Chapter 9
Schizophrenia: Indian Research: I-Epidemiology, Clinical Features Neurobiology and Psychosocial Aspects

Parmanand Kulhara, Sandeep Grover and Natasha Kate

1 Introduction

Schizophrenia as a disorder has fascinated many researchers in India. It is possibly the most researched psychiatric disorder in the Indian context. During the last four or five decades, large numbers of studies have evaluated various aspects of schizophrenia. It is suggested that research on schizophrenia from India far exceeds that done in any developing country from Asia and Africa (Wig 2010). This chapter provides an overview of the research on schizophrenia emerging from India.

2 Epidemiology

In the 1960s and the 1970s, many studies from different parts of the country assessed the prevalence and incidence of schizophrenia (Dube 1979; Elanagar et al. 1971; Issac and Kapur 1980; Nandi et al. 1975; Sethi et al. 1967, 1972, 1974; Surya et al. 1964; Thacore and Gupta 1975; Verghese et al. 1973). These studies have evaluated 1,393–29,648 subjects from the community and reported prevalence rate of schizophrenia to vary from 1.1 to 4.3 per 1,000. Very few studies

---

P. Kulhara, Consultant Psychiatrist; S. Grover, Assistant Professor; N. Kate, Formerly Senior Resident

P. Kulhara (✉)
Fortis Healthcare, Chandigarh, India
e-mail: param_kulhara@yahoo.co.in

P. Kulhara · S. Grover · N. Kate
Department of Psychiatry, Postgraduate Institute of Medical Education and Research (PGIMER), Chandigarh, India

S. Malhotra and S. Chakrabarti (eds.), *Developments in Psychiatry in India*,
DOI 10.1007/978-81-322-1674-2_9

have assessed the incidence rate of schizophrenia. A study from the rural area reported the incidence rate to be 4.2/10,000 population (Sartorius et al. 1986).

A recent World Health Survey (WHS) also covered six states (Assam, Karnataka, Maharashtra, Rajasthan, Uttar Pradesh and West Bengal) in India and provided data about the epidemiology of psychosis in India. Health status was assessed from individual questionnaires administered to 9,994 adult population in ages of 18 and above. This study showed that 0.7–3.7 % of the population was diagnosed with psychosis, but of these, only 36.2–85.2 % received treatment. Higher proportions of patients who received treatment were from the urban areas and from higher income groups (World Health Survey 2003).

3 Clinical Features

Communication and linguistic skills: Some of the studies have focused on communication pattern, linguistic competence and thought disorder, reporting disturbances in communication in the form of inhibition of speech (Murthy 1965) and perseveration, circumstantiality and irrelevancy in speech (Singh 1971). Mazumdar et al. (1988) assessed thought, language and communication disorders and observed that positive and negative thought disorders occurred in equal proportion in patients with positive and negative schizophrenia. Varma et al. (1973) studied concretization of thinking and found that compared to normal controls and subjects with neurosis, patients with schizophrenia had low abstract ability. Abraham et al. (1979) used the repertory grid technique for the assessment of schizophrenic thinking and were able to discriminate patients with schizophrenia from those with neurosis and healthy controls based on this. Giridhar et al. (1992) found a higher linguistic competence in patients with positive schizophrenia, compared to the other groups, and also reported that high linguistic competence was an indicator of poor prognosis in positive schizophrenia and of a better prognosis in negative schizophrenia.

Hallucinations: Studies have also focused on understanding the phenomenology of hallucinations in schizophrenia. Ramanathan (1983) studied auditory hallucinations in patients with schizophrenia and reported that these were more real than unreal for the patients. Other studies have shown that neuroticism scores are positively related to the anxiety prior to the 'voices', anticipation of the voice and interference of activities of the patient by the voice (Ramanathan 1986). Chatterjee and Thakur (1976) found that the Muller-Lyer illusion could be used to distinguish patients with schizophrenia from healthy controls, but not from patients with neurosis. A study by Singh et al. (2003) from PGIMER, Chandigarh studied the phenomenology of hallucinations using factor analysis and identified two factors, i.e., 'reality of hallucinatory perception' and 'immersion in hallucinations'. Thomas et al. (2007) compared the prevalence and correlates of hallucinations in Indians with Americans and found differences in the prevalence of hallucinations in different modalities in the Indian and US samples, though the rank order of frequency was similar.

Delusions: Gupta (1979) reported that different types of delusions occurred in different types of families. A study from NIMHANS evaluated the content of delusions in patients with schizophrenia and affective disorder. The authors reported that the content of delusions remained similar during different episodes in both the disorders. Kulhara et al. (1986a) studied the phenomenology of delusions in 112 patients with schizophrenia using the present state examination (PSE) and found that the delusions of persecution were more common in males and those above the age of 30 years. Educated patients had more delusions of reference, delusional misinterpretation and delusions of thoughts being read. Also, systematization was seen more in younger patients, while married patients had more delusions of reference. Another study which evaluated delusions reported that the delusional content is more consistent in Hindus, those who were married, and those from a rural background in the group with schizophrenia (Sinha and Chaturvedi 1990).

Descriptive studies on subtypes and distinction from other psychotic disorders: Some of the studies have described the clinical picture of different subtypes of schizophrenia. Varma et al. (1977) provided detailed clinical descriptions of 13 cases of 'pseudoneurotic schizophrenia'. Singh and Kulhara (1991) presented four cases of 'simple schizophrenia' and argued in favour of retention of this category. On the basis of clinical criteria, family history, treatment response and follow-up data, a study concluded that schizoaffective schizophrenia was closer to primary affective disorders rather than being considered as a subtype of schizophrenia (Singh and Sachdava 1982). As acute and transient psychosis became a distinct category in ICD-10, Janakiramaiah et al. (1992) successfully used logistic discriminant function analysis to classify patients with schizophrenia or acute psychosis.

Typology of schizophrenia: Many studies have tried to characterize the typology of positive and negative schizophrenia in the Indian context. Kulhara et al. (1986) examined the concept of positive and negative subtyping using principal components analysis and concluded that their data supported the positive and negative symptom complexes. Also, Kota and Kulhara (1988) used a cross-sectional phenomenological approach in 40 patients with schizophrenia and found that on variables such as age, duration of illness and premorbid adjustment, significant differences emerged between positive and negative subtypes. A longitudinal study (Kulhara and Chandiramani 1990) evaluated the stability of positive and negative subtypes of schizophrenia. It was seen that after a follow-up duration of 18–30 months, there was significant reduction in positive symptom scores and the number of patients in the positive subtype of schizophrenia. Further, the mixed subtype of schizophrenia increased in number and at follow-up, and there were significantly more patients with mixed subtypes who did not meet criteria for either the positive or negative subtype, i.e., who had little of either type of symptomatology. However, the number of patients categorized as having negative subtype, as well as negative symptom scores, did not change appreciably over the follow-up period. On the basis of their findings, the authors concluded that compared to positive symptoms, negative symptoms are more stable over a period of time. Borde et al. (1992) reported that negative symptoms and syndromes were more stable over time as compared to positive symptoms, and both positive and negative subtypes were stable. A study from Chennai (Eaton et al. 1995) evaluated the structure and temporal course of the symptoms of schizophrenia. Patients were assessed each month for 10 years following the first hospitalization. Factor analyses revealed positive and negative factors with a slight tendency to merge over time. The prevalence of positive and negative symptoms declined in the year following first hospitalization and was stable thereafter. Positive and negative symptoms in 1 month were highly predictive of the same type of symptoms in the next month. On the basis of this, the authors concluded that positive and negative symptom clusters are independent, both cross-sectionally and longitudinally. Arora et al. (1997) grouped symptoms and signs of schizophrenia by evaluating the patients on the scale for the assessment of positive symptoms (SAPS), the scale for the assessment of negative symptoms (SANS) and the comprehensive psychopathological rating scale (CPRS). However, their analysis did not lead to replication of the positive–negative dichotomy. A study by Tirupati et al. (2006) evaluated psychopathology by using the positive and negative syndrome scale (PANSS), in patients with schizophrenia living in the community never treated with antipsychotic medications. The authors observed that positive symptoms were more frequent than negative symptoms. Factor analysis unfolded a five-factor structure, namely negative, positive, anxiety-depression, motor and excitement. The factor structure resembled that of treated patients reported in most studies except for the identification of a motor symptom cluster. One study compared the onset and course of previously untreated first-episode psychosis in Canada and India (Iyer et al. 2010). Patients with first-episode non-affective psychosis were evaluated for demographic variables, duration of untreated psychosis (DUP), baseline diagnosis, positive, negative and general psychopathology symptoms and overall functioning at baseline and 1 year. The authors reported significant improvement in symptoms and functioning over the 1-year course of treatment. Evaluation of time-by-site interactions showed significant difference between the centres in negative symptoms, with patients in India showing greater improvement over time than their Canadian counterparts. The time-by-site interactions were not significant for positive symptoms and general psychopathology. This relationship of negative symptoms and time-site interaction persisted even after controlling for demographic variables such as age, gender and marital status. On the basis of this, the authors concluded that there is a higher rate of improvement at 1 year in negative symptoms and functioning in patients from India, when compared those receiving similar treatment in Canada. A recent study carried out factor analysis of PANSS ratings done within 1 week of admission and extracted five factors, namely negative, autistic, activation, positive and depression. Negative factors explained the maximum percentage of variance (Kumar and Khess 2012).

Many studies have evaluated the usefulness of different diagnostic systems and rating scales. In a cross-sectional study, Kulhara et al. (1986) evaluated the usefulness, comprehensiveness and concordance between the CATEGO, research diagnostic criteria (RDC), DSM-III criteria, Feighner's criteria, Schneider's first-rank symptoms (FRS) and the ICD-9 diagnosis of schizophrenia. It was found that all the diagnostic systems had good agreement with the ICD-9 diagnosis of schizophrenia. However, the rate of concordance among the different systems varied. In another study, Kulhara et al. (1989a) examined the effect of different diagnostic systems and sociodemographic variables on the outcome of schizophrenia and reported that the DSM-III diagnosis of schizophrenia, duration of illness and the PSE syndrome of non-specific psychosis were important predictors of outcome. The CATEGO and the RDC diagnosis of schizophrenia and the Schneiderian FRS were found to be poor predictors of outcome. Kulhara et al. (1987) also examined the usefulness psychiatric rating scale (BPRS) in positive and negative subtyping of sch Significant differences emerged between the two subtypes on items suc tional withdrawal, guilt feelings, tension, hallucinatory behaviour, motor re blunted affect and excitement. Kota et al. (1986) evaluated the inter-rater for the SANS in schizophrenia and found it to be significant for all items of t

Movement disorders in schizophrenia: A series of studies from Chen evaluated extrapyramidal symptoms in patients with schizophrenia and th tives. One study evaluated the prevalence of abnormal movements in neve cated Indian patients with schizophrenia and reported that dyskinesia were 15 % of normal subjects, 15 % of first-degree blood relatives of younger p with schizophrenia, 38 % of the never-medicated patients and 41 % of med patients. The authors concluded that dyskinesia in elderly patients with sc phrenia was an integral part of the illness and was not associated with ant chotic medications (McCreadie et al. 1996).

One study evaluated the prevalence of spontaneous dyskinesia and Parkinsor in never-medicated, chronically ill patients with schizophrenia at baseline at 18 months of follow-up. Twenty-four per cent of the patients had dyskin at both the assessments, 33 % had the same on one of the assessments and 43 did not have dyskinesia at any time; 35 % had Parkinsonism on at least one occ sion (McCreadie et al. 2002). Another study evaluated the prevalence of spontan ous dyskinesia in first-degree relatives of chronically ill never-treated people wit schizophrenia and reported that 14 % of the relatives had dyskinetic movements i at least one body area, and 3 % had Parkinsonism (McCreadie et al. 2003).

Cenesthesias: According to one study, depersonalization, motor weakness, abnormal pain, numbness and stiffness were the most commonly endorsed cenesthesias. These correlated positively with disturbances of body concept and were present at onset in 40 % of subjects and changed form in 76 % of subjects (Rajender et al. 2009).

Relapse: Studies, which have evaluated the predictors of relapse in schizophrenia, report that regularity of follow-up, presence of affective symptoms, self-neglect and lack of social contacts are associated with relapses (Rajkumar and Thara 1989). Relapse was significantly associated with unemployment, number of psychotic episodes, side effects of medication and life events score (Chabungbam et al. 2007). In a study involving retrospective assessment of life events over a period of 1 year, Das et al. (1997) reported that those who experienced relapses of their illness had experienced a significantly greater number of life events and also had a significantly higher stress score than the 'stable' group. A study, which evaluated the relationship of life events, marriage and social support, concluded that marriage led to experiencing more stress, but there are other psychosocial variables mitigating the same and preventing relapse (Kulhara et al. 1998).

Distinction of depressive and negative symptoms: Studies have also tried to distinguish negative symptoms in schizophrenia from depression. A study revealed that the global ratings for affective flattening, alogia, avolition and inattention were significantly higher in patients with schizophrenia compared to depression, whereas anhedonia–asociality was equally prevalent in patients with schizophrenia and

…haturvedi et al. 1985). Another study compared subjects with schizo-…epression and reported that compared to patients with schizophrenia, …uicide attempts was higher in depressed patients (Gupta et al. 1992).

…*in schizophrenia*: The Indian Council of Medical Research (ICMR) …ollaborative study on course and outcome of schizophrenia reported …e mood was not related to course and outcome of schizophrenia at …of follow-up. At intake, depressed mood was noted in 22.3 % sub-…dropped to 13 % at 2 years of follow-up (ICMR 1988). A prospec-…m Bangalore reported that only 0.5 % of patients with schizophrenia …-psychotic depression (PPD) (Das and Kapur 1980). In another pro-…ly, newly diagnosed patients with schizophrenia were followed for … The findings of this study indicated that depression was either intrin-…phrenia or could be due to neuroleptics. Moreover, this study showed …ortion of patients with depression was high in those who responded to …neuroleptic treatment (Raju 1986). A study, which compared the PSE …f depression in patients with first-episode Feighner's schizophrenia, …ne PSE syndrome of depression was present in 45 % of patients who …se, compared to 19 % of the patients who did not relapse (Rajkumar …1989). A study from Chandigarh, which primarily studied the rela-…tween depressive and negative symptoms, reported depressed mood …tients with schizophrenia (Kulhara et al. 1989). However, none of the …es, rated depressive symptoms on scales used primarily for the assess-…pression. Studies, which have evaluated the role of gender in depres-…reported that at intake simple depression was more common in males, …ıp depressive delusions or hallucinations were also more frequent …nd depressive features at intake and follow-up affected the outcome …However, at 10-year follow-up, no gender differences were noted, and …n was almost non-existent (Thara and Rajkumar 1992; Thara and Joseph …nother prospective longitudinal study evaluated patients with a diagnosis …zophrenia as per DSM-IIIR, with at least 5 years of hospitalization, at the …ıe and after 9 months. This study found that positive and negative subtypes of …ophrenia were stable, whereas depression as assessed on the PANSS was not …d to be stable (Borde et al. 1992). In a cross-sectional study from Chandigarh, …patients with stable chronic schizophrenia as per DSM-III R were rated on the …NS, the SAPS and the CPRS. Factor analysis segregated positive and negative …ymptoms into more than two dimensions. The CPRS led to a factor loading high …on depressive/asthenic items. The authors concluded that depressive symptoms were a salient feature in course of schizophrenia (Arora et al. 1997). Some of the studies have used scales specifically to rate depression. A study from Chandigarh compared two groups of 30 subjects each of PPD and non-PPD in DSM-III-R schizophrenia in remission. Patients with PPD had a longer duration of psychosis, more frequent hospitalizations and more sadness and anxiety-somatisation during florid illness phase. Severity of depression assessed on the Hamilton depression rating scale (HDRS) correlated positively with age of onset, age of patient, number of stressful life events and negatively with social support (Chintalapudi et al. 1993).

attending a drug de-addiction and treatment centre for 13 year period and found that only 1.4 % were diagnosed to have substance-independent psychotic illness, of which only half of the patients had the diagnosis of schizophrenia. The authors ascribed the lower rates to the fact that established cases of psychosis are much more likely to attend (or be referred to) the general psychiatry section rather than a specialized de-addiction centre (Aggarwal et al. 2012).

A study from PGIMER, Chandigarh, compared clinical picture of cannabis psychosis with schizophrenia and reported that compared to patients with schizophrenia, cannabis psychosis is short-lasting, presents with a predominantly polymorphic clinical picture, with more odd and bizarre behaviour, violence and panic but reactive and congruent affect, less evidence of formal thought disorder, and is associated with rapid and complete recovery (Basu et al. 1999). The demographic and clinical correlates of substance abuse in schizophrenia were assessed by Aich et al. (2004). People using substance were predominantly represented by the positive syndrome and non-abusers by the negative syndrome. The same group of authors (Aich et al. 2005) found that psychopathology remitted much faster in the group abusing substances, but after discharge, these patients tended to return back to the preadmission state.

Another study from PGIMER, Chandigarh examined the relationship of the course of substance abuse and schizophrenia symptomatology in patients with 'dual-diagnosis' of substance abuse and schizophrenia and reported that in five out of twenty-two patients, onset of schizophrenia preceded the onset of substance use. In seven out of twenty-two subjects, there was clear temporal relationship between exacerbation of schizophrenia and increase in substance abuse in the preceding 2–12 months. In none of the subjects, decrease in substance use led to a decrease or increase in schizophrenic symptoms (Goswami et al. 2003). A study from Ranchi compared patients with substance dependence with and without psychosis and showed that patients with substance dependence without psychosis attributed both maintenance and relapse to external factors such as nature of work, social milieu or peer pressure, while the 'dual-diagnosis' group attributed them to internal factors such as enhancement of positive mood and alleviation of withdrawal effects (Saddichha et al. 2010).

Srinivasan and Thara (2002) studied the relationship of nicotine use and schizophrenia in urban male patients and found 38 % were current smokers, which was significantly more than in other psychiatric patients studied (major affective disorders and non-psychotic disorders), but not medically ill controls, and was not higher than the rates for the general male population in India.

5 Neurobiology of Schizophrenia

Since the beginning, there have been efforts to study the neurobiology of schizophrenia. However, most of the data have come in last 10–15 years.

Neurochemistry: Various studies have reported biological markers and diagnostic tests in schizophrenia. Kondaiah et al. (1981) found that plasma creatine phosphokinase (CPK) levels were higher in patients with schizophrenia, suggesting diagnostic value of CPK. Ghosh et al. (1981) found that patients with schizophrenia excreted greater amount of vanilmandelic acid (VMA) and lower amounts of steroid fractions as compared to controls. Significantly lower levels of Cerebrospinal fluid (CSF) 5-hydroxy indole acetic acid (5-HIAA) were found in patients as compared to controls by Pandey et al. (1987). Tiwari et al. (1984) found increased levels of serum and cerebrospinal fluid immunoglobulins; whereas Rao et al. (1985) observed no significant differences in immunoglobulin levels between patients with schizophrenia (paranoid and non-paranoid) and normal controls. Platelet monoamine oxidase activity was studied in patients with chronic schizophrenia, and no differences were documented between the patients and normal subjects (Gupta et al. 1985). Serum prolactin level was also studied in treatment-naive and medicated patients, and no differences were found between unmedicated patients and control subjects, refuting the hypothesis that there is a generalized hyper-dopaminergic state in schizophrenia (Kuruvilla et al. 1986). Chatterjee (1988) studied dopamine-related hormones–prolactin, growth hormone and luteinizing hormone in 84 patients with acute schizophrenia, but found that a simple theory of dopamine overactivity was not supported. Radioisotopic techniques were employed to measure platelet monoamine oxidase activity by Sharma et al. (1991), and no differences were found between subjects with schizophrenia, mania and normal subjects. However, the same group also found that the enzyme activity was significantly lower in paranoid schizophrenia, compared to the other groups. Also, significant negative correlations between enzyme activity and severity and duration of illness were found (Sharma et al. 1990). Pradhan et al. (1992) studied plasma homovanillic acid levels in patients with schizophreniform disorder, patients with schizophrenia on medications and patients with schizophrenia off medications. A bimodal distribution of plasma homovanillic acid was seen in schizophreniform disorder, indicating plasticity of the dopaminergic system to neuroleptics. Similarly, concentrations of homovanillic acid and gonadal hormones were studied by Gong et al. (1993). The results suggested that change of gonadal hormones may be related to the pathogenesis of schizophrenia. Kurup et al. (1999) studied serum digoxin levels in 25 patients to support the hypothesis that hypothalamic digoxin dysfunction occurs in schizophrenia. Anand et al. (2002) measured cerebrospinal fluid levels of dopamine, serotonin and their metabolites and attempted to elucidate their relation to various psychopathological dimensions. Serum prolactin levels, when measured in drug-naive patients, were raised, but did not show any relation to severity of psychopathology or prognosis (Shrivastava and Tamhane 2000).

Neuroimaging: In one of the earliest studies, Jayaswal et al. (1987) examined structural changes in brain using computed axial tomography scans (CAT scans) and found that the size of lateral ventricles expressed as the ventricular-brain ratio, and the width of the third ventricle and the sylvian fissure were significantly greater in patients with schizophrenia. Siddharatha et al. (1997) performed CAT scans in 50 patients with schizophrenia and found abnormalities compared to control subjects. Lal et al. (1998) studied neurological soft signs, cognitive dysfunction and ventricular-brain ratio in schizophrenia patients. Minimum of one neurological soft sign was present in all the patients. The positive group had higher memory and IQ scores and lower Bender-Gestalt Test (BGT) scores than the negative group. Negative correlation was seen for memory and BGT scores with ventricular-brain ratio (VBR), and the. soft signs showed positive correlation in the positive subtype only. Raju et al. (2001) carried out magnetic resonance imaging in patients with schizophrenia to measure prefrontal lobe volumes in patients with and without frontal dysfunction, as measured by the Lubria-Nebraska Neuropsychological Battery. They reported that patients with frontal dysfunction had minor frontal structural deficits. Padmavati (2001) studied differences in cerebral morphology in three groups: untreated patients with schizophrenia with dyskinesia, without dyskinesia and normal subjects.

Over the years, schizophrenia has been understood as a neurodevelopmental disorder. Most of the research on neuroimaging from India also suggests this. The National Institute of Mental Health and Neurosciences (NIMHANS) at Bangalore has emerged as the leader in this field. Investigations suggest that compared to healthy control subjects, subjects with schizophrenia have significantly smaller global grey matter, greater global cerebrospinal fluid volumes and smaller regional grey matter volume in superior frontal, inferior frontal, cingulate, post-central, superior temporal and parahippocampal gyri, inferior parietal lobule (IPL), insula, caudate nuclei, thalamus and cerebellum (Jayakumar et al. 2005). It was also seen that positive symptoms have significant negative correlation with left superior temporal gyrus volume. Negative symptoms score have inverse correlation with frontal, cingulate and cerebellar grey matter volumes (Venkatasubramanian et al. 2010). Another study reported negative correlation between negative symptoms score and cerebellar grey matter volumes (Arasappa et al. 2008). Venkatasubramanian et al. (2003) evaluated a new corpus callosum measurement method with a valid neuroanatomical and cytoarchitectural basis and showed a good intraclass correlation coefficient and inter-rater reliability. Studies from NIMHANS have reported significant volume deficits in bilateral lateral orbitofrontal and left medial orbitofrontal cortices as well as bilateral pars triangularis and significant thickness deficit in bilateral medial orbitofrontal cortices in subjects with schizophrenia (Venkatasubramanian et al. 2008; Behere et al. 2009). John et al. (2009) compared frontal pole (FP) grey matter volume in neuroleptic-naïve recent-onset schizophrenia subjects with a matched healthy control group and reported lack of difference in FP grey volumes between the healthy subjects and those with schizophrenia. In a study from Mumbai, Parkar et al. (2006) reported ventricular dilatation and prominent cerebral sulci and cerebellar folia. It has also been found that subjects with schizophrenia have lower phosphocreatine (PCr)/total adenosine tri-phosphate (ATP) ratio in bilateral basal ganglia, and this ratio was least in patients with developmental reflexes suggesting neurodevelopmental aetiology for schizophrenia (Gangadhar et al. 2006). A study from NIMHANS reported that subjects with schizophrenia have significantly smaller caudate volumes than healthy controls. PCr/total phosphorous and PCr/total ATP ratios of both caudate nuclei were significantly lower in patients than controls (Jayakumar et al. 2006). Another study reported that at 1-year follow-up, the difference between healthy controls and subjects with schizophrenia on PCr/total phosphorus ratio became non-significant, and there was significant positive correlation between the magnitude of improvement in PANSS total scores and the extent of change in the PCr/ATP ratio (Jayakumar et al. 2010). McCreadie et al. (2002) studied patients with dyskinesia using magnetic resonance imaging and proposed that there may be a subgroup of schizophrenia associated with dyskinesia and striatal pathology (namely, an enlarged lenticular nucleus, especially on the left side).

Malhotra et al. (2006) studied cerebral perfusion using single photon emission computed tomography (SPECT) in subjects with childhood-onset schizophrenia. Compared to lack of perfusion abnormality in the healthy control group, 9 patients (64 %) showed perfusion anomaly on SPECT scans, specifically in the left temporal and frontal areas of the brain. A cross-sectional study examined the effect of antipsychotics on brain metabolism in individuals with schizophrenia who were in different phases of treatment. Patients underwent an 18F-deoxyglucose positron emission tomography scan in a resting state 12 h after the last dose of antipsychotic. Results showed an immediate increase in cortical uptake followed by a decrease in cortical uptake, while the basal ganglia uptake remained high, albeit with a decreasing trend. Typical antipsychotics were associated with lower frontal cortical and higher basal ganglia and cerebellar uptake as compared to atypical antipsychotics (Seethalakshmi et al. 2007). Another study showed that compared to healthy subjects, genu and body of the corpus callosum were significantly smaller in patients with schizophrenia (Venkatasubramanian et al. 2010). A study from NIMHANS which assessed antipsychotic-naïve schizophrenia patients showed that patients with FRS had significant deficits in the right IPL (specifically angular gyrus), in comparison with patients without FRS and healthy controls. However, there was no difference on the left side, which authors attributed to larger variance in healthy controls (Venkatasubramanian et al. 2011). Another study showed relationship between first-rank symptoms and corpus callosum morphometry with patients having significantly smaller corpus callosum, splenium and isthmus areas than control subjects (Rao et al. 2011).

Family and genetic studies: Sethi et al. (1980) in a family study reported higher incidence of psychiatric morbidity in parents. Ponnudurai (1989) by drawing pedigree charts concluded that the findings favoured a polygenic inheritance. Chaterjee and Basu (1980) by nuclear sexing and karyotyping in patients with schizophrenia showed higher prevalence of chromatin positive compared to controls. Ponnudurai and Jayakar (2010) evaluated ‘parental imprinting’ and the phenomenon of ‘anticipation’ and reported that age of onset in probands was lower in those with family history of psychosis, and the difference was more significant when the paternal side was affected. When the age of onset in the grandparents was compared with either of the parental sides of the probands, no difference emerged, indicating lack of support from this study for the theory of anticipation. Verma et al. (2005) investigated the relationship of MLC1 (putative cation-channel gene on 22q13) with schizophrenia and bipolar disorders and concluded that association of MLC1 with schizophrenia and bipolar disorders suggests involvement of a common pathway. Chowdari et al. (2002) evaluated the role of transcription of the regulator of G-protein signalling 4 (RGS4) in the pathogenesis of schizophrenia, by genetic association and linkage studies using samples ascertained independently in Pittsburgh and New Delhi and by the NIMH Collaborative Genetics Initiative, and reported significant transmission distortion in Pittsburgh and NIMH samples. Tiwari et al. (2005) investigated the significance of CYP3A4*1B and CYP2D6*4 polymorphisms in tardive dyskinesia susceptibility among patients with chronic schizophrenia, but failed to demonstrate significant association of either of the two single nucleotide polymorphisms (SNPs) with tardive dyskinesia. Gangandhar et al. (2002) studied the relationship of reversed gender effect on age at onset (AAO) in schizophrenia in relation to infant mortality rate, but found no difference in age of onset in the samples from lower infant mortality rate. Verma et al. (2005) studied the SYNGR1 gene, located on 22q13.1 in subjects with schizophrenia and bipolar disorders, and found that 9 out of 14 dbSNPs were associated with schizophrenia and bipolar disorder. Mukherjee et al. (2006) reported positive linkage and association finding at 18p11.2 for psychosis (schizophrenia, bipolar disorder and psychosis NOS). Holliday et al. (2006) reported association of dystrobrevin binding protein 1 (dysbindin) gene (DTNBP1) with schizophrenia. Holliday et al. (2009) reported a significant linkage of schizophrenia to chromosome 1p31.1. Talkowski et al. (2006) studied associations between dopamine D3 receptor gene polymorphisms and schizophrenia in two independent samples, one from the US and another from India. In the US samples, significant associations were detected with eight Single nucleotide polymorphisms (SNPs), including rs6280; whereas, in the Indian sample, one SNP was associated (rs10934254, $p = 0.03$) with schizophrenia. Kukreti et al. (2006) investigated the association of synonymous polymorphisms (His313 and Pro319) in the dopamine D2 receptor gene with schizophrenia using a case–control approach and found that genotype distribution for the His313 polymorphism was significantly different between patients with schizophrenia and control subjects, while the Pro319 polymorphism did not show any association with the disease. Debnath et al. (2006) investigated the incidence of human leucocyte antigen (HLA) class I alleles in patients with delusional disorder and paranoid schizophrenia and found that HLA-A*03 gene was significantly associated with delusional disorder as well as with paranoid schizophrenia. Gupta et al. (2009) investigated the role OD16 polymorphisms from three genes, dopamine receptor D2 (DRD2), catechol-O-methyl transferase (COMT) and brain-derived neurotrophic factor (BDNF) in schizophrenia and found significant associations of two SNPs of DRD2 (rs11608185, genotype; rs6275, genotype) and one SNP in the COMT gene (rs4680, genotype). However, when corrections for multiple comparisons were made, a weak association of individual markers of DRD2 and COMT with schizophrenia was seen. Multifactor dimensionality reduction analysis suggested a two locus model (rs6275/DRD2 and rs4680/COMT) as the best model for gene–gene interaction with 90 % cross-validation consistency and 42 % prediction error in predicting disease risk among patients with schizophrenia. Srivastava et al. (2010) studied gene polymorphisms and genetic susceptibility in subjects with schizophrenia and reported a significant allelic association of catechol-O-methyltransferase rs362204 -/G ($p = 0.028$) marker; whereas, nominally significant genotypic associations were seen for tyrosine hydroxylase rs6356 A/G and dopamine beta-hydroxylase rs1108580 A/G with schizophrenia.

Ahmad et al. (2009) reported the role of GRIK3 for susceptibility to schizophrenia in Indian population. Vijayan et al. (2009) reported significant allelic and genotypic associations of rs2066713 (both allelic and genotypic), 5HTTLPR and STin2 polymorphisms with schizophrenia. A haplotype linking these three risk alleles, 5HTTLPR/S-rs2066713/C-STin2/12-repeat, was also significantly associated with schizophrenia. Thara et al. (2009) studied schizophrenia pedigrees and reported very low prevalence of affective psychoses such as schizoaffective disorder in most affected individuals with schizophrenia. Srivastava et al. (2006) reported DRD4 and COMT genes as the most important candidate genes for development of tardive dyskinesia in North Indian subjects with schizophrenia. Thomas et al. (2011) evaluated the associations of selected SNPs with schizophrenia with selected indices of severity and symptom pattern but did not find any significant associations following corrections for multiple comparisons. A recent study showed association of schizophrenia and schizophrenia-related neurocognitive measures with two SNPs (rs35753505 and rs6994992) from the Neuregulin-1 gene promoter region in a North Indian cohort (Kukshal et al. 2013). Singh et al. (2008) showed that compared to age- and gender-matched healthy subjects from the same ethnic group as the patients, patients of schizophrenia have increased frequency of HLA-A*03 as well as decreased frequencies of HLA-A*31 and HLA B*51.

Soft neurological signs and minor physical anomalies: Some genetically determined somatic traits such as ear lobes, finger hair and hairy ear were studied in schizophrenia (Ponnudurai 1989). The proportion of patients with schizophrenia with ear lobes hanging free was much less than the controls. The presence of physical anomalies was investigated in schizophrenia, and the incidence was found to be significantly high (Lal and Sharma 1987). Soft neurological signs (SNS) and minor physical anomalies (MPA) were studied in 107 adult patients with schizophrenia by Nizamie et al. (1989) who found SNS more frequently in patients with chronic schizophrenia compared to normal subjects and also found higher mean MPA score as compared to reported score in normal populations. John et al. (2008) compared MPAs and neurologic soft signs (NSSs) as a composite endophenotype for schizophrenia subjects with a matched healthy control group and noted that subjects with schizophrenia had significantly higher frequencies of MPAs and NSSs than healthy controls. Biswas et al. (2007) compared NSSs in patients with childhood-onset schizophrenia (COS), adolescence onset (AdOS) and adulthood onset (AOS) and reported that NSSs were significantly more frequent in COS and AdOS compared with AOS patients.

Cognitive functions: Ananthnarayan et al. (1993) studied clinically remitted outpatients with schizophrenia on measures of visual information processing and found that they performed poorly when compared to patients with neurotic depression. Borde et al. (1996) used the happy–sad chimeric faces test to elicit left hemifacial bias (LHF bias) and found that patients with mania and schizophrenia did not show significant LHF bias. Another study compared cognitive functions of subjects with schizophrenia with those suffering from bipolar disorder and reported that compared to controls, both bipolar disorder and schizophrenia patients were significantly impaired on different tests of executive function, memory, IQ and perceptuomotor functions. Patients with schizophrenia consistently performed worse than patients with bipolar disorder, but none of the differences between schizophrenia and bipolar disorder were significant (Pradhan et al. 2008). Bhatia et al. (2009) examined cognitive functions of subjects with schizophrenia and schizoaffective disorder and compared them with their parents and a control group and found that subjects with schizophrenia and schizoaffective disorder took significantly more time than controls on Part B of the trail making test (TMT), and there was no significant difference between patients and parents on any of the

TMT parameters. A study, which evaluated the relationship between cognition and work functioning in patients with schizophrenia, found that cognitive deficits did not relate significantly with current employment status or the level of performance at work. Negative symptoms predicted employment status, and poor social functioning predicted poor work performance (Srinivasan and Tirupati 2005). A study evaluated the relationship between insight and executive functions and reported that poor insight was associated with poor executive functioning (Choudhury et al. 2009). Grover et al. (2011) compared the neurocognitive deficits in patients with paranoid schizophrenia and delusional disorder and reported that compared with patients with paranoid schizophrenia, patients with delusional disorder had more impairment on different tests of attention, visual learning and memory, verbal working memory and executive functions. John et al. (2011) examined the pattern of functional magnetic resonance imaging blood oxygen level dependent activations and deactivations during semantic word generation and showed that in addition to the brain regions activated during word generation in healthy individuals, patients with schizophrenia showed additional activations of temporo-parieto-occipital cortical regions as well as subcortical regions, despite significantly poorer behavioural performance than the healthy participants.

Social cognition: A study evaluated the facial emotion recognition deficits in antipsychotic-naïve schizophrenia patients and showed that the patients with schizophrenia made significantly greater number of errors in recognition of negative emotions of fear and disgust compared to normal controls (Behere et al. 2009). In another study, Behere et al. (2011) evaluated the facial emotional recognition deficits in patients with FRS and those without FRS and showed that patients with FRS made significantly greater errors in over-identification as compared to those without FRS.

Dermatoglyphics: Dasgupta et al. (1973) conducted research on dermatoglyphics in schizophrenia and found that the patients had higher indices as compared to normal controls. Eswaraiah (1978) in a study found that patients had higher frequency of single radial base crease than controls. Jhingan and Munjal (1990) studied dermatoglyphics in patients with catatonic schizophrenia; whereas, Jain et al. (1992) studied palmer flexion crease pattern in schizophrenia subjects, their relatives and normal controls. Studies in dermatoglyphics were also reported by Sengupta and Bhuyan (1995) and Ponnudurai et al. (1997) in familial and non-familial schizophrenia.

Neurotropins: Kale et al. (2009) studied the CSF and plasma nerve growth factor (NGF) in drug-naïve patients with psychosis and reported significantly lower levels of NGF in both CSF and plasma.

Oxidative Stress: A study evaluated the levels of malondialdehyde (MDA), superoxide dismutase (SOD), glutathione peroxidase (GSHPx) and reduced glutathione (GSH) in subjects of schizophrenia. Compared to healthy controls, significantly lower levels of SOD, GSHPx and GSH were found in subjects with schizophrenia, along with an increased oxidative stress as indicated by high blood MDA levels (Dadheech et al. 2008). Another study reported lower levels of antioxidants in haloperidol-treated subjects compared to those treated with olanzapine (Singh et al. 2008).

Immunological changes: Significant reduction in interleukin-2 (IL-2) and interleukin-6 (IL-6) was reported in subjects with schizophrenia, irrespective of the medication status, i.e. those on antipsychotics and those not on antipsychotics, suggesting immune dysregulation in pathophysiology of schizophrenia. Further, the medicated patients showed lower level of IL-2 and IL-6 than the psychotropic medication-free patients (Singh et al. 2009).

Lipid metabolites and insulin-like growth factor: A study of antipsychotic-naïve patients with schizophrenia showed significantly lower levels of leptins compared to healthy controls. However, with antipsychotic treatment, leptins levels increased in patients with schizophrenia (Venkatasubramanian et al. 2010). Another study showed significant inverse correlation between total negative syndrome score and serum HDL levels (Venkatasubramanian et al. 2010). A study involving antipsychotic-naïve schizophrenia demonstrated significantly lower levels of insulin-like growth factor (IGF-1) and higher levels of cortisol in patients with schizophrenia, compared to healthy controls. With treatment, IGF-1 levels increased significantly along with significant reduction in cortisol levels (Venkatasubramanian et al. 2010).

6 Psychosocial Issues

Causal or explanatory models: Few studies have evaluated the explanatory models as understood by the patients with schizophrenia themselves and their caregivers (Kulhara et al. 2000; Srinivasan and Thara 2001). It was documented that beliefs in supernatural factors were quite prevalent in caregivers of mentally ill patients and that many patients and their caregivers sought the help of faith healers quite often (Saravanan et al. 2008). It has also been shown that indigenous healing methods are considered complementary to the medical management of mental illness by patients and caregivers (Saravanan et al. 2008). Studies, which have evaluated the patients, suggest that although some patients do subscribe to biomedical models, about two-thirds of the patients have non-biomedical causal models of schizophrenia (Saravanan et al. 2007; Kate et al. 2012). Charles et al. (2007) reported that majority of the patients and their relatives held multiple and contradictory models of illness and its treatment simultaneously. However, in contrast to studies from the South India, a study from the north India suggested that in addition to belief in supernatural causes, many patients also had biological causal models (Kate et al. 2012). Data also suggest that patients who held biomedical concepts of disease had significantly higher scores on the insight scale compared to those who held non-medical beliefs (Saravanan et al. 2007). Multivariate analyses identified three factors associated with spiritual/mystical models (female sex, low education and visits to traditional healers) and a single factor (high level of insight) for the endorsement of biological model. Preserved insight was associated with anxiety, help-seeking and perception of change. Insight was strongly associated with willingness to attribute symptoms to disease in others and in one's self, but not to supernatural forces (Saravanan et al. 2007).

Marriage and related issues: Impact of schizophrenia on marriage had been studied by some researchers. Thara and Srinivasan (1997) followed a cohort of patients with first-episode psychosis for 10 years after the onset of illnesses and reported that 70 % patients with schizophrenia got married, and in 85 % of cases, marriages were intact at follow-up. Compared to females, more men remained single; whereas, more women faced broken marriages. Low marriage rates were associated with a continuous and relapsing course. Thara et al. (2003a, b) evaluated female patients with schizophrenia who had broken marriages and observed that many patients had not separated legally and were not receiving any maintenance from their husbands. It was also observed that even after several years of separation, patients expected to be reunited with their spouse. With regards to the caregivers, most of the families expressed intense distress and concern about the long-term future and security of these women. Further, the families perceived care of children of these women to be an additional problem, due to lack of any financial support from the separated husbands. A recent study evaluated the QOL and marital adjustment in patients with various mental disorders including schizophrenia during the phase of remission in a rural setting and reported that compared to patients with bipolar disorder and recurrent depressive disorder, patients with schizophrenia reported significantly poorer QOL. Patients of schizophrenia also reported greatest marital dissatisfaction. With regards to marital adjustment, patients perceived the same to be poor, but spouses did not endorse the same (Vibha et al. 2013). Bhatia et al. (2004) compared the indices of fertility and fecundity among male and female patients with schizophrenia or schizoaffective disorder from New Delhi with patients from north-eastern United States. In the US sample, male patients were significantly more likely to be single and childless compared with female patients. They also had fewer children. In contrast, there were no significant gender differences among Indian male and female patients with regard to the reproductive indices. Multivariate analyses revealed that the indices of reproduction were associated with different variables in the US and Indian samples.

Stigma: In one of the largest studies from India, Murthy (2005) evaluated stigma in 1,000 patients in four cities, as a part of the Indian initiative of the World Psychiatric Association Programme to reduce the stigma and discrimination because of schizophrenia. He reported that urban respondents in large centres try to hide their illness hoping to remain unnoticed; whereas, rural respondents in smaller regions experience greater ridicule, shame and discrimination, as anonymity is more difficult. Other studies suggest that in women, stigma was related to marriage, pregnancy and childbirth. Both men and women revealed certain cultural myths about their illnesses and how they affected their lives in a negative way (Loganathan and Murthy 2008). Mishra et al. (2009) concluded that those with better insight perceived higher stigma, compared to those with poor insight. With respect to perceived causes of stigma, a strikingly large number of participants (97 %) believed that stigma was caused by a lack of awareness about schizophrenia and the nature of the illness itself. Behavioural symptoms associated with schizophrenia were also thought to be a cause of stigma; whereas, medication-related complications were seen as playing a less causal role in stigma

(Shrivastava et al. 2011). It has also been suggested that stigma in patients is associated with external non-stigmatizing beliefs about illness (karma and evil spirits), the disease model of illness, the total number of causal models, the total number of non-medical causal beliefs, visiting temples or other places of worship for cure, total family stigma score and the relatives' perception of stigma on the patient subscale (Charles et al. 2007). The most common forms, in which stigma was experienced, were through lowered self-esteem. Also prevalent (in approximately half of the patients) were reports of being avoided due to their illness, discrimination suffered in the family, overhearing offensive comments about mental illness, discrimination at the work place, problems coping with their marriage and not receiving proposals for marriage due to their illness (Mishra et al. 2009) and strains in marital relationship (Raguram et al. 2004). Studies of stigma in caregivers suggest that caregivers most frequently have concerns about the social impact of the illness on the affected person in the form of difficulties for the person to marry, problems in an existing marriage, social devaluation and avoidance by others. Other social issues included family concerns about disclosure, feelings of shame and embarrassment about their relative's condition and difficulties for a relative of the patient to marry (Raguram et al. 2004). Raguram et al. (2001) reported that caregivers believe that employability is lower for persons with previous history of schizophrenia and caregivers were likely to hide the history of schizophrenia among patients. Thara and Srinivasan (2000) found that Hindus experience higher level of stigma than Muslims and Christians, and higher level of stigma in caregivers is associated with patient being female and young, and caregiver being younger.

Costs of care: Occasional studies have comprehensively evaluated the cost of care of schizophrenia. Grover et al. (2005) showed that cost of care of schizophrenia is similar to the total cost of care of diabetes mellitus; however, the indirect cost of schizophrenia is significantly more than diabetes mellitus (indirect cost schizophrenia: 63 %, diabetes mellitus 29 %); whereas, direct cost was significantly more in diabetes mellitus compared to schizophrenia (direct cost diabetes mellitus: 71 %, schizophrenia: 37 %). Total cost of schizophrenia was significantly higher in those who were unemployed had higher number of hospital visits and higher psychopathology and higher level of disability (Grover et al. 2005). Another study reported direct cost of treatment of schizophrenia and estimated the drug cost to be about 11 % of the total cost. In this study, development of side effects with treatment was associated with higher treatment cost (Pahuja et al. 2011).

A few studies have compared the cost of care of schizophrenia with cost of care of bipolar disorder (Somaiya et al. 2014a; Deshpande 2005; Thakral et al. 2011). In a comprehensive study, which evaluated multiple aspects of cost of care, Somaiya et al. (2014a) reported that cost of care of schizophrenia is similar to that of bipolar disorder, and the proportion of indirect cost was the main driver of the total cost for both the disorders; it also highlighted the fact that higher total cost of care is associated with total duration of illness and lower level of functioning. Deshpande (2005) compared the cost of care of schizophrenia with bipolar disorder and reported that patients with bipolar disorder spent more on the cost of consultation with faith healers, on travel to reach non-psychiatric services and medications than those with schizophrenia. Thakral et al. (2011) evaluated the direct cost of treatment for patients with schizophrenia, bipolar and major depressive disorder and reported that direct cost of patients with bipolar disorder was more than that that of schizophrenia and major depression, with direct cost for schizophrenia being intermediate between the affective disorders. Thara (2005) assessed the direct cost of treatment with clozapine and reported that after shifting the patients to clozapine from other antipsychotics, despite the costs of blood tests, the total cost of treatment with clozapine had come down by nearly twenty-five per cent. A recent study evaluated the changes in the trends of cost of care of schizophrenia over a decade. It compared the cost of care of schizophrenia as estimated in 2000–2001 and in 2010–2011. Findings suggested that overall cost of care of schizophrenia has doubled. This study also suggested that the indirect cost is the main determinant of total cost of care of schizophrenia. Total direct cost of the treatment had not changed much in last decade, but total indirect cost has increased more than two times. The contribution of the providers' cost (i.e., treating agency) was been minimal, and this proportion has not changed much over the last decade. Cost of care of schizophrenia was more for those with lower levels of functioning, and those who had to visit the hospital more often (Somaiya et al 2014b).

Needs: Some of the studies have attempted to examine health care needs of patients with schizophrenia and their caregivers (Nagaswami et al. 1985; Shankar and Kamath 1991; Elangovan et al. 1997; Nagarajaiah et al. 1997; Shrivastava et al. 2001; Srinivasan 2000; Jagannathan et al. 2008; Gandotra et al. 2004; Kulhara et al. 2010; Neogi 2010; Gopinath et al. 1987; Chadda et al. 2000). Evaluating rehabilitation needs of the patients with schizophrenia, Nagaswami et al. (1985) reported that the most important felt needs for both patients and families were finding a job for the patient and being gainfully employed. In chronically ill patients, Shankar and Kamath (1991) reported that families express needs for information about medication, management of unpredictable or disturbed behaviour and lack of interest in daily activities, assistance with job placement and day care. In patients with chronic schizophrenia, Elangovan et al. (1997) reported that the primary needs expressed were those for patient to participate in meaningful daytime activities. In a rural community, it was reported that there were pressing needs in the form of basic education, money, treatment and benefits; whereas, the need for information was given less importance (Nagarajaiah et al. 1997). Need for information, rehabilitation services, jobs and skills training and financial assistance as the important areas of need were reported by Shrivastava et al. (2001). Others have pointed out that needs in the form of training of patient in daily living skills and vocational activities and facilities for day care are important (Srinivasan 2000). A study from NIMHANS, Bangalore used focused group discussions to understand the needs of the caregivers.

The main needs that emerged were needs regarding managing behaviour of patients (29 %), managing social-vocational problems of patients (21 %), health issues of caregivers (18 %), education about schizophrenia (15 %) and rehabilitation (13 %) and managing sexual and marital problems of patients (5 %). All family caregivers who attended the focus group discussions emphatically stated that they required help in managing all their needs and expressed their willingness to participate in any training that addressed their needs (Jagannathan et al. 2008). A study from Ranchi compared the rehabilitation needs of the inpatients and outpatients and reported significant differences in the needs for help from a voluntary agency, employment, accommodation, leisure activities and help for family. Negative symptoms significantly correlated with rehabilitation needs among both groups of patients (Gandotra et al. 2004).

Kulhara et al. (2010) evaluated the needs of schizophrenia subjects using Camberwell Assessment for Needs instrument and reported 8.12 and 7.13 needs of patients as perceived by patients and caregivers, respectively, of which more than two-third were unmet. The most commonly reported needs by both patients and their caregivers were need for welfare benefits. Government or Non-governmental organizations provided negligible help in the areas of needs. Another study from PGIMER, Chandigarh by using Camberwell Assessment for Needs instrument and a self-designed instrument, assessed the needs of patients with schizophrenia and bipolar disorders and needs of patients as perceived by their caregivers reported that the total number of needs expressed by patients with schizophrenia were significantly more than that reported by patients with bipolar disorder; however, there was no significant difference in the total number of met and unmet needs as perceived by the patients. There was no significant difference in the total number of needs and total number of met and total number of unmet needs of patients as perceived by the caregivers. The most common domain of need as per the patients was that of welfare benefits, which was perceived as not being met at all (Neogi 2010).

Religion: Researchers have looked at the role of religion in psychopathology and help-seeking and in understanding the explanatory models, coping with the illness and influence on QOL. A study from Chennai attempted to understand the reasons why mentally ill patients and their families choose to seek help from a religious site and reported that the main reason for the same was cultural explanation for the illness (Padmavati et al. 2005). One study evaluated the use of religious coping and its relation to psychological well-being among caregivers of patients with schizophrenia and reported that the strength of religious belief was a significant predictor of well-being of the caregivers (Rammohan et al. 2002). In a cross-sectional study, the relationship between coping skills and the WHOQOL-Spirituality, Religiousness and Personal Belief (WHOQOL-SRPB) scale was evaluated, and it was found that positive reappraisal as a coping strategy had significant positive correlation with all the facets of WHOQOL-SRPB and SRPB total domain scores leading to conclusion that a sound spiritual, religious or personal belief system is associated with active and adaptive coping skills in subjects with residual schizophrenia (Shah et al. 2011). A recent study from PGIMER, Chandigarh evaluated the caregivers of patients with schizophrenia and studied QOL, including the spirituality, religiousness and personal beliefs (SRPB) facets and reported significant positive correlation between WHOQOL-BREF and various facets of WHOQOL-SRPB, indicating that SRPB forms an integral component of the concept of QOL (Kate et al. 2013).

Disability: It is well known that schizophrenia, as a disorder is associated with significant disability. As early as in 1970s, the 'PGI Disability Scale' was developed to measure psychiatric disability mainly for use in schizophrenia patients in the community (Murthy et al. 1975; Wig et al. 1979). Later, Thara et al. (1988) developed the Schedule for Assessment of Psychiatric Disability (SAPD) as a modification and Indian adaptation of the WHO-Disability Assessment Schedule II. The SAPD assesses disability in three areas, namely, personal, social and occupational and has a rating for overall disability. The SAPD was found to be reasonably reliable and valid for measuring disability in psychiatric outpatients (Thara et al. 1988). It has been used for studying the course and outcome of schizophrenia, (Thara and Rajkumar 1993) treatment effectiveness, (Singh et al. 2010) relationship of disability with duration of hospitalization in patients with schizophrenia, (Gupta and Chadda 2008) and the association between disability and costs in patients with schizophrenia (Grover et al. 2005). In 2001, the task force of Rehabilitation Committee of the Indian Psychiatric Society developed the Indian Disability Evaluation and Assessment Scale (IDEAS) for measuring and quantifying disability in patients with mental disorders (The Rehabilitation Committee of the Indian Psychiatric Society 2002). The scale was field tested at eight centres across the country and was found to have good internal consistency, face, content and criterion validities (Thara 2005). The scale was later approved by Government of India for the assessment and certification of disability associated with mental illnesses (Ministry of Social Justice and Empowerment, Government of India 2002). In the last decade, about a dozen studies have employed the IDEAS and have focused on prevalence and pattern of psychiatric disabilities in hospital- and community-based samples (Chaudhury et al. 2006; Mohan et al. 2005; Solanki et al. 2010; Kumar et al. 2008; Thirthalli et al. 2009, 2010; Kumar et al. 2006; Balhara et al. 2011; Kashyap et al. 2012; Krishnadas et al. 2007). These studies indicate that schizophrenia is among the most disabling psychiatric disorders (Chaudhury et al. 2006; Mohan et al. 2005; Solanki et al. 2010). Disability in patients with schizophrenia correlates with severity of psychopathology (Chaudhury et al. 2006) and reduces with treatment, (Thirthalli et al. 2010, 2009), and most of the requests for disability certification are for schizophrenia (Kumar et al. 2006; Balhara et al. 2011; Kashyap et al. 2012). However, disability does not correlate with cognitive dysfunction (Krishnadas et al. 2007). One recent study evaluated the internal consistency and validity of IDEAS in patients with schizophrenia and reported that the scale has good internal consistency and construct validity (Grover et al. 2014)

Quality of life: A study compared the QOL of patients with schizophrenia and dysthymia and showed that the QOL of patients with schizophrenia was significantly poorer compared to those with dysthymia, but the duration of illness of schizophrenia did not have significant impact on QOL (Gupta et al. 1998). One study evaluated the convergent validity of quality of life interview—brief version (QOLI) by using it with quality of life scale (QLS) and WHOQOL-BREF in patients of schizophrenia and concluded that QOLI has convergent validity with both a disease-specific (QLS) and a generic (WHOQOL-BREF) scales and also reported that subjective and objective measures of QOL have good correlation (Lobana et al. 2001, 2002). On comparing patients with ICD-10 schizophrenia with and without depression on quality of life (QOL), it emerged that the depressed group had more disability compared to the non-depressed group, but depressive symptoms had no significant correlation with subjective or objective domain of QOL (Dan et al. 2011). Chugh et al. (2013) evaluated the relationship between psychopathology and QOL in patients with first-episode schizophrenia and found that the physical well-being domain of the WHOQOL-BREF to be related significantly to the positive, negative and general psychopathology symptoms of schizophrenia as assessed on PANSS. In remitted patients, significantly better QOL in males compared to females was observed (Kujur et al. 2010).

Studies comparing QOL of patients with schizophrenia with physical illness, like systemic lupus erythematous, suggest that the two disorders differ significantly only the social domain (Radhakrishnan et al. 2012). Studies, which have compared QOL between patients with schizophrenia and obsessive–compulsive disorder, report no statistically significant difference between the two groups (Solanki et al. 2010).

A study, which longitudinally evaluated QOL of patients with schizophrenia on maintenance treatment, reported that patients had lowest QOL scores in social relationships domain and poor QOL in this domain is associated with employment status (Solanki et al. 2008).

7 Conclusions

Over the years there has been significant progress in research on schizophrenia from India. Studies in the early years mainly focused on the epidemiology, clinical features and course and outcome. In recent times, several studies have focused on neurobiology and genetics. Studies evaluating various aspects of caregiving have been carried out, and show that family remains an important support for the patients of schizophrenia. However, except for the early studies, most of the studies have been done at single centres, and on small sample sizes. It is expected that in future multi-centric studies, involving more number of patients and their caregivers, will strengthen the research evidence.

References

Abraham, A., Kuruvilla, K., & Verghese, A. (1979). The use of repertory grid technique in the assessment of schizophrenic thinking disorder. *Indian Journal of Psychiatry, 21*, 51–53.

Aga, V. M., Agarwal, A. K., & Gupta, S. C. (1995). The relationship of insight to psychopathology in schizophrenia: A cross-sectional study. *Indian Journal of Psychiatry, 37*, 129–135.

Ahmad, Y., Bhatia, M. S., Mediratta, P. K., Sharma, K. K., Negi, H., Chosdol, K., et al. (2009). Association between the ionotropic glutamate receptor kainate3 (GRIK3) Ser310Ala polymorphism and schizophrenia in the Indian population. *World Journal of Biological Psychiatry, 10*, 330–333.

Aich, T. K., Sinha, V. K., Khess, C. R., & Singh, S. (2004). Demographic and clinical correlates of substance abuse comorbidity in schizophrenia. *Indian Journal of Psychiatry, 46*, 135–140.

Aich, T. K., Sinha, V. K., Christoday, R., Khess, J., & Singh, S. (2005). Substance abuse comorbidity in schizophrenia: An inpatient study of course and outcome. *Indian Journal of Psychiatry, 47*, 33–39.

Ampalam, P., Deepthi, R., & Vadaparty, P. (2012). Schizophrenia—insight, depression: A correlation study. *Indian Journal of Psychological Medicine, 34*, 44–48.

Anand, L., Sunitha, T. A., & Khanna, S. (2002). CSF amines and their metabolites in first episode drug naive schizophrenic patients and their correlations with dimensions of schizophrenia. *Indian Journal of Psychiatry, 44*, 212–219.

Aggarwal M, Banerjee A., Singh SM., Mattoo SK., Basu D. (2012). Substance-induced psychotic disorders: 13-Year data from a de-addiction centre and their clinical implications. *Asian Journal of Psychiatry, 5*, 220–224.

Ananthanarayanan, C. V., Janakiramaiah, N., Vittals, B. N., Andade, C., & Kumaraiah, V. (1993). Visual information processing deficits in clinically remitted outpatient schizophrenics. *Indian Journal of Psychiatry, 35*, 27–31.

Arasappa, R., Rao, N. P., Venkatasubramanian, G., Jayakumar, P. N., & Gangadhar, B. N. (2008). Structural cerebellar abnormalities in antipsychotic-naive schizophrenia: Evidence for cognitive dysmetria. *Indian Journal of Psychological Medicine, 30*, 83–89.

Armstrongh, K. P., Chandrasekaran, R., & Perme, B. (2002). Insight, psychopathology and schizophrenia. *Indian Journal of Psychiatry, 44*, 332–337.

Arora, A., Avasthi, A., & Kulhara, P. (1997). Subsyndromes of chronic schizophrenia: a phenomeno-logical study. *Acta Psychiatrica Scandinavica, 96*, 225–229.

Bagadia, V. N., Copalani, J., & Shah, L. P. (1976). Habitual use of Cannabis indica in psychiatric patients. *Indian Journal of Psychiatry, 18*, 141–146.

Balhara, Y. P. S., Gauba, D., & Deshpande, S. N. (2011). Profile difference between male and female psychiatric patients seeking certificate of disability. *Oman Medical Journal, 26*, 410–415.

Basu, D., Malhotra, A., Bhagat, A., & Varma, V. K. (1999). Cannabis psychosis and acute schizophrenia: A case-control study from India. *European Addiction Research, 5*, 71–73.

Behere, R. V., Kalmady, S. V., Venkatasubramanian, G., & Gangadhar, B. N. (2009a). Orbitofrontal lobe volume deficits in antipsychotic-naive schizophrenia: A 3-Tesla MRI study. *Indian Journal of Psychological Medicine, 31*, 77–81.

Behere, R. V., Venkatasubramanian, G., Arasappa, R., Reddy, N., & Gangadhar, B. N. (2009b). Effect of risperidone on emotion recognition deficits in antipsychotic-naïve schizophrenia: A short-term follow-up study. *Schizophrenia Research, 113*, 72–76.

Behere, R. V., Venkatasubramanian, G., Arasappa, R., Reddy, N. N., & Gangadhar, B. N. (2011). First rank symptoms & facial emotion recognition deficits in antipsychotic naïve schizophrenia: Implications for social threat perception model. *Progress in Neuropsychopharmacology and Biological Psychiatry, 35*, 1653–1658.

Bharadwaj, B., Arasappa, R., Behere, R. V., Venkatasubramanian, G., Jayakumar, P. N., & Gangadhar, B. N. (2008). Emotion recognition deficits in antipsychotic-naive schizophrenia. *Indian Journal of Psychological medicine, 30*, 90–97.

Bhatia, T., Franzos, M. A., Wood, J. A., Nimgaonkar, V. L., & Deshpande, S. N. (2004). Gender and procreation among patients with schizophrenia. *Schizophrenia Research, 68*, 387–394.

Bhatia, T., Garg, K., Pogue-Geile, M., Nimgaonkar, V. L., & Deshpande, S. N. (2009). Executive functions and cognitive deficits in schizophrenia: Comparisons between probands, parents and controls in India. *Journal of Postgraduate Medicine, 55*, 3–7.

Biswas, P., Malhotra, S., Malhotra, A., & Gupta, N. (2007). Comparative study of neurological soft signs in schizophrenia with onset in childhood, adolescence and adulthood. *Acta Psychiatrica Scandinavica, 115*, 295–303.

Borde, M., Davis, E. J. B., & Sharma, L. N. (1992). The stability of symptoms and syndromes in chronic schizophrenic patients. *Indian Journal of Psychiatry, 34*, 133–139.

Borde, M., Roy, A., Davis, E. J., & Davis, R. (1996). Right hemispheric function in normals, affective disorder and schizophrenia. *Indian Journal of Psychiatry, 38*, 225–230.

Chabungbam, G., Avasthi, A., & Sharan, P. (2007). Sociodemographic and clinical factors associated with relapse in schizophrenia. *Psychiatry and Clinical Neurosciences, 61*, 587–593.

Chadda, R. K., Pradhan, S. C., Bapna, J. S., Singhal, R., & Singh, T. B. (2000). Chronic psychiatric patients: An assessment of treatment and rehabilitation-related needs. *International Journal of Rehabilitation Research, 23*, 55–58.

Chakraborty, R., Chatterjee, A., Chaudhury, S., & Khess, C. R. (2008). Impact of substance abuse on presentation and short term course of schizophrenia. *Indian Journal of Psychiatry, 50*, 4.

Charles, H., Manoranjitham, S. D., & Jacob, K. S. (2007). Stigma and explanatory models among people with schizophrenia and their relatives in Vellore, South India. *International Journal of Social Psychiatry, 53*, 325–332.

Chatterjee, S. B. (1988). Dopamine related hormone levels in acute schizophrenia. *Indian Journal of Psychiatry, 30*, 7–13.

Chatterjee, S. B., & Basu, S. K. (1980). Sex chromosome aberrations in schizophrenia. *Indian Journal of Psychiatry, 22*, 142–153.

Chatterjee, S. B., & Thakur, M. S. (1976). A Comparative study of Muller-Lyer illusion among normal's, neurotics and schizophrenics. *Indian Journal of Psychiatry, 18*, 6–14.

Chaturvedi, S. K., Rao, G. P., Mathai, J. P., Sarmukaddam, S., & Gopinath, P. S. (1985). Negative symptoms in schizophrenia and depression. *Indian Journal of Psychiatry, 27*, 237–242.

Chaudhury, P. K., Deka, K., & Chetia, D. (2006). Disability associated with mental disorders. *Indian Journal of Psychiatry, 48*, 95–101.

Chintalapudi, M., Kulhara, P., & Avasthi, A. (1993). Post-psychotic depression in schizophrenia. *European Archives of Psychiatry and Clinical Neuroscience, 243*, 103–108.

Choudhury, S., Khess, C. R. J., Bhattacharyya, R., & Sanyal, D. (2009). Insight in schizophrenia and its association with executive functions. *Indian Journal of Psychological Medicine, 31*, 71–76.

Chowdari, K. V., Mirnics, K., Semwal, P., Wood, J., Lawrence, E., Bhatia, T., et al. (2002). Association and linkage analyses of RGS4 polymorphisms in schizophrenia. *Human Molecular Genetics, 11*, 1373–1380.

Chugh, P. K., Rehan, H. S., Unni, K. E., & Sah, R. K. (2013). Predictive value of symptoms for quality of life in first-episode schizophrenia. *Nordic Journal of Psychiatry, 67*, 153–158.

Dadheech, G., Mishra, S., Gautam, S., & Sharma, P. (2008). Evaluation of antioxidant deficit in schizophrenia. *Indian Journal of Psychiatry, 50*, 16–20.

Dan, A., Kumar, S., Avasthi, A., & Grover, S. (2011). A comparative study on quality of life of patients of schizophrenia with and without depression. *Psychiatry Research, 189*, 185–189.

Das, P., & Kapur, R. L. (1980). Post psychotic depression in schizophrenics: A prospective study. *Indian Journal of Psychiatry, 22*, 277–282.

Das, M. K., Kulhara, P. L., & Verma, S. K. (1997). Life events preceding relapse of schizophrenia. *International Journal of Social Psychiatry, 43*, 56–63.

Dasgupta, J., Dasgupta, D., & Balasubrahmanyan, M. (1973). Dermatoglyphics in the diagnosis of schizophrenia. *Indian Journal of Psychiatry, 15*, 104–122.

Debnath, M., Das, S. K., Bera, N. K., Nayak, C. R., & Chaudhuri, T. K. (2006). Genetic associations between delusional disorder and paranoid schizophrenia: A novel etiologic approach. *Canadian Journal of Psychiatry, 51*, 342–349.

Deshpande, S. (2005). Cost of illness in schizophrenia—perspective from a GHPU. *Indian Journal Psychiatry, 47*, 205–217.

Dube, K. C. (1979). A study of prevalence and biological variables in mental illness in rural urban community in Uttar Pradesh. *India Acta Psychiatr Scand, 46*, 327–342.

Dube, K. C., & Handa, S. K. (1971). Drug use in health and mental illness in an Indian population. *British Journal of Psychiatry, 118*, 345–346.

Eaton, W. W., Thara, R., Federman, B., Melton, B., & Liang, K. Y. (1995). Structure and course of positive and negative symptoms in schizophrenia. *Archives of General Psychiatry, 52*, 127–134.

Elanagar, M. N., Maitra, P., & Rao, M. N. (1971). Mental health in an Indian rural community. *British Journal of Psychiatry, 118*, 499.

Elangovan, S., Verghese, M., & Murali, T. (1997). Assessment of needs and disability in chronic schizophrenia and bipolar affective disorder. *NIMHANS Journal, 15*, 199–200.

Eswaraiah, G. (1978). Palm prints and schizophrenia. *Indian Journal of Psychiatry, 20*, 349–353.

Gandotra, S., Paul, S. E., Daniel, M., Kumar, K., Raj, H. A., & Sujeetha, B. (2004). A preliminary study of rehabilitation needs of in-patients and out-patients with schizophrenia. *Indian Journal of Psychiatry, 46*, 244–255.

Kumar, S. G., Das, A., Bhandary, P. V., Soans, S. J., Harsha Kumar, H. N., & Kotian, M. S. (2008). Prevalence and pattern of mental disability using Indian disability evaluation assessment scale in a rural community of Karnataka. *Indian Journal of Psychiatry, 50*, 21–23.

Gangadhar, B. N., Panner Selvan, C., Subbakrishna, D. K., & Janakiramaiah, N. (2002). Age-at-onset and schizophrenia: Reversed gender effect. *Acta Psychiatrica Scandinavica, 105*, 317–319.

Gangadhar, B. N., Jayakumar, P. N., Venkatasubramanian, G., Janakiramaiah, N., & Keshavan, S. (2006). Developmental reflexes and 31P magnetic resonance spectroscopy of basal ganglia in antipsychotic-naive schizophrenia. *Progress in Neuropsychopharmacology and Biological Psychiatry, 30*, 910–913.

Ghosh, A., Varma, V. K., & Amma, M. K. P. (1981). Correlation between psychopathology and urinary steroid and biogenic amine metabolites in male schizophrenics. *Indian Journal of Psychiatry, 23*, 298–303.

Giridhar, C., Kulhara, P., & Varma, V. K. (1992). Linguistic compentence in positive and negative subtypes of schizophrenia. *Indian Journal of Psychiatry., 34*, 311–320.

Goel, D. S., & D'Netto, T. B. (1975). Cannabis: The habit and psychosis. *Indian Journal of Psychiatry, 17*, 238–243.

Gong, S. L., Wei, J., Ramchand, C. N., Ramchand, R., & Hemmings, G. P. (1993). Concentrations of homovanillic acid and gonadal hormones in the serum of male schizophrenic patients. *Indian Journal of Psychiatry, 35*, 181–184.

Gopinath, P. S., Sharma, P. S. V. N., & Reddy, M. V. (1987). Patients who discontinue day hospitalization—An analysis. *Indian Journal of Psychiatry, 29*, 197–201.

Goswami, S., Singh, G., Mattoo, S. K., & Basu, D. (2003). Courses of substance use and schizophrenia in dual diagnosis patients. *Indian Journal of Medical Sciences, 57*, 338–346.

Grover, S., Avasthi, A., Chakrabarti, S., Bhansali, A., & Kulhara, P. (2005). Cost of care of schizophrenia: A study of Indian outpatient attenders. *Acta Psychiatrica Scandinavica, 112*, 54–63.

Grover, S., Nehra, R., Bhateja, G., Kulhara, P., & Kumar, S. (2011). A comparative study of cognitive deficits in patients with delusional disorder and paranoid schizophrenia. *Industrial Psychiatry Journal, 20*, 107–114.

Grover S., Shah R., Kulhara P., Malhotra R. (2014). Internal consistency and validity of Indian Disability Evaluation and Assessment Scale (IDEAS) in patients with schizophrenia. *Indian Journal of Medical Research* (in press).

Gupta, S. (1979). Socio clinical aspects of delusions in schizophrenia. *Indian Journal of Psychiatry, 21*, 169–175.

Gupta, A., & Chadda, R. K. (2008). Disability in schizophrenia: Do short hospitalizations have a role? *International Journal of Psychosoc Rehabilitation, 13*, 91–96.

Gupta, A. K., Sethi, B. B., & Trivedi, J. K. (1985). Platelet MAO activity in chronic schizophrenia. *Indian Journal of Psychiatry, 27*, 279–287.

Gupta, S. C., Singh, H., & Trivedi, J. K. (1992). Evaluation of suicidal risk in depressives and schizophrenics: A 2-year follow-up study. *Indian Journal of Psychiatry, 34*, 298–310.

Gupta, S., Kulhara, P., & Verma, S. K. (1998). Quality of life in schizophrenia and dysthymia. *Acta Psychiatrica Scandinavica, 97*, 290–296.

Gupta, M., Chauhan, C., Bhatnagar, P., Gupta, S., Grover, S., Singh, P. K., et al. (2009). Genetic susceptibility to schizophrenia: Role of dopaminergic pathway gene polymorphisms. *Pharmacogenomics, 10*, 277–291.

Hemrom, S., Pushpa, D. P., Jahan, M., Jahan, A. R., & Kenswar, D. K. (2009). Prevalence of obsessive compulsive symptoms in patients with schizophrenia. *Industrial Psychiatry Journal, 18*, 77–80.

Holliday, E. G., Handoko, H. Y., James, M. R., McGrath, J. J., Nertney, D. A., Tirupati, S., et al. (2006). Association study of the dystrobrevin-binding gene with schizophrenia in Australian and Indian samples. *Twin Research and Human Genetics, 9*, 531–539.

Holliday, E. G., Nyholt, D. R., Tirupati, S., John, S., Ramachandran, P., Ramamurti, M., et al. (2009). Strong evidence for a novel schizophrenia risk locus on chromosome 1p31.1 in homogeneous pedigrees from Tamil Nadu, India. *American Journal of Psychiatry, 166*, 206–215.

Indian Council of Medical Research-ICMR. (1988). *Factors associated with the course and outcome of schizophrenia: ICMR-multicentred collaborative study*. New Delhi: ICMR.

Issac, M. K., & Kapur, R. L. (1980). A cost effectiveness analysis of three different methods of psychiatric case finding in the general population. *British Journal of Psychiatry, 137*, 540–546.

Iyer, S. N., Mangala, R., Thara, R., & Malla, A. K. (2010). Preliminary findings from a study of first-episode psychosis in Montreal, Canada and Chennai, India: Comparison of outcomes. *Schizophrenia Research, 121*, 227–233.

Jagannathan, A., Hamza, A., Thirthahalli, J., Nagendra, H. R., Hapipraqsad, V. R., & Gangadhar, B. N. (2008). Need of family caregivers of inpatients with schizophrenia in India. In Poster Presentation at the Third International Conference on Schizophrenia (p. 48). October 17–19, 2008, Chennai.

Jain, R., Jain, R. K., & Gurunani, K. C. (1992). Palmar flexion crease in male schizophrenics and their first degree relatives. *Indian Journal of Psychiatry, 34*, 148–154.

Janakiramaiah, N., Gururaj, G., Subbakrishna, D. K., Gangadhar, B. N., Rao, S., & Joseph, M. (1992). Acute psychosis diagnosed as schizophrenia in ICD 9: A discriminant validity study. *Indian Journal of Psychiatry, 34*, 344–346.

Jangid, R. K., & Verma, S. M. (1989). Schizophrenia and season of birth. *Indian Journal of Psychiatry, 31*, 238–241.

Jayakumar, P. N., Venkatasubramanian, G., Gangadhar, B. N., Janakiramaiah, N., & Keshavan, M. S. (2005). Optimized voxel-based morphometry of gray matter volume in first-episode, antipsychotic-naive schizophrenia. *Progress in Neuropsychopharmacology and Biological Psychiatry, 29*, 587–591.

Jayakumar, P. N., Venkatasubramanian, G., Keshavan, M. S., Srinivas, J. S., & Gangadhar, B. N. (2006). MRI volumetric and 31P MRS metabolic correlates of caudate nucleus in antipsychotic-naïve schizophrenia. *Acta Psychiatrica Scandinavica, 114*, 346–351.

Jayakumar, P. N., Gangadhar, B. N., Venkatasubramanian, G., Desai, S., Velayudhan, L., Subbakrishna, D., et al. (2010). High energy phosphate abnormalities normalize after antipsychotic treatment in schizophrenia: a longitudinal 31P MRS study of basal ganglia. *Psychiatry Research, 181*, 237–240.

Jayaswal, S. K., Chawla, H. M., Goulatia, R. K., & Rao, G. S. (1987). Structural changes in the brain in schizophrenia a computed tomographic study. *Indian Journal of Psychiatry, 29*, 229–234.

Jaydeokar, S., Gore, Y., Diwan, P., Deshpande, P., & Desai, N. (1997). Obsessive-compulsive symptoms in chronic schizophrenia: A new idea or an old belief? *Indian Journal of Psychiatry, 39*, 324–328.

Jhingan, H. P., & Munjal, G. C. (1990). Dermatoglyphics in male catatonic schizophrenics. *Indian Journal of Psychiatry, 32*, 198–201.

John, J. P., Shakeel, M. K., & Jain, S. (2008). Corpus callosal area differences and gender dimorphism in neuroleptic-naïve, recent-onset schizophrenia and healthy control subjects. *Schizophrenia Research, 103*, 11–21.

John, J. P., Burgess, P. W., Yashavantha, B. S., Shakeel, M. K., Halahalli, H. N., & Jain, S. (2009). Differential relationship of frontal pole and whole brain volumetric measures with age in neuroleptic-naïve schizophrenia and healthy subjects. *Schizophrenia Research, 109*, 148–158.

John, J. P., Halahalli, H. N., Vasudev, M. K., Jayakumar, P. N., & Jain, S. (2011). Regional brain activation/deactivation during word generation in schizophrenia: fMRI study. *British Journal of Psychiatry, 198*, 213–222.

Kale, A., Joshi, S., Pillai, A., Naphade, N., Raju, M., Nasrallah, H., et al. (2009). Reduced cerebrospinal fluid and plasma nerve growth factor in drug-naïve psychotic patients. *Schizophrenia Research, 115*, 209–214.

Kashyap, K., Thunga, R., Rao, A. K., & Balamurali, N. P. (2012). Trends of utilization of government disability benefits among chronic mentally ill. *Indian Journal of Psychiatry, 54*, 54–58.

Kate, N., Grover, S., Kulhara, P., & Nehra, R. (2012). Supernatural beliefs, aetiological models and help seeking behaviour in patients with schizophrenia. *Industrial Journal of Psychiatry, 21*, 49–54.

Kate, N., Grover, S., Kulhara, P., Nehra, R. (2013) Relationship of quality of life with coping and burden in primary caregivers of patients with schizophrenia. International Journal of Social Psychiatry. January 3, 2013 (Epub ahead of print).

Kisore, P., Lal, N., Trivedi, J. K., Dalal, P. K., & Aga, V. M. (1994). A study of comorbidity in psychoactive substance dependence patients. *Indian Journal of Psychiatry, 36*, 133–137.

Kondaiah, P., Murthy, K. K., & Reddy, O. S. (1981). Plasma creatine Phosphokinase in schizophrenia. *Indian Journal of Psychiatry, 23*, 351–352.

Kota, S. K., & Kulhara, P. (1988). A clinical study of positive and negative subtypes of schizophrenia. *Indian Journal of Psychiatry, 30*, 355–361.

Kota, S. K., Kulhara, P., Joseph, S., & Nagpal, R. S. (1986). Inter-rater reliability of the scale for assessment of negative symptoms in schizophrenia. *Indian Journal of Psychiatry, 28*, 349–350.

Krishnadas, R., Moore, B. P., Nayak, A., & Patel, R. R. (2007). Relationship of cognitive function in patients with schizophrenia in remission to disability: A cross-sectional study in an Indian sample. *Annals of General Psychiatry, 30*, 6–19.

Kujur, N. S., Kumar, R., & Verma, A. N. (2010). Differences in levels of disability and quality of life between genders in schizophrenia remission. *Indian Psychiatry Journal, 19*, 50–54.

Kukreti, R., Tripathi, S., Bhatnagar, P., Gupta, S., Chauhan, C., Kubendran, S., et al. (2006). Association of DRD2 gene variant with schizophrenia. *Neuroscience Letters, 392*, 68–71.

Kukshal, P., Bhatia, T., Bhagwat, A. M., Gur, R. E., Gur, R. C., Deshpande, S. N., et al. (2013). Association study of neuregulin-1 gene polymorphisms in a north Indian schizophrenia sample. *Schizophrenia Research, 144*, 24–30.

Kulhara, P., & Avasthi, A. (2003). Influence of depressive symptoms and premorbid adjustment on factor structure of phenomenology of schizophrenia: A study from India. *European Psychiatry, 18*, 226–232.

Kulhara, P., & Chandiramani, K. (1990). Positive and negative subtypes of schizophrenia. A follow-up study from India. *Schizophrenia Research, 3*, 107–116.

Kulhara, P., Chandiramani, K., Mattoo, S. K., & Awasthi, A. (1986a). A phenomenological study of delusions in schizophrenia. *Indian Journal of Psychiatry, 28*, 281–286.

Kulhara, P., Kota, S. K., & Joseph, S. (1986b). Positive and negative subtypes of schizophrenia. A study from India. *Acta Psychiatrica Scandinavica, 74*, 353–359.

Kulhara, P., Mattoo, S. K., Chandiramani, K., Bhave, S., & Avasthi, A. (1986c). Diagnostic systems for schizophrenia. A cross-sectional study of concordance from India. *Acta Psychiatrica Scandinavica, 74*, 55–61.

Kulhara, P., Mattoo, S. K., Awasthi, A., & Chandiramani, K. (1987). Psychiatric manifestations of Catego class + schizophrenia. *Indian Journal of Psychiatry, 29*, 307–313.

Kulhara, P., Avasthi, A., & Chandiramani, K. (1989a). Prognostic variables in schizophrenia. *Indian Journal of Psychiatry, 31*, 51–62.

Kulhara, P., Avasthi, A., Chadda, R., Chandiramani, K., Mattoo, S. K., Kota, S. K., et al. (1989b). Negative and depressive symptoms in schizophrenia. *British Journal of Psychiatry, 154*, 207–211.

Kulhara, P., Avasthi, A., Gupta, N., Das, M. K., Nehra, R., Rao, S. A., et al. (1998). Life events and social support in married schizophrenics. *Indian Journal of Psychiatry, 40*, 376–382.

Kulhara, P., Avasthi, A., & Sharma, A. (2000). Magico-religious beliefs in schizophrenia: A study from north India. *Psychopathology, 33*, 62–68.

Kulhara, P., Avasthi, A., Grover, S., Sharan, P., Sharma, P., Malhotra, S., et al. (2010). Needs of schizophrenia patients. *Social Psychiatry and Psychiatric Epidemiology, 45*, 809–818.

Kumar, A., & Khess, C. R. (2012). Factor analysis of positive and negative syndrome scale in schizophrenia: An exploratory study. *Indian Journal of Psychiatry, 54*, 233–238.

Kumar, S., Kulhara, P., Grover, S., & Malhotra, R. (2006). Preliminary experiences with use of disability assessment scales at mental disability clinic, PGIMER, Chandigarh. *Journal of Mental Health and Human Behavior, 11*, 39–43.

Kurup, R. A., Augustine, J., & Kurup, P. A. (1999). Hypothalamic digoxin and schizophrenia—a model for conscious and subliminal perception and its dysfunction in schizophrenia. *Indian Journal of Psychiatry, 41*, 197–203.

Kuruvilla, K., Kuruvilla, A., & Kanagasabapathy, A. S. (1986). Serum prolactin levels in schizophrenia effects of neuroleptic medication—a preliminary study. *Indian Journal of Psychiatry, 28*, 237–243.

Lal, R., & Sharma, S. (1987). Minor physical anomalies in schizophrenia. *Indian Journal of Psychiatry, 29*, 119–123.

Lal, N., Tiwari, S. C., Srivastava, S., Khalid, A., & Siddharatha, K. N. (1998). Neurological soft signs, cognitive dysfunction and ventricular brain ratio in schizophrenics. *Indian Journal of Psychiatry, 40*, 180–185.

Lobana, A., Mattoo, S. K., Basu, D., & Gupta, N. (2001). Quality of life in schizophrenia in India: comparison of three approaches. *Acta Psychiatrica Scandinavica, 104*, 51–55.

Lobana, A., Mattoo, S. K., Basu, D., & Gupta, N. (2002). Convergent validity of quality of life interview (qoli) in an Indian setting: preliminary findings. *Indian Journal of Psychiatry, 44*, 118–124.

Loganathan, S., & Murthy, S. R. (2008). Experiences of stigma and discrimination endured by people suffering from schizophrenia. *Indian Journal of Psychiatry, 50*, 39–46.

Malhotra, S., Gupta, N., Bhattacharya, A., & Kapoor, M. (2006). Study of childhood onset schizophrenia (COS) using SPECT and neuropsychological assessment. *Indian Journal of Psychiatry, 48*, 215–223.

Mazumdar, P. K., Chaturvedi, S. K., & Gopinath, P. S. (1988). A study of thought, language and communication (T.L.C) disorders in schizophrnia. *Indian Journal of Psychiatry, 30*, 263–275.

McCreadie, R. G., Thara, R., Kamath, S., Padmavathy, R., Latha, S., Mathrubootham, N., et al. (1996). Abnormal movements in never-medicated Indian patients with schizophrenia. *British Journal of Psychiatry, 168*, 221–226.

McCreadie, R. G., Padmavati, R., Thara, R., & Srinivasan, T. N. (2002). Spontaneous dyskinesia and parkinsonism in never-medicated, chronically ill patients with schizophrenia: 18-month follow-up. *British Journal of Psychiatry, 181*, 135–137.

McCreadie, R. G., Thara, R., Srinivasan, T. N., & Padmavathi, R. (2003). Spontaneous dyskinesia in first-degree relatives of chronically ill, never-treated people with schizophrenia. *British Journal of Psychiatry, 183*, 45–49.

McLean, D., John, S., Barrett, R., McGrath, J., Loa, P., Thara, R., et al. (2012). Refining clinical phenotypes by contrasting ethnically different populations with schizophrenia from Australia, India and Sarawak. *Psychiatry Research, 196*, 194–200.

Ministry of Social Justice and Empowerment, Government of India. (2002). Guidelines for evaluation and assessment of mental illness and procedure for certification. (No. 16-18/97-NI). Available at: http://www.ccdisabilities.nic.in/page.php?s=reg&p=guidemental&t=pb#maincont.

Mishra, D. K., Alreja, S., Sengar, K. S., et al. (2009). Insight and its relationship with stigma in psychiatric patients. *Indian Psychiatry Journal, 18*, 39–42.

Mohan, I., Tandon, R., Kalra, H., & Trivedi, J. K. (2005). Disability assessment in mental illnesses using Indian disability evaluation assessment scale (IDEAS). *Indian Journal of Medical Research, 121*, 759–763.

Mukherjee, O., Meera, P., Ghosh, S., Kubendran, S., Kiran, K., Manjunath, K. R., et al. (2006). Evidence of linkage and association on 18p11.2 for psychosis. *American Journal of Medical Genetics B Neuropsychiatr Genetics, 141*, 868–873.

Murthy, N. (1965). Disturbances in communication in the schizophrenic. *Indian Journal of Psychiatry, 7*, 167–171.

Murthy, S. R. (2005). *Perspectives on the stigma of mental illness. Stigma of mental illness in the third world.* Geneva: World Psychiatric Association.

Murthy, R. S., Anuradha, D., Pershad, D., & Wig, N. N. (1975). Psychiatric disability Scale. Preliminary report. *Indian Journal of Clinical Psychology, 2*, 183.

Nagarajaiah, P., Murthy, R. S., Sekar, K., Puttamma, M., Moily, S., & Kishore Kumar, K. V. (1997). Needs of persons with schizophrenia in a rural community. *Indian Journal of Psychiatry, 39*(Suppl), 23.

Nagaswami, V., Valecha, V., Thara, R., Rajkumar, S., & Menon, M. S. (1985). Rehabilitation needs of schizophrenic patients: A preliminary report. *Indian Journal of Psychiatry, 27*, 213–220.

Nandi, D. N., Ajmany, S., Ganguly, H., et al. (1975). Psychiatric disorder in a rural community in West Bengal—an epidemiological study. *Indian Journal Psychiatry, 17*, 87–90.

Neogi, R. (2010). Health care needs of patients with bipolar disorder. MD Thesis submitted to PGIMER.

Nizamie, S. H., Nizamie, A., Sangma, M. W., & Sharma, P. L. (1989). Soft neurological signs and minor physical anomalies in schizophrenia. *Indian Journal of Psychiatry, 31*, 230–238.

Padmavati, R. (2001). Structural (MRI) brain differences between never treated schizophrenia patients with and without dyskinesia and normal control subjects. *Indian Journal of Psychiatry, 43*, 1.

Padmavati, R., Thara, R., & Corin, E. (2005). A qualitative study of religious practices by chronic mentally ill and their caregivers in South India. *International Journal of Social Psychiatry, 51*, 139–149.

Pahuja, S., Aboobacker, S., & Shini, V. K. (2011). Schizophrenia—cost of illness. *International Journal of Pharmaceutical Sciences Review and Research, 6*, 55–59.

Pandey, R. S., Rao, B. S. S., Subash, M. N., Krishna, D. K., & Srinivas, K. N. (1987). Central dopamine and serotonin turnover in schizophrenia. *Indian Journal of Psychiatry, 29*, 203–213.

Parkar, S. R., Seethalakshmi, R., & Shah, H. (2006). Structural brain lesions in schizophrenia—magnetic resonance imaging on a mid field magnet. *Indian Journal of Radiology Imaging, 16*(3), 299–301.

Ponnudurai, R. (1989). Schizophrenia—a genetic study. *Indian Journal of Psychiatry, 31*, 219–221.

Ponnudurai, R., & Jayakar, J. (2010). Mode of transmission of schizophrenia. *Asian Journal of Psychiatry, 3*, 67–72.

Ponnudurai, R., Menon, S., & Muthu, M. (1997). Dermatoglyphic fluctuating asymmetry and symmetry in familial and non familial schizophrenia. *Indian Journal of Psychiatry, 39*, 205–211.

Pradhan, N., Harihar, C., Das, P., & Andrade, C. (1992). Heterogeneity in plasma homovanillic acid levels in schizophreniform disorder. *Indian Journal of Psychiatry, 34*, 128–132.

Pradhan, B. K., Chakrabarti, S., Nehra, R., & Mankotia, A. (2008). Cognitive functions in bipolar affective disorder and schizophrenia: comparison. *Psychiatry and Clinical Neurosciences, 62*, 515–525.

Radhakrishnan, R., Menon, J., Kanigere, M., Ashok, M., Shobha, V., & Galgali, R. B. (2012). Domains and determinants of quality of life in schizophrenia and systemic lupus erythematosus. *Indian Journal of Psychological Medicine, 34*, 49–55.

Raguram, R., Weiss, M. G., Keval, H., et al. (2001). Cultural dimensions of clinical depression in Bangalore, India. *Anthropology and Medicine, 8*, 31.

Raguram, R., Raghu, T. M., Vounatsou, P., et al. (2004). Schizophrenia and the cultural epidemiology of stigma in Bangalore, India. *Journal of Nervous and Mental Disease, 192*, 734–744.

Raj, S. M., & Raguram, R. (2001). Neurotic symptoms in schizophrenia. *Indian Journal of Psychiatry, 43*, 4.

Rajender, G., Kanwal, K., Rathore, D. M., & Chaudhary, D. (2009). Study of cenesthesias and body image aberration in schizophrenia. *Indian Journal of Psychiatry, 51*, 195–199.

Rajkumar, S., & Thara, R. (1989). Factors affecting relapse in schizophrenia. *Schizophrenia Research, 2*, 403–409.

Rajkumar, R. P., Reddy, Y. C., & Kandavel, T. (2008). Clinical profile of "schizo-obsessive" disorder: A comparative study. *Comprehensive Psychiatry, 49*, 262–268.

Raju, S. S. (1986). Depressive disorders in schizophrenia. *Indian Journal of Psychiatry, 28*, 109–118.

Ramanathan, A. (1983). A study of experienced reality of auditory hallucinations in schizophe-renics. *Indian Journal of Psychiatry, 25*, 148–154.

Ramanathan, A. (1986). An exploratory study on the relation between neuroticism and certain aspects of auditory hallucinations in schizophrenics. *Indian Journal of Psychiatry, 28*, 69–73.

Rammohan, A., Rao, K., & Subbakrishna, D. K. (2002). Religious coping and psychological well-being in carers of relatives with schizophrenia. *Acta Psychiatrica Scandinavica, 105*, 356–362.

Rao, N., Gopinath, P. S., Jayasimha, N., Rao, B. S. S., & Subbakrishna, D. K. (1985). Serum immunoglobulins and schizophrenia. *Indian Journal of Psychiatry, 27*, 325–329.

Rao, N. P., Venkatasubramanian, G., Arasappa, R., & Gangadhar, B. N. (2011). Relationship between corpus callosum abnormalities and schneiderian first-rank symptoms in antipsychotic-naive schizophrenia patients. *Journal of Neuropsychiatry and Clinical Neurosciences, 23*, 155–162.

Saddichha, S., Sur, S., Sinha, B. N., & Khess, C. R. (2010). How is substance use linked to psychosis? A study of the course and patterns of substance dependence in psychosis. *Substance Abuse, 31*, 58–67.

Saravanan, B., Jacob, K. S., Johnson, S., Prince, M., Bhugra, D., & David, A. S. (2007). Belief models in first episode schizophrenia in South India. *Social Psychiatry and Psychiatric Epidemiology, 42*, 446–451.

Saravanan, B., Jacob, K. S., Deepak, M. G., Prince, M., David, A. S., & Bhugra, D. (2008). Perceptions about psychosis and psychiatric services: A qualitative study from Vellore, India. *Social Psychiatry and Psychiatric Epidemiology, 43*, 231–238.

Sartorius, N., Jablensky, A., Korten, A., et al. (1986). Early manifestations and first contact incidence of schizophrenia in different cultures. *Psychological Medicine, 16*, 909–928.

Seethalakshmi, R., Parkar, S. R., Nair, N., Batra, S. A., Pandit, A. G., Adarkar, S. A., et al. (2007). Regional brain metabolism in schizophrenia: The influence of antipsychotics. *Journal of Postgraduate Medicine, 53*, 241–246.

Sengupta, S., & Bhuyan, S. D. (1995). Palmar dermatoglyphics in schizophrenia. *Indian Journal of Psychiatry, 37*, 86–90.

Sethi, B. B., Gupta, S. C., & Kumar, R. (1967). A psychiatric study of 300 urban families. *Indian Journal of Psychiatry, 9*, 280–302.

Sethi, B. B., Gupta, S. C., & Kumar, R. (1972). A psychiatric survey of 500 rural families. *Indian Journal of Psychiatry, 14*, 183–186.

Sethi, B. B., Gupta, S. C., Mahendru, R. K., et al. (1974). Mental health and urban life. A study of 850 families. *British Journal of Psychiatry, 124*, 293.

Sethi, B. B., Gupta, S. C., & Trivedi, J. K. (1980). Psychiatric morbidity among parents of schizophrenic patients. *Indian Journal of Psychiatry, 22*, 217–224.

Shah, R., Kulhara, P., Grover, S., Kumar, S., Malhotra, R., & Tyagi, S. (2011). Relationship between spirituality/religiousness and coping in patients with residual schizophrenia. *Quality of Life Research, 20*, 1053–1060.

Shankar, R., Kamath, S. (1991). Needs based interventions with families of the chronic mentally ill. Presented at the Congress of the World Association of Psychosocial Rehabilitation, Montreal. October 14–18, 1991.

Sharma, I., Kumar, A., & Chansouria, J. P. (1990). Platelet MAO activity in subgroups of schizophrenia. *Indian Journal of Psychiatry, 32*, 324–330.

Sharma, I., Kumar, A., Chansouria, J. N., & Varma, S. L. (1991). Clinical variables and platelet MAO in schizophrenia. *Indian Journal of Psychiatry, 33*, 271–280.

Shrivastava, A., & Tamhane, M. (2000). Serum prolactin level and severity of psychopathology in patients of schizophrenia. *Indian Journal of Psychiatry, 42*, 49–51.

Shrivastava, A., Sarkel, G., & Iyer, S. (2001). Experience of working with relatives of schizophrenia: evolving caregivers program for advocacy and intervention. *Indian Journal of Psychiatry, 43*(Suppl), 105.

Shrivastava, A., Johnston, M. E., Thakar, M., et al. (2011). Origin and impact of stigma and discrimination in schizophrenia—patients' perception: Mumbai study. *Stigma Research and Action, 1*, 67–72.

Siddharatha, N. L., Tewari, S. C., Dalal, P. K., Kohli, N., & Srivastava, S. (1997). A computed tomographic study of schizophrenia. *Indian Journal of Psychiatry, 39*, 115–121.

Singh, M. V. (1971). A psychometric approach to schizophrenic thought disorders. *Indian Journal of Psychiatry, 13*, 113–118.

Singh, S. P., & Kulhara, P. (1991). Simple schizophrenia: Patients in search of a diagnosis. *Indian Journal of Psychiatry, 33*, 266–270.

Singh, G., & Sachdava, J. S. (1982). Schizo affective psychoses—are they schizophrenic? *Indian Journal of Psychiatry, 24*, 42–49.

Singh, G., Sharan, P., & Kulhara, P. (2003). Phenomenology of hallucinations: A factor analytic approach. *Psychiatry and Clinical Neurosciences, 57*, 333–336.

Singh, N. H., Sharma, S. G., & Pasweth, A. M. (2005). Psychiatric co-morbidity among alcohol dependents. *Indian Journal of Psychiatry, 47*, 222–224.

Singh, B., Banerjee, S., Bera, N. K., Nayak, C. R., & Chaudhuri, T. K. (2008a). Analysis of the role of human leukocyte antigen class-I genes to understand the etiopathology of schizophrenia. *Indian Journal of Psychiatry, 50*, 166–171.

Singh, O. P., Chakraborty, I., Dasgupta, A., & Datta, S. (2008b). A comparative study of oxidative stress and interrelationship of important antioxidants in haloperidol and olanzapine treated patients suffering from schizophrenia. *Indian Journal of Psychiatry., 50*, 171–176.

Singh, B., Bera, N. K., Nayak, C. R., & Chaudhuri, T. K. (2009). Decreased serum levels of interleukin-2 and interleukin-6 in Indian Bengalee schizophrenic patients. *Cytokine, 47*, 1–5.

Singh, T. B., Kaloiya, G. S., Kumar, S., & Chadda, R. K. (2010). Rehabilitation need assessment of severely mentally ill and effect of intervention. *Delhi Psychiatry Journal, 13*, 109–116.

Sinha, V. K., & Chaturvedi, S. K. (1990). Consistency of delusions in schizophrenia and affective disorder. *Schizophrenia Research, 3*, 347–350.

Solanki, R. K., Singh, P., Midha, A., & Chugh, K. (2008). Schizophrenia: Impact on quality of life. *Indian Journal of Psychiatry, 50*, 181–186.

Solanki, R. K., Singh, P., Midha, A., Chugh, K., & Swami, M. K. (2010a). Disability and quality of life in schizophrenia and obsessive compulsive disorder: A cross-sectional comparative study. *East Asian Archives of Psychiatry, 20*, 7–13.

Solanki, R. K., Singh, P., Midha, A., Chugh, K., & Swami, M. K. (2010b). Disability and quality of life in schizophrenia and obsessive compulsive disorder: A cross-sectional comparative study. *East Asian Archives Psychiatry, 20*, 7–13.

Somaiya, M., Grover, S., Avasthi, A., & Chakrabarti, S. (2014a). Comparative study of cost of care of Bipolar disorder and schizophrenia: A study from India. *Asian J Psychiatr*. 2014 Aug 19. pii: S1876-2018(14)00191-9. doi: 10.1016/j.ajp.2014.08.003. [Epub ahead of print]

Somaiya, M., Grover, S., Avasthi, A., & Chakrabarti, S. (2014b). Changes in the cost of treating schizophrenia in India: A comparison of two studies done a decade apart. Psychiatry Research, *215*, 547–553

Sovani, A., Thatte, S., & Deshpande, C. G. (2005). Felt affect in good- and poor-outcome schizophrenia. *Indian Journal of Psychiatry, 47*, 27–30.

Srinivasan, N. (2000). Families as partners in care. Perspectives from AMEND. *Indian Journal of Social Work, 61*, 352–365.

Srinivasan, T. N., & Thara, R. (2001). Beliefs about causation of schizophrenia: Do Indian families believe in supernatural causes? *Social Psychiatry and Psychiatric Epidemiology, 36*, 134–140.

Srinivasan, T. N., & Thara, R. (2002). Smoking in schizophrenia—all is not biological. *Schizophrenia Research, 56*, 67–74.

Srinivasan, L., & Tirupati, S. (2005). Relationship between cognition and work functioning among patients with schizophrenia in an urban area of India. *Psychiatric Services, 56*, 1423–1428.

Srivastava, V., Varma, P. G., Prasad, S., Semwal, P., Nimgaonkar, V. L., Lerer, B., et al. (2006). Genetic susceptibility to tardive dyskinesia among schizophrenia subjects: IV. Role of dopaminergic pathway gene polymorphisms. *Pharmacogenetics and Genomics, 16*, 111–117.

Srivastava, V., Deshpande, S. N., & Thelma, B. K. (2010). Dopaminergic pathway gene polymorphisms and genetic susceptibility to schizophrenia among north Indians. *Neuropsychobiology, 61*, 64–70.

Surya, N. C., Datta, S. P., Gopalakrishna, R., et al. (1964). *Mental morbidity in Pondicherry* (pp. 50–61). Transaction of All India Institute of Mental Health: Bangalore.

Talkowski, M. E., Mansour, H., Chowdari, K. V., Wood, J., Butler, A., Varma, P. G., et al. (2006). Novel, replicated associations between dopamine D3 receptor gene polymorphisms and schizophrenia in two independent samples. *Biological Psychiatry, 60*, 570–577.

Thacore, V. R., & Gupta, S. (1975). Psychiatric morbidity in a North Indian Community. *British Journal of Psychiatry, 126*, 364.

Thakral, S., Mishra, N., & Bhatia, T. (2011). Cost of major mental disorders in Delhi India. *Asian Journal of Psychiatry, 4*, 155–156.

Thara, R. (2005a). Perspective from an NGO. *Indian Journal of Psychiatry, 47*, 212–214.

Thara, R. (2005b). Measurement of psychiatric disability. *Indian Journal of Medical Research, 121*, 723–724.

Thara, R., & Joseph, A. A. (1995). Gender differences in symptoms and course of schizophrenia of schizophrenia. *Indian Journal of Psychiatry, 37*, 124–128.
Thara, R., & Rajkumar, S. (1992). Gender differences in schizophrenia. Results of a follow-up study from India. *Schizophrenia Research, 7*, 65–70.
Thara, R., & Rajkumar, S. (1993). Nature and course of disability in schizophrenia. *Indian Journal of Psychiatry, 35*, 33–35.
Thara, R., & Srinivasan, T. N. (1997). Marriage and gender in schizophrenia. *Indian Journal of Psychiatry, 39*, 64–69.
Thara, R., & Srinivasan, T. N. (2000). How stigmatizing is schizophrenia in India? *International Journal of Social Psychiatry, 46*, 135–141.
Thara, R., Rajkumar, S., & Valecha, V. (1988). The schedule for assessment of psychiatric disability—a modification of the DAS-II. *Indian Journal of Psychiatry, 30*, 47–55.
Thara, R., Kamath, S., & Kumar, S. (2003a). Women with schizophrenia and broken marriages-doubly disadvantaged? Part I: Patient perspective. *International Journal of Social Psychiatry, 49*, 225–232.
Thara, R., Kamath, S., & Kumar, S. (2003b). Women with schizophrenia and broken marriages –doubly disadvantaged? Part I: Family perspective. *International Journal of Social Psychiatry, 49*, 233–240.
Thara, R., Srinivasan, T., John, S., Nancarrow, D., Chant, D., Holliday, E., et al. (2009). Design and clinical characteristics of a homogeneous schizophrenia pedigree sample from Tamil Nadu. *Indian, Australian, New Zealand Journal of Psychiatry, 43*, 561–570.
Tharyan, P., & Kuruvilla, K. (1994). The correlates of the syndrome of depression in schizophrenia. *Indian Journal of Psychiatry, 36*, 74–78.
Tharyan, A., & Saravanan, B. (2000). Insight and psychopathology in schizophrenia. *Indian Journal of Psychiatry, 42*, 421–426.
The Rehabilitation Committee of the Indian Psychiatric Society. (2002). *IDEAS (Indian disability evaluation and assessment scale)—A scale for measuring and quantifying disability in mental disorders*. India: Indian Psychiatric Society.
Thirthalli, J., Venkatesh, B. K., Kishorekumar, K. V., Arunachala, U., Venkatasubramanian, G., Subbakrishna, D. K., et al. (2009). Prospective comparison of course of disability in antipsychotic-treated and untreated schizophrenia patients. *Acta Psychiatrica Scandinavica, 119*, 209–217.
Thirthalli, J., Venkatesh, B. K., Naveen, M. N., Venkatasubramanian, G., Arunachala, U., Kishore Kumar, K. V., et al. (2010). Do antipsychotics limit disability in schizophrenia? A naturalistic comparative study in the community. *Indian Journal of Psychiatry, 52*, 37–41.
Thomas, P., Mathur, P., Gottesman, I. I., Nagpal, R., Nimgaonkar, V. L., & Deshpande, S. N. (2007). Correlates of hallucinations in schizophrenia: A cross-cultural evaluation. *Schizophrenia Research, 92*, 41–49.
Thomas, P., Chandra, A., Bhatia, T., Mishra, N. N., Sharma, V. R., Gauba, D., et al. (2011). Clinical and genetic correlates of severity in schizophrenia in India: an ordinal logistic regression approach. *Psychiatry Research, 189*, 321–323.
Tirupati, N. S., Rangaswamy, T., & Raman, P. (2004). Duration of untreated psychosis and treatment outcome in schizophrenia patients untreated for many years. *Australian and New Zealand Journal of Psychiatry, 38*, 339–343.
Tirupati, S. N., Padmavati, R., Thara, R., & McCreadie, R. G. (2006). Psychopathology in never-treated schizophrenia. *Comprehensive Psychiatry, 47*, 1–6.
Tiwari, S. G., Lal, N., Trivedi, J. K., Sayeed, J., & Bahauguna, L. M. (1984). Immunoglobulin patterns in schizophrenic patients. *Indian Journal of Psychiatry, 26*, 223–229.
Tiwari, A. K., Deshpande, S. N., Rao, A. R., Bhatia, T., Mukit, S. R., Shriharsh, V., et al. (2005). Genetic susceptibility to tardive dyskinesia in chronic schizophrenia subjects: I. Association of CYP1A2 gene polymorphism. *Pharmacogenomics J, 5*, 60–69.
Trivedi, J. K., & Sethi, B. B. (1978). Drug abuse in psychiatric patients. *Indian Journal of Psychiatry, 21*, 345–348.
Varma, V. K., Suri, A. K., & Kaushal, P. (1973). Abstract thinking in schizophrenia. *Indian Journal of Psychiatry, 15*, 123–131.

Varma, V. K., Ghosh, A., & Murthy, R. S. (1977). Pseudo-neurotic schizophrenia: Incidence and phenomenology in India. *Indian Journal of Psychiatry, 19*, 24–30.

Venkatasubramanian, G., Jayakumar, P. N., Gangadhar, B. N., Janakiramaiah, N., Subbakrishna, D. K., & Keshavan, M. S. (2003). Measuring the corpus callosum in schizophrenia: A technique with neuroanatomical and cytoarchtectural basis. *Neurol India, 51*, 189–192.

Venkatasubramanian, G., Jayakumar, P. N., Gangadhar, B. N., & Keshavan, M. S. (2008). Automated MRI parcellation study of regional volume and thickness of prefrontal cortex (PFC) in antipsychotic-naïve schizophrenia. *Acta Psychiatrica Scandinavica, 117*, 420–431.

Venkatasubramanian, G., Jayakumar, P. N., Reddy, V. V., Reddy, U. S., Gangadhar, B. N., & Keshavan, M. S. (2010a). Corpus callosum deficits in antipsychotic-naïve schizophrenia: Evidence for neurodevelopmental pathogenesis. *Psychiatry Research, 182*, 141–145.

Venkatasubramanian, G., Chittiprol, S., Neelakantachar, N., Shetty, T. K., & Gangadhar, B. N. (2010b). A longitudinal study on the impact of antipsychotic treatment on serum leptin in schizophrenia. *Clinical Neuropharmacology, 33*, 288–292.

Venkatasubramanian, G., Arasappa, R., Rao, N. P., Behere, R. V., Kalmady, S., & Gangadhar, B. N. (2010c). Inverse relationship between serum high density lipoprotein and negative syndrome in antipsychotic-naive schizophrenia. *Clinical Chemistry and Laboratory Medicine, 48*, 95–98.

Venkatasubramanian, G., Chittiprol, S., Neelakantachar, N., Shetty, T., & Gangadhar, B. N. (2010d). Effect of antipsychotic treatment on insulin-like growth factor-1 and cortisol in schizophrenia: A longitudinal study. *Schizophrenia Research, 119*, 131–137.

Venkatasubramanian, G., Jayakumar, P. N., Keshavan, M. S., & Gangadhar, B. N. (2011). Schneiderian first rank symptoms and inferior parietal lobule cortical thickness in antipsychotic-naïve schizophrenia. *Progress in Neuropsychopharmacology and Biological Psychiatry, 35*, 40–46.

Venkatesan, J., & Suresh, S. S. D. (2008). Substance dependence: decades apart in a teaching hospital. *Indian Journal of Psychiatry, 50*, 100–105.

Verghese, A., Beig, A., Senseman, L. A., et al. (1973). A social psychiatric study of a representative group of families in Vellore town. *Indian Journal of Medical Research, 61*, 608–620.

Verma, R., Mukerji, M., Grover, D., B-Rao, C., Das, S. K., Kubendran, S., et al. (2005a). MLC1 gene is associated with schizophrenia and bipolar disorder in Southern India. *Biological Psychiatry, 58*, 16–22.

Verma, R., Kubendran, S., Das, S. K., Jain, S., & Brahmachari, S. K. (2005b). SYNGR1 is associated with schizophrenia and bipolar disorder in southern India. *Journal of Human Genetics, 50*(635–40), 37.

Vibha, P., Saddichha, S., Khan, N., & Akhtar, S. (2013). Quality of life and marital adjustment in remitted psychiatric illness: An exploratory study in a rural setting. *Journal of Nervous Mental Disease, 201*, 334–338.

Vijayan, N. N., Iwayama, Y., Koshy, L. V., Natarajan, C., Nair, C., Allencherry, P. M., et al. (2009). Evidence of association of serotonin transporter gene polymorphisms with schizophrenia in a South Indian population. *Journal of Human Genetics, 54*, 538–542.

Vohra, A. K., Yadav, B. S., & Khurana, H. (2003). A study of psychiatric morbidity in alcohol dependence. *Indian Journal of Psychiatry, 45*, 247–250.

Wig, N. N. (2010). Schizophrenia: The Indian scene keynote address. In P. Kulhara, A. A. Vasthi, & S. Grover (Eds.), *Schizophrenia Indian scene* (2nd ed.). Chandigarh: PSYPROM, PGIMER.

Wig, N. N., Murthy, R. S., & Pershad, D. (1979). Relationship of disability with psychiatric diagnosis and treatment acceptance patterns. *Indian Journal of Psychiatry, 21*, 355–358.

World Health Survey, India. (2003). Health system Performance Assessment, International Institute for Population Sciences (IIPS), Mumbai, World Health Organisation, Geneva, World Health Organisation-India-WR Office, New Delhi. July 2006.

Chapter 10
Schizophrenia: Indian Research: II—Treatment Issues

Parmanand Kulhara, Sandeep Grover and Natasha Kate

1 Treatment and Related Issues

Researchers from India have kept pace with rest of the world to evaluate the efficacy and effectiveness of various treatments used in the management of schizophrenia. Additionally, the research has also focused on other treatment-related issues such as treatment compliance/adherence, attitude towards treatment and side effects of various treatments. It is very difficult to discuss in detail about all the aspects, and we would discuss most of the issues in brief and present the recent trends in research on various treatment-related issues.

Antipsychotics: Over the years, many researchers from India have evaluated the efficacy and effectiveness of various antipsychotic medications. Additionally, authors have also reported on the side effects of various antipsychotic medications in the Indian context. The research focusing the usefulness of antipsychotics in India has more or less followed the trends in the West; however, some of the newer antipsychotics drugs, which are currently marketed, have not been evaluated as thoroughly as others. Moreover, the quality of studies in terms of research design, sample size and duration of evaluation has been in general below the level of satisfaction. Various studies, which have evaluated antipsychotics in India, have been reviewed earlier (Avasthi et al. 2010). This review suggests that first-generation antipsychotics have been mostly evaluated in open-label trials, with occasional double-blind randomized controlled trials. However, available data suggest that typical antipsychotics are useful for the treatment of schizophrenia, typical

P. Kulhara, Consultant Psychiatrist; S. Grover, Assistant Professor; N. Kate, Formerly Senior Resident

P. Kulhara (✉) · S. Grover · N. Kate
Department of Psychiatry, Postgraduate Institute of Medical Education and Research, Chandigarh, India
e-mail: paramkulhara@yahoo.co.in

S. Malhotra and S. Chakrabarti (eds.), *Developments in Psychiatry in India*,
DOI 10.1007/978-81-322-1674-2_10

antipsychotics are more efficacious than placebo in the treatment of schizophrenia, and improvement is seen more in paranoid and catatonic symptoms and aggression and less so in depressive symptoms. Data also suggest that extrapyramidal symptoms are common with typical antipsychotics (Avasthi et al. 2010).

Some of the open-label non-comparative trials have also evaluated the efficacy of depot first-generation antipsychotics in schizophrenia. Most of these trials included subjects who were non-complaint to oral medications and had frequent relapses. These studies have shown that depot antipsychotics are useful in the management of schizophrenia in the acute phase and are also useful for maintenance treatment. However, most of these trials have been of short duration (2–4 weeks), except for one which evaluated the outcome at 1–3 years (Shukla 1981).

Studies, which have compared the efficacy/effectiveness of typical antipsychotics with either electroconvulsive therapy (ECT) alone or a combination of ECT and typical antipsychotic medication, suggest that typical antipsychotic alone, or when used in combination with ECT, produces similar response rate in short term; however, addition of ECT leads to a faster response. The only study that evaluated the efficacy of ECT and chlorpromazine in treatment-resistant schizophrenia (TRS) showed that augmentation with ECT in TRS may be a worthwhile option (Goswami et al. 2003).

Studies evaluating the efficacy/effectiveness of second-generation antipsychotics have, in general, used better study designs than studies evaluating the efficacy of first-generation antipsychotics. Among the various second-generation antipsychotics, risperidone has been evaluated more frequently than other medications, followed by clozapine. Occasional studies have also looked at the usefulness of olanzapine, aripiprazole and quetiapine. However, most of these trials have been of short duration, with exception of one trial, which evaluated the outcome on risperidone at 1 year (Shrivastava and Gopa 2000), and two studies, which followed up subjects on clozapine for 20 months and 3 years, respectively (Srivastava et al. 2002; Raguraman et al. 2005). All the studies, which have evaluated clozapine, have done so in patients with TRS and have reported it to be useful in both short and long terms. Data also suggest that risperidone is efficacious in the treatment of schizophrenia in short term. Studies, which have compared risperidone with other antipsychotics, have shown it to be more efficacious than quetiapine, but as efficacious as haloperidol and centbutindole. Agarwal and Chadda (2001) demonstrated that there was no difference in efficacy of once-daily dose versus twice-daily dose of risperidone. The study, which followed up the subjects on risperidone for 1 year, showed that compared to haloperidol, more subjects on risperidone had better social functioning, productivity and education, and significantly fewer patients had suicidal ideation or attempts and needed rehospitalization. Srivastava et al. (2001) showed that half of the subjects with schizophrenia in India required 3–4 mg/day of risperidone and another one-third improve with dose ranging from 1 to 2 mg/day. Data also suggest that olanzapine is as efficacious as haloperidol (Avasthi et al. 2001). The study, which evaluated the efficacy of different doses of aripiprazole, suggested that there were no differences in efficacy of 10 and 15 mg/day of aripiprazole (Sarin et al.

2004). One small study evaluated the usefulness of clozapine in childhood-onset schizophrenia (Malhotra et al. 2000).

Besides the efficacy or usefulness studies, some studies have specifically evaluated the side effects and tolerability issues with antipsychotics (Avasthi et al. 2010). In one of the earliest studies, Sarada Menon and Rarnachandra (1972) reported side effects of subjects who participated in two of their drug trials and had received either trifluoperazine or trifluperidol. Other studies have evaluated the rates of skin pigmentation with phenothiazines (Ananth et al. 1972), rise in prolactin levels with chlorpromazine and trifluoperazine and changes in serum electrolytes (Kuruvilla et al. 1986). Studies have reported prevalence rates of akathisia (25–28 %), tardive dyskinesia (5–25.5 %) and dystonia (17 %) in subjects receiving typical antipsychotics (Pandurangi et al. 1978; Ray et al. 1992; Datta et al. 1994; Suresh Kumar and Manoj Kumar 1997). Studies have also evaluated the incidence of neuroleptic malignant syndrome (Chopra et al. 1999; Sarkar et al. 2009) and extrapyramidal side effects with risperidone (Basu et al. 2000). A study by Pandey et al. (1992) compared the rate of neuroleptic-induced acute dystonia and reported that there was no difference in vulnerability to develop dystonias in subjects with mania or schizophrenia. A recent study showed that clozapine dose, caffeine intake and valproate comedication influence the serum clozapine levels. Further, this study showed that serum clozapine levels above 750 ng/ml increased the risk of seizures (odds ratio 5.15; $p = 0.03$) (Rajkumar et al. 2013). Studies have also shown that use of typical antipsychotics leads to higher rates of sexual dysfunction (Nagaraj et al. 2004; Nebhinani et al. 2012), and among the atypical antipsychotics, sexual desire is more frequently impaired in subjects on risperidone and erectile dysfunction is more prevalent in subjects on olanzapine (Nagaraj et al. 2001).

Metabolic syndrome: Metabolic syndrome (MS) has emerged as an important area of research in the recent years. Many studies from India have evaluated the prevalence of MS in patients with schizophrenia. Cross-sectional studies from India, which have evaluated drug-naïve patients with schizophrenia, have reported prevalence rates to vary from 4 to 26 % among them (Padmawati et al. 2010; Pallava et al. 2012; Grover et al. 2012d). Studies, which have compared drug-naïve patients with healthy control groups, have in general reported lower prevalence in the drug-naïve patients compared to healthy control groups (Grover et al. 2012d). Besides MS, occasional studies have evaluated the prevalence of subthreshold MS (i.e. patients fulfilling one to two criteria of MS) and have reported that 30 % patients fulfilled two criteria and 41 % fulfilled one criterion of MS (Grover et al. 2012). These studies also show that prevalence of MS is high in those who are married, of higher age and have higher level of education (Grover et al. 2012d). In a series of longitudinal studies involving drug-naïve patients with schizophrenia, authors reported baseline prevalence of MS to vary from 3.3 to 9.5 %, which increased to 32–52 % after 3 months of antipsychotic treatment (Sahoo et al. 2007a, b; 2008), with the highest increase seen in patients receiving olanzapine, followed by risperidone, and least with haloperidol (Sahoo et al. 2008). Cross-sectional studies, which have evaluated the patients with schizophrenia on treatment, have reported prevalence rates of MS to be in the range of 34–47 % (Grover et al. 2011b,

2012a, 2013; Kagal et al. 2012; Subashini et al. 2011). Studies, which have used comparison groups, suggest that prevalence rate in patients with schizophrenia is higher than that seen in the healthy controls (Subashini et al. 2011), but lower than that seen in patients with bipolar disorder (Grover et al. 2013). Correlates of MS in patients on treatment include urban locality, being employed, longer duration of illness, higher age and higher education (Grover et al. 2011b, 2012a). The most common abnormalities noted include high waist circumference, followed by raised blood pressure/lipid abnormalities, and raised blood glucose level is the least common abnormality noted (Grover et al. 2011b, 2012).

Longitudinal studies, which have evaluated the patients on treatment, suggest that with 4 months of treatment, the highest incidence of MS is seen in those who are receiving olanzapine (23 %), followed by clozapine (13 %), risperidone (10 %) and none in the haloperidol group (Gautam and Meena 2011). One study specifically assessed the incidence and prevalence of MS in patients considered for clozapine. Prior to starting clozapine, the prevalence of MS was 33 %, which increased to 53 % after 3 months of clozapine treatment (Nebhinani et al. 2013). In one of the longest longitudinal study from India, the authors noted an increase in prevalence rate by 9 % among patients (Malhotra et al. 2013). These longitudinal studies have also shown that there is high rate of conversion to MS in those with pre-existing abnormalities (Nebhinani et al. 2013; Malhotra et al. 2013).

From the above research, it can be concluded that prevalence of MS increases in drug-naïve patients with use of antipsychotics and prevalence increases after switching to clozapine. Prevalence also increases significantly in those receiving olanzapine and risperidone. Further, the evidence suggests a high rate of conversion to MS in those with subthreshold symptoms. Hence, clinicians must be judicious while choosing antipsychotic medications in patients with schizophrenia. A 12-week double-blind, parallel-group study showed that topiramate may be useful in the prevention of olanzapine-associated weight gain and metabolic abnormalities in patients with schizophrenia (Narula et al. 2010).

Pharmacogenomics: With increasing interest in the role of genetic factors in the treatment response and side effects of medications, studies from India have tried to address the genetic links of tardive dyskinesia, treatment response and severity of psychopathology (Tiwari et al. 2005; Vijayan et al. 2007; Thomas et al. 2008; Gupta et al. 2009, 2013). However, the findings are preliminary and inconclusive. Tiwari et al. (2005) evaluated the role of six single nucleotide polymorphisms (SNP) in tardive dyskinesia and showed that CYP1A2 1545 C > T SNP was associated with tardive dyskinesia and schizophrenia, but the association was rendered insignificant after corrections for multiple comparisons. Vijayan et al. (2007) studied various alleles, genotypes, haplotypes and their linkage disequilibrium and observed that H313HTT genotype was associated with schizophrenia and TaqIB1B1 genotype was significantly associated with higher psychopathology scores. Subjects with H313HCC, TaqIA2A2 and Taq1D1D1 had higher mean improvement scores. Distinct shift in the linkage disequilibrium pattern of responder and non-responder groups was observed. Thomas et al. (2008) reported that average olanzapine dose, baseline weight and dopamine receptor D4

(DRD4-120 bp) duplication marker had significant associations with the efficacy index. Gupta et al. (2009) reported significant allelic associations of two SNPs (rs4633 and rs4680) with drug response. Gupta et al. (2013) attempted to elucidate a genetic signature, which could predict patients' response to atypical monotherapy, and showed that 76 % patients carrying a combination of four SNPs did not show favourable response to atypical antipsychotics. A recent study evaluated the role P-glycoprotein (ABCB1) polymorphism in understanding the effectiveness of antipsychotic medications in schizophrenia and reported that patients with favourable homozygous genotypes of rs1045642 and rs2032582 display better response with increased dosage, while those carrying the risk genotype manifest refractoriness on increased dosage (Vijayan et al. 2012).

Predictors of treatment response: A study reported that subjects, who showed initial dysphoric response to a test dose of neuroleptic, later respond poorly to the neuroleptics (Borde et al. 1991). Shrivastava et al. (2012) evaluated antipsychotic-naïve patients with schizophrenia at baseline and at 5-year follow-up and showed that higher baseline serum prolactin levels were associated with better outcome at 5 years. In a recent study, the authors showed a possible relationship between clinical improvement in symptoms of schizophrenia and antipsychotic-induced neuroleptic dysphoria as well as metabolic side effects in schizophrenia (Venkatasubramanian et al. 2013).

Impact of antipsychotics on disability: In a recently published study, which compared three groups of community-dwelling subjects with schizophrenia, mean disability scores remained virtually unchanged in those who remained untreated, but showed a significant decline (indicating decrement in disability) in those who continued to receive antipsychotics and in those in whom antipsychotic treatment was initiated. The proportion of patients classified as "disabled" declined significantly in the treated group, but remained the same in the untreated group (Thirthalli et al. 2009).

Prescription patterns: Some studies have focused on the antipsychotic prescription patterns, and these suggest that antipsychotic prescriptions vary from centre to centre and possibly have changed over the years. In one of the earliest studies, Khanna et al. (1990) evaluated the psychotropic drug prescription pattern in chronic long-stay patients at Ranchi and compared the prescription trends in 1984 and 1988. Most of the patients whose prescriptions were reviewed were suffering from schizophrenia. More than one antipsychotic medication was prescribed in 13 % of patients in 1984, which fell down to 7 % in 1988. Moreover, it was seen that very few patients received anticholinergic agents, and the use of benzodiazepines increased over the years (4 % in 1984 and 10 % in 1988), which the authors attributed to the development of distressing tardive dyskinesia over the years (Khanna et al. 1990). Another study from St. Johns Medical College, Bangalore, reviewed the discharge prescription of all patients of schizophrenia during the period January 2003–December 2003. Risperidone was the most commonly prescribed antipsychotic (56 %), followed by olanzapine (21 %) and quetiapine (4 %). Typical antipsychotics were used only in 16 % of the patients, and polypharmacy (concurrent use of more than one antipsychotic) was seen in 9 % of the patients

(Padmini et al. 2007). In contrast to most of the studies from other parts of India, a study from Jammu evaluated the prescription of 270 outpatients, during the period January 2004 to June 2004, and reported that a fixed-dose formulation of trifluoperazine, chlorpromazine and trihexyphenidyl (parkinforte) was most commonly used drug, and this was followed by chlorpromazine and quetiapine. The authors also found that typical antipsychotics were used in 83 % of the patients and polypharmacy was seen in 73 % of the patients (Sawhney et al. 2005). Trivedi et al. (2010) from Lucknow reviewed the prescription of 100 outpatients and reported that olanzapine was the most commonly used antipsychotic medication (64 %), followed by risperidone (48 %) and flupenthixol decanoate injections (17 %). Typical antipsychotics were used in 41 % of the patients, and polypharmacy was seen in 55 % of the patients (Trivedi et al. 2010). Another study evaluated the prescription patterns in 118 stable subjects with schizophrenia and reported that on average, 2.8 medications were prescribed to each subject and olanzapine was the most commonly prescribed antipsychotic, followed by haloperidol and risperidone. About half of the subjects were receiving more than one antipsychotic (Dutta et al. 2005). In a recent study, Grover et al. (2012c) evaluated the first prescription handed over to more than 10,000 patients attending the psychiatry outpatient clinic of a tertiary care hospital. Irrespective of the diagnosis, olanzapine was the most commonly prescribed antipsychotic, followed by risperidone. Very few patients (8 %) received typical antipsychotic medications. A survey evaluated 168 psychiatrists across India regarding their antipsychotic prescription pattern reported that three most commonly prescribed antipsychotics were risperidone, olanzapine and haloperidol. It was also found that typical antipsychotics are comprised of 25 % (SD = 21.66; range 0–100) of all prescriptions, and in about 23 % of the patients, the psychiatrists were using more than one antipsychotic in the same patient (Grover and Avasthi 2010). A survey specifically assessed the prescribing practices of clozapine. In this survey, only 28 % of psychiatrists reported that their prescription of clozapine was guided by their knowledge about the efficacy of clozapine. Majority of the psychiatrists opined that clozapine leads to symptom reduction to the extent of 40–70 % and the average dose required for stabilization was between 75 and 300 mg/day. Only 16 % of psychiatrists preferred to combine clozapine with other antipsychotics. In terms of blood monitoring, 80 % of the psychiatrists monitored the blood counts weekly in the first month of therapy and then once monthly for the next 6 months, and further monitoring was done as required (Shrivastava and Shah 2009).

Compliance and attitudes towards treatment: Occasional studies have evaluated compliance with appointments and medications, and attitude of patients and their relatives towards medications. Most of the studies evaluating the compliance with appointments have come from PGIMER, Chandigarh. Kulhara (1974) reported that one-fourth of patients with schizophrenia do not come for follow-up after 6 months of detailed assessment and diagnostic clarification, and another one-fourth do not seek any medical help in the next 5 years. Murthy et al. (1974) studied a mixed group of patients (which included subjects with psychosis) and reported that a duration of illness more than 6 months, residence at a distance of more than 50 km from the hospital and psychiatric diagnosis other than functional psychosis favoured treatment discontinuation. With regard to medication adherence, one of the older studies that evaluated the compliance with phenothiazines in patients with psychosis reported a non-adherence rate of 19 % (Ponnudurai et al. 1983). Another study from SCARF, Chennai, reported non-compliance rate of 58 % in patients with schizophrenia during the course of the illness, and half of these subjects were given oral medications at least once without their knowledge by the family members under the psychiatrist's advice (Srinivasan and Thara 2002). It was seen that surreptitious administration of antipsychotic leads to reduction in symptoms in 91 % of subjects and helped convince the patient to take oral medications subsequently. Half of the caregivers who participated in the study felt that surreptitious administration of antipsychotic was the right action under the circumstances (Srinivasan and Thara 2002).

A study from Delhi evaluated the rate of non-compliance with medications and reported that 39 % of patients with schizophrenia were non-compliant with medication. The authors also reported that a majority of the patients and family members had a positive attitude towards medication and treatment. Further, family members were able to identify the compliance status of the patients and the reasons for the non-compliance better than the patients. The factors, which had significant influence on the medication compliance, included perceived daily benefit from medication, positive relationship with the psychiatrist, pressure from the family and the health system and positive family beliefs about the illness and its treatment. Significant reasons for non-compliance were no perceived daily benefit from medications, difficulty in gaining access to treatment and medications, financial obstacles, embarrassment or stigma related to treatment and medications and medicines currently not perceived as necessary (Baby et al. 2009). In another study from Delhi, 120 patients of schizophrenia were evaluated for non-compliance which was defined as the extent to which a person's behaviour did not coincide with medical or nursing advice in the last 6 months. It was found that about 40 % of the patients were non-complaint. Non-compliance was more common in males, in those who were on paid work, were residing in rural areas and were using substances (most common being nicotine, followed by alcohol) (Maheshwari et al. 2009). In a study from Ranchi, which evaluated 100 non-complaint patients with psychiatric disorders (bipolar disorder—42 %; schizophrenia—32 %; psychosis—18 %; obsessive-compulsive disorder—3 %; and epilepsy—5 %), the common reasons for the treatment of non-compliance were financial problems (41 %), distance from the hospital (35 %), improvement in previous symptoms (28 %), side effects of medications (16 %) and older age of caregivers or lack of caregivers (15 %) (Roy et al. 2005). Sharma et al. (2012) showed that among patients with mental disorders, the rate of non-adherence was 38 %, and compared to other disorders, the rate of non-adherence in patients with schizophrenia was higher, i.e. 50 %. Younger patients with good social support had good adherence, whereas those with more severe illnesses and who were sedated were more likely to be non-adherent.

Expectations of patients and caregivers from treatment: Balaji et al. (2012) evaluated the expectations of patients with schizophrenia and their primary caregivers with respect to treatment and reported that social functioning, employment or education, and activity were the most important expected outcomes of both patients and the caregivers. Symptom control and cognitive ability were more important expected outcomes of patients with schizophrenia, while independent functioning and fulfilment of duties were more important from the caregiver's perspective.

Electroconvulsive therapy (ECT): Different surveys done across India and Asia have shown that schizophrenia is the most common indication for ECT in India (Chanpattana et al. 2005, 2010). A recent study that compared ECT practices in Bengaluru and London suggested that compared to London, more inpatients in Bengaluru site were referred for ECT (8 % vs. 0.8 %) and a higher proportion of patients at the Bengaluru site had a diagnosis of schizophrenia (Eranti et al. 2011). Many studies have evaluated the efficacy of ECT in acute-phase treatment of patients with schizophrenia in India. A review and meta-analysis of studies from India, which evaluated the usefulness of a combination of ECT and antipsychotics, included 11 studies and four controlled trials. The review of the 11 studies suggested that combined treatment with ECT and antipsychotics was more efficacious than antipsychotics alone in the initial few weeks of treatment. Meta-analysis of the controlled trials showed that combination of ECT and antipsychotic medications had an advantage over antipsychotics alone during the first four to five weeks of treatment (Painuly and Chakrabarti 2006). A recent study evaluated the effect of ECT on QOL in patients with TRS and showed that ECT leads to significant improvement in all the domains of quality of life, except the domain named satisfaction with social relations (Garg et al. 2011). In patients with schizophrenia, greater intensity of seizures (higher fractional dimension) during initial sessions of ECT is associated with better response at the end of 2 weeks (Abhishekh et al. 2013).

Non-pharmacological interventions: Beneficial effects of add-on yoga therapy on positive and negative symptoms, socio-occupational functioning and facial recognition deficits were noted by Behere et al. (2011). Bhatia et al. (2012) evaluated the role of adjunctive yoga treatment on cognitive remediation in patients with schizophrenia and showed that yoga led to significantly greater improvement with regard to measures of attention following corrections for multiple comparisons; the changes were more prominent among men. A partial double-blind, placebo-controlled, parallel-group design trial concluded that d-serine and computerized cognitive retraining does not have any significant effect on the Global Cognitive Index (D'Souza et al. 2013). In a study, in which more than half of the patients eligible for yoga did not consent to the study, the authors evaluated the barriers to add-on yoga therapy for patients with schizophrenia and suggested that the reasons for refusal were distance from the centre, lack of relative or attendant to accompany the patient for training, busy work schedule, unwillingness to come for 1 month, not willing for yoga therapy, personal reasons and religious reasons (Baspure et al. 2012). Balaji et al. (2012) found an intervention package comprising of five components (psychoeducation; adherence management; rehabilitation; referral to community agencies; and health promotion) for people with schizophrenia delivered by trained lay health workers under the supervision of specialists to be acceptable by the patients as well as beneficial to them.

2 Rehabilitation

Chatterjee et al. (2003) compared community-based rehabilitation (CBR) with outpatient care (OPC) for chronic schizophrenia in the Indian setting. At the end of 1 year, compliance was significantly better in the CBR group; 63 % were fully compliant, compared to 46 % in the outpatient care group. Treatment completer analyses showed that clinical and disability outcomes were superior for the CBR group. This study of community-based rehabilitation for people with chronic schizophrenia provides evidence that CBR is a feasible model of rehabilitation for people with schizophrenia even in economically deprived settings and that outcomes are better, at least for those who are treatment compliant. Murthy et al. (2005) assessed the costs and effects of a community-based outreach programme in rural Karnataka. They visited eight rural communities and identified cases of drug-naive or currently untreated schizophrenia. Summary scores for psychotic symptoms, disability and family burden reduced significantly, with improvement being observed at the first follow-up assessment. Increases in treatment and community outreach costs over the follow-up period were accompanied by reductions in the costs of informal-care sector visits and family care-giving time. The authors concluded that organizing community-based care can bring substantial benefits to patients and families alike. The impact of vocational rehabilitation was studied in 34 patients with chronic schizophrenia, and significant improvement was found in social functioning, cognitive functioning and psychopathology (Suresh Kumar 2008). Chatterjee et al. (2009) evaluated the impact of a CBR programme for people with psychotic disorders in a very-low-resource setting and reported that at 46 months of follow-up, there was a significant reduction in levels of disability with vast majority (83 %) of subjects engaged in the programme. On multivariate analyses, it was seen that lower baseline disability scores, family engagement with the programme, medication adherence and being a member of a self-help group were independent determinants of good outcomes. As part of a project called "Operation Oasis", Banerjee et al. (2009) studied the outcome of major psychiatric illness at 3 years in prison subjects and reported that 10 % of the subjects had major mental illness at baseline. These patients were provided psychiatric treatment and rehabilitation. At 3 years of follow-up, there was significant improvement in the global assessment of functioning compared to baseline. Thara et al. (2008) evaluated the outcome of community care and found that of the 185 patients followed up, 15 % had continued treatment, 35 % had stopped treatment, 21 % had died, 12 % had wandered away from home, and 17 % were untraceable. Of the patients who had discontinued treatment, 25 % were asymptomatic, while 75 % were acutely psychotic. The referral service was used only by 15 % of the patients, and mental health services provided by the primary health centre stopped within a year. The authors concluded that community-based initiatives in the management of mental disorders were not sustainable unless the family and the community are involved in the intervention programme and mental health professionals render regular support.

3 Caregivers' Issues

Caregiver burden: Caregiver burden in schizophrenia is one of the well-researched areas in India. Commonly used instruments to assess the caregiver burden in the Indian context include the Family Burden Interview Schedule (FBI) (Pai and Kapur 1981) and the Burden Assessment Schedule (BAS) (Thara et al. 1998). Recently, some of the studies have also used the Hindi version of Involvement Evaluation Questionnaire (IEQ) (Grover et al. 2011a). Most of the studies have been cross-sectional in design with occasional studies following up the patients. Most of the studies have been conducted among patients and caregivers attending hospitals. Majority of the studies have included patients with chronic illnesses (Rammohan et al. 2002; Agarwal and Chandhok 2007; Ali and Bhatti 1988; Chadda et al. 2007; Chakrabarti and Gill 2002; Chakrabarti and Kulhara 1999; Chakrabarti et al. 1995; Chandrasekaran et al. 2002; Creado et al. 2006; Gautam and Nijhawan 1984; Giel et al. 1983; Gururaj et al. 2008; Jayakumar et al. 2002; Kalra et al. 2009; Kataria et al. 2002; Kiran 2004; Kumar and Mohanty 2007; Kumari et al. 2009; Moily et al. 1997; Nehra et al. 2005, 2006; Nirmala et al. 2011; Pai and Kapur 1982; Raj et al. 1991; Ranga Rao 1988; Rao et al. 1988; Roychaudhuri et al. 1995; Saldanha et al. 2002; Sekaran et al. 2001; Sreeja et al. 2009; Srivastava 2005; Thomas 2004; Vohra et al. 2000). In general, studies have reported high levels of burden perceived by the caregivers of patients with schizophrenia (Agarwal and Chandhok 2007; Ali and Bhatti 1988; Chadda et al. 2007; Chakrabarti and Gill 2002; Chakrabarti and Kulhara 1999; Chakrabarti et al. 1995; Chandrasekaran et al. 2002; Creado et al. 2006; Gautam and Nijhawan 1984; Giel et al. 1983; Gururaj et al. 2008; Jayakumar et al. 2002; Kalra et al. 2009; Kataria et al. 2002; Kiran 2004; Kumar and Mohanty 2007; Kumari et al. 2009; Moily et al. 1997; Nehra et al. 2005, 2006; Nirmala et al. 2011; Pai and Kapur 1982; Raj et al. 1991; Rammohan et al. 2002; Ranga Rao 1988; Rao et al. 1988; Roychaudhuri et al. 1995; Saldanha et al. 2002; Sekaran et al. 2001; Sreeja et al. 2009; Srivastava 2005; Thomas et al. 2008; Vohra et al. 2000). Longitudinal studies show that the burden, though high initially, declines with treatment over 3–6 months (Chadda et al. 2007; Pai and Kapur 1982; Raj et al. 1991; Rao et al. 1988). With regard to various domains of burden, studies have reported high burden in the area of financial burden, effect on family routine and family leisure (Gautam and Nijhawan 1984; Giel et al. 1983; Raj et al. 1991; Saldanha et al. 2002). In many of the studies, the effect on the family is far greater than the financial burden (Chakrabarti et al. 1995; Gururaj et al. 2008; Kiran 2004; Nehra et al. 2006; Raj et al. 1991; Rammohan et al. 2002; Saldanha et al. 2002; Vohra et al. 2000). With regard to the effect of patients' illness on the caregivers' mental and physical health, in general, caregivers report it to be of lesser importance compared to the impact on the family and the financial consequences of care (Chakrabarti et al. 1995; Gautam and Nijhawan 1984; Moily et al. 1997; Nehra et al. 2006; Raj et al. 1991; Roychaudhuri et al. 1995; Saldanha et al. 2002). Studies, which have compared the burden perceived by the caregivers of schizophrenia, have reported this to be higher than the burden perceived by the caregivers of patients with chronic lung disease (Gautam and Nijhawan 1984), affective disorders, (Chakrabarti and Kulhara 1999; Chakrabarti et al. 1995), bipolar disorder, (Chakrabarti and Gill 2002; Roychaudhuri et al. 1995), neurotic disorders (Chakrabarti and Kulhara 1999) and obsessive-compulsive disorder (Agarwal and Chandhok 2007; Gururaj et al. 2008; 2004). However, occasional studies have reported that burden of schizophrenia is comparable to affective disorders (Chadda et al. 2007; Nehra et al. 2006), obsessive-compulsive disorder (Jayakumar et al. 2002; Kalra et al. Thomas et al. 2008), substance dependence (Kiran 2004) and epilepsy (Sreeja et al. 2009). Subjective aspects of burden have been examined far less often, though certain studies have found pattern of high objective and low subjective burden reflecting the caregivers' tolerance and acceptance of the patients' problems (Chakrabarti et al. 1995; Kiran 2004; Nehra et al. 2005; Roychaudhuri et al. 1995). In terms of correlation between high burden and age of the patients, the findings have been inconsistent with some studies reporting high burden to be associated with older age of the patient (Rammohan et al. 2002), whereas others report high burden when the patient is young (Srivastava 2005). Higher burden is associated with patient being male (Roychaudhuri et al. 1995), less educated (Rammohan et al. 2002) and unemployed (Roychaudhuri et al. 1995). With regard to the age of the caregivers, studies suggest that higher burden in perceived by the older caregivers (Rammohan et al. 2002). With regard to gender of the caregivers, studies have reported higher burden in female caregivers (Nehra et al. 2006). Other caregiver variables associated with higher burden include unemployed carers (Jayakumar et al. 2002; Nehra et al. 2006) and those from urban locality (Ranga Rao1988; Srivastava 2005), nuclear families (Kumar and Mohanty 2007), caregivers being unaware about illness (Nehra et al. 2006) and disturbed relationship between patients and the caregiver (Giel et al. 1983).

In terms of clinical correlates of burden, high burden has been most consistently associated with higher levels of dysfunction or disability (Chakrabarti et al. 1995; Creado et al. 2006; Kalra et al. 2009; Kataria et al. 2002; Kiran 2004; Nehra et al. 2005; Pai and Kapur 1982; Raj et al. 1991; Rammohan 2002; Ranga Rao 1988; Sreeja et al. 2009; Thomas 2004), higher severity of symptoms, (Creado et al. 2006; Kalra et al. 2009; Kiran 2004; Pai and Kapur 1982; Raj et al. 1991), higher severity of negative symptoms (Chakrabarti et al. 1995) and longer duration of illness (Vohra et al. 2000).

With regard to various coping strategies, higher burden has been reported to be associated with denial (Rammohan et al. 2002), resignation (Chandrasekaran et al. 2002; Sekaran et al. 2001), avoidance, coercion (Sekaran et al. 2001), emotion-focused coping, (Chakrabarti and Gill 2002; Creado et al. 2006), maladaptive coping (Kiran 2004) and avoidant coping (Chadda et al. 2007). Use of problem-focused coping has been in general associated with lower burden (Rammohan et al. 2002; Creado et al. 2006). Some studies, which have evaluated burden with regard to relationship with patients, have reported that compared to parents, spouses report higher burden (Jayakumar et al. 2002; Rammohan et al. 2002).

Recently, studies have evaluated burden in the stress–appraisal–coping framework by using instruments such as Experience of Caregiving Inventory (ECI) (Szmukler et al. 1996) and the IEQ (Grover et al. 2011a). A study from PGIMER, Chandigarh, which assessed the caregivers on the ECI, reported that caregivers had maximum scores in the domains of handling the difficult behaviour followed by negative symptoms, loss and dependency. This study also for the first time reflected that caregiving can also be associated with positive experiences. Further, this study showed that those caregivers who experienced higher negative consequences of caregiving also reported higher positive caregiving experiences (Aggarwal et al. 2011). Grover et al. (2012b) compared the caregiving experience of caregivers of patients with schizophrenia and bipolar disorder and reported that compared to caregivers of patients with bipolar affective disorder, caregivers of patients with schizophrenia had overall more positive and negative appraisal of caregiving experience, while caring for their ill relatives. There were significant differences too for the total positive personal experience subscore. There was a significant positive correlation between the negative and positive caregiving experience score for both schizophrenia and bipolar groups.

Caregiver distress with symptoms: Few studies have assessed distress in the caregivers associated with specific symptoms of patients. Some of the studies have reported inactivity, not working, lack of participation in household chores, slowness and poor personal hygiene to be more distressing for the relatives, than aggressive or assaultive behaviours (Saldanha et al. 2002; Gopinath and Chaturvedi 1986, 1992), whereas others have reported that florid symptoms, unpredictable and disturbed behaviour, aggression, substance abuse and psychotic symptoms cause greater distress, than the less obvious ones such as depressive, negative or somatic symptoms (Shankar and Kamath 1991; Chakrabarti et al. 2003).

Positive aspects of caregiving: Recently, some of the studies have also evaluated the positive aspects of the caregiving. The first step in this direction was development of a comprehensive scale. From PGIMER, Chandigarh, Kate et al. (2012) developed the "Scale for Positive Aspects of Caregiving Experience (SPACE)" and assessed its psychometric properties. Later, the same group of authors assessed positive aspect of caregiving in a cohort of caregivers of patients with schizophrenia and reported that caregivers had the highest mean score in the domains of motivation for the caregiving role, followed by that of caregiver satisfaction domain, caregiver gains and least in the domain of self-esteem and social aspect of caring. The researchers did not find any relationship between total SPACE score and socio-demographic variables, clinical variables, FBI (except for financial burden), IEQ, social support and coping strategies. There was a negative correlation between the financial burden as assessed by the FBI and the total SPACE score. However, the total SPACE score correlated with quality of life as assessed by WHOQOL-BREF and WHOQOL-SRPB (Kate et al. 2013).

Coping strategies: Studies have evaluated different coping mechanisms used by the caregivers of patients with schizophrenia. Commonly used coping strategies by the caregivers of patients with schizophrenia include help seeking, diversion, religious coping, positive thinking and avoidance (Nagarajaiah et al. 1998), positive communication, increasing patient's social involvement (Bhargava et al. 2001), resignation (Chakrabarti and Kulhara 1999), negative distraction (among spouses), denial (among parents) (Padmavati et al. 2005), problem-solving (Thara et al. 2008; Creado et al. 2006; Rammohan et al. 2002), emotion-focused coping (Chakrabarti and Gill 2002; Nehra et al. 2005), consulting doctors, talking to friends or family and seeking practical help (Nehra et al. 2005), positive reappraisal, escape avoidance (Kiran 2004) and fatalism (Creado et al. 2006). Studies comparing coping strategies used by the caregivers of patients with schizophrenia with other disorders suggest lack of difference between schizophrenia and physical illnesses (Nagarajaiah et al. 1998) and obsessive-compulsive disorder (Agarwal and Chandhok 2007). Another study done on caregivers of patients with bipolar disorder and schizophrenia revealed that emotion-focused strategies were more commonly employed in caregivers of patients with schizophrenia (Chakrabarti and Gill 2002). Caregiver's gender, patient dysfunction and caregiver neuroticism had a significant influence on coping patterns (Nehra et al. 2005). Singh et al. (2003) evaluated distress related to auditory hallucinations and coping strategies used and concluded that distress due to hallucinations in schizophrenia is determined by severity of hallucinations (stressor) and problem-solving coping strategies. Studies also suggest that higher caregiver burden is associated with the use of resignation, (Chandrasekaran et al. 2002; Sekaran et al. 2001), coercion, (Chandrasekaran et al. 2002) denial (Rammohan et al. 2002), emotion-focused coping (Chakrabarti and Gill 2002; Creado et al. 2006), maladaptive coping (Kiran 2004), and avoidance (Chadda et al. 2007).

Expressed Emotions: Wig et al. (1987) and Leff et al. (1987) studied expressed emotions (EE) in relatives of patients with schizophrenia in India (Chandigarh), Denmark (Aarhus) and the UK (London) and sought to explore its relationship with relapse over a follow-up period of 1 year. It was observed that greater numbers of relatives of schizophrenia patients in Chandigarh were categorized as low EE, as compared to relatives of similar patients in Denmark or the UK. Also, relatives of Chandigarh patients were less critical, less overinvolved than the Anglo-Danish relatives. It was further observed that over a period of 1-year follow-up, significantly more relapses occurred in the high EE families compared with low EE families.

Family intervention: Many studies have evaluated the efficacy and effectiveness of family intervention in schizophrenia (Chacko 1967; Narayanan et al. 1972, 1988; Pai and Kapur 1983; Pai and Roberts 1983; Pai et al. 1985; Verghese 1988; Ismail Shihabuddeen and Gopinath 2005; Thara et al. 2005; Kulhara et al. 2009; Sovani 1993; Devaramane et al. 2011; Patra et al. 2011). These studies have used different kinds of interventions such as home-based treatment by nurse, treatment in the family ward, family psychoeducation, brief inpatient intervention and single-session psychoeducation. Some of the studies have compared the structured family education versus flexible need-based intervention (Thara et al. 2005), psychoeducation versus standard outpatient care (Kulhara et al. 2009) and home-based treatment versus inpatient treatment (Pai and Roberts 1983; Pai et al. 1985). Other studies have used the unique method of 1-day psychoeducation programme (Sovani 1993), or single-session psychoeducation programme (Patra et al. 2011), and three 1-h sessions (Devaramane et al. 2011). These studies reflect that family psychoeducation for schizophrenia (addressing optimal medication management and addressing the family's feelings of loss) leads to reduction in the rates of relapse, which is significantly more than that seen in the control groups. Benefits are also noted in the form of reduction in burden, functioning, symptom reduction, rate of hospitalization, knowledge and attitude, use of better coping skills, treatment adherence, drug compliance, disability, caregiver satisfaction and caregiver support (Chacko 1967; Narayanan et al. 1972, 1988; Pai and Kapur 1983; Pai and Roberts 1983; Pai et al. 1985; Verghese 1988; Ismail Shihabuddeen and Gopinath 2005; Thara et al. 2005; Kulhara et al. 2009; Sovani 1993; Devaramane et al. 2011).

4 Course and Outcome

Studies from different centres of India, in general, suggest that compared to the Western countries, the course and outcome of schizophrenia are better in the Indian context. In one of the first studies from India, Kulhara and Wig (1978) reported 5-year outcome of patients with schizophrenia attending the psychiatric unit in the setting of a general hospital and showed that 29 % of patients had no disturbance, 16 % were improving, 23 % patients had episodic course, and 32 % had continued to be ill. India was part of the World Health Organization (WHO)-funded International Pilot Study of Schizophrenia (IPSS) (World Health Organisation 1979), the Determinants of Outcome of Severe Mental Disorders (DOSMeD) study (Sartorius et al. 1986) and the International Study of Schizophrenia (Hopper and Wanderling 2000). Few studies were funded by Indian Council of Medical Research (ICMR 1988), and many researchers followed up the original cohorts of the WHO-funded studies from time to time to understand the outcome of schizophrenia in the Indian context. In the IPSS study, 2-year follow-up revealed that centres at Agra, Cali and Ibadan had more asymptomatic patients compared to Aarhus, London and Washington patients. Patients in Agra, Cali and Ibadan had spent less period of follow-up in psychotic episodes compared to patients from Aarhus, Washington and London. Agra, Cali and Ibadan had more patients who fell in the category of "best course", and patients in Aarhus, London and Washington had more patients belonging to "worst course" category. Greater number of patients in Aarhus, Washington and London had severe social impairment compared with patients in Agra, Cali and Ibadan. Overall outcome was remarkably more favourable for patients in developing countries, i.e. in patients from India, Nigeria and Colombia. Five-year follow-up of the IPSS cohort confirmed that the outcome of schizophrenia in developing countries continued to be better than that in developed countries (Sartorius et al. 1987; Leff et al. 1992). The DOSMeD study was launched with a view to obtain accurate estimates of prevalence and incidence of schizophrenia in different cultures and evidence about the outcome of this disorder in different countries of the world. It recruited first-contact patients from 12 centres in 10 different countries, and some centres were in developing countries (India–Chandigarh and Agra, Colombia, Nigeria) and some in developed countries (Denmark, Ireland, USA, Japan, UK, USSR and Czechoslovakia). Chandigarh had 2 field centres, one for urban population and the other for rural. At 2-year follow-up, 54 % of patients in Agra, 42 % of Chandigarh (rural) patients and 27 % of Chandigarh (urban) patients had single episode, followed by complete remission. Continuous psychotic illness was seen in 18 % of Agra patients, 4 % of Chandigarh (rural) patients and 10 % of Chandigarh (urban) patients. Compared with patients in developed countries, Agra and Chandigarh patients had more favourable 2-year course and outcome. Agra and Chandigarh (both urban and rural) patients had less impairment of social functioning compared with patients from developed countries. The findings from India were comparable to other developing countries, and more patients in these countries fell in the category of "best possible" outcome compared with patients from developed countries (Sartorius et al. 1986). After the IPSS and the DOSMeD, the WHO launched the International Study of Schizophrenia (ISoS) (Hopper and Wanderling 2000; Harrison et al. 2001; Sartorius et al. 1996), which provided the opportunity to follow up the cohorts from the DOSMeD and Assessment and Reduction of Psychiatric Disability (RAPyD) studies after 15 years and those from the IPSS after 25 years from intake assessments. Results of the ISoS showed that outcome of schizophrenia was poor compared to other psychoses across all domains; still, 50 % of them were rated as "recovered", and only one-third of them were continuously ill. In terms of predictors of outcome, it was seen that the "percentage of time experiencing psychotic symptoms in first 2 years of illness after onset" was the strongest predictor of symptoms and disability scores at follow-up; the less the percentage of time with psychotic symptoms, the better the longer-term symptoms and disability scores, as well as overall course of the illness. A CART analysis of the data also showed that pattern of course in the first 2 years was also related to long-term pattern of course (Hopper and Wanderling 2000; Wiersma et al. 2000).

The ICMR (ICMR 1988; Verghese et al. 1989)-sponsored study had three centres at Vellore and Madras in South India and at Lucknow in North India. At 2-year follow-up, it was seen that most of the patients (62 %) had spent 15 % or less of the follow-up period in the psychotic state, and only about 4 % had spent more than 75 % of the follow-up period in psychotic state. "Best" pattern of course was observed in 45 % of the patients, and "worst" pattern of course was seen in only 10 % of the patients. As regards occupational outcome, 40 % of the patients were rated to have no occupational impairment. Social outcome was also observed to be more favourable with nearly 34 % of the patients displaying no social impairment. Assessment of overall outcome revealed that 66 % of the patients had favourable overall outcome and only 4 % of the patients had unfavourable outcome. The rest had intermediate outcome. Intercentre comparison did not show any significant variability (ICMR 1988).

Besides these studies, many individual research groups have attempted to study the course and outcome of schizophrenia. Kulhara and Chandiramani (1988) published the results of 18–30 months of follow-up of patients with diagnosis of schizophrenia according to ICD-9 and other definitions of schizophrenia. At follow-up, 66 % of the patients had improved, and the rest had either no change or had worsened. Similarly, 66 % of the patients had improving or episodic course, and the rest had a static or deteriorating course; 56 % were working with or without impairment, and the rest were not working. Overall, there were only minor differences in outcome across different diagnostic criteria for schizophrenia. On the basis of this, the authors concluded that outcome does not distinguish diagnostic systems for schizophrenia, implying that the course and outcome are not dependent on the conceptual framework of diagnosis, but are influenced more by clinical and background variables. Mojtabai et al. (2001) followed up the two incidence cohorts of the DOSMeD study in urban and rural Chandigarh at 15 years by using the life chart schedule and found that patients with a poor 2-year course (a continuous psychotic illness) had very poor prognosis in the long term. It was further seen that the effect of a poor 2-year course on poor long-term outcome persisted even after controlling for the potential effects of gender, urban/rural setting, narrow versus broad definitions of schizophrenia and the interval between onset and intake into the study. In addition, high rate of morality (47 %) was seen among those with a poor 2-year course. Dube et al. (1984) re-evaluated the IPSS, and a cohort of patients of schizophrenia was recruited from Agra after 13–14 years in an attempt to delineate the long-term course and outcome of the patients. They found that nearly 60 % of the patients were normal. In addition, it was found even those who did not recover completely, did have periods of recovery, and in those with a continuous course, the disorder usually lost its intensity.

Thara et al. (1994) reported extended 10-year follow-up of patients of first-onset patients with schizophrenia, who were originally recruited for the ICMR multicentred collaborative study. Various types of patterns of course were described, complete remission after the initial psychotic episode (11 out of 76 patients), two patients had no relapses but continued to have residual symptoms, 37 patients had one or more relapses with complete remissions, 21 patients had one or more relapses, but incomplete recovery, and 5 patients were described to have been continuously ill. The authors concluded that the pattern of course was largely favourable. The authors also noted that there was a general decline in both positive and negative symptoms during the 10-year period of follow-up. One study prospectively evaluated patients with schizophrenia every year over a period of 10 years with occupational outcome as an indicator of the functional status of patients. Overall, 53 % of the patients had good occupational outcome (Srinivasan and Thara 1997). Thara (2004) also followed up the same cohort after 20 years to assess the course of symptomatology, work, social functioning and pattern of illness. Of the initial cohort of 96 patients, 67 % of the sample was assessed at 20 years. After 20 years, 5 patients had recovered completely, another 5 were continuously ill, and most of the cohort had multiple relapses with or without complete remission between them. The Global Assessment of Functioning Scale showed that symptoms and social functioning in this sample were much better than those observed in developed nations. Marriage and occupational rates were higher than those observed in many published reports. The authors concluded that clinical and social outcomes were still distinctly superior to those observed in developed countries. Recently, 25-year follow-up of the same cohort was presented. Out of the original cohort of 96 patients, 47 could be reassessed. Twenty-five had died, and 18 were lost to follow-up; 32 of the 47 of the followed-up patients were in partial or total remission. Outcome was good in 28 %, intermediate in 52 % and poor in 19 %. More men were single, and more women were either married or separated. In a 10-year longitudinal follow up study, Shrivastava et al. (2010) showed that compared to non-recovered group, mean duration of untreated psychosis was longer for a group, which showed clinical recovery as assessed on the Clinical Global Impression Scale. A recent study evaluated the predictors of 5-year outcome of patients with schizophrenia and reported that level of insight, number of non-medical explanatory models and individual explanatory models held during the later course of the illness have a significant impact on the outcome (Johnson et al. 2012).

Other outcome measures: Ponnudurai et al. (2006) followed up 121 patients with schizophrenia, of which 60 were reassessed at 13 years with regard to mortality and cause of death. Seven deaths were recorded, and the standardized mortality ratio for all the age groups was 54.2. Unnatural causes of death accounted for 2 out of 7 deaths, one of which was accidental and other was suicide. A recent study reported the long-term outcome (10 year) of schizophrenia and did not find any relationship between duration of untreated psychosis and good clinical or social outcome (Shrivastava et al. 2010). Similar were the observations of Gupta et al. (2010). In a recent study, the authors evaluated the 4-year outcome of schizophrenia in the form of work functioning by using the "Work" section of the Indian Disability Evaluation and Assessment Scale (IDEAS) in a rural South Indian community. They reported that 27 % were working as agriculturists, 29 % were pursuing household jobs, 14 % were working as daily wage labourers, and 13 % were not doing any sort of work. Further, the authors noted that there was a significant reduction in disability. Regression analysis showed that work-related disability was significantly associated with male gender, longer duration of illness, higher psychopathology and poor treatment adherence (Suresh et al. 2012). Using open-ended questions regarding patient's perceptions of indicators of recovery, Thara (2012) showed that most of the patients (88 % of the respondents) equate recovery with the absence of symptoms and not having any more relapses (73 %). Other common themes associated with recovery were getting back to their regular lives in terms of functioning (70 %), being able to handle the associated responsibilities (62 %) and lack of further need to take medications (65 %).

5 Research on Special Populations

Childhood-onset schizophrenia: In the recent times, many studies have evaluated various aspects of schizophrenia having onset in childhood and adolescence. With regard to epidemiology, clinic-based studies suggest a prevalence rate of

2.4–7.5 % for schizophrenia and other related psychotic disorders (Malhotra et al. 2007; Sagar et al. 2012). Many studies from different centres across the country have described the socio-demographic and clinical profile of childhood-onset schizophrenia (COS) (Sagar et al. 2012; Reddy et al. 1996; Thakur et al. 2003; Srivastava et al. 1988; Sharma et al. 2005). A study from Ranchi evaluated children and adolescents with schizophrenia and related disorders, or mood disorders on the PANSS; factor analysis of the scales showed a four-factor model comprising primary negative, secondary negative, manic and paranoid factors (Thakur et al. 2003). A study from PGIMER compared three groups of patients with schizophrenia, i.e. childhood-onset schizophrenia (COS), adolescent-onset schizophrenia (AdOS) and adult-onset schizophrenia (AOS). Compared to the other groups, patients with COS had significantly higher rate of socio-economic dependence, poorer academic performance, non-paranoid subtype, poorer outcome, poorer response to typical antipsychotics, significantly more number of soft neurological signs, significantly greater deficits on scales of IQ, memory and perceptuomotor skills, the highest PANSS score and more somatic and obsessive symptoms (John et al. 2008; Biswas et al. 2006a, b). A study from PGIMER, Chandigarh, also evaluated the cerebral cortical perfusion defects by using single-photon emission computed tomography (SPECT) imaging in patients with childhood-onset schizophrenia (COS) and showed that a majority of patients had perfusion anomaly specifically in the left temporal and frontal areas of the brain (Malhotra et al. 2006).

Late-onset schizophrenia: Kulhara et al. (1999) compared the clinical features of late-onset schizophrenia (LOS) and early-onset schizophrenia (EOS) and found that the LOS group had higher scores only on “persecutory delusions”, which led them to conclude that the findings did not support the diagnostic validity of LOS. Similarly, Harish et al. (1996) showed that the commonest symptoms were persecutory delusions, followed by delusions of influence, and hallucinations in any modality in a group of patients with LOS.

6 Conclusions

Over the years, there has been significant progress in research on schizophrenia from India. With the emergence of pharmacotherapy, many studies evaluated the efficacy of various antipsychotics in patients with schizophrenia. Studies evaluating various aspects of caregivers and family have been done and show that family remains an important support for the patients of schizophrenia. However, except for the early studies, most of the studies have been done at single centres and on small sample sizes. It is expected that in future, multicentric studies involving more number of patients and their caregivers will strengthen the research evidence.

References

Abhishekh, H. A., Thirthalli, J., Manjegowda, A., Phutane, V. H., Muralidharan, K., & Gangadhar, B. N. (2013). Ictal EEG fractal dimension in ECT predicts outcome at 2 weeks in schizophrenia. *Psychiatry Research, 209*, 155–159.

Agarwal, V., & Chadda, R. K. (2001). Once daily dose in treatment of schizophrenia. *Indian Journal of Psychiatry, 43*, 32–35.

Agarwal, K. M., & Chandhok, R. (2007). Comparison of burden and coping in caregivers of persons with schizophrenia and obsessive compulsive disorder. *Indian Journal of Psychiatry, 49*(Suppl), 16.

Aggarwal, M., Avasthi, A., Kumar, S., & Grover, S. (2011). Caregiving experience in Schizophrenia: A study from India. *International Journal of Social Psychiatry, 57*, 224–236.

Ali, R. M., & Bhatti, R. S. (1988). Social support system and family burden due to chronic schizophrenia in rural and urban background. *Indian Journal of Psychiatry, 30*, 349–353.

Ananth, J. V., Ban, T. A., Lehmann, H. E., & Rizvi, F. A. (1972). A survey of phenothiazine induced skin pigmentation. *Indian Journal of Psychiatry, 14*, 76–80.

Avasthi, A., Agarwal, M., Grover, S., & Khan, M. K. R. (2010). Research on antipsychotics in India. *Indian Journal of Psychiatry, 52*(Suppl), S317–S340.

Avasthi, A., Kulhara, P., & Kakkar, N. (2001). Olanzapine in treatment of schizophrenia: An open label comparative clinical trial from India. *Indian Journal of Psychiatry, 43*, 257–263.

Baby, R. S., Gupta, S., & Sagar, R. (2009). *Attitudes and subjective reasons of medication compliance and noncompliance among outpatients with schizophrenia in India* (p. 7). Internet: Internet Journal of Epidemiology.

Balaji, M., Chatterjee, S., Koschorke, M., Rangaswamy, T., Chavan, A., Dabholkar, H., et al. (2012). The development of a lay health worker delivered collaborative community based intervention for people with schizophrenia in India. *BMC Health Services Research, 12*, 42.

Banerjee, A., Sengupta, P., & Ray, T. K. (2009). Persons with major psychiatric illness in prisons—A three years study. *Journal of the Indian Medical Association, 107*, 14–16.

Baspure, S., Jagannathan, A., Kumar, S., Varambally, S., Thirthalli, J., Venkatasubramanain, G., et al. (2012). Barriers to yoga therapy as an add-on treatment for schizophrenia in India. *International Journal of Yoga, 5*, 70–73.

Basu, D., Mattoo, S. K., Khurana, H., Malhotra, S., & Kulhara, P. (2000). Risperidone—Truly non-cataleptogenic? *Hong Kong Journal of Psychiatry, 10*, 2–5.

Behere, R. V., Arasappa, R., Jagannathan, A., Varambally, S., Venkatasubramanian, G., Thirthalli, J., et al. (2011). Effect of yoga therapy on facial emotion recognition deficits, symptoms and functioning in patients with schizophrenia. *Acta Psychiatrica Scandinavica, 123*, 147–153.

Bhargava, S. C., Kataria, D. K., & Vohra, A. K. (2001). The coping strategies in the families of schizophrenic patients. *Indian Journal of Psychiatry, 43*(Suppl), 113.

Bhatia, T., Agarwal, A., Shah, G., Wood, J., Richard, J., Gur, R. E., et al. (2012). Adjunctive cognitive remediation for schizophrenia using yoga: An open, non-randomized trial. *Acta Neuropsychiatry, 24*, 91–100.

Biswas, P., Malhotra, S., Malhotra, A., & Gupta, N. (2006a). Comparative study of neuropsychological correlates in schizophrenia with onset in childhood, adolescence and adulthood. *European Child and Adolescent Psychiatry, 15*, 360–366.

Biswas, P., Malhotra, S., Malhotra, A., & Gupta, N. (2006b). A Comparative Study of Clinical Correlates in Schizophrenia with Onset in Childhood, Adolescence and Adulthood. *Journal of Indian Association for Child and Adolescent Mental Health, 2*, 18–30.

Borde, M., Davis, E. J. B., & Sharma, L. N. (1991). Prediction of outcome in schizophrenia using the subjective response to a test dose of a neuroleptic. *Indian Journal of Psychiatry, 33*, 58–61.

Chacko, R. (1967). Family participation in the treatment and rehabilitation of the mentally ill. *Indian Journal of Psychiatry, 9*, 328–333.

Chadda, R. K., Singh, T. B., & Ganguly, K. K. (2007). Caregiver burden and coping. A prospective study of relationship between burden and coping in caregivers of patients with schizophrenia and bipolar affective disorder. *Social Psychiatry and Psychiatric Epidemiology, 42*, 923–930.

Chakrabarti, S., & Gill, S. (2002). Coping and its correlates among caregivers of patients with bipolar disorder: A preliminary study. *Bipolar Disorders, 4*, 50–60.

Chakrabarti, S., & Kulhara, P. (1999). Family burden of caring for people with mental illness. *British Journal of Psychiatry, 174*, 463.

Chakrabarti, S., Nehra, R., & Sharma, S. (2003). Distress associated with symptoms of schizophrenia and bipolar disorder: The caregiver's perspective. *Journal of Mental Health Human Behaviour, 8*, 39–50.

Chakrabarti, S., Raj, L., Kulhara, P., Avasthi, A., & Verma, S. K. (1995). A comparison of the extent and pattern of family burden in affective disorders and schizophrenia. *Indian Journal of Psychiatry, 37*, 105–112.

Chandrasekaran, R., Sivaprakash, B., & Jayestri, S. R. (2002). Coping strategies of the relatives of schizophrenia patients. *Indian Journal of Psychiatry, 44*, 9–13.

Chanpattana, W., Kramer, B. A., Kunigiri, G., Gangadhar, B. N., Kitphati, R., & Andrade, C. (2010). A survey of the practice of electroconvulsive therapy in Asia. *The Journal of ECT, 26*, 5–10.

Chanpattana, W., Kunigiri, G., Kramer, B. A., & Gangadhar, B. N. (2005). Survey of the practice of electroconvulsive therapy in teaching hospitals in India. *The Journal of ECT, 21*, 100–104.

Chatterjee, S., Patel, V., Chatterjee, A., & Weiss, H. A. (2003). Evaluation of a community-based rehabilitation model for chronic schizophrenia in rural India. *British Journal of Psychiatry, 182*, 57–62.

Chatterjee, S., Pillai, A., Jain, S., Cohen, A., & Patel, V. (2009). Outcomes of people with psychotic disorders in a community-based rehabilitation programme in rural India. *British Journal of Psychiatry, 195*, 433–439.

Chopra, M. P., Prakash, S. S., & Raguram, R. (1999). The neuroleptic malignant syndrome: An indian experience. *Comprehensive Psychiatry, 40*, 19–23.

Creado, D. N., Parkar, S. R., & Kamath, R. M. (2006). A comparison of the level of functioning in chronic schizophrenia with coping and burden in caregivers. *Indian Journal of Psychiatry, 48*, 27–33.

Datta, S., Subhalakshmi, T. P., Jeyaseelan, L., & Kuruvilla, K. (1994). Risk factors for tardive dyskinesia. *Indian Journal of Psychiatry, 36*, 22–24.

Devaramane, V., Pai, N. B., & Vella, S. L. (2011). The effect of a brief family intervention on primary carer's functioning and their schizophrenic relatives levels of psychopathology in India. *Asian Journal of Psychiatry, 4*, 183–187.

D'Souza, D. C., Radhakrishnan, R., Perry, E., Bhakta, S., Singh, N. M., Yadav, R., et al. (2013). Feasibility, safety, and efficacy of the combination of D-serine and computerized cognitive retraining in schizophrenia: An international collaborative pilot study. *Neuropsychopharmacology, 38*, 492–503.

Dube, K. C., Kumar, N., & Dube, S. (1984). Long term course and outcome of the Agra cases in the International Pilot Study of schizophrenia. *Acta Psychiatrica Scandinavica, 70*, 170–179.

Dutta, S. B., Dhasmana, D. C., & Bhardwaj, R. (2005). Psychotropic drug utilization pattern among patients with schizophrenia. *Indian Journal of Psychiatry, 47*, 243–244.

Eranti, S. V., Thirthalli, J., Pattan, V., Mogg, A., Pluck, G., Velayudhan, L., et al. (2011). Comparison of electroconvulsive therapy practice between London and Bengaluru. *The Journal of ECT, 27*, 275–280.

Garg, R., Chavan, B. S., & Arun, P. (2011). Quality of life after electroconvulsive therapy in persons with treatment resistant schizophrenia. *Indian Journal of Medical Research, 133*, 641–644.

Gautam, S., & Meena, P. S. (2011). Drug-emergent metabolic syndrome in patients with schizophrenia receiving atypical (second-generation) antipsychotics. *Indian Journal of Psychiatry, 53*, 128–133.

Gautam, S., & Nijhawan, M. (1984). Burden on families of schizophrenic and chronic lung disease patients. *Indian Journal of Psychiatry, 26*, 156–159.

Giel, R., DeArango, M. V., Hafeiz-Babikir, A., et al. (1983). The burden of mental illness on the family: results of observations in four developing countries. *Acta Psychiatrica Scandinavica, 68*, 186–201.

Gopinath, P. S., & Chaturvedi, S. K. (1986). Measurement of distressful psychotic symptoms perceived by the family: preliminary findings. *Indian Journal of Psychiatry, 28*, 343–345.

Gopinath, P. S., & Chaturvedi, S. K. (1992). Distressing behaviour of schizophrenics at home. *Acta Psychiatrica Scandinavica, 86*, 185–188.

Goswami, U., Kumar, U., & Singh, B. (2003). Efficacy of electroconvulsive therapy in treatment resistant schizophrenia: A double-blind study. *Indian Journal of Psychiatry, 45*, 26–29.

Grover, S., Aggarwal, M., Dutt, A., Chakrabarti, S., Avasthi, A., Kulhara, P., et al. (2012a). Prevalence of metabolic syndrome in patients with schizophrenia in India. *Psychiatry Research, 200*, 1035–1037.

Grover, S., & Avasthi, A. (2010). Antipsychotic prescription pattern: A preliminary survey of Psychiatrists in India. *Indian Journal of Psychiatry, 52*, 257–259.

Grover, S., Chakrabarti, S., Aggarwal, M., Avasthi, A., Kulhara, P., Sharma, S., et al. (2012b). Comparative study of the experience of caregiving in bipolar affective disorder and schizophrenia. *International Journal of Social Psychiatry, 58*, 614–622.

Grover, S., Chakrabarti, S., Ghormode, D., Dutt, A., Kate, N., & Kulhara, P. (2011a). An Indian adaptation of the Involvement Evaluation Questionnaire: similarities and differences in assessment of caregiver-burden. *East Asian Archives of Psychiatry, 21*, 142–151.

Grover, S., Kumar, V., Avasthi, A., & Kulhara, P. (2012c). First prescription of new elderly patients attending the psychiatry outpatient of a tertiary care Institute in North India. *Geriatrics and Gerontology International, 12*, 284–291.

Grover, S., Nebhinani, N., Chakrabarti, S., Avasthi, A., & Kulhara, P. (2011b). Metabolic syndrome among patients receiving clozapine: A preliminary estimate. *Indian Journal of Pharmacology, 43*, 591–595.

Grover, S., Nebhinani, N., Chakrabarti, S., Avasthi, A., Kulhara, P., Basu, D., et al. (2013, Jan 7) Comparative study of prevalence of metabolic syndrome in bipolar disorder and schizophrenia from North India. Nordic Journal of Psychiatry (Epub ahead of print).

Grover, S., Nebhinani, N., Chakrabarti, S., Parakh, P., & Ghormode, D. (2012d). Metabolic syndrome in antipsychotic naïve patients diagnosed with schizophrenia. *Early Intervention in Psychiatry, 6*, 326–331.

Gupta, M., Bhatnagar, P., Grover, S., Kaur, H., Baghel, R., Bhasin, Y., et al. (2009). Association studies of catechol-O-methyltransferase (COMT) gene with schizophrenia and response to antipsychotic treatment. *Pharmacogenomics, 10*, 385–397.

Gupta, P. R., Chakrabarti, S., & Kulhara, P. (2010). Lack of association between duration of untreated psychosis and outcome in an Indian cohort. *World Psychiatry, 9*, 124–125.

Gupta, M., Moily, N. S., Kaur, H., Jajodia, A., Jain, S., Kukreti, R. (2013 Feb 9). Identifying a predictive model for response to atypical antipsychotic monotherapy treatment in south Indian schizophrenia patients. *Genomics*. doi:10.1016/j.ygeno.2013.02.002 (Epub ahead of print) (pii: S0888-7543(13)00018-9).

Gururaj, G. P., Math, S. B., Reddy, J. Y. C., & Chandrashekar, C. R. (2008). Family burden, quality of life and disability in obsessive compulsive disorder: An Indian perspective. *Journal of Postgraduate Medicine, 54*, 91–97.

Harish, M. G., Suresh, K., Rajan, I., Reddy, Y. C., & Khanna, S. (1996). Phenomenological study of late-onset schizophrenia. *Indian Journal of Psychiatry, 38*, 231–235.

Harrison, G., Hopper, K., Craig, T., et al. (2001). Recovery from psychotic illness: A 15- and 25-year international follow-up study. *British Journal of Psychiatry, 178*, 506–517.

Hopper, K., & Wanderling, J. (2000). Revisiting the developing versus developed country distinction in course and outcome in Schizophrenia: Results from ISoS, the WHO collaborative follow up project. *International Study of Schizophrenia. Schizophrenia Bulletin, 26*, 835–846.

Indian Council of Medical Research-ICMR. (1988). *Factors associated with the course and outcome of schizophrenia: ICMR-multicentred collaborative study*. New Delhi: ICMR.

Ismail Shihabuddeen, T. M., & Gopinath, P. S. (2005). Group meetings of caretakers of patients with schizophrenia and bipolar mood disorder. *Indian Journal of Psychiatry, 47*, 153–156.

Jayakumar, C., Jagadheesan, K., & Verma, A. N. (2002). Caregiver's burden: A comparison between obsessive compulsive disorder and schizophrenia. *Indian Journal of Psychiatry, 44*, 337–342.

John, J. P., Shakeel, M. K., & Jain, S. (2008). Corpus callosal area differences and gender dimorphism in neuroleptic-naïve, recent-onset schizophrenia and healthy control subjects. *Schizophrenia Research, 103*, 11–21.

Johnson, S., Sathyaseelan, M., Charles, H., Jeyaseelan, V., & Jacob, K. S. (2012). Insight, psychopathology, explanatory models and outcome of schizophrenia in India: A prospective 5-year cohort study. *BMC Psychiatry, 12*, 159.

Kagal, U. A., Torgal, S. S., Patil, N. M., & Malleshappa, A. (2012). Prevalence of the metabolic syndrome in schizophrenic patients receiving second-generation antipsychotic agents—A cross-sectional study. *Journal of Pharmacy Practice, 25*, 368–373.

Kalra, H., Nischal, A., Trivedi, J. K., Dalal, P. K., & Sinha, P. K. (2009). Extent and determinants of burden of care in Indian families: a comparison between obsessive compulsive disorder and schizophrenia. *International Journal of Social Psychiatry, 55*, 28–38.

Kataria, D., Bhargava, S. C., & Vohra, A. K. (2002). A correlational study between psychiatric disability and family burden in schizophrenia. *Indian Journal of Psychiatry, 44*(Suppl), 54.

Kate, N., Grover, S., Kulhara, P., & Nehra, R. (2012). Scale for positive aspects of caregiving experience: Development, reliability and factor structure. *East Asian Archives Psychiatry, 22*, 62–69.

Kate, N., Grover, S., Kulhara, P. & Nehra, R. (2013). Positive aspects of caregiving and its correlates in caregivers of schizophrenia: a study from North India. *East Asian Archives of Psychiatry, 23*, 45–55.

Khanna, R., Bhandari, S. N., & Das, A. (1990). Survey of psychotropic drug prescribing patterns for long stay patients. *Indian Journal of Psychiatry, 32*, 162–165.

Kiran, C. N. (2004). Burden and coping in caregivers of men with alcohol and opioid dependence. MD thesis. Chandigarh: Department of Psychiatry, PGIMER.

Kulhara, P. N. (1974). Long term follow-up study of schizophrenia. MD thesis. Chandigarh: PGIMER.

Kulhara, P., Avasthi, A., Sharan, P., Gupta, N., & Rao, S. A. (1999). Late Onset Schizophrenia Versus Early Onset Schizophrenia: A Comparison of Clinical Features. *Indian Journal of Psychiatry, 41*, 333–335.

Kulhara, P., Chakrabarti, S., Avasthi, A., Sharma, A., & Sharma, S. (2009). Psychoeducational intervention for caregivers of Indian patients with schizophrenia: A randomised-controlled trial. *Acta Psychiatrica Scandinavica, 119*, 472–483.

Kulhara, P., & Chandiramani, K. (1988). Outcome of schizophrenia in India using various diagnostic systems. *Schizophrenia Research, 1*, 339–349.

Kulhara, P., & Wig, N. N. (1978). The chronicity of schizophrenia in north-west India: results of a follow-up study. *British Journal of Psychiatry, 132*, 186–190.

Kumar, S., & Mohanty, S. (2007). Spousal burden of care in schizophrenia. *Journal of Indian Academy Applied Psychology, 33*, 189–194.

Kumari, S., Singh, A. R., Verma, A. N., Verma, P. K., & Chaudhury, S. (2009). Subjective burden on spouses of schizophrenia patients. *Industrial Psychiatry Journal, 18*, 97–100.

Kuruvilla, K., Kuruvulla, A., & Kanagasbapthy, A. S. (1986). Serum prolactin levels in schizophrenia: Effects of neuroleptics medication: A preliminary study. *Indian Journal of Psychiatry, 28*, 237–247.

Leff, J., Sartorius, N., Jablensky, A., Korten, A., & Ernberg, E. (1992). The International pilot study of schizophrenia: five-year follow-up findings. *Psychological Medicine, 22*, 131–145.

Leff, J., Wig, N. N., Ghosh, I., et al. (1987). Expressed emotion and schizophrenia in north India III: Influence of relatives' expressed emotion on the course of schizophrenia in Chandigarh. *British Journal of Psychiatry, 151*, 165–173.

Maheshwari, S. K., Gupta, S., & Sharan, P. (2009). Medication non-compliance and substance abuse in schizophrenia. *Nursing Journal of India, 100*, 201–203.

Malhotra, S., Biswas, P., Sharan, P., & Grover, S. (2007). Characteristics of patients visiting the Child & Adolescent Psychiatric Clinic: A 26-year study from North India. *Journal of Indian Association for Child and Adolescent Mental Health, 3*, 53–60.

Malhotra, S., Gupta, N., Bhattacharya, A., & Kapoor, M. (2006). Study of childhood onset schizophrenia (COS) using SPECT and neuropsychological assessment. *Indian Journal of Psychiatry, 48*, 215–223.

Malhotra, S., Gupta, N., & Singh, G. (2000). Clozapine in childhood-onset schizophrenia: a report of five cases. *Clinical Child Psychology and Psychiatry, 5*, 403–410.

Malhotra, N., Kulhara, P., Chakrabarti, S. & Grover, S. (2013 Apr 19). A prospective, longitudinal study of metabolic syndrome in patients with bipolar disorder and schizophrenia. *Journal of Affective Disorders*. [Epub ahead of print].

Moily, S., Murthy, R. S., Nagarajaiah, B., et al. (1997). Burden in families with schizophrenic patients in a rural community. *Indian Journal of Psychiatry, 39*(Suppl), 48.

Mojtabai, R., Varma, V. K., Malhotra, S., Mattoo, S. K., Misra, A., Wig, N. N., et al. (2001). Mortality and long-term course in schizophrenia with a poor 2-year course. A study in a developing country. *British Journal of Psychiatry, 178*, 71–75.

Murthy, S. R., Ghosh, A., & Wig, N. N. (1974). Treatment acceptance patterns in a psychiatric out-patient clinic: Study of demographic and clinical variables. *Indian Journal of Psychiatry, 16*, 323–329.

Murthy, R. S., Kishore Kumar, K. V., Chisholm, D., Thomas, T., Sekar, K., & Chandrashekari, C. R. (2005). Community outreach for untreated schizophrenia in rural India: A follow-up study of symptoms, disability, family burden and costs. *Psychological Medicine, 35*, 341–351.

Nagaraj, A. K. M., Haque Nizamie, S., Akhtar, S., Sinha, B. N. P., & Goyal, S. (2004). A comparative study of sexual dysfunction due to typical and atypical antipsychotics in remitted bipolar-I disorder. *Indian Journal of Psychiatry, 46*, 261–267.

Nagaraj, A. K. M., Pai, N. B., & Rao, S. (2001). A comparative study of sexual dysfunction involving risperidone, quetiapine, and olanzapine. *Indian Journal of Psychiatry, 51*, 265–271.

Nagarajaiah, P., Moily, S., Murthy, R. S., & Shymala, S. (1998). A comparative study of coping strategies in families of chronic schizophrenic and medically ill patients. *Indian Journal of Psychiatry, 40*(Suppl), 63.

Narayanan, H. S., Embar, P., & Reddy, G. N. (1972). Review of treatment in a family ward. *Indian Journal of Psychiatry, 14*, 123–126.

Narayanan, H. S., Girimaji, S. R., Gandhi, D. H., Maruthai, R. K., Rao, M. P., & Nardev, G. (1988). Brief in-patient family intervention in mental retardation. *Indian J Psychiatry, 30*, 275–281.

Narula, P. K., Rehan, H. S., Unni, K. E., & Gupta, N. (2010). Topiramate for prevention of olanzapine associated weight gain and metabolic dysfunction in schizophrenia: a double-blind, placebo-controlled trial. *Schizophrenia Research, 118*, 218–223.

Nebhinani, N., Grover, S., & Avasthi, A. (2012). Sexual dysfunction in male subjects receiving trifluoperazine, risperidone & olanzapine: Does the rate of sexual dysfunction vary with assessment questionnaire? *Primary Care Companion for CNS Disorders, 14*, e1–e7.

Nebhinani, N., Grover, S., Chakrabarti, S., Kate, N. & Avasthi, A. (2013). A longitudinal study of change in prevalence of metabolic syndrome and metabolic disturbances 3 months after Clozapine therapy. *Journal of Human Behaviour and Mental Health, 18*, 9–17.

Nehra, R., Chakrabarti, S., Kulhara, P., & Sharma, R. (2005). Caregiver coping in bipolar disorder and schizophrenia A re-examination. *Social Psychiatry and Psychiatric Epidemiology, 40*, 329–336.

Nehra, R., Chakrabarti, S., Kulhara, P., & Sharma, R. (2006). Family burden and its correlates among caregivers of schizophrenia and bipolar affective disorder. *Journal of Mental Health Human Behaviour, 11*, 78–84.

Nirmala, B. P., Vranda, M. N., & Reddy, S. (2011). Expressed emotion and caregiver burden in patients with schizophrenia. *Indian journal of psychological medicine, 33*, 119–122.

Padmavati, R., Thara, R., & Corin, E. (2005). A qualitative study of religious practices by chronic mentally ill and their caregivers in South India. *International Journal of Social Psychiatry, 51*, 139–149.

Padmawati, R., McCreadle, R. G., & Tirupati, S. (2010). Low prevalence of obesity and metabolic syndrome in never treated chronic schizophrenia. *Schizophrenia Research, 121*, 199–202.

Padmini, D. D., Amarjeeth, R., Sushma, M., & Guido, S. (2007). Prescription patterns of psychotropic drugs in hospitalized schizophrenic patients in a tertiary care hospital. *Calicut Medical Journal, 5*, e3.

Pai, S., Channabasavanna, S. M., Nagarajaiah, S., & Raghuram, R. (1985). Home care for chronic mental illness in Bangalore. An experiment in prevention of repeated hospitalization. *British Journal of Psychiatry, 147*, 175–179.

Pai, S., & Kapur, R. L. (1981). The burden on the family of a psychiatric patient: development of an assessment scale. *British Journal of Psychiatry, 138*, 332–335.

Pai, S., & Kapur, R. L. (1982). Impact of treatment intervention on the relationship between dimensions of clinical psychopathology, social dysfunction and burden on the family of psychiatric patients. *Psychological Medicine, 12*, 651–658.

Pai, S., & Kapur, R. L. (1983). Evaluation of home-care treatment of schizophrenic patients. *Acta Psychiatrica Scandinavica, 67*, 80–88.

Pai, S., & Roberts, E. J. (1983). Follow-up study of schizophrenic patients initially treated with home care. *British Journal of Psychiatry, 143*, 447–450.

Painuly, N., & Chakrabarti, S. (2006). Combined use of electroconvulsive therapy and antipsychotics in schizophrenia: The Indian evidence. A review and a meta-analysis. *The Journal of ECT, 22*, 59–66.

Pallava, A., Chadda, R. K., Sood, M., & Lakshmy, R. (2012). Metabolic syndrome in schizophrenia: A comparative study of antipsychotic-free/naïve and antipsychotic-treated patients from India. *Nordic Journal of Psychiatry, 66*, 215–221.

Pandey, R. S., Sreenivas, K. N., & Subbakrishna, D. K. (1992). Neuroleptic—induced acute dystonia in schizophrenia and mania. *Indian Journal of Psychiatry, 34*, 331–333.

Pandurangi, A. K., Ananth, J., & Channabavasanna, S. M. (1978). Dyskinesia in an Indian mental hospital. *Indian Journal of Psychiatry, 20*, 339–342.

Patra, S., Kar, N., Mishra, A., & Singh, S. P. (2011). Single-session psychoeducation in schizophrenia: a feasibility and effectiveness study in an Indian patient population. *Clinical Schizophrenia and Related Psychoses, 5*, 107–108.

Ponnudurai, R., Jayakar, J., & Sekaran, S. (2006). Assessment of mortality and marital status of schizophrenic patients over a period of 13 years. *Indian Journal of Psychiatry, 48*, 84–88.

Ponnudurai, R., Vijayasekaran, V., Kameswaran, L., Somasundaram, O., & Rajendran, A. J. (1983). Therapeutic compliance of patients on phenothiazines. *Indian Journal of Psychiatry, 25*, 239–242.

Raguraman, J., Vijay Sagar, K. J., & Chandrasekaran, R. (2005). Effectiveness of clozapine in treatment-resistant schizophrenia. *Indian Journal of Psychiatry, 47*, 102–105.

Raj, L., Kulhara, P., & Avasthi, A. (1991). Social burden of positive and negative schizophrenia. *International Journal of Social Psychiatry, 37*, 242–250.

Rajkumar, A. P., Poonkuzhali, B., Kuruvilla, A., Jacob, M., & Jacob, K. S. (2013). Clinical predictors of serum clozapine levels in patients with treatment-resistant schizophrenia. *International Clinical Psychopharmacology, 28*, 50–56.

Rammohan, A., Rao, K., & Subbakrishna, D. K. (2002). Religious coping and psychological well-being in carers of relatives with schizophrenia. *Acta Psychiatrica Scandinavica, 105*, 356–362.

Ranga Rao, N. V. S. S. (1988). Comparative study of disability and family burden in rural and urban areas. MD thesis. Bangalore: Bangalore University.

Rao, K., Barnabas, I. P., & Gopinath, P. S. (1988). Family burden in chronic schizophrenia: The role of the day hospital. *Indian Journal of Psychological Medicine, 11*, 131–135.

Ray, D., Samajdar, J., & Khanna, R. (1992). Drug induced akathisia: Preliminary report. *Indian Journal of Psychiatry, 34*, 159–161.

Reddy, Y. C. J., Srinath, S., Sathyanarayana, V., Girimaji, S., & Seshadri, S. (1996). Clinical profile of early onset schizophrenia: A review of 43 cases. *NIMHANS Journal, 14*, 93–98.

Roy, R., Jahan, M., Kumari, S., & Chakraborty, P. K. (2005). Reasons for drug non-compliance of psychiatric patients: A centre based study. *Journal of the Indian Academy of Applied Psychology, 31*, 24–28.

Roychaudhuri, J., Mondal, D., Boral, A., & Bhattacharya, D. (1995). Family burden among long-term psychiatric patients. *Indian Journal of Psychiatry, 37*, 81–85.

Sagar, R., Pattanayak, R. D., & Mehta, M. (2012). Clinical profile of child and adolescent ($\leq$16 years) psychotic disorders at a tertiary care centre in India. *Journal of Basic and Applied Sciences, 8*, 139–144.

Sahoo, S., Ameen, S., & Akhtar, S. (2007a). Incidence of new onset metabolic syndrome with atypical antipsychotics in first episode schizophrenia: A six-week prospective study in Indian female patients. *Schizophrenia Research, 95*, 247.

Sahoo, S., Ameen, S., & Akhtar, S. (2007b). Metabolic syndrome in drug-naïve first episode psychosis treated with atypical antipsychotics. *Australian and New Zealand Journal of Psychiatry, 4*, 628–629.

Sahoo, S., Manjunatha, N., Ameen, S., & Akhtar, S. (2008). Metabolic syndrome in first episode schizophrenia—a randomized double-blind controlled, short-term prospective study. *Schizophrenia Research, 101*, 266–272.

Saldanha, P., Pai, N., & Krishnamurthy, K. (2002). A study of family burden and family distress in schizophrenia. *Indian Journal of Social Psychiatry, 18*, 63–68.

Sarada Menon, M. & Rarnachandra, V. (1972). Trifluperidol-therapeutic response and extra pyramidal symptoms. *Indian Journal of Psychiatry, 14*, 289–292.

Sarin, A., Nagpal, J., Bohra, N. K., Jiloha, R. C., Rao, G. P., Sharma, S. K., et al. (2004). Open labeled, randomized, switch-over study of two fixed doses (10/15 mg) of aripiprazole: to evaluate its safety and efficacy in the treatment of Indian patients of schizophrenia. *Indian Journal of Psychiatry, 46*, 64–71.

Sarkar, P., Natarajan, C., & Gode, N. (2009). Prevalence of neuroleptic malignant syndrome in 672 consecutive male in-patients. *Indian Journal of Psychiatry, 51*, 208–211.

Sartorius, N., Gulbinat, W., Harrison, G., Laska, E., & Siegel, C. (1996). Long-term follow-up of schizophrenia in 16 countries: A description of the international study of schizophrenia conducted by the World Health Organisation. *Social Psychiatry and Psychiatric Epidemiology, 31*, 249–258.

Sartorius, N., Jablensky, A., Ernberg, G., et al. (1987). Course of schizophrenia in different cultures: some results of a WHO International comparative five year follow-up study. In: H. Hafner, W. F. Gattaz, & W. Janzarik (Eds.), *Search for the Cause a of Schizophrenia* 9th. Berlin: Springer.

Sartorius, N., Jablensky, A., Korten, A., et al. (1986). Early manifestations and first-contact incidence of schizophrenia in different cultures. A preliminary report on the initial evaluation phase of the WHO collaborative study on determinants of outcome of severe mental disorders. *Psychological Medicine, 16*, 909–928.

Sawhney, V., Chopra, V., Kapoor, B., Thappa, J. R., & Tandon, V. R. (2005). Prescription trends in schizophrenia and manic depressive psychosis. *J K Science, 7*, 156–158.

Sekaran, R. C., Jayashree, S. R., & Sivaprakash, B. (2001). Family burden and coping strategies in relatives of schizophrenic patients. *Indian Journal of Psychiatry, 43*(Suppl), 36.

Shankar, R. & Kamath, S. (1991, October). Needs based interventions with families of the chronic mentally ill. Presented at the Congress of the World Association of Psychosocial Rehabilitation, Montreal (pp. 14–18).

Sharma, I., Giri, D., Dutta, A., Mazumder, P., & Anuradha, M. (2005). Clinical profile of childhood onset schizophrenia in India. *Journal of Indian Association of Child and Adolescent Mental Health, 1*, 6.

Sharma, S., Kumar, N., Chakraborti, S., Sinha, S., Kumari, S., & Gajendragad, J. M. (2012). Prevalence and factors associated with medication compliance in Indian patients suffering from mental disorders. *Tropical Doctor, 42*, 28–31.

Shrivastava, A., & Gopa, S. (2000). Comparative study of risperidone and haloperidol on clinical and psychosocial parameters in treatment of schizophrenia: A randomised open trial. *Indian Journal of Psychiatry, 42*, 52–56.

Shrivastava, A., Johnston, M., Bureau, Y., & Shah, N. (2012). Baseline serum prolactin in drug-naive, first-episode schizophrenia and outcome at five years: Is it a predictive factor? *Innovations in Clinical Neuroscience, 9*, 17–21.

Shrivastava, A., & Shah, N. (2009). Prescribing practices of clozapine in India: Results of a opinion survey of psychiatrists. *Indian Journal of Psychiatry, 51*, 225–226.

Shrivastava, A., Shah, N., Johnston, M., Stitt, L., Thakar, M., & Chinnasamy, G. (2010). Effects of duration of untreated psychosis on long-term outcome of people hospitalized with first episode schizophrenia. *Indian Journal of Psychiatry, 52*, 164–167.

Shukla, G. D. (1981). Fluphenazine decanoate in chronic schizophrenia. *Indian Journal of Psychiatry, 23*, 234–236.

Singh, G., Sharan, P., & Kulhara, P. (2003). Role of coping strategies and attitudes in mediating distress due to hallucinations in schizophrenia. *Psychiatry and Clinical Neurosciences, 57*, 517–522.

Sovani, A. (1993). Understanding schizophrenia: A family psychoeducational approach. *Indian Journal of Psychiatry, 35*, 97–98.

Sreeja, I., Gupta, S., Rakesh, L. & Singh, M. B. (2009). Comparison of burden between family caregivers of patients having schizophrenia and epilepsy. *Internet Journal of Epidemiology, 6*(2).

Srinivasan, T. N., & Thara, R. (1997). How do men with schizophrenia fare at work? A follow-up study from India. *Schizophrenia Research, 25*, 149–154.

Srinivasan, T. N., & Thara, R. (2002). At issue: Management of medication noncompliance in schizophrenia by families in India. *Schizophrenia Bulletin, 28*, 531–535.

Srivastava, S. (2005). Perception of burden by caregivers of patients with schizophrenia. *Indian Journal of Psychiatry, 47*, 148–152.

Srivastava, S., Agarwal, A. K., & Sharma, M. (2002). A three-year naturalistic follow-up of patients receiving clozapine: Report from India. *International Journal of Psychiatry in Clinical Practice, 6*, 167–171.

Srivastava, A. K., Gupta, S., & Srinivasan, N. (2001). Risperidone: Dosing pattern and efficacy in clinical practice—A post-marketing survey. *Indian Journal of Psychiatry, 43*, 147–151.

Srivastava, V. K., Sitholey, P., Dwivedi, C. M., & Tripathi, S. K. (1988). Influence of socio-cultural factors on delusions: A study on children and adolescents. *Child Psychiatry Quarterly, 21*, 121–128.

Subashini, R., Deepa, M., Padmavati, R., Thara, R., & Mohan, V. (2011). Prevalence of diabetes, obesity, and metabolic syndrome in subjects with and without schizophrenia (CURES-104). *Journal of Postgraduate Medicine, 57*, 272–277.

Suresh Kumar, P. N. (2008). Impact of vocational rehabilitation on social functioning, cognitive functioning, and psychopathology in patients with chronic schizophrenia. *Indian Journal of Psychiatry, 50*, 257–261.

Suresh Kumar, P. N., & Manoj Kumar, T. (1997). A comparative study of neuroleptic induced neurological side effects in schizophrenia and mood disorder. *Indian Journal of Psychiatry, 39*, 110–114.

Suresh, K. K., Kumar, C. N., Thirthalli, J., Bijjal, S., Venkatesh, B. K., Arunachala, U., et al. (2012). Work functioning of schizophrenia patients in a rural south Indian community: Status at 4-year follow-up. *Social Psychiatry and Psychiatric Epidemiology, 47*, 1865–1871.

Szmukler, G. I., Burgess, P., Herrman, H., Benson, A., Colusa, S., & Bloch, S. (1996). Caring for relatives with serious mental illness: The development of the Experience of Caregiving Inventory. *Social Psychiatry and Psychiatric Epidemiology, 31*, 137–148.

Thakur, A., Jagadheesan, K., & Sinha, V. K. (2003). Psychopathological dimensions in childhood and adolescent psychoses: a confirmatory factor analytical study. *Psychopathology, 36*, 190–194.

Thara, R. (2004). Twenty-year course of schizophrenia: the Madras longitudinal study. *Canadian Journal of Psychiatry, 49*, 564–569.

Thara, R. (2012). Consumer perceptions of recovery: An Indian perspective. *World Psychiatry, 11*, 169–170.

Thara, R., Henerietta, M., Joseph, A., Rajkumar, S., & Eaton, W. W. (1994). Ten year course of schizophrenia—the Madras longitudinal study. *Acta Psychiatrica Scandinavica, 90*, 329–336.

Thara, R., Padmavati, R., Aynkran, J. R., & John, S. (2008). Community mental health in India: A rethink. *International Journal of Mental Health System, 2*, 11.

Thara, R., Padmavati, R., Kumar, S., & Srinivasan, L. (1998). Burden assessment schedule: an instrument to assess burden on caregivers of chronic mentally ill. *Indian Journal of Psychiatry, 40*, 21–29.

Thara, R., Padmavati, R., Lakshmi, A., & Karpagavalli, P. (2005). Family education in schizophrenia: A comparison of two approaches. *Indian Journal of Psychiatry, 47*, 218–221.

Thirthalli, J., Venkatesh, B. K., Kishorekumar, K. V., Arunachala, U., Venkatasubramanian, G., Subbakrishna, D. K., et al. (2009). Prospective comparison of course of disability in antipsychotic-treated and untreated schizophrenia patients. *Acta Psychiatrica Scandinavica, 119*, 209–217.

Thomas, J. K. (2004). Suresh Kumar PN, Verma AN, Sinha VK, Andrade C. Psychosocial dysfunction and family burden in schizophrenia and obsessive compulsive disorder. *Indian Journal of Psychiatry, 46*, 238–243.

Thomas, P., Srivastava, V., Singh, A., Mathur, P., Nimgaonkar, V. L., Lerer, B., et al. (2008). Correlates of response to olanzapine in a north indian schizophrenia sample. *Psychiatry Research, 161*, 275–283.

Tiwari, A. K., Deshpande, S. N., Rao, A. R., Bhatia, T., Mukit, S. R., Shriharsh, V., et al. (2005). Genetic susceptibility to tardive dyskinesia in chronic schizophrenia subjects: I. Association of CYP1A2 gene polymorphism. *Pharmacogenomics Journal, 5*, 60–69.

Trivedi, J. K., Dhyani, M., Yadav, V. S., Rai, S. B., Sinha, P. K. (2010). Anti psychotic drug prescription pattern for schizophrenia: An Indian perspective. (Personal Communication) Indian Journal of Psychiatry.

Venkatasubramanian, G., Rao, N. P., Arasappa, R., Kalmady, S. V., & Gangadhar, B. N. (2013). A longitudinal study of relation between side-effects and clinical improvement in schizophrenia: Is there a neuro-metabolic threshold for second generation antipsychotics? *Clinical Psychopharmacology and Neuroscience, 11*(1), 24–27.

Verghese, A. (1988). Family participation in mental health care—The Vellore experiment. *Indian Journal Psychiatry, 30*, 117–121.

Verghese, A., John, J. K., Rajkumar, S., Richard, J., Sethi, B., & Trivedi, J. K. (1989). Factors associated with the course and outcome of schizophrenia in India: Results of a two-year multicenter follow-up study. *British Journal of Psychiatry, 154*, 499–503.

Vijayan, N. N., Bhaskaran, S., Koshy, L. V., Natarajan, C., Srinivas, L., Nair, C. M., et al. (2007). Association of dopamine receptor polymorphisms with schizophrenia and antipsychotic response in a South Indian population. *Behavioral and Brain Functions, 3*, 34–45.

Vijayan, N. N., Mathew, A., Balan, S., Natarajan, C., Nair, C. M., Allencherry, P. M., et al. (2012). Antipsychotic drug dosage and therapeutic response in schizophrenia is influenced by ABCB1 genotypes: A study from a south Indian perspective. *Pharmacogenomics, 13*, 1119–1127.

Vohra, A. K., Garg, S., & Gaur, D. R. (2000). A study of burden on families of schizophrenia and depressive disorder. *Indian Journal of Psychiatry, 42*(Suppl), 33.

Wiersma, D., Wanderling, E., Dragomireck, E., et al. (2000). Social disability in schizophrenia: Its development and prediction over 15 years in incidence cohorts in six European centres. *Psychological Medicine, 30*, 1155–1167.
Wig, N. N., Menon, D. K., Bedi, H., et al. (1987). Expressed emotion and schizophrenia in north India, II: Distribution of expressed emotion components among relatives of schizophrenic patients in Aarhus and Chandigarh. *British Journal of Psychiatry, 151*, 160–165.
World Health Organisation. (1979). *Schizophrenia: An international follow-up study*. Chichester: Wiley.

Chapter 11
Suicide Studies in India

P.B. Behere, M.C. Bhise and A.P. Behere

1 Introduction

Suicide is known since birth of humanity. In India, Ramayana and Mahabharata have recorded instances of suicide. During Vedic and Upanishadic times, death by drowning at the confluence of rivers to achieve *"punya"*, the self-destruction for incurable diseases and ascetics by undertaking a great journey towards last years of life (mahaprasthan) were allowed. Subsequently over the years, "Sutee pratha" became a common practice in India. This is an example of "altruistic" suicide, in which the suicide is expected, almost required rather than an outcome of personal sorrow or guilt. Buddhist, Confucian and Shintoist ethics accepted suicide and euthanasia in case of incurable illness.

First, we have addressed the issues how suicides can be studied, and then, we have discussed findings from some important studies and our own studies.

P.B. Behere, Director Research and Development (R & D), Professor and Head; M.C. Bhise, Assistant Professor; A.P. Behere, Child Psychiatry Fellow

---

P.B. Behere (✉)
Department of Psychiatry, Jawaharlal Nehru Medical College,
Datta Meghe Institute of Medical Sciences, Sawangi (Meghe), Wardha,
Maharashtra, India
e-mail: pbbehere@gmail.com

M.C. Bhise
Department of Psychiatry, MGM'S Medical College, Aurangabad,
N-6, CIDCO, Aurangabad, Maharashtra, India

A.P. Behere
Department of Child and Adolescent Psychiatry, Mid Coast Mental Health Centre,
Rockland, ME, USA

A.P. Behere
Pen Bay Psychiatry, Belfast, ME, USA

S. Malhotra and S. Chakrabarti (eds.), *Developments in Psychiatry in India*,
DOI 10.1007/978-81-322-1674-2_11

While working in rural areas in Maharashtra, we realised that farmers' suicide is very big and burning issue. We became more interested to research in this field, and finally, we started working on survivors of farmers' suicide and their mental health issues, which needed to be addressed. Luckily at this stage, government of Maharashtra took interest and asked for our help. This was the turning point when we got government support for this community work.

World scenario: Currently, worldwide every year, almost one million people die from suicide. Globally, mortality rate from suicide is 16 per 100,000 or one death every 20 s (WHO 2010). In the last 45 years, suicide rates have increased by 60 % worldwide. Suicide is one of the three leading causes of death among those aged 15–44 years in some countries and the second leading cause of death in the 10–24 years age group; these figures do not include suicide attempts which are up to 20 times more frequent than completed suicide. Suicide worldwide is estimated to represent 1.8 % of the total global burden of disease in 1998, and 2.4 % in countries with market economies and former socialist economies in 2020. The WHO estimates that worldwide every year, approximately 873,000 people commit suicide. Estimates for the year 2020 suggest that approximately 1.53 million people will die from suicide and 10–20 times more people than this will attempt suicide worldwide. Highest suicide rates for both men and women are found in Europe, more particularly in Eastern Europe (e.g. Estonia, Latvia and Lithuania). Lowest suicide rates are found in the Eastern Mediterranean Region, which comprises mostly countries that follow Islamic traditions (WHO 1999). With only exception of China (Male/Female = 14.3:17.9), suicide rates in males are consistently higher than suicide rates in females. This male predominance of suicide rates has been a relatively constant phenomenon over the years. In 1950, male-to-female ratio was 3.2:1; in 1995, it was 3.6:1; and in 2020, it is projected to be 3.9:1. In Europe, the highest suicide rate is in Lithuania (45.6 per 100,000), while the highest number of suicides occur in China (195,000 per year). India stands second in total number of suicides (87,000 per year). Although traditionally suicide rates have been highest among elderly males, rates among young people have been increasing to such an extent that they are now the group at highest risk in a third of countries, in both developed and developing countries. Mental disorders (particularly depression and alcohol-use disorders) are a major risk factor for suicide in Europe and North America; however, in Asian countries, impulsiveness plays an important role.

1.1 Scenario in Asia

Asian countries are the major contributors to the global suicide, accounting for approximately 60 % cases in the world. Suicides in China and India make up 30 % of the suicides in the world. The number of suicides in China alone is 30 % greater than total number of suicides in the whole Europe (Bertolote and Fleischmann 2002). These figures should be viewed in the light of the fact that many Asian countries do not report suicide data to the WHO (Vijaykumar 2005). A few Asian countries rank highest in the world in terms of suicide rates, e.g. Japan (24 per 100,000 per year of population), South Korea (23.8 per 100,000 per year of population) and Sri Lanka (21.6 per

100,000 per year of population), while others such as Philippines have rates as low as 2.1 per 100,000 per year (Wei and Chua 2008).

There has been a steep increase in suicides in some countries such as Japan, South Korea and Hong Kong. Other countries in this region such as Australia, Malaysia, New Zealand and Singapore have low to medium suicide rates between 9.9 and 13.1 per 100,000 (Hendin et al. 2008). It has been hypothesised that in family-centric Asian societies which place a higher value on collectivism, intact marriages and families play a crucial role in social integration. They are therefore important protective factors against suicide in Asian countries. Male-to-female ratio in most of the Asian countries is much lower as compared to European countries. In Pakistan, Sri Lanka and Thailand, young people have the highest rates; in China, Hong Kong SAR, Japan, Malaysia, the Republic of Korea and Singapore, suicide is a relatively greater problem for older people; in China and New Zealand, there are high rates in both the young and the old; and in India, middle-aged individuals have the highest rates. Rural rates of suicide are higher than urban rates in Australia, China, India, the Republic of Korea and Sri Lanka, but in New Zealand, urban rates are higher than rural rates.

1.2 Indian Scenario

India ranks second highest in terms of the total number of suicides in the world. More than one lakh (one hundred thousand) lives are lost every year to suicide in our country. Most recent data are available for year 2011 from the National Crime Records Bureau (2011). According to it, 135,585 persons in the country lost their lives by committing suicide during the year 2011. This indicates 2010 an increase of 0.7 % over the previous year's figure (1,34,599). The number of suicides in the country during the decade (2001–2011) has recorded an increase of 25.0 % (from 1,08,506 in 2001 to 1, and 35,585 in 2010). The increase in incidence of suicides was reported each year during the decade. The population has increased by 17.8 % during the decade, but the suicide rate in 2011 was 11.2 which are marginally greater than 10.6 recorded in 2001. The rate of suicides has shown a declining trend since 2001–2003. An increasing trend is observed during 2007–2010. There is a wide variation of suicide rates and numbers within country (Fig. 1). In year 2011, five states with highest percentage contribution to national suicides were West Bengal (12.2 %) followed by Tamil Nadu (11.8 %), Maharashtra (11.8 %), Andhra Pradesh (11.1 %) and Karnataka (9.3 %) of the total suicides in the country. These five states have been constantly on top five lists in last few years. The all-India rate of suicides was 11.2 during the year 2011, which is marginally lower than 11.4 reported in the year 2010. Within the country, suicide rates vary widely. Puducherry reported the highest rate of suicide (44.8) followed by Andaman and Nicobar Islands (35.8), Sikkim (30.3), Chhattisgarh (26.5) and Kerala (25.3). Maharashtra ranked 13th in this list, with a suicide rate of 14.2 per one lakh population. Among causes of suicide "family problems" and "illness", accounting for 24.3 and 19.6 % respectively, were the major causes of suicides among the specified causes. "Love affairs" (3.4 %), "bankruptcy" (2.2 %), "dowry dispute" (2.4 %) and "poverty" (1.7 %) were the other causes driving people towards suicides. Suicides due

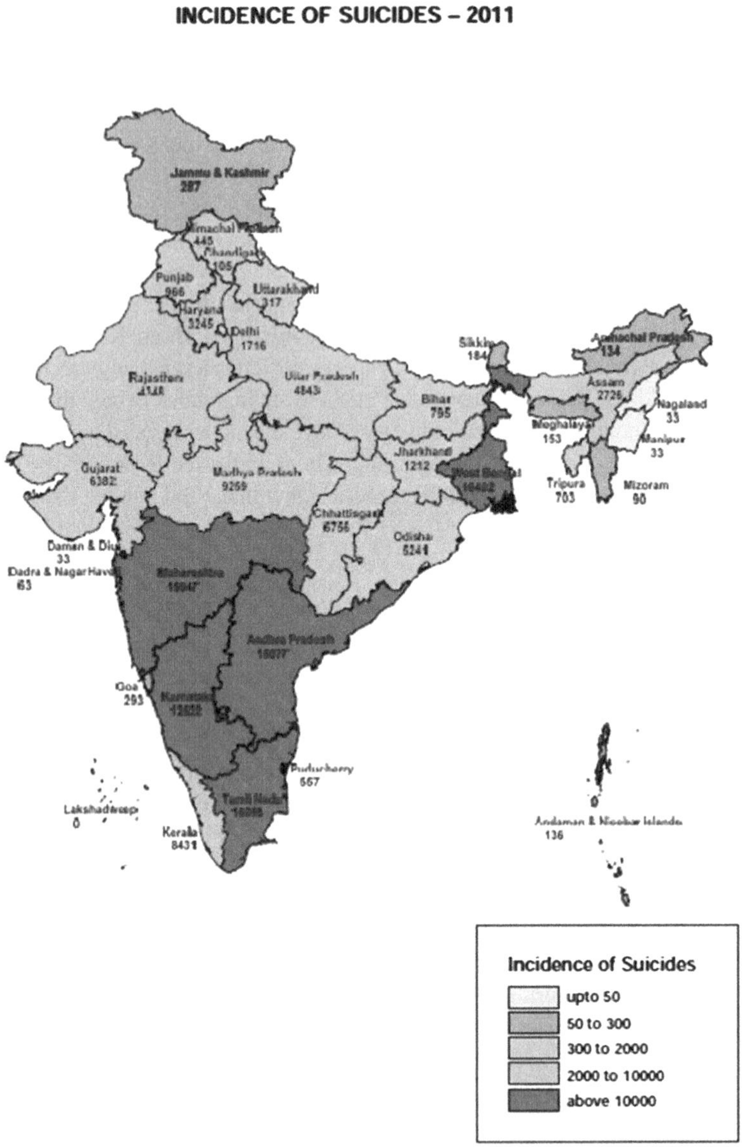
INCIDENCE OF SUICIDES - 2011
Jammu & Kashmir
287
Punjab
Uttarakhand
Delhi
1716
Rajasthan
Uttar Pradesh
4843
Bihar
795
Sikkim
184
Assam
2726
Nagaland
33
Meghalaya
153
Manipur
33
Tripura
703
Mizoram
90
Jharkhand
1212
Gujarat
6382
Madhya Pradesh
9259
Chhattisgarh
6756
Odisha
5241
Daman & Diu
33
Dadra & Nagar Haveli
63
Goa
293
Puducherry
567
Lakshadweep
0
Kerala
8431
136
Incidence of Suicides
upto 50
50 to 300
300 to 2000
2000 to 10000
above 10000

Fig. 1 Suicide rate in different states in India for year 2011 (*Source* NCRB India-2011)

to "illness", "drug abuse/addiction" and "poverty" have shown an increasing trend during last 3 years.

In the last two decades, the suicide rate has increased from 7.9 to 10.3 per 100,000 (Vijaykumar 2002). Higher literacy, a better reporting system, lower external aggression, higher socio-economic status and higher expectations are the possible explanations for higher suicide rates in the southern states of India. In India, young

(15–29 years) and lower middle-aged people (30–44 years) were the prime groups taking recourse to the path of suicide. Around 35 % suicide victims were youths in the age group of 15–29 years, and 34 % were middle-aged persons in the age group 30–44 years. This leads to a huge social, emotional and economic burden on the society. Male-to-female suicide ratio has been consistently narrow in India (1.4:1). Hanging (33.2 %), poisoning (32.3 %) and self-immolation (8.8 %) are the commonest methods of suicide in India. There is gross under reporting of suicides in India. Verbal autopsy studies in rural Tamil Nadu have revealed that the annual suicide rate is 6–9 times the official suicide rate (Joseph et al. 2003; Gajalakshmi and Peto 2007).

The presence of mental illness in suicide victims varies among different studies in India. Two case–control studies using psychological autopsy approach have been done in Chennai (Vijaykumar and Rajkumar 1999) and Bangalore (Gururaj et al. 2004). In Bangalore, 88 % and, in Chennai, 43 % of the suicide victims had diagnosable mental illness. In Chennai, 25 % of suicides were found to be due to mood disorders. This rate increased to 35 % when suicide cases with adjustment disorder with depressed mood were also counted. Although social drinking is not a way of life in India, alcoholism plays a significant role in suicides in India. In Chennai, alcohol dependence was found in 35 % of the suicide cases and 30–50 % victims were under the influence of alcohol at the time of suicide. Modernisation has led to sweeping changes in socio-economic, socio-philosophical and cultural arenas of peoples' lives in India. This has greatly added to the stress in life, leading to substantially higher rates of suicide (Gehelot and Nathawat 1983). On the other hand, religiosity and belief on god act as protective factors for suicide in India (Vijaykumar 2002). Other protective factors are intact marriages, supportive families and stigma against suicide per se in India. The assessment of suicide is dealt in great detail (Behere and Reddy 2010a).

2 Farmers' Suicides with Special Reference to Maharashtra

Suicide of farmers is not only seen in India, but it is observed worldwide and across the cultures (Behere and Bhise 2009b). Farming is the one of the oldest industries in world. As civilisations have set in, man has learned cultivation to meet the demands of food. Farming made previously wandering human beings settle at one place. It has been one of the most respected professions and has a popular image as a peaceful and healthy way of life. Despite this fact, agriculture has one of the highest rates of mortality than any other industries (McCurdy and Carroll 2000). Although farming practices, production systems and type of farms are diverse, there are commonalities across the farms that are important to health (Behere and Bhise 2009a). Most farms continue to be family-owned and family-operated businesses and are exposed to volatility of commodity markets, the variability of weather patterns and the influence of governmental regulations (Fraser et al. 2005). This exposes farmers to a high level of stress. Economic concerns and government bureaucracy have been consistently identified as a major cause of stress and contributor to suicide (Malmberg et al. 1999). There is no customary or mandatory retirement age for farmers all over the world, and many tend to work beyond the customary retirement age, placing the younger generation in a dependent relationship with their parents for much longer than usual. This can lead to tension between the two generations on the farm. Roles between work, home and family are often blurred with farming operating as an occupation and way of life for many farmers (Melberg 2003). Research had shown a relationship between monetary and family problems with suicide. British farmers were more concerned about family problems (Thomas et al. 2003), while indebtedness and monetary concerns were reported to be major reason for suicide among Indian farmers (Behere and Behere 2008). From an early age, those in the farming families can be exposed to a range of risks to their physical and mental health, which continue in adulthood and later life. Many studies have found higher rates of depression and anxiety among farmers when compared with the general population (Eisner et al. 1998; Peck et al. 2002). A study in England found that even in the absence of psychiatric morbidity, farmers were more likely to report that life is not worth living compared with general population (Thomas et al. 2003), and suicide in them was an end point to a series of difficulties that accumulated over time.

In its seventh decade of independence, our nation is losing its vey sons of soil, our food growers. After the independence, according to Gandhiji's vision of *Gram Swaraj*, villages and specially farmers were to be the main focus of any development plan of India. India consists of 16 % of world's population, which is sustained on only on 2.4 % of the world land resource. The agriculture sector is the only livelihood to the two-third of its population, which gives employment to the 57 % of work force, and is a raw material source to large number of industries (Behere and Behere 2008). In the 1990s, India woke up to a spate of suicide by farmers. Since then, suicide by farmers has figured in the newspapers, the state assemblies and the parliament. It has been included in some of the election manifestos. According to the analysis by K. Nagraja of Madras Institute of Development Studies, between the years 1997 and 2006, about 200,000 farmers have committed suicide. Thus, on an average, nearly 16,000 farmers' committed suicide every year, putting every seventh suicide in country as farmers' suicide. Farmers' suicides have increased at annual compound growth rate of about 2.5 % per annum over this time period. There is a high degree of variation in farmers' suicide across different states in country. According to 2001 census of India, top five states in number of farmer suicides were Maharashtra, Karnataka, Andhra Pradesh, Chhattisgarh and Madhya Pradesh. In these, farmers' suicide rate is nearly 60 % higher than the general suicide rate, indicating a very distressing situation in these states. For the state of Maharashtra, picture is even bleaker. Between years 1997 and 2006, the number of farmers' suicide has more than doubled with annual compound growth rate of 9.8 % (Nagraja 2007). During this decade, every fifth farmers' suicide committed in country had occurred in Maharashtra. Vidarbha region of Maharashtra, which lies in centre of India, is a particularly vulnerable pocket for farmers' suicide making a continuous suicide belt with Telangana region of Andhra Pradesh (Behere and Bansal 2009). With much of media and political uproar on this issue, various steps were taken to mitigate this crisis. Most of the interventions done by states were directed towards survivors of farmers' suicide. With politicisation of issue, especially prior to elections, various packages were announced for survivors by state governments. These mostly included financial ex gratia help to affected families. Media and government initiatives together led to the projection of farmers' suicide as a mere economical and debt-driven crisis and adopted policy of only providing financial help to the bereaved (Behere and Bhise 2011).

Studies show that suicide in general is an outcome of multiple factors. At a given time, there are many forces that drive the people to commit suicide. Same forces apply to farmers who end their lives. Roles between work, home and family are often blurred with farming operating as an occupation and way of life for many farmers. Research had shown a relationship between monetary and family problems with suicide. On the other hand, farmers' suicides also differ in some aspects from general suicides. Farmers are more likely to be in their middle ages, married with children in schools, living with family. Most are the sole bread earners for the family. Majority have small to marginal farms of 1–2 ha. Farmers who commit suicide tend to use methods to which they have easy access because of their occupation. In India, pesticides are easily available, and hence, its consumption is the most common method of suicide (Behere and Bhise 2012). Family of famers who committed suicide are under great stress and needs help (Behere and Reddy 2010; Behere 2010a). These factors need special attention when it comes to prevention of suicides and provision of help to survivors. This makes identification of persons at risk more difficult, as even under stress, most of them would be functioning normally. Family members often fail to recognise any minor changes in their behaviours that usually precede the suicide.

Female farmers' suicide: Suicide among female farmers is on rise. Studies of women in farming have found high levels of stress, fatigue and depression (Walker and Walker 1988). Explanations most commonly given are role conflicts and high work load. Farm women, unlike men, experience stress not only related to the farm operations but also to the impact of farming stressors on the physical, social and financial well-being of all family members. As farming has become less profitable, women are taking more and more on- and off-farm work to supplement the family income (Gallagher and Delworth 2003). Farming women in this position often become stressed and fatigued due to multiple tasks, and the conflict between their traditional role as a house-makers and the need for off-farm income. Female farmers have to bear the additional burden of doing household chores apart from farming. This makes farm women a high-risk category for suicide. England, Australia and, now, India had reported suicide among female farmers. In India, the State Government's report on farmers' suicide in Karnataka State shows that approximately 20 % of victims were females (Veeresh 2002), while Kerala figures were 26 % of all farmers' suicides. Surviving suicides is more common among females. As most of the farmers' suicide victims are married and have families, spouses are more vulnerable to psychological distress (Behere and Bhise 2011).

In one of the study we found that 30 % of the study group (i.e. farmers included in the study exposed to pesticide) was having suicidal ideation as compared to control group, (8 % of the sample had suicidal ideation). It is also noticed that those who got suicidal ideation were having depressive symptoms as well on the Self-Reporting Questionnaire (SRQ), as compared to controls. These raised important question whether exposure to pesticide causes suicidal ideas and depressive symptoms (Behere et al. 2013).

3 Suggested Action Plan and Recommendations

"Farmers" suicides are preventable! This is the basic concept that needs to be understood when we think of any policies to reduce the suicide numbers (Behere and Bhise 2012). Studies across world have revealed that a strategic policy for prevention with a multifaceted prevention approach involving community participation is the most effective method in suicide prevention. Most of the developed countries have devised their national suicide prevention policies, which have been effective in reducing suicides. The United Kingdom had witnessed high rates of suicide by farmers in 1980s and implemented its national suicide prevention strategy. As part of prevention programme, the Firearms Act was amended in 1988, making rules more stringent. Studies have found that suicide rate had declined significantly after this act was implemented, highlighting the importance of restriction of availability of means to commit suicide. Another inspiring example is from our neighbouring country, Sri Lanka. Suicide rates among farmers have declined by 50 % in a decade in Sri Lanka. This was an outcome of series of legislative activities that systematically banned the most highly toxic pesticides that had been responsible for the majority of pesticide deaths in the preceding two decades (Jayewardene and Saravanabananthan 1966). In addition to restricting or withdrawing a number of pesticides, Sri Lanka has also actively pursued a number of initiatives to reduce use and increase the safety of pesticide use by farmers, e.g. integrated pest management, use of lockable boxes to restrict access to pesticides (Hawton et al. 2009). Furthermore, there has been considerable research interest in Sri Lanka in the medical management of self-poisoning, and so it is possible that the improved management of pesticide self-poisoning has also contributed to the favourable trends observed in terms of suicide incidences. There are many similarities in farmers' suicides in India and Sri Lanka, implying that in India, we can also reduce the burden of farmers' suicides by significant numbers. The following are the few suggested strategies on various aspect of farmers' suicide prevention:

1. Primary prevention:

   This involves the identification of high-risk individuals and training community gate keepers. Among the farmers, those at high risk for suicide are those with depression, alcoholism, bank loan defaulters and previous suicide attempters (Xavier et al. 2007). In addition to these, we have found a significant association between crop failures, marriage of sister or daughter and suicide by farmers. Early detection of at-risk groups is very important in suicide prevention. A more humane and scientific approach needs to be evolved to deal with loan defaulters. Bank personnel need to be trained in this approach. Psychological help may be provided when dealing with defaulters. Alcoholism is another important contributor to farmers' suicides. Alcoholism should not be projected only as a moral problem of individual. Medical facilities and professional help of psychiatrists should be made available to those who are alcohol dependant at free of cost. Training should be imparted to all medical and paramedical professionals for early detection and treatment of mental illnesses. Depression in community is often undiagnosed, and simple tools such as the SRQ-20 may be useful in detecting those suffering from psychological distress (WHO 1994).

Awareness programmes for the general public and high-risk individuals can focus on the promotion of better mental health, stress management and coping skills, proper financial planning, life skills development, and early identification and treatment of mental illnesses. Community gatekeepers such as representatives of local bodies, teachers, spiritual leaders, Aanganwadi and ASHA workers should be trained in suicide prevention strategies. Apart from these, some of the specific primary prevention measures for farmers' suicide could be the following:

- Restriction of access to pesticides: Pesticide consumption is the most common method of suicide among farmers in the country. An essential pesticide list needs to be built that excludes extremely lethal compounds and regulate their formulation, packaging and sale (Jacob 2008). A simple intervention like providing a lockable storage box to keep pesticides safe and out of reach is also effective. A study in Sri Lanka on the introduction of *lockable boxes* for storing pesticides to farming households was found to be acceptable. Most households used the boxes responsibly, although there was some decline in the proper usage over time. Most informants regarded the box as useful with convenience for storage, security, avoiding wastage and protection of children being major factors (Hawton et al. 2009). A message on the box about how to deal with bad feelings and the importance of safer storage was well received. We, in India, need to consider this measure more seriously.
- Macroeconomic policies: Policies to protect failing industries including agriculture should be devised taking into consideration social cost. Crop loans issued to the farmers need to be revised. State should ensure fresh crop loans to every farmer at the beginning of each season. Loans should carry a minimal interest, and for non-irrigated farmers, this may be interest free as is done in China (Sainath 2006). Crop insurance needs to be covered well so that like other industries when a yield failure occurs, economy of poor farmers does not collapse all of a sudden. Suicide prevention campaign in Sri Lanka had slogan "Agricultural loans only for agricultural purpose", which suits the Indian scenario as well.
- Coping skills: Farming is one of the most uncertain industries when it comes to yielding results. Indian farmers heavily rely on things beyond their control such as good rains and pests, making this uncertainty many folded. Farmers need to be trained in coping skills so that they can adopt favourable defence mechanisms in the face of adversities. It is important to make them aware of availability of mental health services nearby, so that they can seek round the clock help when in distress.
- Training farmers in new agricultural practices: Most of the farms in India are family-run businesses that adopt the farming practices prevalent since many years. Newer technologies in this field should be made available to farmers at low cost. There should be proper information portals that will provide information to villages rather than in cities. When it comes to new technology, cost is often a barrier. Poor farmers will need subsidies on these so that it is affordable to common man.

2. Secondary prevention:

   This involves early intervention and treatment of high-risk individuals and attempters. For this, we suggest the use of the existing three-tier system of health care infrastructure in India. At primary health centre and the sub-centre level, health workers and other voluntary workers should be provided with simple questionnaires for screening of mental illness. They should be advised to screen the population covered by them with these instruments. Those found to be disturbed and at risk should be treated at the primary health centre by medical officer who should have received some training in mental health. A team should be formed under the leadership of a psychiatrist at district hospitals, which serve as second level in the current infrastructure. Those found to have mental illness and also all those who attempt suicide or threaten to do so should be evaluated and treated here. Proper follow-up and monitoring of treatment of suicide attempters should be ensured in the community. Private sector and nursing homes may also be involved in providing specialist help at this level with proper incentives to them. If patients require further management, they may be referred to psychiatry departments in medical colleges and mental hospitals which serve as third level institutes in the current health care structure. These institutes can also be utilised efficiently as training centres for professionals at the primary health centre level and grass root workers.

3. Tertiary prevention:

   This involves rehabilitation of rescued attempters and helping the survivors of the victims. A psychological autopsy should be performed on all farmers' suicides as this objectively brings out relationship between suicides and socio-demographic, psychological factors, and stressful life events. This is particularly important in case of farmers' suicides as there are many unscientific speculative reports in the media, which may mislead the administrators and public as well. Any preventive strategy is productive only if it is based on sound research. Furthermore, reaching out to the families by mental health professionals can ensure psychological support to the survivors. Those families affected by farmers' suicides should receive compensation. But, only financial support is not enough in itself for the survivors. Long-term strategies are required to help the survivors cope with the loss of a bread earner for them. Children of the victims are particularly at risk and should be offered free education and other facilities. Compensation should always be accompanied by mental health package through which mental health services are delivered.

Given the complexities of factors driving farmers to suicide, strategies to deal with problem of farmers' suicide need to be systematic and well planned. India is facing problem of farmers' suicide along with other suicides in significant numbers for quite a long time now. It is time to devise a National Suicide Prevention Policy. Countries such as the United Kingdom had high rates of farmers' suicide. It was tackled through systematic research by psychiatrists and social scientists that came out with brilliant suicide prevention policies. Today, this problem is well tackled there. It is high time now to take necessary steps in India also; otherwise, we may be facing extinction of another group from earth, this time a class from our own *homo sapiens* species, our food growers: *the farmers.*

References

Barraclough, B. M., & Pallis, D. J. (1975). Depression followed by suicide: A comparison of depressed suicides with living depressives. *Psychological Medicine, 5*, 55–61.

Behere, P. B., & Behere, A. P. (2008). Farmers' suicide in vidarbha region of Maharashtra State: A myth or reality? *Indian Journal of Psychiatry, 50*, 124–127.

Behere, P. B., & Bansal, A. (2009). Farmers' suicide in vidarbha: Everybody's concern. *Journal of MGIMS, 4*, iii–v.

Behere, P. B., & Bhise, M. C. (2009). Farmers' suicide: Across culture. *Indian Journal of Psychiatry, 51*, 242–243.

Behere, P. B., & Reddy, S. (2010). Clinical Evaluation of Suicide and Related issues, Psychiatry in India. Training & Training Centers. T. S. S. Rao (Ed.), Publisher Indian Psychiatric Society. p. 457.

Behere, P. B. (2010a). Families take years to cope with loss. Times of India Nagpur edition, May 11th, 2010.

Behere, P. B. (2010b). Families of Farmers who killed self also distressed. Times of India Nagpur edition. May 11th, 2010.

Behere, P. B., & Bhise, M. C. (2011). Psychological distress in survivors of farmers' suicides: A cross sectional comparative study from central part of rural India. In *Proceedings of 63rd Annual National Conference of Indian Psychiatric Society*. January 16th–19th, New Delhi, India.

Behere, P. B., & Bhise, M. C. (2012). Farmers' suicides in central rural India. In B. S. Chavan, N. Gupta, P. Arun, A. Sidana, & S. Jadhav (Eds.), *Community mental health in India* (pp. 231–240). New Delhi: Jaypee Publications.

Behere, P. B., Das, A., & Behere, M. (2013). Pesticide exposure and suicidal ideation in rural communities of Wardha district of Central India. In *Proceedings bridging south North South East and West in joint ISEE, ISES and ISIAQ Environmental Health Conference 2013*. in Basel, Switzerland (19–23 August).

Beautrais, A. L. (2004). Further suicidal behaviour amongst medically serious suicide attempters. *Suicide and Life-Threatening Behaviour., 34*, 1–11.

Beautrais, A. L. (2003a). Suicide and serious suicide attempts in young people: a multiple group case control study. *American Journal of Psychiatry, 160*, 1093–1099.

Beautrais, A. L. (2003b). Suicides and serious suicide attempts: two populations or one? *Psychological Medicine, 31*, 837–845.

Bertolote, J. M., & Fleischmann, A. (2002). A global perspective of the epidemiology of suicide. *Suicidologi, 7*, 6–8.

Eisner, C. S., Neal, R. D., & Scaife, B. (1998). Depression and anxiety in farmers. *Primary Care Psychiatry, 4*, 101–105.

Eklind, P. D., Carlson, J. E., & Schanbel, B. (1998). Agricultural hazards reduction through stress management. *Journal of Agromedicine, 39*(2), 159–165.

Fraser, C. E., Smith, K. B., & Judd, F. (2005). Farming and mental health problems and mental illness. *International Journal of Social Psychiatry, 51*(4), 340–349.

Gajlakshmi, V., & Peto, R. (2007). Suicide rates in Tamil Nadu, South India: Verbal autopsy of 39000 deaths in 1997-98. *International Journal of Epidemiology, 36*(1), 203–207.

Gallagher, E., Delworth, U. (2003). The third shift: Juggling employment, family and the farm. Family farm business in a changing rural society. (Rep No. 95/8). Canberra: RIRDC Research.

Gehelot, P. S., & Nathawat, S. S. (1983). Suicide and family constellation in India. *American Journal of Psychotherapy, 37*, 273–278.

Gururaj, G., Issac, M., Subhakrishna, D. K., & Ranjani, R. (2004). Risk factors for completed suicides: A case control study from Bangalore, India. *Injury Control and Safety Promotion, 11*, 183–191.

Hawton, K., Rantnanayke, L., Simkins., Harriss, L., & Scott, V. (2009). Evaluation of acceptability and use of lockable storage devices for pesticides in Sri Lanka that might assist prevention of self-poisoning. *BMC Public Health, 9*, 69–71.

Hendin, H., Phillips, M. R., Vijayakumar, L., Pirkis, J., Wang, H., Yip, P., et al. (2008). Epidemiology of suicide in Asia. In H. Hendin, L. Vijayakumar, J. M. Bertolote, H. Wang, M. R. Phillips, & J. Pirkis (Eds.), *Suicide prevention in asia* (pp. 7–18). Geneva: World Health Organisation.

Jayewardene, C. H., & Saravanabavananthan, N. (1966). Insecticide poisoning. *Ceylon Medical Journal, 11*, 143–152.

Jacob, K.S. (2008). Public health strategies for suicide prevention. The Hindu, Bangalore Edition. 15th December 2008.

Joseph, A., Abraham, S., Mullyl, J. P., George, K., Prasad, J., Minz, S., et al. (2003). Evaluation of suicide rates in rural India using verbal autopsies- 1994-1999. *British Medical Journal, 326*, 1121–1122.

Malmberg, A., Simkin, S., & Howton, K. (1999). Suicide in farmers. *British Journal of Psychiatry, 175*, 103–105.

McCurdy, S., & Carroll, D. J. (2000). Agricultural injury. *American Journal of Industrial Medicine, 38*, 463–480.

Melberg, K. (2003). Farming, stress and psychological well-being: the case of Norwegian spouses. *Sociologia Ruralis, 43*(1), 56–76.

Nagaraja, K. (2007). Farmers' suicides in India: Magnitude, trends and partial patterns. Madras Institute of Development studies (Cited July, 10, 2008). Available at http://macroscan.com/anl/mar08/pdf/farmers_suicides.pdf.

National Crime Records Bureau (2011). Accidental Deaths and Suicide in India. Ministry of Home Affairs. Government of India 2011. Accessed from Feb, 09, 2013. Available at http://ncrb.nic.in/.

Peck, D., Grant, S., McArthur, W., & Godden, D. (2002). Psychological impact of foot and mouth disease on farmers. *Journal of Mental Health, 11*(5), 523–531.

Sainath, P.(2006). Vidarbha: Slowing down the suicides. The Hindu, Bangalore Edition dated 12th June 2006.

Thomas, H. V., Lewis, G., Thomas, R., Salmon, R. L., Chalmers, R. M., Coleman, T. J., et al. (2003). Mental health of British farmers. *Occupational and Environmental Medicine, 60*(3), 181–185.

Vijaykumar, L., & Rajkumar, S. (1999). Are risk factors for suicide universal? A case control study in India. *Acta Psychiatrica Scandinavia, 99*, 407–411.

Vijaykumar, L. (2002). Religion: A protective factor in suicide. *Sociology, 2*, 9–12.

Vijaykumar, L. (2005). Suicide and mental disorders in Asia. *International Review of Psychiatry, 17*, 109–114.

Veeresh, G. K. (2002). *Farmers' suicides in Karnataka—A scientific analysis*. Bangalore: Report of expert committee for study on farmers' suicides.

Walker, J. L., & Walker, L. S. (1988). Self-reported stress symptoms in farmers. *Journal of Clinical Psychology, 44*(1), 10–16.

Wei, K. C., & Chua, H. C. (2008). Suicide in Asia. *International Review of Psychiatry, 3*(3), 103–109.

World Health Organisation (WHO) (1994). User's guide to the self reporting questionnaire. In world Health organisation, Division of mental health Geneva: WHO/MHN/MBD/99.1.

World Health Organisation (1999). Figures and facts about suicide. Doc. WHO/MNH/MBD/99.1. WHO: Geneva.

World Health Organisation (2010). Suicide prevention (SUPRE). Available: http://www.who.int/mental_health/prevention/suicide/suicideprevent/en/print.html Accessed on 10th June.

Xavier, P. V., Dinesh, N., John, A. J., Radhakrishnan, V. K., Suresh Kumar, P. N., & Ali, A. (2007). Position paper and action plan on farmers' suicide: presentation to chief minister and health minister. *Kerala Journal of Psychiatry, 22*, 68–75.

Part IV
Developments in Child Psychiatry

Chapter 12
Research Endeavors in Child Psychiatry in India-I

Savita Malhotra and Natasha Kate

1 Introduction

The impact of early childhood on the development and evolution of an individual as he/she matures into adulthood has been recognized since ages. That the mental state of the child and childhood experiences shall be paramount in the mental health of the adult was further exemplified in the psychoanalytic concepts and movement. While it was Freud who talked about child mental disorders in his case of Little Hans, analysts like Anna Freud and Melanie Klein were further instrumental in further developing psychoanalysis of children and using it in their treatment. Bowlby's Attachment theory and the description of anaclitic depression by Spitz showed that infants and very young children too can understand and feel, and therefore have a mental life as complex and as rich as an adult. The origins of "child psychiatry" as a concept can possibly be traced to the mental hygiene movement in the United States of America, wherein the focus of care included a multi-disciplinary emphasis, a child welfare approach, and an inclusion of environmental causes. In 1935, Kanner's textbook provided the first English language systematic account of child psychiatry (Kanner 1935), although several earlier works have alluded to the same. Later, the Isle of Wight epidemiological studies the late 1960s and early 1970s (Rutter et al. 1976, 1979) demonstrated the feasibility of systematic studies on children, the use of standardized methods of interviewing children, and elucidated the important psychopathological risks associated with family dysfunction.

India, as a nation, has a more than 450 million children and adolescents in the present day, and yet, Child psychiatry in India is a fledgling field. Research in child psychiatry, in India, is at a nascent stage and has picked up only in the last few decades and these have followed developments in adult psychiatry in general in the post

S. Malhotra, Professor and Head; N. Kate, Formerly Senior Resident

S. Malhotra (✉) · N. Kate
Department of Psychiatry, PGIMER, Chandigarh, India
e-mail: savita.pgi@gmail.com

S. Malhotra and S. Chakrabarti (eds.), *Developments in Psychiatry in India*,
DOI 10.1007/978-81-322-1674-2_12

independent era. It is only when general adult psychiatry got itself established as an independent medical discipline with several postgraduate training centers and courses that the need for child psychiatry training and research was recognized. There are only a few academic and research centers in the country that exhibit a significant focus on this special population and hence available literature in child psychiatry in India is fragmented and patchy. Despite this, it is evident that Indian researchers are now beginning to take large leaps in the field of child psychiatry. An attempt is made to review broad.

Areas in which significant or substantial research is currently available in child and adolescent psychiatry (CAP) in India. This chapter covers research in India, in the areas of epidemiology and temperament; whereas Chap. 2 includes other major areas of research understood in the context of world literature.

2 Temperament

Individual differences in how infants behave, react, interact, what they like or dislike—to eat or play, are instrumental in identifying the uniqueness of the child. These characteristics often form the template for the future, shaping adult personality, and behavior. Each child is born with these individual differences in emotional reactivity and regulation that appear early in life, are relatively stable, and are at least partly biologically based (Rothbart and Bates 2006). These characteristics are termed as temperament (Rothbart and Bates 2006).

2.1 Laying Down the Framework

Evidence supports the heritability and stability/continuity of temperamental traits, particularly from age three onward (Gagne et al. 2009; Roberts and DelVecchio 2000). Temperament has been found to impact the developing personality of the individual and certain temperamental characteristics have also been found to increase the risk for development of psychopathology during childhood, adolescence, and adulthood (Malhotra and Varma 1986; Narang et al. 1997).

One of the major challenges in temperament research is the existence of multiple systems of organization, each with partially overlapping dimensions that are given different names and load onto slightly different factors. The original work of Thomas and Chess in their New York Longitudinal Study (Thomas and Chess 1977) postulated nine continuous dimensions of temperament in addition to three higher-order categories of "difficult," "easy," and "slow to warm up". A temperament measurement schedule for children was developed and standardized for use in India by Malhotra et al. (1988). Questions in simple Hindi and English were devised from the published descriptions of behavior associated with each of the nine dimensions of Thomas et al. (1963, 1968) and also with some help from Temperament Characteristics Schedule of Graham et al. (1973) and from authors own clinical experience taking behavioral items considered logically consistent with the category definitions. Since its standardization, Temperament Measurement Schedule has been used extensively in India. Temperament has been found to be a valid concept applicable to Indian populations that could discriminate between the emotionally disturbed and healthy groups of children (Malhotra and Randhawa 1983). Temperamental differences were seen between boys and girls, in the domains of activity, and threshold for responsiveness. Earlier studies have shown significant differences in mood between the two genders (Maccoby and Jacklin 1974; Eaton and Enns 1986). However, a recent meta-analysis (Else-Quest et al. 2006) which compared the temperamental characteristics of boys and girls demonstrated differences in the domains of persistence, intensity of emotion, activity, approach-withdrawal, and mood. Additionally, temperament also varies with socioeconomic status, as demonstrated by a study that assessed the temperament of school going children of New England and found significant differences in temperamental characteristics of children belonging to different socioeconomic classes, but no difference were found in the temperaments among different age groups (McClowry 2002). Temperament factors that constitute risk for development of psychopathology in Indian children differ to some extent from those described for Western children (Maccoby and Jacklin 1974) and moreover, studies from India have shown that temperament is not merely a general risk factor, but it is specific for certain disorders (Malhotra and Chaturvedi 1983; Malhotra 1989).

It should come as a little surprise that temperamental characteristics including dimensions such as a higher activity level, short attention span, high intensity of reaction with low threshold of responsiveness as well as impulsivity have been strongly associated with childhood disorders like conduct disorder (CD) and ADHD (Foley et al. 2008). Indian studies which have evaluated the temperamental characteristics of children, show that compared to those with conversion disorder and normal controls, children with CD showed a temperament profile of high activity and intensity of reactions, as well persistently negative mood (Malhotra 1989). In another retrospective Indian study of ADHD and CD, children with ADHD had temperamental deviance in the form of inattention and increased distractibility (Foley et al. 2008).

With regard to the internalizing spectrum of disorders, it has been proposed that both anxiety and depressive disorders share the relation to high negative affectivity and mood (Watson and Clark 1992). Studies have found an association between conversion disorders and temperamental traits like low emotionality, low threshold of responsiveness (Malhotra 1999a), and low distractibility (Malhotra 1989). In another study that compared the temperament of children and adolescents presenting with unexplained physical symptoms that included somatoform and conversion disorders (Raghuthaman and Cherian 2003), the authors found that that children with these disorders had characteristic temperaments of low activity, low emotionality, low rhythmicity, and low distractibility. Children with somatoform disorder were less approachable than children with conversion disorder; otherwise temperamentally there were no differences between these two disorders.

MR too has been found to be associated with certain temperamental correlates, namely low emotionality and a study from India found that the relationship between intelligence and emotionality variable of temperament was linear in the mentally retarded children (Malhotra and Malhotra 1990). Temperament also impacts physical disorders, as demonstrated by study that looked at children with persistent asthma and reported than children with asthma had significantly lower score on the temperament dimension of rhythmicity as compared to normal children (Rajesh et al. 2008).

Children of parents with mental disorders too seem to have certain temperamental characteristics that are different from children whose parents do not have mental illness. Malhotra and Kaur (1997) studied the temperament of children of parents with psychotic, affective, neurotic disorders as well as those without mental illness.

They found that the children of parents with mental illness were less sociable, withdrawing and less adaptable to negative emotions, had low activity and intensity of emotional reactions as well as low distractibility and low rhythmicity. Children of parents with depression were found to have significantly lower threshold of responsiveness, lower intensity of response, sociability, activity but more negative affect, withdrawal, and distractibility (Kalra et al. 2012). This is in line with Western data that show that children born to mothers who were suffering from psychiatric disorders before pregnancy were more likely to have negative mood, low rhythmicity, poor frustration tolerance, and emotional instability (Worland et al. 1984). Sons of alcohol-dependent males have been found to be low on rhythmicity, persistence, and manifest more negative mood compared to sons of non-alcohol-dependent fathers (Narang et al. 1997).

Hence, it is apparent that from the early childhood; there are temperamental differences that seem to set apart children who are impacted by mental illness, either in themselves or their parents. Temperament being an innate, constitutional characteristic would be considered as a vulnerability marker. More longitudinal research shall possibly throw light on the complex interaction between the temperament and the environment, thereby illuminating the role of temperament as a key factor impinging on the development of child and adult psychiatric disorders.

3 Epidemiology

In the early part of the twentieth century, most clinicians and researchers gave scant importance to diagnostic distinctions, but this changed with the work of Robins and O'Neal (1953) and Hewitt and Jenkins' (1946) important factor analytic study of patterns of emotional and behavioral disturbance (which they termed "maladjustment"). This led to an acceptance of the need to differentiate between emotional disturbances on the one hand and disorders of disruptive behavior on the other. This resulted in clinicians accepting that phenomenology can be used for distinguishing diagnoses. However, while children exhibiting behavioral extremes would be considered as disordered around the world, it is often the children who lie close to the median who shuttle between diagnostic categories. Present day nosological systems are often heatedly debated, and diagnoses and their criteria often undergo a sea change with each new edition. This is understandable as nosological systems often give importance to disability and dysfunction in the patient, which might be especially difficult to identify and characterize in children. Changes in disorder prevalence (especially the increase in the prevalence of autism) are often believed to be secondary to changes in the diagnostic criteria. The use of the Feighner criteria is delineating diagnosis has lead to the inclusion of new disorders and nosological identity of some disorders have been discarded in the diagnostic systems (Robins et al. 1981; Kaplan et al. 2009). The use of the multi-axial diagnoses has helped capture the psychosocial factors in the child's illness, thereby promoting the bio-psycho-social model of understanding mental health and mental health disorders. Yet, like in all of psychiatry, the debate on what decides the line between normalcy and illness continues unabated in child psychiatric disorders as well.

3.1 Magnitude of the Problem

Psychiatric epidemiology is the study of the prevalence and distribution of psychiatric disorders in a population or in a community. What makes that information so valuable is that the frequency and burden of psychiatric disorders in a community can be estimated and hence intervention strategies can also be planned. Before the late 1960s, there were no data on the epidemiology of child and adolescent psychiatric disorders until the landmark Isle of Wight studies that were led by Tizard, Whitmore, and Rutter (1976, 1979). These studies were conceptualized and therefore planned in a manner as to identify disorders, comorbidities, causal factors, and possible interventions. They were instrumental in identifying the reality of comorbidities, they also demonstrated the role of family functioning and impact of family conflict on the psychological functioning of the child. Additionally, and possible equally importantly, they showed that children and their families could be systematically interviewed, and demonstrated the value of standardized methods of measurement. Another study of significance that followed was the Waltham Forest Study (Richman et al. 1982) that demonstrated that psychopathology in young children, including preschoolers often preceded later psychiatric disorders. Present day epidemiological studies have demonstrated that 3-month prevalence of any disorder averaged 13.3 % (Costello et al. 2003a). As the child moved into adolescence, some disorders (social anxiety, panic, depression, and substance abuse) increase in prevalence, whereas others, including separation anxiety disorder and ADHD decrease. Children, as they grow, also have different disorders and change from one diagnosis to another included change from depression to anxiety and vice versa, from ADHD to oppositional defiant disorder, and from anxiety and CD to substance abuse (Costello et al. 2003a). Other studies that have been primarily conducted in Great Britain and the USA have found the median prevalence estimate of functionally impairing child and adolescent psychiatric disorders is 12 %, although the range of estimates is wide, varying from 9.5 % (Costello et al. 2003a, b) to 16 % (Ford et al. 2003). Literature from middle and low income countries have shown prevalence rates of 17.7 % in 1–15 years old in Ethopia (Maccoby and Jacklin 1974; Esser et al. 1990) 15 % among 5–10 years old from Bangladesh (Thomas et al. 1963; Tadesse et al. 1999) 7 % in 7–14 years olds urban Brazilian school sample (Mullick and Goodman 2005) and 7 % in 7–14 years rural Brazilian school (Flietlich-Bilyk and Goodman 2004) and 6.9 % in 4–17 years Puerto Rican community-based sample (Goodman 2005).

While the studies were published by Michael Rutter and colleagues in the 1970s, epidemiological data regarding the prevalence of childhood mental disorders in India first came from a WHO collaborative study (Canino et al. 2004) that looked at childhood mental disorders in primary care. The study had four centers in different countries and the Indian center was at Raipur Rani. Following a screening and detailed evaluation process, a clinical psychiatric syndrome was present in 22 % of the children evaluated, with intellectual impairment present in 12 % of children (intellectual impairment was not included in other epidemiological studies). The study presented an overall mental morbidity of 22 % which was much more than that seen in Sudan (10 %) and Philippines (14 %) but less than that seen in Columbia (29 %). However, the authors attributed the lower rates of mental illness in Sudan and Philippines to lower sensitivity of the diagnostic instruments and noted that prevalence figures in the

Indian study were similar to international data. However, indigenous research focusing of the epidemiology of childhood psychiatric disorders came to the fore when the Indian Council of Medical Research (ICMR) decided to focus on the same. Under its aegis, Malhotra et al. (2002) studied the prevalence of childhood psychiatric disorder in 963 school children, aged 4–11 year, in the city of Chandigarh, using multi-stage random sampling, and multi-informant assessment procedure. Psychiatric morbidity as per the ICD-10 criteria was seen in 6.33 % of the children. Teacher's estimation of the prevalence rates was higher, i.e., 10.17 % as compared to parent's estimate, i.e., 7.48 %. The most prevalent disorder in this population was enuresis. Later, in another ICMR funded study, Srinath et al. (2005) revealed a prevalence rate of 12.5 % in children aged 0–16 years. There were no significant differences among prevalence rates in urban middle class, slum, and rural areas. The psychiatric morbidity among 0–3 year old children was 13.8 % with the most common diagnoses being breath holding spells, pica, behavior disorder NOS, expressive language disorder, and MR. The prevalence rate in the 4–16 year old children was 12 %. Enuresis, specific phobia, hyperkinetic disorders, stuttering, and oppositional defiant disorder were the most frequent diagnoses. When impairment associated with the disorder was assessed, significant disability was found in 5.3 % of participants aged 4–16 year. However, this study included both breath holding spells (not an ICD 10 Diagnostic category) and epilepsy (conventionally included in neurological disorders), and excluded possible learning disorders, all of which could significantly impact the prevalence figures. A recent study evaluated psychopathology in 982 school going children in the age group of 10–15 years found that 20.2 % of the children to have a psychiatric disorder as per ICD-10 criteria. In another community-based study from Calicut, Hackett et al. (1999) (Bansal and Barman 2011) found the prevalence of childhood psychiatric disorders to be 9.4 % among the 1,403 children aged 8–12 years selected by random cluster sampling. Presence of psychiatric disorder was associated with male gender, Muslim religion, lower social class, less parental education, school failure, and impaired reading and vocabulary.

While there have been Indian and Western studies that have evaluated the prevalence of mental disorders in children, data on the incidence of these disorders are sorely lacking. In a collective expert report on mental illness in children and adolescents in 2001–2002, incidence of mental illness in children in France was reported to be 1 in (Cohen et al. 1993; Narang et al. 1997). An Indian study that throws light on the incidence of childhood psychiatric disorders (Giel et al. 1981) has estimated it to be 18 per 1,000/year. While this study was novel in its design and execution and attempted to fill a large epidemiological void, more studies and data are essential before we can conclusively estimate the incidence of childhood psychiatric disorders in India.

3.2 *Epidemiological Studies of major psychiatric disorders are reviewed below:*

3.2.1 Mental Retardation

Across the world, MR is recognized as a disability and a common mental health problem. It has been estimated that the prevalence of MR in the non-institutionalized population of the United States to be 7.8 people per 1,000 (Malhotra et al. 2009). Studies have found the prevalence rate for severe MR in children of school age is relatively stable, varying around an average value of 3.8 per 1,000 (Larson et al. 1994). However, the prevalence rate for severe MR is age dependent, as prevalence data show an increasing prevalence up to age of 15 which indicates that severe MR may not be fully assessed in the first few years of life. The male: female ratio shows a 20 % excess of males, probably due to sex-linked genetic factors. Sociodemographics do not seem to impact the prevalence of severe MR (Larson et al. 1994). The average prevalence rate for mild MR in children of school age is about 29.8 per 1,000. Some studies have found the prevalence to be more in males or in urban areas, while other studies have conflicting results. Additionally, the prevalence of mild MR increases in children belonging to lower socioeconomic class. Prevalence of MR ranges from 4 per 1,000 in the Philippines, 138 per 1,000 in Bangladesh (Malhotra and Kaur 1997; Roeleveld and Zielhuis 2008) per 1,000 in Pakistan (Stein et al. 1986).

MR has been well established as a common mental health problem in our country as well, with prevalence being as high as 6.9 per 1,000 in the general population as established in meta-analysis by Reddy and Chandrashekar (1998, Hasan 1981). In a multi-centric study done by the ICMR on 1,314 children with MR without an obvious environmental cause was carried out at Bangalore, Bombay, Delhi, and Lucknow, it was seen that in all, 42.3 % patients had mild, 25.3 % moderate, 19.2 % severe, and 13.1 % profound MR.

4 Autism and Autistic Spectrum Disorder

The epidemiological data of autistic spectrum disorders (ASD) are often subject to a great degree of heterogeneity. Data from meta-analysis have revealed the overall estimate of prevalence of typical autism was 7.1 per 10,000 and of all ASD was 20.0 per 10,000 (Kaplan et al. 2009). Diagnostic criteria used (ICD-10 or DSM-IV vs. other), age of the children screened, and study location all impacted the prevalence of typical autism.

Possibly, the earliest published study from India that looked at the clinic prevalence of infantile autism was funded by the ICMR, at a private missionary hospital where it was found that 2.9 % child cases seen were of infantile autism. However, this study did not use any diagnostic criteria, relying chiefly on clinical assessments (Hoch 1967). 11 years later, a case series of seven cases of autism from the MR clinic at NIMHANS, Bangalore described autism (Narayanan 1978). In a retrospective chart review, Malhotra and Chaturvedi (1983) found only 4 cases from 1980 to 1982, which met ICD-9 criteria for childhood psychotic disorders, wherein cases of infantile autism were included. In another retrospective chart review of cases seen during 1981-1984, from NIMHANS, Bangalore (Robins and O'Neal 1953; Srinath and Chowdhury 1989) cases met the ICD-9 diagnosis for autism in the child psychiatry clinic. The cases were aged from 2.5 to 14 years, with males outnumbering the female children (M:F = 7.5:1), with most belonging to well to do families.

Clinic-based studies to understand the prevalence of autism have also come from non-psychiatric settings. In a retrospective review of the case notes of the children less than 5 years of age done in the pediatric neurology clinic of PGIMER, Chandigarh, Singhi, and Malhi (2001) found 16 children DSM IV criteria for autism, in a 2-year period. The cases were primarily referred to them for speech, and/or developmental delay. Males were only slightly more than females (M:F = 1.3:1) which is contrary to both Indian and Western data, but this can be due to the fact that most children assessed by them were severely autistic, as the score on Childhood Autism Rating Scale's score was in the severely autistic range in 62.5 % of cases. About one-fourth of the cases had normal development up to at least 18 months of age and after that there was regression of milestones in the areas of language and behavior. The authors did not, however, differentiate between infantile autism and other ASD like Rett's syndrome and childhood disintegrative disorder (CDD).

If we are to look at other ASD separately, epidemiological data are sparse. A study from PGIMER, Chandigarh (Malhotra and Singh 1993) described 5 cases of CDDs registered at CAP clinic from 1980 to 1989. These cases constituted 0.22 % of the total cases registered during this period. In a later study, Malhotra and Gupta (2002), in a retrospective chart review of cases registered at CAP clinic between 1989 and 1999 found 12 cases of CDD, which was 0.45 % of all the cases registered in CAP clinic. Average age at onset was 3.76 years and average age of the patients at the time of assessments was 7.46 years. Sex ratio of 5:1 (F > M) is concordant with international literature. Again, a rapid onset of illness was noted which was unusual, as a gradual onset is much more widely seen and reported internationally. Presently, there is also one case report on Asperger's syndrome with comorbid social anxiety disorder (SAD) in Indian literature from PGIMER (Subodh et al. 2006). Malhotra et al. (2002) also reported two cases of Rett's syndrome.

4.1 Unipolar Depression

Numerous studies have estimated the prevalence of Major Depression (MDD) in children and adolescents in community samples. A review showed a median prevalence estimate of 4.0 % (range 0.2–17 %) (Costello et al. 2004). Prevalence rates of dysthymia in this population are lower than that for depression (Kim-Cohen et al. 2003; Verhulst et al. 1997). In contrast, prevalence estimates of subthreshold depressive disorders and syndromes, including minor depression and depression not otherwise specified (NOS), are generally higher than those of MDD across all age groups (Gonzalez-Tejera et al. 2005; Angold et al. 2002). Longitudinal studies of community samples of children and adolescents found the average age of onset between 11 and 14 years for MDD and depressive disorder (DD) (Lewinsohn et al. 1993). The Oregon Adolescent Depression Project showed that the rates of onset of depression increased from 1 to 2 % at age 13 and from 3 to 7 % at age 15 (Lewinsohn et al. 2000).

In India, many studies have evaluated the prevalence of depression in children and adolescents in different settings and these studies suggest that the prevalence of depression in children and adolescents in community setting is 0.1–0.5 %, with higher prevalence in adolescent and no case of depression seen in children up to 3 years of age (Malhotra et al. 2002; Pillai et al. 2008). The clinic-based studies suggest that the prevalence of depression/affective disorders varies from 1.2 to 9.2 %, however, in some of the studies these prevalence rates are inclusive of bipolar disorder. A recent study from PGIMER, Chandigarh, which looked at the trend of various diagnoses in clinic population, reported an increase in prevalence of affective disorders from 2 to 13.49 % in children up to the age of 14 years attending the psychiatric outpatient clinics (Malhotra and Chakrabarti 1992; Malhotra et al. 1999b; Malhotra et al. 2007). Studies have also evaluated special population like school drop outs, school aged children, high school girls, etc. for depression and have reported prevalence rate as high as 60.8 % (Mohanraj and Subbhiah 2010). A study evaluated the prevalence of depression among adolescents and reported that 11.2 % of school dropouts had severe and extreme grades of depression as assessed by BDI compared to prevalence of 3 % in those attending the school regularly and none of the college going adolescents having depression (Nair et al. 2004). A lot of variation in the prevalence can be understood in the light of differences in the instrument used for assessment and the diagnostic criteria used for affective disorders. Only one study has evaluated the incidence of depression in children and adolescents and reported an annual incidence rate of 1.61/1,000 children in a community-based study on school children from Chandigarh (Inserm Collective Expert Report on Mental Illness 2007).

Risk factors for unipolar depression: Studies from the West suggests that among children, there are no gender differences in rates of depression or report higher rates in preadolescent boys (Merikangas and Avenevoli 2002). During adolescence, however, rates of depression are greater among females than among males (Wittchen et al. 1998; Kessler and Walters 1998; Lewinsohn et al. 1993).

Studies of adults suggest that depression is seen more frequently in the lower socioeconomic classes (Kessler et al. 2003), findings in children and adolescents are less consistent. Some researchers have found no association between depression and social class (Costello et al. 2003a), and others have found a significant association (Costello et al. 1996; Reinherz et al. 1993). Some studies have found that African-Americans have lower rates of depression than whites (Angold et al. 2002) and an increased depressive symptoms among Hispanics and Mexican-Americans, compared with their white and African-American counterparts (Roberts et al. 2007; McLaughlin et al. 2007).

Very few Indian studies have evaluated the relationship of depression in children and adolescents with risk factors. These studies suggest that perceived stressful life events and daily hassles are associated with increased risk for depression (Mohanraj et al. 2010) and about half of the patients had an identifiable stressor (Sagar et al. 2012). The life events which have been shown to be associated with depression include death of a family member, change in residence, failure in examination, end of a relationship and serious illness (Patel et al. 1998), stress at school and family, and family history of mental illness (Krishnakumar and Geeta 2006). One of the older studies failed to find a link between childhood bereavement and depression (Venkoba 1970). However, one of the recent studies from Rohtak which evaluated the children and adolescents who had experienced a suicidal death in the family reported that these children and adolescents were at elevated risk for major depressive disorder, posttraumatic disorder, and impaired social adjustment (Sethi and Bhargava 2003).

Other risk factors which have been found as significant predictors of depression in school going children include age, class attendance, family history of psychiatric illness, and birth complications (Sarkar et al. 2012). The risk factors identified in adolescents include female gender, being in the board classes, poor academic performance, and higher number of adverse events (Bhasin et al. 2010). Studies have shown there is a high family history of psychiatric illness with prevalence as high as 67.8 % for girls and 52.5 % for boys (Sagar et al. 2012; Krishnakumar and Geeta 2006). Studies also report that high self-esteem, good family relationships, and peer acceptance act as protective factors against depression (Mohanraj et al. 2010).

4.1.1 Bipolar Disorder

While most adults with bipolar disorder report their first affective episode in adolescence, epidemiological data on bipolar disorder in this population are sparse. The prevalence rates of mania, hypomania, and bipolar disorder in population-based studies in this population range from 0 to 0.9 % in adolescents. Lifetime prevalence rates for bipolar disorder among youth range from 0 to 2.1 %, and the lifetime prevalence rate for hypomania ranges between 0 and 0.4 % (Lewinsohn et al. 1993). The results of most community surveys find nearly equal rates of bipolar disorder in males and females. Also, the incidence of bipolar disorder peaks at age 14 in both males and females and decreases gradually thereafter (Lewinsohn et al. 2002). Presently, there is no Indian data that the authors were aware of that describes the epidemiology of childhood bipolar disorders.

4.2 Childhood Anxiety Disorders

During the past decade, the results of international epidemiologic surveys have revealed that anxiety disorders are the most prevalent class of mental disorders in adults. Similar to community studies of adults, anxiety disorders are also quite prevalent in the general population of children and adolescents. The median prevalence rate of all anxiety disorders in a recent review was 8 % with an extremely wide range of estimates (e.g., 2–24 %) (Costello et al. 2005). Current or 12-month rates of anxiety disorders range from 2.2 % in North Carolina (Costello et al. 2005) to 9.5 % in Puerto Rico (Goodman 2005). Generalized Anxiety Disorder (GAD) and SAD are the two most prevalence disorders in youth (Merikangas et al. 2009). In contrast, panic disorder and OCD are both quite rare in children under age of 12. Similar to the gender ratio for adults, girls tend to have more of all subtypes of anxiety disorders, irrespective of the age composition of the sample. However, it has also been reported that, despite the greater rates of anxiety in girls across all ages, there is no significant difference between boys and girls in the average age at onset of anxiety (Merikangas and Avenevoli 2002).

One of the earliest studies from Hyderabad reported a prevalence rate of childhood neurosis to be 9.7 % in outpatient population and 9.3 % in inpatients with higher preponderance of females (Female:Male ratio 2:1) (Nagaraja 1966). Other older clinic-based studies have reported prevalence of 3.71 % for neurotic disorders in children and a prevalence rate of 2.7 % for the hysterical disorders (Raju et al. 1969). A recent clinic-based study which evaluated the prevalence of various psychiatric disorders in children aged 0–14 years over the period of 26 years revealed that neurotic/anxiety disorders formed the most common psychiatric diagnosis in this group of children with clinic prevalence rate of 37.33–45.69 % (Inserm Collective Expert Report on Mental Illness 2007). Studies from other centers report a prevalence rate of 0.5 and 0.9 % among outdoor and indoor patients, respectively (Gupta et al. 2011).

There are few community-based studies from India which have evaluated the epidemiology of childhood anxiety disorders. In a community-based study, 11.0 % of the children were found to have various neurotic disorders, however, the clinical states mentioned therein varied and did not follow any classificatory scheme (Lal and Sethi 1977). Another epidemiological study conducted by Manchanda and Manchanda

(1978) reported incidence of neuroses was reported to be 1.1 % among pediatric inpatients and 8.2 % in CGC outpatient clinics with female preponderance and most common psychiatric diagnosis being that of hysteria. The recent community-based study from Bangalore noted a prevalence rate of 4.4 % for various anxiety disorders with highest prevalence rate for specific isolated phobia (2.9 %), followed by social phobia (0.3 %), GAD (0.3 %), separation anxiety disorder of childhood (0.2 %), OCD (0.1 %), SAD (0.1 %), panic disorder (0.1 %), and agoraphobia (0.1 %). A study from Kolkata evaluated the prevalence of anxiety among adolescents (13–17 years) by using state-trait anxiety inventory revealed that 20.1 % of boys and 17.9 % of girls had high anxiety, with significantly higher prevalence rate in boys. Adolescents from Bengali medium schools were more anxious than adolescents from English medium schools and those belonging to the middle socioeconomic class suffered from more anxiety than those from both high and low socioeconomic class. Further, it was seen that severity of anxiety correlated with working status of the mothers (Deb et al. 2010).

4.3 Childhood Externalizing Disorders (ADHD and Conduct Disorders)

The point prevalence of ADHD in 5- to 15-year-olds was 2.23 % (Costello et al. 2003a), and the 12-month prevalence ranged between 2 and 8.7 % for ages 4–17 years (Costello et al. 2003a, b; Goodman 2005; Roberts et al. 2007). Rates of ADHD in recent surveys consistently show a male preponderance of ADHD as follows: 2.0 % for boys and 0.5 % for girls (Goodman 2005), and 1.5 % for boys and 0.3 % for girls (Costello et al. 2003a). There is conflicting evidence linking ADHD with socioeconomic status. While one study found a twofold increase in ADHD for the poorest children when compared with the wealthiest children (Froehlich et al. 2007), two other studies found no association between family income or education and rates of ADHD (Goodman 2005; Roberts et al. 2007).

Estimates of current or point prevalence in the UK are 2.3 % for ODD and 1.5 % for CD (Costello et al. 2003a), whereas somewhat higher rates were found in recent U.S. studies with ranges of 2.8–5.5 % for ODD and 2.0–3.32 % for CD (Goodman 2005; Roberts et al. 2007). Similar to ADHD, CD is also more prevalent in boys than girls, with many studies showing a difference of 3–4 times higher for boys.

Asian children in the UK had lower rates of ODD than non-Asian youth (Costello et al. 2003a). Age of onset of disruptive behavior disorders appears to be an important predictor of outcome, with earlier onset associated with more aggressive behaviors, and boys who have a diagnosis of ADHD being more likely to have an early onset of CD (Loeber et al. 2000). Community studies of youth have shown a high degree of co-occurrence of CD and ADHD (Loeber et al. 2000).

While epidemiological studies on externalizing spectrum of childhood psychiatric disorders (ADHD, CD) are plentiful in the Western countries, the epidemiology of these disorders has been explored only by a few Indian authors. Bhatia et al. (1991) found a prevalence of 11 % for ADHD in the pediatric outpatient and found that the prevalence of ADHD increased with age, from 5.2 % in those aged 3–4 years, up to 29.2 % in those aged 11–12 years, with a male to female ratio of 4:1. Additionally, ADHD was most common in first born children and those from a lower social class, and these children had a higher rate of complications during pregnancy and delivery relative to a comparison group. Delayed development, temper-tantrums, enuresis, tics, broken homes, persistent parental discord, and psychiatric illness in parents were all more common in children with ADHD. In another clinic-based study, Malhi and Singhi (2000) found that 8.1 % of the children referred to the child outpatient department were found to meet the DSM IV criteria for ADHD. The male to female ratio in children with ADHD was 5:1. With regard to CD, a school-based study found that 4.58 % of the children had CD and identified lying, bullying, and cruelty to animals as the most frequent symptoms. Boys significantly outnumbered the girls, and childhood onset was found in 73 % and adolescent onset in 27 %. Comorbid ADHD was found in 36 %, hyperactive-impulsive subtype being predominant (Sarkhel et al. 2006). However, in other community-based studies, prevalence of CD, however, is found to be quite low (Malhotra and Chaturvedi 1983; Pillai et al. 2008) with rates being less than 1 % among children and adolescents.

4.4 Childhood Psychotic Disorders

Childhood onset schizophrenia is clinically widely accepted and relatively uncommon diagnostic entity. It is no surprise that no systematic epidemiological data are available from the West or India. Whatever little data are available shows that 0.1–1 % of all schizophrenic disorders manifest before age 10, and this increases to 4 % before age 15. Point prevalence of schizophrenia among children is approximately 1 per 10,000 (Kaplan et al. 2009), though this figure increases sharply following adolescence. However, more community-based data are required to further understand this disorder.

5 Conclusion

Child psychiatry is much needed but yet underdeveloped branch of psychiatry in India. Its importance is exemplified by various India epidemiological studies that show that child psychiatric disorders as common in India as reported in western countries. There is need to pursue more focused incidence studies, multi-centric research with standardized methodologies to get the true profile of child psychiatric disorders in India needed for planning and resource allocation for developing services and intervention strategies at the national level. At the same time, the role of temperament and developmental processes cannot be understated and both clinicians and researchers need to focus their energies on the same. Hopefully, with greater awareness coupled with greater demand for psychiatric services for children, the planners and policy makers of India would be pushed into framing of a child mental health policy and development of more academic centers for mental health of children and adolescents.

References

Angold, A., Erkanli, A., Farmer, E. M., et al. (2002). Psychiatric disorder, impairment, and service use in rural African American and white youth. *Archives of General Psychiatry, 59*, 893–901.

Bansal, P. D., & Barman, R. (2011). Psychopathology of school going children in the age group of 10–14 years. *International Journal of Applied and Basic Medical Research, 1*, 43–47.

Bhasin, S. K., Sharma, R., & Saini, N. K. (2010). Depression, anxiety and stress among adolescent students belonging to affluent families: A school-based study. *Indian Journal of Pediatrics, 77*, 161–165.

Bhatia, M. S., Nigam, V. R., Bohra, N., & Malik, S. C. (1991). Attention deficit disorder with hyperactivity among paediatric outpatients. *Journal of Child Psychology and Psychiatry, 32*, 297–306.

Canino, G., Shrout, P. E., Rubio-Stipec, M., Bird, H. R., Bravo, M., Ramirez, R., et al. (2004). The DSM-IV rates of child and adolescent disorders in Puerto Rico: Prevalence, correlates, service use, and the effects of impairment. *Archives of General Psychiatry, 61*, 85–93.

Cohen, P., Cohen, J., Kasen, S., et al. (1993). An epidemiological study of disorders in late childhood and adolescence-I. Age- and gender-specific prevalence. *Journal of Child Psychology and Psychiatry, 34*, 851–867.

Costello, E., Angold, A., Burns, B., Erkanli, A., Stangl, D., & Tweed, D. (1996). The Great Smoky Mountains Study of Youth. Functional impairment and serious emotional disturbance. *Archives of General Psychiatry, 53*, 1137–1143.

Costello, E., Egger, H., & Angold, A. (2005). 10-year research update review: The epidemiology of child and adolescent psychiatric disorders: I. Methods and public health burden. *Journal of the American Academy of Child & Adolescent Psychiatry, 44*, 972–986.

Costello, E. J., Mustillo, S., Erkanli, A., Keeler, G., & Angold, A. (2003a). Prevalence and development of psychiatric disorders in childhood and adolescence. *Archives of General Psychiatry, 60*(8), 837–844.

Costello, E. J., Mustillo, S., Erkanli, A., Keeler, G., & Angold, A. (2003b). Prevalence and development of psychiatric disorders in childhood and adolescence. *Archives of General Psychiatry, 60*(8), 837–844.

Costello, E. J., Mustillo, S., Keller, G., & Angold, A. (2004). Prevalence of psychiatric disorders in childhood and adolescence. In B. L. Levin, J. Petrila, & K. D. Hennessy (Eds.), *Mental health services: A public health perspective* (2nd ed., pp. 111–128). Oxford, UK: Oxford University Press.

Deb, S., Chaterjee, P., & Walsh, K. (2010). Anxiety among high school students in India: Comparisons across gender, school type, social strata and perceptions of quality time with parents. *Australian Journal of Educational & Developmental Psychology, 10*, 18–31.

Eaton, W. C., & Enns, L. R. (1986). Sex differences in human motor activity level. *Psychological Bulletin, 100*, 19–28.

Else-Quest, N. M., Hyde, J. S., Goldsmith, H. H., & Van Hulle, C. A. (2006). Gender differences in temperament: A meta-analysis. *Psychological Bulletin, 132*, 33–72.

Esser, G., Schmidt, M. H., & Woerner, W. (1990). Epidemiology and course of psychiatric disorders in school-age children—Results of a longitudinal study. *Journal of Child Psychology and Psychiatry, 31*, 243–263.

Flietlich-Bilyk, B., & Goodman, R. (2004). Prevalence of child and adolescent psychiatric disorders in southeast Brazil. *Journal of American Academy of Child Adolescent Psychiatry, 43*, 727–734.

Foley, M., McClowry, S. G., & Castellanos, F. X. (2008). The relationship between attention deficit hyperactivity disorder and child temperament. *Journal of Applied Developmental Psychology, 29*, 157–169.

Ford, T., Goodman, R., & Meltzer, H. (2003). The British child and adolescent mental health survey 1999: The prevalence of DSM-IV disorders. *Journal of the American Academy of Child and Adolescent Psychiatry, 42*, 1203–1211.

Froehlich, T. E., Lanphear, B. P., Epstein, J. N., Barbaresi, W. J., Katusic, S. K., & Kahn, R. S. (2007). Prevalence, recognition, and treatment of attention-deficit/hyperactivity disorder in a national sample of US children. *Archives of Pediatrics and Adolescent Medicine, 161*, 857–864.

Gagne, J. R., Vendlinski, M. K.& Goldsmith, H. H. (2009). The genetics of childhood temperament. In: Y.-K. Kim (Ed.), *Handbook of behavior genetics* (pp. 251–267). New York: Springer.

Giel, R., de Arango, M. V., Climent, C. E., Harding, T. W., Ibrahim, H. H., Ladrido-Ignacio, L., et al. (1981). Childhood mental disorders in primary health care: Results of observations in four developing countries. A report from the WHO collaborative study on strategies for extending mental health care. *Pediatrics*. 68:677–683.

Gonzalez-Tejera, G., Canino, G., Ramirez, R., et al. (2005). Examining minor and major depression in adolescents. *Journal of Child Psychology and Psychiatry, 46*, 888–899.

Goodman, R., Neves dos Santos, D., Robatto Nunes, N. P., Pereira de Miranda, D., Fleitlich-Bilyk, B., & Almeida Filho, N. (2005). The Ilha de Mare study: A survey of child mental health problems in a predominantly African-Brazilian rural community. *Social Psychiatry and Psychiatric Epidemiology, 40*, 11–17.

Graham, P., Rutter, M., & George, S. (1973). Temperamental characteristics as predictors of behavior disorders in children. *American Journal of Orthopsychiatry, 43*, 329–339.

Gupta, V., Singh, A., Upadhyay, S., & Bhatia, B. (2011). Clinical profile of somatoform disorders in children. *Indian Journal of Pediatrics, 78*, 283–286.

Hackett, R., Hackett, L., Bhakta, P., & Gowers, S. (1999). The prevalence and associations of psychiatric disorder in children in Kerala, South India. *Journal of Child Psychology and Psychiatry, 40*, 801–807.

Hasan, Z., & Hasan, A. (1981). Report on a population survey of mental retardation in Pakistan. *International Journal of Mental Health, 10*, 23–27.

Hewitt, L. E., & Jenkins, R. L. (1946). *Fundamental patterns of maladjustment; the dynamics of their origin; a statistical analysis based upon five hundred case records of children examined at the Michigan Child Guidance Institute*. Springfield: Illinois.

Hoch, E. M. (1967). *Indian children on psychiatrist's playground*. New Delhi: Indian Council of Medical Research.

Inserm Collective Expert Report on Mental Illness (2007). Detections and prevention in children and adolescents. Available from: http://www.inserm.fr [cited in 2007].

Kalra, I., Jhanjee, A., Unni, K. E. S., & Bhatia, M. S. (2012). A comparative study of temperament in children of patients suffering from depression in comparison to normal controls. *Delhi Psychiatry Bulletin, 15*, 64–71.

Kanner, L. (1935). *Child psychiatry*. London: Bailliere, Tindal and Cox.

Kaplan, B. J., Sadock, V. A., & Ruiz, P. (2009). *Kaplan and Sadock's comprehensive textbook of psychiatry* (9th ed.). Philadelphia: Lippincott Williams & Wilkins.

Kessler, R. C., Berglund, P., Demler, O., et al. (2003). The epidemiology of major depressive disorder: Results from the National Comorbidity Survey Replication (NCS-R). *JAMA, 289*, 3095–3105.

Kessler, R. C., & Walters, E. E. (1998). Epidemiology of DSM-III-R major depression and minor depression among adolescents and young adults in the National Comorbidity Survey. *Depression and Anxiety, 7*, 3–14.

Kim-Cohen, J., Caspi, A., Moffitt, T. E., Harrington, H., Milne, B. J., & Poulton, R. (2003). Prior juvenile diagnoses in adults with mental disorder: Developmental follow-back of a prospective-longitudinal cohort. *Archives of General Psychiatry, 60*, 709–717.

Krishnakumar, P., & Geeta, M. G. (2006). Clinical profile of depressive disorder in children. *Indian Pediatrics, 43*, 521–526.

Lal, N., & Sethi, B. B. (1977). Estimate of mental ill health in children of an urban community. *Indian Journal of Pediatrics, 44*, 55–64.

Larson, S. A., Lakin, K. C., Anderson, L., Lee, N. K., Lee, J. H., Anderson, D. (2001). Prevalence of mental retardation and developmental disabilities: Estimates from the 1994/1995 national health interview survey disability supplements. *American journal of mental retardation*. 106(3).

Lewinsohn, P. M., Moerk, K. C., & Klein, D. N. (2000). Epidemiology of adolescent depression. *Economics Neuroscience, 2*, 52–68.

Lewinsohn, P. M., Rohde, P., Seeley, J. R., & Fischer, S. A. (1993). Age-cohort changes in the lifetime occurrence of depression and other mental disorders. *Journal of Abnormal Psychology, 102*, 110–120.

Lewinsohn, P., Seeley, J., Buckley, M., & Klein, D. (2002). Bipolar disorder in adolescence and young adulthood. *Child and adolescent psychiatric clinics of North America, 11*, 461–475.

Loeber, R., Burke, J. D., Lahey, B. B., Winters, A., & Zera, M. (2000). Oppositional defiant and conduct disorder: a review of the past 10 years, part I. *Journal of the American Academy of Child and Adolescent Psychiatry, 39*, 1468–1484.

Maccoby, E. E., & Jacklin, C. N. (1974). *The psychology of sex differences*. Stanford: Stanford University Press.

Malhi, P., & Singhi, P. (2000). Spectrum of attention deficit hyperactivity disorders in children among referrals to psychology services. *Indian Pediatrics, 37*, 1256–1260.

Malhotra, S. (1988). Stability of temperament characteristics over time. *Child Psychiatry Quarterly, 21*, 43–49.

Malhotra, S. (1989). Temperament characteristics of children with conduct and conversion disorders. *Indian Journal of Psychiatry, 31*, 168–172.

Malhotra, S., Aga, V. M., Balraj, & Gupta, N. (1999a). Comparison of conduct disorder and hyperkinetic conduct disorder : A retrospective clinical study from north India. *Indian Journal of Psychiatry, 41*, 111–121.

Malhotra, S., Biswas, P., Sharan, P., & Grover, S. (2007). Characteristics of patients visiting the child and adolescent psychiatric clinic: A 26-year study from North India. *JIACAM, 3*, 53–60.

Malhotra, S., & Chakrabarti, S. (1992). A clinical profile of depression in children. *Indian Journal of Social Psychiatry, 8*, 54–58.

Malhotra, S., & Chaturvedi, S. K. (1983). Patterns of childhood psychiatric disorders in India. *Indian Journal Paediatrics, 51*, 235–240.

Malhotra, S., & Gupta, N. (2002). Childhood disintegrative disorder—Re examination of the current concept. *European Child and Adolescent Psychiatry, 11*, 108–114.

Malhotra, S., Gupta, N., & Singh, G. (1999b). Retrospective study of affective disorders in children attending a child psychiatry clinic. *Indian Journal of Medical Research, 109*, 71–75.

Malhotra, S., & Kaur, R. P. (1997). Temperament study on the children of mentally ill patients. *Hong Kong Journal of Psychiatry, 7*(1), 39–45.

Malhotra, S., Kohli, A., & Arun, P. (2002a). Prevalence of psychiatric disorders in school children in Chandigarh India. *Indian Journal of Medicinal Research, 116*, 21–28.

Malhotra, S., Kohli, A., Kapoor, M., & Pradhan, B. (2009). Incidence of childhood psychiatric disorders in India. *Indian Journal of Psychiatry, 51*, 101–107.

Malhotra, S., Kumar, D., & Gupta, N. (2002b). Rett's syndrome. A neurodevelopmental disorder: Report of two cases. *Neurology India, 50*, 330–333.

Malhotra, S., & Malhotra, A. (1990). Psychological adjustment of physically sick children: Relationship with temperament. *Indian Pediatrics, 27*, 577–584.

Malhotra, S., & Randhawa, A. (1983). A schedule for measuring temperament in children: Preliminary data on development and standardization. *Indian Journal of Clinical Psychology, 9*, 203–210.

Malhotra, S., & Singh, S. P. (1993). Disintegrative psychosis of childhood: An appraisal and case study. *Acta Paedopsychiatrica, 56*, 37–40.

Malhotra, S., Varma, V. K., & Verma, S. K. (1986). Temperament as determinant of phenomenology of childhood psychiatric disorders. *Indian Journal of Psychiatry, 28*, 263–276.

Manchanda, M., & Manchanda, R. (1978). Neuroses in children: Epidemiological aspect. *Indian Journal of Psychiatry, 20*, 161–165.

McClowry, S. G. (2002). Transforming temperament profile statistics into puppets and other visual media. *Journal of Pediatric Nursing, 17*, 11–17.

McLaughlin, K. A., Hilt, L. M., & Nolen-Hoeksema, S. (2007). Racial/ethnic differences in internalizing and externalizing symptoms in adolescents. *Journal of Abnormal Child Psychology, 35*, 801–816.

Merikangas, K. R., & Avenevoli, S. (2002). Epidemiology of mood and anxiety disorders in children and adolescents. In M. T. Tsaung & M. Tohen (Eds.), *Textbook in psychiatric epidemiology* (2nd ed., pp. 657–704). New York, NY: Wiley-Liss.

Merikangas, K. R., Nakamura, E. F., & Kessler, R. C. (2009). Epidemiology of mental disorders in children and adolescents. *Dialogues in Clinical Neuroscience, 11*(1), 7.

Mohanraj, R., & Subbhiah, K. (2010). Prevalence of depressive symptoms among urban adolescents in South India. *JIACAM, 6*, 33–43.

Mohanraj, R., Subbhiah, K., & Watson, B. (2010). Risk and protective factors to depressive symptoms in school-going adolescents. *JIACAM, 6*, 101–119.

Mullick, M. S., & Goodman, R. (2005). The prevalence of psychiatric disorders among 5–10 year olds in rural, urban and slum areas in Bangladesh: An exploratory study. *Social Psychiatry and Psychiatric Epidemiology, 40*, 663–671.

Nagaraja, J. (1966). Seven years of child psychiatry at Hyderabad. A review. *Indian Journal of Psychiatry, 8*, 291.

Nair, M. K., Paul, M. K., & John, R. (2004). Prevalence of depression among adolescents. *Indian Journal of Pediatrics, 71*, 523–524.

Narang, R. L., Gupta, R., Mishra, B. P., & Mahajan, R. (1997). Temperamental characteristics and psychopathology among children of alcoholics. *Indian Journal of Psychiatry, 39*(3), 226–231.

Narayanan, H. S. (1978). A report of clinical observations and management in 7 cases of childhood autism. *Indian Journal of Psychiatry, 20*, 93–97.

Patel, S., Shah, R., Patel, H., Tilwani, M., & Vankar, G. K. (1998). Depressive symptomatology among adolescent school girls. *Indian Journal of Psychiatry, 40*, s35.

Pillai, A., Patel, V., Cardozo, P., Goodman, R., Weiss, H. A., & Andrew, G. (2008). Nontraditional lifestyles and prevalence of mental disorders in adolescents in Goa, India. *The British Journal of Psychiatry, 192*, 45–51.

Raghuthaman, G., & Cherian, A. (2003). Temperament of children and adolescents presenting with unexplained physical symptoms. *Indian Journal of Psychiatry, 45*, 43–47.

Rajesh, T. V., Krishnakumar, P., & Mathews, L. (2008). Temperamental traits and psychological problems of children with bronchial asthma. *Indian Pediatrics, 45*, 772–774.

Raju, V. B., Sundaravalli, N., Somasundaram, O., & Raghavan, V. G. (1969). Neurotic disorders in children. *Indian Paediatrics, 6*, 296.

Reddy, V. M., & Chandrashekar, C. R. (1998). Prevalence of mental and behavioral disorders in India: A meta-analysis. *Indian Journal of Psychiatry, 40*, 149–157.

Reinherz, H. Z., Giaconia, R. M., Pakiz, B., Silverman, A. B., Frost, A. K., & Lefkowitz, E. S. (1993). Psychosocial risks for major depression in late adolescence: A longitudinal community study. *Journal of the American Academy of Child and Adolescent Psychiatry, 32*, 1155–1163.

Richman, N., Stevenson, J., & Graham, P. (1982). *Preschool to school: A behavioural study*. London: Academic Press.

Roberts, B. W., & DelVecchio, W. F. (2000). The rank-order consistency of personality traits from childhood to old age: A quantitative review of longitudinal studies. *Psychological Bulletin, 126*, 3–25.

Roberts, R. E., Roberts, C. R., & Xing, Y. (2007). Rates of DSM-IV psychiatric disorders among adolescents in a large metropolitan area. *Journal of Psychiatric Research, 41*, 959–967.

Robins, L. N., Helzer, J. E., Croughan, J., & Ratcliff, K. S. (1981). National Institute of Mental Health diagnostic interview schedule: Its history, characteristics, and validity. *Archives of General Psychiatry, 38*(4), 381.

Robins, E., & O'Neal, P. (1953). Clinical features of hysteria in children, with a note on prognosis; a two to seventeen year follow-up study of 41 patients. *The Nervous Child, 10*(2), 246.

Roeleveld, N., Zielhuis, G. A. (2008). The prevalence of mental retardation: A critical review of recent literature. *Developmental Medicine and Child Neurology, 39*.

Rothbart, M. K., & Bates, J. E. (2006). Temperament. In W. Damon & R. Lerner (Eds.), *Handbook of child psychology, Social, emotional, and personality development* (6th ed., pp. 99–166). New York: Wiley.

Rutter, M., Maughan, B., Mortimore, P., & Ouston, J. (1979). *Fifteen thousand hours: Secondary schools and their effects on children*. Cambridge: Harvard University Press.

Rutter, M., Tizard, J., Yule, W., Graham, P., & Whitmore, K. (1976). Research report: Isle of Wight studies, 1964–1974. *Psychological Medicine, 6*, 313–332.

Sagar, R., Pattanayak, R. D., & Mehta, M. (2012). Clinical profile of mood disorders in children. *Indian Pediatrics, 49*, 21–23.

Sarkar, S., Sinha, V. K., & Praharaj, S. K. (2012). Depressive disorders in school children of suburban India: an epidemiological study. *Social Psychiatry and Psychiatric Epidemiology, 47*, 783–788.

Sarkhel, S., Sinha, V. K., Arora, M., & DeSarkar, P. (2006). Prevalence of conduct disorder in schoolchildren of Kanke. *Indian Journal of Psychiatry, 48*, 159–164.

Sethi, S., & Bhargava, S. C. (2003). Child and adolescent survivors of suicide. *Crisis, 24*, 4–6.

Singhi, P., & Malhi, P. (2001). Clinical and neurodevelopmental profile of young children with autism. *Indian Paediatrics, 38*, 384–390.

Srinath, S., Chowdhury, J., Bhide, A. V., Narayanan, H. S., & Shivaprakash, Z. Z. (1989). Descriptive study of infantile autism. *Nimhans Journal, 7*(1), 77–81.

Srinath, S., Girimaji, S. C., Gururaj, G., Seshadri, S., Subbakrishna, D. K., Bhola, P., et al. (2005). Epidemiological study of child & adolescent psychiatric disorders in urban and rural areas of Bangalore, India. *Indian Journal of Medicinal Research, 122*, 67–79.

Stein, Z., Durkin, A., & Belmont, I. (1986). 'Serious' mental retardation in developing countries: An epidemiologic approach. *Annals of New York Academy of Science, 477*, 8–41.

Subodh, B. N., Grover, S., & Sharan, P. (2006). Asperger's disorder with co-morbid social anxiety disorder: A case report. *Journal of Indian Association. Child Adolescence Mental Health, 2*, 68–69.

Tadesse, B., Kebede, D., Tegegne, T., & Alem, A. (1999). Childhood behavioural disorders in the ambo district, western Ethopia: I, Prevlaence estimates. *Acta psychiatrica Scandinavica, 397*, 92–97.

Thomas, S., & Chess, S. (1977). *Temperament and Development*. New York: Brunner/Mazel.

Thomas, A., Chess, S., & Birch, H. G. (1968). *Temperament and behavior disorders in children*. New York: New York University Press.

Thomas, A., Chess, S., Birch, H. G., Hertzig, M. E., & Korn, S. (1963). *Behavioral individuality in early childhood*. New York: New York University Press.

Venkoba Rao, A. (1970). Broken home (in particular reference to parental deaths) and its relationship to depressive illness. *Indian Journal of Psychiatry*, 12, 23–32.

Verhulst, F. C., van der Ende, J., Ferdinand, R. F., & Kasius, M. C. (1997). The prevalence of DSM-III-R diagnoses in a national sample of Dutch adolescents. *Archives of General Psychiatry, 54*, 329–336.

Watson, D., & Clark, L. A. (1992). Affects separable and inseparable: On the hierarchical arrangement of the negative affects. *Journal of Personality and Social Psychology, 62*, 489–505.

Wittchen, H. U., Nelson, C. B., & Lachner, G. (1998). Prevalence of mental disorders and psychosocial impairments in adolescents and young adults. *Psychological Medicine, 28*, 109–126.

Worland, J., Weeks, D. G., Janes, C. L., & Strock, B. D. (1984). Intelligence, classroom behavior, and academic achievement in children at high and low risk for psychopathology: A structural equation analysis. *Journal of Abnormal Child Psychology, 12*(3), 437–454.

Chapter 13
Research Endeavors in Child Psychiatry in India-II

Savita Malhotra and Natasha Kate

Following an upsurge in neurobiological research psychiatry, genetics and neuroimaging have provided great insights into our understanding of childhood psychiatric disorders as well.

1 Genetic Studies

Mental retardation: Mental retardation in a child is accepted to be mutlifactorial in its causality. However, the frequency of chromosome anomalies identified by high-resolution karyotyping varies between 9 and 36 % (Schreppers-Tijdink et al. 1988). In a review of the frequency of cytogenetic abnormalities in patients with mental retardation (Van Karnebeek et al. 2002a), the authors found the median frequency of detected chromosome abnormalities was nearly 1 in 10 patients. This review noted a wide range of reported frequencies of chromosome abnormalities causing mental retardation—from 2 to 50 % depending on the type of studies. Chromosome abnormalities were found in all categories of mental retardation (mild to profound) and in both genders. In a prospective study which evaluated the etiology of mental retardation by using karyotyping, abnormalities were reported in 8.3 % of children (Van Karnebeek et al. 2002b). These authors also found that there was a relationship between the number of minor anomalies and the likelihood of a chromosomal abnormality: A higher number of anomalies indicated a

S. Malhotra, Professor and Head; N. Kate, Formerly Senior Resident

S. Malhotra (✉) · N. Kate
Department of Psychiatry, Postgraduate Institute of Medical Education and Research, Chandigarh, India
e-mail: savita.pgi@gmail.com

S. Malhotra and S. Chakrabarti (eds.), *Developments in Psychiatry in India*,
DOI 10.1007/978-81-322-1674-2_13

significantly higher likelihood to find a chromosomal abnormality, and they concluded that karyotyping should be performed in all cases in whom no known cause is detected. Van Karnebeek et al. (2005) found that those with more significant mental retardation are more likely to have positive results of fragile X testing (4.1 %), compared with those with milder delays or borderline intelligence testing results (1.0 %).

Among Indians, consanguinity is a common cause for genetic abnormalities and consanguinity among parents is often considered as a cause of mental retardation in their children. Madhavan and Narayan (1991) indicated that when there is a history of mental retardation in the family and if the parents are consanguineously married, the risk of mental retardation in the offspring is significantly high. Among the consanguineously married families, the blood relationship of uncle-niece seems to have the highest risk of affecting the offsprings. The influence of genetic factors like Fragile X has also been looked at in Indian patients with MR. In a large study from AIIMS, New Delhi, 29.8 % boys fulfilled defined clinical criteria to be screened for fragile X syndrome by chromosomal studies and 6.38 % of them were found to be positive for fragile X syndrome using cytogenetic techniques (Jain et al. 1998). Agarwal (1991) found that chromosomal anomalies were found in 23.7 %, metabolic defects in 5.0 %, and an identifiable genetic syndrome in 11.6 % of the patients with mental retardation. In the remaining 59.7 % patients, no known genetic cause could be identified. However, 66.5 % of these patients had one or more of the following conditions: (i) congenital malformation with or without neurological deficit, (ii) history of consanguinity, (iii) positive family history of mental retardation, or (iv) a positive screening test but without a confirmed diagnosis of metabolic defect (suggesting that there may be additional unidentified genetic causes of mental retardation). In a more recent study (Eggers and Bunk 1997), it was found that the various aetiological categories for mental retardation included were chromosomal disorders (33.1 %) and nonchromosomal syndromes (9.5 %) with genetic syndromes identified including Down's syndrome, microdeletion syndromes like William's syndrome, Prader–Willi syndrome, and unbalanced karyotypes.

Autism and Autistic Spectrum Disorders: Genetic studies in autism and autistic spectrum disorders have shown an association of these disorders with abnormalities of X-chromosomes, especially Fragile X syndrome. Other mutations seen include CACNA1C, calcium channel voltage-dependent L-type alpha 1C subunit; CNTNAP2, contactin-associated protein-like 2; FMR1, fragile X mental retardation 1; and SHANK3, SH3, and multiple ankyrin repeat domains (Abrahams and Geschwind 2008). Manjunatha et al. (1989) did a cryptogenetic investigation in autistic children with the aim of finding the association and prevalence of fragile X syndrome in autistic children. Though none of the six cases studied had fragile X chromosome, fragile sites were noted in autosomes 1, 2, 3, 5, and 6. However, significance of this finding is limited as these sites are also observed in general population and mentally retarded subjects (Manjunatha et al. 1989; Fryns 1984). In Tamil Nadu, cytogenetic analysis of the peripheral blood samples of patients who have been diagnosed positive for autism was performed to identify the structural or numerical chromosomal abnormalities by karyotyping (Selvi et al. 2010). The study showed no complex rearrangements or other chromosomal abnormalities. In view of the negative results obtained in this study, the authors hypothesized that autism develops due to the influence of some environmental factors during embryogenesis.

Glutaminergic abnormalities have also been proposed in autism, and it is observed that reduction of GluR5 gene dosage can decrease ASD-like features in fragile X mice (Abrahams and Geschwind 2008). The gene coding for glutamate receptor 6 (GluR6 or GRIK2) has also been suggested as a candidate gene for autism based on its localization in the autism-specific region on chromosome 6q21 and the involvement of receptor protein in cognitive functions like learning and memory. In a study from West Bengal, Dutta et al. (2007) performed genetic analysis of three markers of GluR6 (SNP1: rs2227281, SNP2: rs2227283, SNP3: rs2235076) for possible association with autism through population and family-based approaches. DSM-IV criteria and CARS were utilized for diagnosis. Genotyping analysis for the SNPs was carried out in 101 probands with ASD, 180 parents, and 152 controls from different regions of India. This study could not find any biased transmission of alleles or haplotypes in those affected with autism. They suggested that these markers of GluR6 were unlikely to be associated with autism in the Indian population. In another large sample study, it was found that less that 10 % of children with ASD had a normal karyotype, with the most common chromosomal aberration being Fragile X syndrome. Inborn errors of metabolism were found to be rare (Balasubramanian et al. 2009). In order to understand the neurochemical changes in autism, cerebrospinal fluid (CSF) concentrations of the serotonin and dopamine metabolites, 5-hydroxyindoleacetic acid (5HIAA), and homovanillic acid (HVA), respectively, have also been measured by researchers. Studies have found no difference in the CSF levels of 5HIAA or HVA in children with autistic disorder as compared to those without the disorder, suggesting that consistent, marked alterations in central serotonin and dopamine turnover are not present in the autistic subjects, though larger sample sizes are required to come to any conclusions (Narayan et al. 1993).

ADHD: Attention-deficit hyperkinetic disorder (ADHD) and related disorders have a very high heritability, as demonstrated by family studies. ADHD linkage studies have identified a number of genetic loci (potentially) harboring genes for ADHD, and some chromosome regions such as 5p13, 14q12, and 17p11 have been indicated in multiple studies (Banaschewski et al. 2010). Additionally, most of the present-day studies have focused on genes involved in the dopaminergic system, including DRD4, DRD5, DAT1/SLC6A3, DBH, and DDC. Genes associated with the noradrenergic (such as NET1/SLC6A2, ADRA2A, ADRA2C) and serotonergic systems (such as 5-HTT/SLC6A4, HTR1B, HTR2A, TPH2) have also been implicated. Additionally, research is now looking at the genes that control neurotransmission and neuronal plasticity including SNAP25, CHRNA4, NMDA, BDNF, NGF, NTF3, NTF4/5, and GDNF. An Indian study showed significant difference in the frequency of 3.5 repeat allele of the MAO-A promoter gene in children with ADHD and preferential transmission of this short allele from mothers to male ADHD children, and the authors concluded that the short 3.5 repeat allele of the *MAO-A* is probably associated with ADHD in our population and could be the reason for making boys prone to ADHD as compared to girls (Das et al. 2006). Other genetic changes shown to be associated with ADHD include dopamine beta hydroxylase (DBH) polymorphisms (Bhaduri et al. 2010). Das et al. (2011) additionally found interaction between ten functional polymorphisms in DRD4, DAT1, MAOA, COMT, and DBH genes in Indian children with ADHD, and this corelation was found especially in male children with ADHD.

There is very little literature regarding genetic abnormalities seen in other childhood disorders, and it chiefly centers on case reports of genetic syndromes with associated psychopathology and hence are not elaborated upon in this section.

2 Neuroimaging: Neurostructural and Neurophysiological Studies

Mental Retardation: The neurobiology of mental retardation is dependent on the cause for the retardation. However, given that mental retardation should suggest obligate brain abnormality, it is surprising that the percentage of individuals in imaging studies who are positive for abnormality is as low as 9 % in some studies (Kaplan et al. 2009). The results also depend on the modality of neuroimaging used in the study. Some studies have shown dorsal stream abnormalities were associated with visuospatial deficits in Williams' syndrome, and aberrant frontal–striatal connections were implicated in the executive function and attention impairments in individuals with fragile X syndrome (Kaplan et al. 2009). In a mental retardation clinic in Bangalore (Narayanan 1981), it was seen that aetiology for mental retardation was discernible in 77.1 %, and a majority had associated physical disorders such as cerebral palsy, seizures, and hearing and/or visual impairment. In a more recent study (Aggarwal et al. 2012), it was found that the various aetiological categories for mental retardation included were chromosomal disorders (33.1 %), nonchromosomal syndromes (9.5 %), neurometabolic disorders (10.1 %), central nervous system structural defects (7.4 %), cerebral palsy (12.7 %), and environmental insults (2 %). A significant number of children with MR (25.2 %) had no discernible cause for their developmental delay, highlighting the fact that at times, no single abnormality can be identified as causality for mental retardation.

Autism and Autistic Spectrum Disorders: No single neurobiological cause can be attributed to the autism spectrum disorders and entail heterogeneity of the causative mechanisms, and autistic disorder is associated with cerebellar changes, greater total brain and lateral ventricle volume, and asymmetry (Hendren et al. 2000). Postmortem studies of a small number of individuals with autism have revealed a range of abnormalities, including a significant decrease in the number of Purkinje cells and granule cells in the cerebellum. MRI studies focusing on the cerebellar vermis have revealed an initial finding of a decrease in the midsagittal area of vermal lobules VI and VII (Kaplan et al. 2009; Minshew and Williams 2007). Studies that look at the limbic system have found decreased neuronal size, decreased dendritic arborization, and increased neuronal packing density of neurons in the amygdala, hippocampus, septum, anterior cingulate, and mammillary bodies. The best replicated functional finding concerns underactivation of a region of the fusiform gyrus on the ventral surface of the temporal lobe during face perception tasks (Kaplan et al. 2009; Minshew and Williams 2007). Neuroimaging studies from India have been fairly recent in autism. A single-photon emission computed tomography (SPECT) study that assessed the cerebral perfusion in children with autism and mental retardation found generalized hypoperfusion of brain frontal and prefrontal regions revealed maximum hypoperfusion (Gupta and Ratnam 2009). Subcortical areas also indicated hypoperfusion. On the basis of the findings, the authors concluded that children with autism have varying levels of perfusion abnormities in brain which may lead to neurophysiologic dysfunction that presents as cognitive and neuropsychological defects. In another study from PGIMER (Singhi et al. 2008), 22 children with primary autism with varying degrees of severity were studied using SPECT. Fifteen children had no perfusion abnormalities on SPECT imaging. Of the remaining seven, decreased perfusion in the left frontoparietal cortex was seen in three, and in the left inferior and medial frontal cortex in two children. No correlation could be found between SPECT, electroencephalography, and magnetic resonance imaging findings. In another neuroimaging study from PGIMER (Anil 2011), using FDG-PET, an attempt was made to study the rCGM in patients with autism and to study relationship, if any, between behavioral and neuropsychological deficits and rCGM. It was found that out of ten, four patients had abnormal brain functioning on positron emission tomography (PET) scan and bilateral cerebellar hypometabolism being the most consistent finding. Bilateral cerebellar hypometabolism as a consistent finding reflects the role of cerebellum in cognitive and emotional functioning which is impaired in subjects with ASD. Disturbed metabolism in temporal, frontal, and occipital cortex was also found in some patients, reflecting the complex nature of abnormal brain functioning in ASD which accounts for its clinical heterogeneity. When PET scan findings and the symptom profile was looked at, it was found that higher abnormal behavior in the form of clumsiness, repetitive movements, poor coordination, and strange finger/body movements point toward the cerebellar functional abnormalities.

ADHD: Authors have described neuroanatomical correlations for the superior and temporal cortices with the focusing of attention; external parietal and corpus striatal regions with motor executive function; the hippocampus with the encoding of memory traces; the prefrontal cortex with the act of shifting from one salient stimulus to another; and brainstem areas such as reticular thalamic nuclei with the sustaining of attention (Castellanos and Tannock 2002). Also, evidence suggests decreased volume and activity in prefrontal areas, anterior cingulate, globus pallidus, caudate, thalamus, hippocampus, and cerebellum in children with ADHD (Kaplan et al. 2009).

Other disorders: Neurobiology of other childhood disorders is not as well characterized as in adult disorders. Overall, childhood-onset schizophrenia shows progressive ventricular enlargement, reduction in total brain and thalamus volume, changes in temporal lobe structures, and reductions in frontal metabolism (Hendren et al. 2000). Neuroimaging studies of depressed youth have found smaller left subgenual prefrontal cortex, smaller frontal white matter volumes, larger frontal gray matter volumes, and larger lateral ventricular volumes than normal children (Kaplan et al. 2009). Pediatric bipolar disorder shows the presence of white matter hyperintensities and decreased amygdala volume. Studies of youth with early-onset bipolar disorder have decreased neuronal density in the prefrontal cortex and decreased neuronal homeostasis in the anterior cingulate cortex (Kaplan et al. 2009). Reduced globus pallidus volume and gray matter volumetric abnormalities in the anterior cingulated gyrus have been seen in pediatric patients with obsessive-compulsive disorder (OCD). PET studies in OCD have shown increased glucose metabolism in orbitofrontal cortex, right caudate nucleus, and anterior cingulate gyrus, at rest and in response to symptom provocation (Kaplan et al. 2009). However, neuroimaging studies in India are in their infancy, and hence, literature on these disorders from India is scant.

3 Phenomenology

Psychiatric disorders in children and adolescents are often different in their phenomenology in comparison with adults. Due to their atypical presentation, childhood psychiatric disorders are often misdiagnosed and therefore incorrectly treated leading to further dysfunction. Hence, we shall review the available literature with regard to childhood psychiatric disorders.

Childhood depressive disorder: Many studies from the West have evaluated the symptomatology of depression in children and adolescents. Earlier studies suggested that depression in children often presents as "masked depression," but the recent data suggest that children more often manifest typical presentation, and the masked symptoms, most of which was somatization (seen in about 40 % of subjects), occurred less frequently than typical symptoms (Luby et al. 2003; Kashani and Carlson 1987). Comparison of phenomenology across different age groups suggests that adolescent may display more vegetative symptoms in the form of sleep and appetite disturbances along with suicidal ideations and attempts and more impairment than younger children, but less than adults (Birmaher et al. 1998). Psychotic symptoms as part of the depressive episode more frequently manifest as auditory hallucinations in children, whereas delusions are more common in adolescents (Kowatch et al. 2005). Studies from India suggest that children and adolescents with depression most commonly present with multiple somatic complaints (Tharoor et al. 2002) and such a manifestation is more common in children compared to adults (Bhargava and Sethi 2005). Further, it is seen that predominant mood symptom in children is that of irritability in contrast to sadness in adults (Bhargava and Sethi 2005; Sagar et al. 2012). Other commonly reported symptoms of depression across studies include low mood, diminished interest in play and activities, excessive tiredness, low self-esteem, problems with concentration, behavior symptoms like anger and aggression, decreased interest in school and recent deterioration in school performance, death wish, suicidal behavior, anhedonia, sleep or appetite disturbances, concentration difficulty, and anxiety (Bhargava and Sethi 2005; Sagar et al. 2012; Krishnakumar and Geeta 2006). In terms of dysfunction, when compared with adults, children present exclusively with poor scholastic performance and reduced play activity, whereas adults presented with the poor work performance (Bhargava and Sethi 2005).

Comorbidity in childhood and adolescent depression is a rule rather than exception. It has been reported that about 40–70 % of depressed adolescent patients have at least one concomitant condition, and 20–50 % patients have two or more comorbid conditions (Fleming and Offord 1990; Angold and Costello 1993). The most common comorbid conditions in adolescents include anxiety (30–75 %), conduct disorder (CD) (10–80 %), substance abuse (20–30 %), and personality disorder (60 %) (Fleming and Offord 1990; Angold and Costello 1993). According to the meta-analysis by Angold and Costello (1993), anxiety disorders, conduct and oppositional disorders, and attention-deficit hyperactivity disorder are 8.2, 6.6, and 5.5 times more common in depressed children and adolescents, respectively. Further, it is suggested that onset of unipolar depression is known to follow the onset of other disorders, except for substance abuse and panic disorder, which have their onset in adolescence. Studies which have evaluated the comorbidity pattern in preschool depressed children report comorbid conditions like attention-deficit hyperactivity disorder (42 %), oppositional defiant disorder (ODD) (62 %), and both attention-deficit hyperactivity disorder and ODD (41 %) and only 28 % had comorbid anxiety disorders (Luby et al. 2003). Studies from India suggest that about one-fourth (28.5 %) of children and adolescents with mood disorders have comorbid psychiatric disorder (Sagar et al. 2012). The commonly and consistently reported psychiatric comorbidities in children with depression include anxiety and conversion/dissociative disorder (Bhargava and Sethi 2005; Sagar et al. 2012; Angold and Costello 1993). Other comorbid conditions include dysthymia, adjustment disorder, CD, and attention-deficit hyperactivity disorder (Bhargava and Sethi 2005; Sagar et al. 2012; Angold and Costello 1993). Studies which have compared children and adolescents with adults report that there is difference in comorbidity profile with substance abuse and anxiety disorder being more common in adults (Bhargava and Sethi 2005).

Childhood bipolar disorder: Western studies have suggested that mania in children and adolescents manifests with typical symptoms. However, understanding the developmental perspective in evaluating is very important. The school-going child, besides some of the typical features, may manifest with symptoms like harassment of the teacher, and slightly older children may manifest with sexually disinhibited behavior if they are brought up in conservative families (Geller and Luby 1997). Studies from India too have described typical clinical picture of mania in children and adolescents (Reddy et al. 1997; Bhargava Raman et al. 2007).

As with unipolar depression, comorbidity is very common in bipolar disorders in children and adolescents and many a times, the comorbidity impedes the proper evaluation of manic symptoms (Geller and Luby 1997). The common comorbid conditions which are known to coexist in children and adolescents with bipolar disorder and to be considered as differential diagnosis too include ADHD, ODD, CD, and sexual abuse. Additionally, specific learning disorders should be considered in children and a psychotic disorder and substance abuse must be kept in mind while evaluating adolescents (Geller and Luby 1997). Studies from India too suggest that disruptive behavior disorders (DBD), i.e., ADHD, ODD, and CD in patients with juvenile bipolar disorder are common, and it was noted that those with DBD had earlier onset of bipolar disorder and spent more time ill compared to those without DBD (Bhargava Raman 2007). With regard to the course of bipolar disorders in children and adolescents, data suggest that the initial episodes are that of depressive episodes followed by mixed episodes and a rapid cycling course without clear-cut episodes (Geller and Luby 1997). In contrast studies from India which have evaluated patients of mania suggest that almost all patients with juvenile bipolar disorder in the manic phase recover from the index episode (Srinath et al. 1998; Jairam et al. 2004; Rajeev et al. 2003). However, a significant proportion (33–72.4 %) (Srinath et al. 1998; Jairam et al. 2004; Rajeev et al. 2003, 2004; Malhotra et al. 2007) of patients experience relapse during the initial 2 years of recovery despite being on treatment (Srinath et al. 1998) and the mean duration to relapse is 18 (SD-16.4) months (Jairam et al. 2004).

Childhood schizophrenia: Childhood-onset schizophrenia is considered to be more severe form of schizophrenia. Earlier studies tried to establish the link between childhood schizophrenia and autism. Rutter (1972) followed up children of autism and concluded that these children do not show clinical features of schizophrenia in adulthood. Other studies showed that patients with childhood-onset schizophrenia show typical delusions and hallucinations as seen in adults; however, these are not seen in those with autism (Kolvin 1971). These studies laid the foundation of recognition of schizophrenia as a distinct entity in childhood.

Over the years, studies have shown that majority of the patients with childhood-onset schizophrenia have premorbid difficulties in the form of social withdrawal, language disturbances, academic difficulties, and developmental delays. The symptoms usually appear insidiously, especially in those manifesting with negative symptoms. In terms of positive symptoms, studies have consistently reported the presence of hallucinations, delusions, and formal thought disorder; however, the prevalence of these has varied in different studies. The prevalence of various symptoms reported in different studies is as follows: auditory hallucinations (25–84 %), delusions (50–63 %), formal thought disorder (40–100 %), visual hallucinations (30–47 %), and flat affect (74–84 %). Other common symptoms include suicidal ideations, suicide attempts, anxiety symptoms, and depressive symptoms (Kolvin 1971; Kimura et al. 1978; Green et al. 1992; Eggers and Bunk 1997; Krausz and Müller-Thomsen 1993; Yang et al. 1995). Studies from India have also reported presence of hallucinations, delusions, and thought disorder in most patients (Srivastava et al. 1988; Thakur et al. 2003; Sharma et al. 2005; Biswas et al. 2006). Further, the data suggest that except for minor differences, there is lack of difference in the symptom profile in patients with childhood-onset schizophrenia, adolescent-onset schizophrenia, and adult-onset schizophrenia (Biswas et al. 2006). This study suggested that patients with COS have more somatic and obsessive symptoms, whereas those of adolescent onset have more self-injurious behavior and suicidal attempts (Biswas et al. 2006). In terms of subtype of schizophrenia, studies from India suggest that paranoid and undifferentiated schizophrenia (Srivastava et al. 1988) are the most common subtypes and this is in keeping with the literature from other parts of the world.

Childhood obsessive-compulsive disorder: Despite the typical symptoms, OCD having onset in childhood and adolescence, commonly known as juvenile-onset OCD, is considered to have certain unique features and risk factors. Data suggest that compared to adult-onset OCD, juvenile OCD is characterized by male preponderance (Kimura et al. 1978; Green et al. 1992; Eggers and Bunk 1997; Krausz and Müller-Thomsen 1993; Yang et al. 1995; Srivastava et al. 1988; Thakur et al. 2003; Sharma et al. 2005; Biswas et al. 2006; Hanna 1995; Masi et al. 2005, 2006; Swedo et al. 1989), familial aggregation of OCD with tic disorder (Chabane et al. 2005; Lenane et al. 1990; Nestadt et al. 2000; Pauls et al. 1995), higher rates of comorbidity, especially ADHD and non-OCD anxiety disorders (Chabane et al. 2005; Lenane et al. 1990; Nestadt et al. 2000; Pauls et al. 1995; Chowdhury et al. 2004; Geller et al. 1996; Leonard et al. 1992; Rosario-Campos et al. 2005; Jans et al. 2007; Coskun et al. 2012), presence of compulsions only (Swedo et al. 1989; Geller et al. 1996, 1998; Rettew et al. 1992), higher rates of aggressive obsessions, and higher rates of hoarding (Geller et al. 2001). Few studies from India have also addressed OCD in children and adolescents. A study from NIMHANS evaluated 54 patients with juvenile OCD for various comorbid psychiatric disorders and reported that more than two-third (69 %) of patients had a comorbid psychiatric disorder with 22 % having disruptive disorders, 20 % having mood disorders, 19 % having anxiety disorders, and 17 % having tic disorder. Only 1 subject had bipolar disorder, and none had psychosis (Reddy et al. 2000). Another study from the same center compared patients with juvenile OCD ($\leq$18 years N = 39), juvenile-onset adult OCD (age of onset $\leq$ 18 years), and adult-onset OCD (age of onset $\geq$ 18 years). The findings of the study revealed that after controlling for age and gender, patients with juvenile OCD were more frequently male having comorbid attention-deficit hyperactivity disorder, chronic tics, body dysmorphic disorder, and major depression. Patients of juvenile-onset adult OCD differed from juvenile OCD by having later age at onset and low rate of comorbid ADHD (Jaisoorya et al. 2003). Compared to adult-onset OCD, patients of juvenile-onset adult OCD more frequently had comorbid social phobia and chronic tics. Based on these findings, the authors concluded that patients with juvenile OCD appear to differ from others and juvenile OCD could be a developmental subtype of the disorder.

4 Psychopharmacology

The story of modern child psychopharmacology began in 1937 when Charles Bradley reported the effects of administering racemic amphetamine sulfate to 30 children 5–14 years of age with various behavioral disturbances. Following this, there had been slow but steady research in this field, though researchers have focused their efforts chiefly on ADHD. However, it is essential to realize that children are not miniature adults. Their metabolizing capacities as well as their sensitivity to medication can be quite different from that of an adult, and differences in body weights make it difficult to set doses among children and in the same child over a period of time.

Stimulants and related medication: Indeed, ADHD is the only disorder that has medications that were developed specifically for, while the psychopharmacological agents used in other disorders are largely chosen following extrapolation from adult disorders. ADHD is possibly the most commonly medicated diagnosis, with 8–10 % of children in the USA (LeFever et al. 1999) receiving medication for the same. Presently, stimulants are the most widely used and also most useful medication in the management of ADHD. Most children (88 %) who are started on methylphenidate would continue medication (Vitiello et al. 2001), and the response rates to stimulant medication are as high as 60–70 % (Kaplan et al. 2009). However, the short half-life of amphetamines have resulted in the development of their sustained release versions that are now growing in popularity, given their reported ability to control symptoms with a once-daily dose. Atomoxetine is the second-line drug approved for children and adults with ADHD (Coghill 2003), followed by alpha-adrenergic agonists (like clonidine), and then other drugs such as bupropion, antipsychotics, tricyclic antidepressants (TCAs), and buspirone, though the evidence for them is small. However, the use of stimulants and clonidine has come under a cloud following reports of sudden cardiac death with their use (Cantwell et al. 1997). Though this has occurred in children with previous cardiac malformations, it brings to light the problems with indiscriminate use of medication.

Presently, stimulants are the first-line pharmacological agents in the management of ADHD around the world. However, in developing countries like India, costs of stimulants may be prohibitive for more common use. Hence, cheaper alternatives are often looked for. This reality is possibly reflected in the present state of research on psychopharmacological agents in ADHD. While there seem to be no Indian studies that evaluate the efficacy of stimulants in ADHD, Malhotra and Santosh (1998) showed that buspirone had a favorable side effect profile and significantly reduced the symptoms of ADHD.

Stimulants have been the flagship compounds for pediatric psychopharmacology. Reports of sudden cardiac death have not dimmed their popularity. However, cost and related concerns may affect management plans.

Antidepressants: A Cochrane review (Hazell and Mirzaie 2013) has demonstrated that TCAs (unlike in adults) are unlikely to be of much benefit in managing depression in preadolescent children and there might be only marginal efficacy in adolescents. Additionally, there have been case reports of death of adolescents while receiving desimipramine (Popper and Zimnitzky 1995), prompting clinician to seriously consider the risk benefit ratios of using TCAs in conditions like ADHD where other drugs are available. Selective serotonin reuptake inhibitors (SSRIs) are now being increasingly used for childhood depressive and anxiety disorders, with fluoxetine being licensed by the FDA for major depression in this age group and clomipramine, fluoxetine, and sertraline being licensed for OCD. However, there is a recent black box warning issued by the US FDA, in view of the risk on increase in suicidal ideation and suicide attempts in adolescents with severe depression being treated with SSRIs (Olfson et al. 2006). TCAs have also been used in the management of enuresis, often in treatment-resistant cases as well (Monda and Husmann 1995).

From India, two open-label trials evaluated the usefulness of imipramine in enuresis (Chatterjee and Khandpur 1965) and behaviorally disturbed children (Mahendru et al. 1970) and reported positive results with few side effects. Surprisingly, there is lack of data with respect to efficacy and effectiveness of antidepressants in patients with depression. One study evaluated the usefulness of loading dose of imipramine in treatment of depression in children and adolescents. The study included 16 children and adolescents diagnosed with depression as per DSM-IIIR criteria. Using a double-blind randomized control design, these patients were administered conventional dosing versus loading dose of imipramine and it was seen that high bolus doses of imipramine led to reduction in depressive features within 72 h (Malhotra and Santosh 1996). Hence, it is evident that antidepressants do play a role in the management of pediatric psychiatric disorders in India and the world, but caution needs to be exercised during their use especially among depressed children.

Antipsychotics: Antipsychotic use in children and adolescents increased from 1987 to 1996, ranging from a 1.6-fold to 5.5-fold increase (Zito et al. 2003). In the USA, children and adolescents accounted for 15 % of the patient use in 2004–2005, as compared with 7 % in 1996–1997 (Domino and Swartz 2008). Additionally, the overall duration of treatment with antipsychotics has also increased (Kalverdijk et al. 2008; Rani et al. 2008). There are a few short-term, placebo-controlled trials supporting the efficacy of risperidone, aripiprazole, olanzapine, and quetiapine in psychotic symptoms of schizophrenia in adolescents and manic symptoms of pediatric bipolar disorder (Sikich 2008; Chang 2008; Findling et al. 2008; Kryzhanovskaya et al. 2009). Based on this, the US FDA has approved both risperidone and aripiprazole for the treatment of adolescents with schizophrenia and of 10–17-year-olds with mania or mixed episodes. In addition, risperidone has been shown to be effective in decreasing behavioral problems, such as aggression and self-injury in autistic children (Research Units on Pediatric Psychopharmacology Autism Network 2002) and is approved for use in these children. In Europe, risperidone is approved for children with aggression in the context of CD following positive results in some studies (Aman et al. 2002; Snyder et al. 2002; Buitelaar et al. 2001). In children, few controlled studies have directly compared the effects of first- and second-generation antipsychotics. Clozapine has been shown to be better than haloperidol or olanzapine in children and adolescents with schizophrenia (Kumra et al. 2008a, b; Shaw et al. 2006). However, no evidence of differences in efficacy among the remaining antipsychotics has emerged. There are indications that children are more sensitive than adults to the metabolic adverse effects of SGA, as well as to the extrapyramidal effects of the first-generation antipsychotics (Correll et al. 2006).

Few studies from India have evaluated the efficacy of different antipsychotics in children and adolescents. In one of the first such studies, Doongaji et al. (1961) evaluated the efficacy of Prothipendyl in children with mental retardation and found that children who received prothipendyl showed significant improvement in restlessness without any reported side effects. Bagadia et al. (1972) found trifluperidol to be useful in children with emotional disturbance, epilepsy, and mental retardation along with aggression and hyperkinesis though side effects were reported. One recent study from PGIMER, Chandigarh, evaluated the usefulness of risperidone in children with autism (Nagaraj et al. 2006). In a double-blind randomized placebo-controlled trial of children with autism, it was found that children in risperidone group showed improvement in the symptoms of social responsiveness, nonverbal communication, hyperactivity, and aggression with few side effects. With regard to antipsychotics in schizophrenia, in a small case series of 5 subjects, Malhotra et al. (2000) reported usefulness of clozapine in childhood-onset schizophrenia. Positive symptoms improved more than the negative symptoms; however, there was no benefit in the ritualistic behavior. No serious side effects like seizures or neutropenia were noted. Agarwal and Sitholey (2006) evaluated the efficacy of olanzapine in patients with acute and transient psychosis and found improvement in BPRS and CGI scores with olanzapine with side effects like dryness of mouth, increase in appetite, weight gain, drowsiness, and others. No patient developed EPS though significant weight gain was observed. Banerjee et al. (2007) carried out an open-label trial comparing aripiprazole to haloperidol and found these to be equally efficacious. Aripiprazole led to significantly lower rates of extrapyramidal symptoms and weight gain. Additionally, studies have reported usefulness of haloperidol in children with delirium (Grover et al. 2009).

Hence, antipsychotics are useful in both psychotic and non-psychotic behaviorally disturbed children. Both first- and second-generation antipsychotics seem equally efficacious (except clozapine), and the choice of drug may be dictated by side effect profile or cost.

5 Somatic Treatment

Electroconvulsive therapy (ECT) is a well-known and accepted treatment modality for severe mental disorders in adults. Since its first clinical description in 1934 by Cerletti and Bini, it has undergone a great degree of chance and improvement (with the use of brief pulse therapy, unilateral electrode placement techniques, anesthetic agents). However, today, the place of ECT in psychiatric treatment protocols is heavily debated, given the ethical issues involved in its use. Yet, today, the most use of ECT in the child and adolescent population is in catatonia in children with autism (Zaw et al. 1999; Dhossche et al. 2009). ECT has been found to be effective for the treatment of catatonia and catatonia-related conditions of intractable compulsions, tics, and self-injury in people with autism. ECT has been shown to be a safe and effective option in adolescent depression (Griesemer et al. 1997) and has also been used in children with intractable seizures (Walter and Rey 1997). As per a review (Rey and Walter 1997), rates of improvement across studies focusing on young patients were 63 % for depression, 80 % for mania, 42 % for schizophrenia, and 80 % for catatonia. However, despite the efficacy of ECT, its use has been steadily declining. This could be partly due to inadequate knowledge of ECT in clinicians who deal with children and adolescents. When awareness was assessed, around forty percent for child and adolescent psychiatrists rated their knowledge about ECT in the young as nil or negligible and believed ECT to be unsafe in children compared to adults, quite contrary to the available literature.

In India, like in the West, data with respect to use of ECT in children and adolescents are limited. One large survey which included 19,632 patients who received 1,14,111 instances of use of ECT from 316 psychiatrists revealed that only 1.4 % of the total ECTs are administered to persons less than 18 years (Chanpattana et al. 2005). One recent study from PGIMER, Chandigarh, evaluated the effectiveness of ECT in adolescents (aged 13–18 years) (Grover et al. 2013). The authors reviewed the treatment record of all patients who received ECT during the period of 1999–2011. Only 6 % of patients who received ECT were aged 18 or less. Schizophrenia was the commonest indication for ECT in this group, followed by depression. Catatonic symptoms were the most common symptoms among these subjects, and in three-forth of the patients, the treating clinicians considered ECT as the treatment of choice in view of the clinical picture. On average, each patient received 10 ECTs, and the response rate according to diagnosis was 76.3 % for schizophrenia, 87.2 % for depression, 81.8 % for Psychosis (NOS), and 77.7 % for acute and transient psychosis. Response rate in patients with catatonic features was 91.6 %. Very few patients developed side effects in the form of prolonged seizures, nausea and vomiting, and headache (Grover et al. 2013). Hence, the presently available data clearly put ECT as a potentially useful treatment in children and adolescents.

6 Non-Pharmacological Management

As described previously, children often react differently to medication compared to adults and have more side effects than adults. Given this, there is often a question that arises in parents and clinicians mind—whether we can mange psychiatric ailments in children through non-pharmacological means.

Behavioral management can aid the management of multiple psychiatric disorders. This is because parenting impacts child's learned behavior irrespective of the illness, and hence, modifying improper parenting practices is of great importance, as poor parenting is one of the predictors of negative long-term outcomes in children with behavior disorders (Chamberlain et al. 1995). Behavioral parent training (BPT) is one of the techniques described to change parenting patterns and hence manage ADHD (Pelham et al. 1998), ODD and CD (Brestan and Eyberg 1998), anxiety disorders (Silverman et al. 1999), and other childhood disorders. Attentional training was also found to be effective in patients with ADHD (Rapport et al. 1996). Intensive behavioral therapy may improve the intellectual, language, and adaptive functions of children with autistic spectrum disorder (Eikeseth et al. 2002; Harris and Handleman 2000; Sheinkopf and Siegel 1998; Smith et al. 2000; Weiss 1999). Parent training programmes have also been shown to be effective in children with CD and ODD (Webster-Stratton et al. 2004). Yoga as a mode of intervention is being increasingly recognized for children with ADHD, CD, and other behavioral problems. Despite yoga originating from India, a large part of international literature comes from non-Indian countries (Krisanaprakornkit et al. 2010). Mehta et al. (2011) showed children could successfully learn both yoga and meditation irrespective of their age, ADHD type, or initial performance impairment. Additionally, they found that multimodal intervention, including yoga, was found to be beneficial in a large number of children with ADHD (90.5 %) and this improvement was noted both by parents and teachers. Additionally, the same authors found that following continued intervention, these gains were reportedly sustained over a year (Mehta et al. 2012). Dogra and Veeraraghavan (1994) found that an 8-week intervention consisting of play therapy and parental counseling produced significant improvement in children with aggressive CD and helped improve their overall adjustment and family environment.

Studies have also showed the usefulness of Yoga in autism and autistic spectrum disorder in increasing the imitation skills (Radhakrishna et al. 2010). One of the major goals of an intervention program for children with autism is to provide them a method of functional communication and to control problem behaviors. To manage these, authors have proposed an number of behavioral management models like Una Breccia nel Muro (UBM)—A Comprehensive Behavioral Model (Favaa et al. 2012), applied behavioral analysis (Griffith et al. 2012), applied behavior analysis with stimulus control (Green 2001), and so on. In an Indian study that looked at parent-based behavioral intervention, Juneja et al., (2012) found significant improvement in 16 children in the areas of development, social, expressive, and receptive language quotients following months of individualized intervention. Lal (2010) assessed the effectiveness of Makaton Vocabulary Language Program, a system of alternative and augmentative communication (AAC), on development of language and social behavior of children with autism and found a significant change in receptive, expressive language and social behavior. A novel method of speech intervention 'Communication developmental eclectic approach to language learning (DEALL)' was assessed by Karanth et al (2010). Significant improvement was seen in the domains of gross motor skills, fine motor skills, activities of daily life skills, receptive language, and expressive language, cognitive, social, and emotional skills, and a significant decrease in behavioral symptoms was also seen.

As seen above, non-pharmacological means of managing childhood psychiatric disorders are also being increasingly looked at as methods to deal with such problems. Given the complex interaction between the environmental milieu (that non-pharmacological methods try to address), and the neurobiological pathology (that medication tries to impact), it is evident that non-pharmacological interventions have an essential role to play in child psychiatric disorders.

7 Future of Child Psychiatry

Despite a huge paucity of trained child and adolescent psychiatrists in India, systematic research in child psychiatry has begun and there is gradual trickle of research data on various aspects of childhood psychiatric disorders. One of the major and landmark studies relates to development and implementation of a model telepsychiatry application for delivering mental health care to remote areas, using medical knowledge-based decision support system, through the agency of non-specialist doctors and paramedics (Malhotra et al. 2014). In this Net-based computerized system of psychiatric diagnosis and management, the paramedic and the general physician or a pediatrician or a general adult psychiatrist can treat children and adolescents with psychiatric disorders in the remote areas. The system is currently being piloted at three hill states in north India and will soon become available for wider implementation.

There is concern that thrust of research in child psychiatry world over is propelled by psychopharmacology, and psychosocial and behavioral interventions have been pushed into the background. Additionally, demands for "quick fix" cure, increasing public awareness and expectations, and the need of the society for addressing holistic development (in place of simple symptom amelioration) put additional pressures on child psychiatrists.

Presently, child psychiatry in India is at a crucial juncture, pushing for an identity, clamoring for recognition, asserting for resource allocation, in order to steer and strengthen not only its research base but also for establishing comprehensive service and training infrastructure. Concerted efforts, by clinicians, researchers, and policy makers will be essential for it to become an academic superspecialty with prime public health focus.

References

Abrahams, B. S., & Geschwind, D. H. (2008). Advances in autism genetics: On the threshold of a new neurobiology. *Nature Reviews Genetics, 9*(5), 341–355.

Agarwal, S. S. (1991). Multicentric study on genetic causes of mental retardation in India. *Indian Journal of Medical Research, 94*, 161–169.

Agarwal, V., & Sitholey, P. (2006). A preliminary open trial of olanzapine in pediatric acute and transient psychotic disorders. *Indian Journal of Psychiatry, 48*, 43–46.

Aggarwal, S., Bogula, V. R., Mandal, K., Kumar, R., & Phadke, S. R. (2012). Aetiologic spectrum of mental retardation and developmental delay in India. *Indian Journal of Medical Research, 136*, 436–444.

Aman, M. G., De Smedt, G., Derivan, A., Lyons, B., Findling, R. L., Risperidone Disruptive Behavior Study Group (2002). Doubleblind, placebo-controlled study of risperidone for the treatment of disruptive behaviors in children with subaverage intelligence. *American Journal of Psychiatry, 159*, 1337–1346.

Angold, A., & Costello, E. J. (1993). Depressive comorbidity in children and adolescents: empirical, theoretical, and methodological issues. *American Journal of Psychiatry, 150*, 1779–1791.

Anil, B. N. (2011). A study of the regional cerebral glucose metabolism (rCGM) in patients with ASD using PET scan and to study their neuropsychological correlates. Thesis submitted to Post Graduate Institute of Medical Education and Research, December 2011.

Bagadia, V. N., Kotwani, P. N., Dave, K. P., Saraf, K. R., & Shah, L. P. (1972). Fluphenthixol in certain psychiatric illness (a clinical trial). *Indian Journal of Psychiatry, 14*, 19–23.

Balasubramanian, B., Bhatt, C. V., & Goyel, N. A. (2009). Genetic studies in children with intellectual disability and autistic spectrum of disorders. *Indian Journal of Human Genetics, 15*, 103–107.

Banaschewski, T., Becker, K., Scherag, S., Franke, B., & Coghill, D. (2010). Molecular genetics of attention-deficit/hyperactivity disorder: An overview. *European Child and Adolescent Psychiatry, 19*(3), 237–257.

Banerjee, M., Ram, D., & Das, A. (2007). An open label comparison of aripiprazole versus haloperidol for the treatment of childhood and adolescent psychiatric disorders. *Indian Journal of Psychiatry, 49*(Suppl), 3.

Bhaduri, N., Sarkar, K., Sinha, S., Chattopadhyay, A., & Mukhopadhyay, K. (2010). Study on DBH genetic polymorphisms and plasma activity in attention deficit hyperactivity disorder patients from Eastern India. *Cellular and Molecular Neurobiology, 30*, 265–274.

Bhargava Raman, R. P., Sheshadri, S. P., Janardhan Reddy, Y. C., Girimaji, S. C., Srinath, S., & Raghunandan, V. N. (2007). Is bipolar II disorder misdiagnosed as major depressive disorder in children? *Journal of Affective Disorders, 98*, 263–266.

Bhargava, S. C., & Sethi, S. (2005). Depressive disorder in children. *JIACAM, 1*, 4.

Birmaher, B., Brent, D. A., & Benson, R. S. (1998). Practice parameters for the assessment and treatment of children and adolescents with depressive disorders. *Journal of the American Academy of Child and Adolescent Psychiatry, 37*(10 Suppl), 63S–83S.

Biswas, P., Malhotra, S., Malhotra, A., & Gupta, N. (2006). Comparative study of neuropsychological correlates in schizophrenia with onset in childhood, adolescence and adulthood. *European Child and Adolescent Psychiatry, 15*, 360–366.

Brestan, E. V., & Eyberg, S. M. (1998). Effective psychosocial treatments of conduct-disordered children and adolescents: 29 years, 82 studies, and 5,272 kids. *Journal of clinical child psychology, 27*(2), 180–189.

Buitelaar, J. K., vander Gaag, R. J., Cohen-Kettenis, P., & Melman, C. T. (2001). A randomized controlled trial of risperidone in the treatment of aggression in hospitalized adolescents with subaverage cognitive abilities. *The Journal of Clinical Psychiatry, 62*, 239–248.

Cantwell, D. P., Swanson, J., & Connor, D. F. (1997). Case study: Adverse response to clonidine. *Journal of the American Academy of Child and Adolescent Psychiatry, 36*(4), 539–544.

Castellanos, F. X., & Tannock, R. (2002). Neuroscience of attention-deficit/hyperactivity disorder: The search for endophenotypes. *Nature Reviews Neuroscience, 3*(8), 617–628.

Chabane, N., Delorme, R., Millet, B., Mouren, M. C., Leboyer, M., & Pauls, D. (2005). Early-onset obsessive–compulsive disorder: A subgroup with a specific clinical and familial pattern? *Journal of Child Psychology and Psychiatry and Allied Disciplines, 46*(8), 881–887.

Chamberlain, P., Patterson, G. R., & Bornstein, M. (Eds.). (1995). *Handbook of parenting: Vol. 4. Applied and practical parenting* (pp. 205–225). Mahwah, NJ: Lawrence Erlbaum Associates.

Chang, K. D. (2008). The use of atypical antipsychotics in pediatric bipolar disorder. *Journal of Clinical Psychiatry, 69*(4), 4–8.

Chanpattana, W., Kunigiri, G., Kramer, B. A., & Gangadhar, B. N. (2005). Survey of the practice of electroconvulsive therapy in teaching hospitals in India. *The Journal of ECT, 21*, 100–104.

Chatterjee, A. K., & Khandpur, S. S. (1965). Tofranil in enuresis of children. *Indian Journal of Psychiatry, 7*, 243–245.

Chowdhury, U., Frampton, I., & Heyman, I. (2004). Clinical characteristics of young people referred to an obsessive compulsive disorder clinic in the United Kingdom. *Clinical Child Psychology and Psychiatry, 9*(3), 395–401.

Coghill, D. (2003). Current issues in child and adolescent psychopharmacology. Part 1: Attention-deficit hyperactivity and affective disorders. *Advances in Psychiatric Treatment, 9*(2), 86–94.

Correll, C. U., Penzner, J. B., Parikh, U. H., Mughal, T., Javed, T., Carbon, M., et al. (2006). Recognizing and monitoring adverse events of second-generation antipsychotics in children and adolescents. *Child and Adolescent Psychiatric Clinics of North America, 15*, 177–206.

Coskun, M., Zoroglu, S., & Ozturk, M. (2012). Phenomenology, psychiatric comorbidity and family history in referred preschool children with obsessive-compulsive disorder. *Child and Adolescent Psychiatry and Mental Health, 6*, 36.

Das, M., Das Bhowmik, A., Bhaduri, N., Sarkar, K., Ghosh, P., Sinha, S., et al. (2011). Role of gene-gene/gene-environment interaction in the etiology of eastern Indian ADHD probands. *Progress in Neuro-Psychopharmacology and Biological Psychiatry, 35*(2), 577–587.

Das, M., Das Bhowmik, A., Sinha, S., Chattopadhyay, A., Chaudhuri, K., Singh, M., et al. (2006). MAOA Promoter Polymorphism and Attention Deficit Hyperactivity Disorder (ADHD) in Indian Children. *American Journal of Medical Genetics Part B, 141B*, 637–642.

Dhossche, D., Reti, I. M., & Wachtel, L. E. (2009). Catatonia and Autism: A historical review, with implications for electroconvulsive therapy. *Journal of ECT, 25*, 19–22.

Dogra, A., & Veeraraghavan, V. (1994). A study of psychological intervention of children with aggressive conduct disorder. *Indian Journal of Clinical Psychology, 21*, 28–32.

Domino, M. E., & Swartz, M. S. (2008). Who are the new users of antipsychotic medications? *Psychiatric Services, 59*, 507–514.

Doongaji, D. R., Bagadia, V. N., & Vahia, N. S. (1961). Clinical experience with prothipendyl hydrochloride (dominal)—A new tranquiliser. *Indian Journal of Psychiatry, 3*, 228–234.

Dutta, S., Das, S., Guhathakurta, S., Sen, B., Sinha, S., Chatterjee, A., et al. (2007). Glutamate receptor 6 gene (GluR6 or GRIK2) polymorphisms in the Indian population: A genetic association study on autism spectrum disorder. *Cellular and Molecular Neurobiology, 27*, 1035–1047.

Eggers, C., & Bunk, D. (1997). The long-term course of childhood-onset schizophrenia: A 42-year follow up. *Schizophrenia Bulletin, 23*, 105–117.

Eikeseth, S., Smith, T., Jahr, E., & Eldevik, S. (2002). Intensive behavioral treatment at school for 4- to 7-year-old children with autism: A 1-year comparison controlled study. *Behavior Modification, 26*(1), 49–68.

Favaa, L., Vicarib, S., Valeri, G., D'Elia, L., Arimad, S., & Strauss, K. (2012). Intensive Behavioral Intervention for school-aged children with autism: Una Breccia nel Muro (UBM)—A Comprehensive Behavioral Model. *Research in Autism Spectrum Disorders, 6*, 1273–1288.

Findling, R. L., Robb, A., Nyilas, M., Forbes, R. A., Jin, N., Ivanova, S., et al. (2008). A multiple-center, randomized, double-blind, placebo-controlled study of oral aripiprazole for treatment of adolescents with schizophrenia. *American Journal of Psychiatry, 165*, 1432–1441.

Fleming, J., & Offord, D. (1990). Epidemiology of childhood depressive disorders: A critical review. *Journal of the American Academy of Child and Adolescent Psychiatry, 29*, 571–580.

Fryns, J. P. (1984). The fragile X syndrome: A study of 83 families. *Clinical Genetics, 26*, 497–528.

Geller, D. A., Biederman, J., Faraone, S., Agranat, A., Cradock, K., Hagermoser, L., et al. (2001). Developmental aspects of obsessive compulsive disorder: Findings in children, adolescents, and adults. *Journal of Nervous and Mental Disease, 189*(7), 471–477.

Geller, D. A., Biederman, J., Griffin, S., Jones, J., & Lefkowitz, T. R. (1996). Comorbidity of juvenile obsessive–compulsive disorder with disruptive behavior disorders. *Journal of the American Academy of Child and Adolescent Psychiatry, 35*(12), 1637–1646.

Geller, D. A., Biederman, J., Jones, J., Park, K., Schwartz, S., Shapiro, S., et al. (1998). Is juvenile obsessive–compulsive disorder a developmental subtype of the disorder? A review of the pediatric literature. *Journal of the American Academy of Child and Adolescent Psychiatry, 37*(4), 420–427.

Geller, B., & Luby, J. (1997). Child and Adolescent Bipolar Disorder: A Review of the Past 10 Years. *Journal of the American Academy of Child and Adolescent Psychiatry, 36*, 1168–1176.

Green, G. (2001). Behavior analytic instruction for learners with autism advances in stimulus control technology. *Focus on Autism and Other Developmental Disabilities, 16*(2), 72–85.

Green, W. H., Padron-Gayol, M., Hardesty, A. S., & Bassiri, M. (1992). Schizophrenia with childhood onset: a phenomenological study of 38 cases. *Journal of the American Academy of Child and Adolescent Psychiatry, 31*, 968–976.

Griesemer, D. A., Kellner, C. H., Beale, M. D., et al. (1997). Electroconvulsive therapy for the treatment of intractable seizures. Initial findings in two children. *Neurology, 49*, 1389–1392.

Griffith, G. M., Fletcher, R., & Hastings, R. P. (2012). A national UK census of Applied Behavior Analysis school provision for children with autism. *Research in Autism Spectrum Disorders, 6*, 798–805.

Grover, S., Malhotra, S., Bharadwaj, R., Subodh, B. N., & Kumar, S. (2009). Delirium in children and adolescents. *International Journal of Psychiatry in Medicine, 39*, 179–187.

Grover, S., Malhotra, S., Varma, S., Chakrabarti, S., Avasthi, A., & Mattoo, S. K. (2013). Electroconvulsive therapy in adolescents: A retrospective study from north India. *Journal of ECT, 29*, 122–126.

Gupta, S. K., & Ratnam, B. V. (2009). Cerebral Perfusion Abnormalities in Children with Autism and Mental Retardation: A Segmental Quantitative SPECT Study. *Indian Pediatr, 46*, 161–164.

Hanna, G. L. (1995). Demographic and clinical features of obsessive–compulsive disorder in children and adolescents. *Journal of the American Academy of Child and Adolescent Psychiatry, 34*(1), 19–27.

Harris, S. L., & Handleman, J. S. (2000). Age and IQ at intake as predictors of placement for young children with autism: A four- to six-year follow-up. *Journal of Autism and Developmental Disorders, 30*(2), 137–142.

Hazell, P., & Mirzaie, M. (2013). Tricyclic drugs for depression in children and adolescents. *Cochrane Database of Systematic Reviews, 6*, CD002317.

Hendren, R. L., De Backer, I., & Pandina, G. J. (2000). Review of neuroimaging studies of child and adolescent psychiatric disorders from the past 10 years. *Journal of the American Academy of Child and Adolescent Psychiatry, 39*(7), 815–828.

Jain, U., Verma, I. C., & Kapoor, A. K. (1998). Prevalence of fragile X(A) syndrome in mentally retarded children at a genetics referral centre in Delhi, India. *Indian Journal of Medical Research, 108*, 12–16.

Jairam, R., Srinath, S., Girimaji, S. C., & Seshadri, S. P. (2004). A prospective 4–5 year follow-up of juvenile onset bipolar disorder. *Bipolar Disorders, 6*, 386–394.

Jaisoorya, T. S., Janardhan Reddy, Y. C., & Srinath, S. (2003). Is juvenile obsessive-compulsive disorder a developmental subtype of the disorder?—Findings from an Indian study. *European Child and Adolescent Psychiatry, 12*, 290–297.

Jans, T., Wewetzer, C., Klampfl, K., Schulz, E., Herpertz-Dahlmann, B., Remschmidt, H., et al. (2007). Phenomenology and co-morbidity of childhood onset obsessive compulsive disorder. *Zeitschrift fur Kinder-und Jugendpsychiatrie und Psychotherapie, 35*(1), 41–50.

Juneja, M., Mukherjee, S., Sharma, S., Jain, R., Das, B., & Sabu, P. (2012). Evaluation of a parent-based behavioral intervention program for children with autism in a low-resource setting. *Journal of Pediatric Neurosciences, 7*, 16–18.

Kalverdijk, L., Tobi, H., van den Berg, P., Buiskool, J., Wagenaar, L., Minderaa, R., et al. (2008). Use of antipsychotic drugs among Dutch youths between 1997 and 2005. *Psychiatric Services, 59*(5), 554–560.

Kaplan, B. J., Sadock, V. A., & Ruiz, P. (2009). *Kaplan and Sadock's comprehensive textbook of psychiatry (9th edition)*. Philadelphia: Lippincott Williams & Wilkins.

Karanth, P., Shaista, S., & Srikanth, N. (2010). Efficacy of communication DEALL—An indigenous early intervention program for children with autism spectrum disorders. *The Indian Journal of Pediatrics, 77*, 957–962.

Kashani, J. H., & Carlson, G. A. (1987). Seriously depressed preschoolers. *American Journal of Psychiatry, 144*, 348–350.

Kimura, S., Asai, S., Wakeno, M., & Aoki, N. (1978). On early and mid-onset schizophrenia, Part 1: Phenomenological aspects. *Folia Psychiatrica et Neurologica Japonica, 32*, 41–56.

Kolvin, I. (1971). Studies in the childhood psychoses. I. Diagnostic criteria and classification. *British Journal of Psychiatry, 118*, 381–384.

Kowatch, R. A., Emslie, G. J., Wilkaitis, J., Dingle, A. D. (2005). Mood disorders, In S. B. Sexson (Ed.), *Child and adolescent psychiatry* (pp. 132–153). Massachusetts: Blackwell Publishing Ltd.

Krausz, M., & Müller-Thomsen, T. (1993). Schizophrenia with onset in adolescence: An 11-year follow up. *Schizophrenia Bulletin, 19*, 831–841.

Krisanaprakornkit, T., Ngamjarus, C., Witoonchart, C., & Piyavhatkul, N. (2010). Meditation therapies for attention-deficit/hyperactivity disorder (ADHD). *Cochrane Database Systematic Reviews, 6*, CD006507.

Krishnakumar, P., & Geeta, M. G. (2006). Clinical profile of depressive disorder in children. *Indian Pediatrics, 43*, 521–526.

Kryzhanovskaya, L., Schultz, S. C., McDougle, C., Frazier, J., Dittman, R., Robertson-Plouch, C., et al. (2009). Olanzapine versus placebo in adolescents with schizophrenia: A 6-week, randomized, double-blind, placebo-controlled trial. *Journal of the American Academy of Child and Adolescent Psychiatry, 48*, 60–70.

Kumra, S., Kranzler, H., Gerbino-Rosen, G., Kester, H. M., DeThomas, C., Kafantaris, V., et al. (2008a). Clozapine and "high-dose" olanzapine in refractory early-onset schizophrenia: A 12-week randomized and double-blind comparison. *Biological Psychiatry, 63*, 524–529.

Kumra, S., Oberstar, J. V., Sikich, L., Findling, R. L., McClellan, J. M., Vinogradov, S., et al. (2008b). Efficacy and tolerability of second-generation antipsychotics in children and adolescents with schizophrenia. *Schizophrenia Bulletin, 34*, 60–71.

Lal, R. (2010). Effect of alternative and augmentative communication on language and social behavior of children with autism. *Educational Research and Reviews, 5*(3), 119–125.

LeFever, G. B., Dawson, K. V., & Morrow, A. L. (1999). The extent of drug therapy for attention deficit-hyperactivity disorder among children in public schools. *American Journal of Public Health, 89*(9), 1359–1364.

Lenane, M. C., Swedo, S. E., Leonard, H. L., Pauls, D., Sceery, W., & Rapoport, J. L. (1990). Psychiatric disorders in first degree relatives of children and adolescents with obsessive compulsive disorder. *Journal of the American Academy of Child and Adolescent Psychiatry, 29*(3), 407–412.

Leonard, H. L., Lenane, M. C., Swedo, S. E., Rettew, D. C., Gershon, E. S., & Rapoport, J. L. (1992). Tics and Tourette's disorder: A 2- to 7-year follow up of 54 obsessive–compulsive children. *American Journal of Psychiatry, 149*(9), 1244–1251.

Luby, J. L., Heffelfinger, A. K., Mrakotsky, C., et al. (2003). The clinical picture of depression in preschool children. *Journal of the American Academy of Child and Adolescent Psychiatry, 42*, 340–348.

Madhavan, T., & Narayan, J. (1991). Consanguinity and mental retardation. *Journal of Intellectual Disability Research, 35*, 133–139.

Mahendru, B. K., Gupta, S. C., Agarwal, A. K., & Sethi, B. B. (1970). Imipramine as an effective tool in the management of behavioural disorders in children. *Indian Journal of Psychiatry, 12*, 238–243.

Malhotra, S., Biswas, P., Sharan, P., & Grover, S. (2007). Characteristics of patients visiting the child and adolescent psychiatric clinic: A 26-year study from North India. *Journal of Indian Association for Child and Adolescent Mental Health, 3*, 53–60.

Malhotra, S., Gupta, N., & Singh, G. (2000). Clozapine in childhood-onset schizophrenia: A report of five cases. *Clinical Child Psychology and Psychiatry, 5*, 403–410.

Malhotra, S., Chakrabarti, S., Shah, R., Gupta, G., Mehta, A., Nithya, B. et al. (2014). Development of a novel diagnostic system for a telepsychiatry application: A pilot study. *BMC Research Notes, 7*, 508. doi: 10.1186/1756-1500-7-508. http://www.biomedcentral.com/1756-1500-7-508

Malhotra, S., & Santosh, P. J. (1996). Loading dose imipramine—New approach to pharmacotherapy of melancholic depression. *Journal of Psychiatric Research, 30*, 51–58.

Malhotra, S., & Santosh, P. J. (1998). An open clinical trial of buspirone in children with attention-deficit/hyperactivity disorder. *Journal of the American Academy of Child and Adolescent Psychiatry, 37*(4), 364–371.

Manjunatha, K. R., Narayanan, H. S., Rao, B. S. S. R., Srinath, S., & Girimaji, S. R. (1989). Cryptogenetic investigations in autistic children: A preliminary study on the detection of fragile X chromosome. *NIMHANS Journal, 7*, 163–167.

Masi, G., Millepiedi, S., Mucci, M., Bertini, N., Milantoni, L., & Arcangeli, F. (2005). A naturalistic study of referred children and adolescents with obsessive–compulsive disorder. *Journal of the American Academy of Child and Adolescent Psychiatry, 44*(7), 673–681.

Masi, G., Millepiedi, S., Mucci, M., Bertini, N., Pfanner, C., & Arcangeli, F. (2006). Cormorbidity of obsessive–compulsive disorder and attention-deficit/hyperactivity disorder in referred children and adolescents. *Comprehensive Psychiatry, 47*, 42–47.

Mehta, S., Mehta, V., Mehta, S., Shah, D., Motiwala, A., Vardhan, J., et al. (2011). Multimodal behavior program for ADHD incorporating yoga and implemented by high school volunteers: A pilot study. *ISRN Pediatr, 2011*, 780745.

Mehta, S., Shah, D., Shah, K., Mehta, S., Mehta, N., Mehta, V., et al. (2012). Peer-mediated multimodal intervention program for the treatment of children with ADHD in India: One-year follow up. *ISRN Pediatric, 2012*, 419168.

Minshew, N. J., & Williams, D. L. (2007). The new neurobiology of autism: Cortex, connectivity, and neuronal organization. *Archives of Neurology, 64*(7), 945.

Monda, J. M., & Husmann, D. A. (1995). Primary nocturnal enuresis: A comparison among observation, imipramine, desmopressin acetate and bed-wetting alarm systems. *Journal of Urology, 154*, 745–748.

Nagaraj, R., Singhi, P., & Malhi, P. (2006). Risperidone in children with autism: Randomized, placebo-controlled, double-blind study. *Journal of Child Neurology, 21*, 450–455.

Narayan, M., Srinath, S., Anderson, G. M., & Meundi, D. B. (1993). Cerebrospinal fluid levels of homovanillic acid and 5-hydroxyindoleacetic acid in autism. *Biological Psychiatry, 33*, 630–635.

Narayanan, H. S. (1981). A study of the prevalence of mental retardation in Southern India. *International Journal of Mental Health, 10*, 28–36.

Nestadt, G., Samuels, J., Riddle, M., Bienvenu, O. J., Liang, K. Y., LaBuda, M., et al. (2000). A family study of obsessive–compulsive disorder. *Archives of General Psychiatry, 57*, 358–363.

Olfson, M., Marcus, S., & Shaffer, D. (2006). Antidepressant drug therapy and suicide in severely depressed children and adults a case-control study. *Archives of General Psychiatry, 63*(8), 865–872.

Pauls, D., Alsobrook, J. P., Goodman, W. K., Rasmussen, S. A., & Leckman, J. F. (1995). A family study of obsessive–compulsive disorder. *American Journal of Psychiatry, 152*(1), 76–84.

Pelham, W. E, Jr, Wheeler, T., & Chronis, A. (1998). Empirically supported psychosocial treatments for attention deficit hyperactivity disorder. *Journal of clinical child psychology, 27*(2), 190–205.

Popper, C. W., & Zimnitzky, B. (1995). Sudden death putatively related to desipramine treatment in youth: A fifth case and a review of speculative mechanisms. *Journal of Child and Adolescent Psychopharmacology, 5*(4), 283–300.

Radhakrishna, S., Nagarathna, R., & Nagendra, H. R. (2010). Integrated approach to yoga therapy and autism spectrum disorders. *Journal of Ayurveda and Integrative Medicine, 1*, 120–124.

Rajeev, J., Srinath, S., Girimaji, S., Seshadri, S. P., & Singh, P. (2004). A systematic chart review of the naturalistic course and treatment of early-onset bipolar disorder in a child and adolescent psychiatry center. *Comprehensive Psychiatry, 45*, 148–154.

Rajeev, J., Srinath, S., Reddy, Y. C., Shashikiran, M. G., Girimaji, S. C., Seshadri, S. P., et al. (2003). The index manic episode in juvenile-onset bipolar disorder: The pattern of recovery. *Canadian Journal of Psychiatry, 48*, 52–55.

Rani, F., Murray, M. L., Byrne, P. J., & Wong, I. C. (2008). Epidemiologic features of antipsychotic prescribing to children and adolescents in primary care in the United Kingdom. *Pediatrics, 121*(5), 1002–1009.

Rapport, M. D., Loo, S., Issacs, P., Goya, S., Denney, C., & Scanlan, S. (1996). Methylphenidate and attentional training: Comparative effects on behavior and neurocognitive performance in twin girls with attention-deficit/hyperactivity disorder. *Behavior Modification, 20*, 428–450.

Reddy, Y. C., Girimaji, S., & Srinath, S. (1997). Clinical profile of mania in children and adolescents from the Indian subcontinent. *Canadian Journal of Psychiatry, 42*, 841–846.

Reddy, Y. C., Reddy, P. S., Srinath, S., Khanna, S., Sheshadri, S. P., & Girimaji, S. C. (2000). Comorbidity in juvenile obsessive-compulsive disorder: A report from India. *Canadian Journal of Psychiatry, 45*, 274–278.

Research Units on Pediatric Psychopharmacology Autism Network. (2002). Risperidone in children with autism and serious behavioral problems. *New England Journal of Medicine, 347*, 314–321.

Rettew, D. C., Swedo, S. E., Leonard, H. L., Lenane, M. C., & Rapoport, J. L. (1992). Obsessions and compulsions across time in 79 children and adolescents with obsessive–compulsive disorder. *Journal of the American Academy of Child and Adolescent Psychiatry, 31*, 1050–1056.

Rey, J. M., & Walter, G. (1997). Half a century of ECT use in young people. *American Journal of Psychiatry, 154*, 595–602.

Rosario-Campos, M. C., Leckman, J. F., Curi, M., Quatrano, S., Katsovitch, L., Miguel, E. C., et al. (2005). A family study of early-onset obsessive compulsive disorder. *American Journal of Genetics, 136B*, 92–97.

Rutter, M. (1972). Childhood schizophrenia reconsidered. *Journal of Autism and Childhood Schizophrenia, 2*, 315–337.

Sagar, R., Pattanayak, R. D., & Mehta, M. (2012). Clinical profile of mood disorders in children. *Indian Pediatrics, 49*, 21–23.

Schreppers-Tijdink, G. A., Curfs, L. M., Wiegers, A., Kleczkowska, A., & Fryns, J. P. (1988). A systematic cytogenetic study of a population of 1170 mentally retarded and/or behaviourally disturbed patients including fragile X-screening. The Hondsberg experience. *Journal De Genetique Humaine, 36*, 425–446.

Selvi, R., Vineeta, N., & Paul, S. F. D. (2010). Cytogenetics in Autism. *Sri Ramachandra Journal of Medicine, 3*, 5–8.

Sharma, I., Giri, D., Dutta, A., Mazumder, P., Anuradha (2005). Clinical profile of childhood onset schizophrenia in India. *Journal of Indian Association of Child and Adolescent Mental Health, 1*(3), 6.

Shaw, P., Sporn, A., Gogtay, N., Overman, G. P., Greenstein, D., Gochman, P., et al. (2006). Childhood-onset schizophrenia: A double-blind, randomized clozapine–olanzapine comparison. *Archives of General Psychiatry, 63*, 721–730.

Sheinkopf, S. J., & Siegel, B. (1998). Home based behavioral treatment of young children with autism. *Journal of Autism and Developmental Disorders, 28*(1), 15–23.

Sikich, L. (2008). Efficacy of atypical antipsychotics in early-onset schizophrenia and other psychotic disorders. *Journal of Clinical Psychiatry, 69*(Suppl. 4), 21–25.

Silverman, W. K., Kurtines, W. M., Ginsburg, G. S., Weems, C. F., Lumpkin, P. W., & Carmichael, D. H. (1999). Treating anxiety disorders in children with group cognitive-behavioral therapy: A randomized clinical trial. *Journal of Consulting and Clinical Psychology, 67*(6), 995.

Singhi, P., Mittal, B. R., Nagaraj, R., & Malhi, P. (2008). Single photon emission tomography in children with autism. *Journal of Pediatric Neurology, 6*, 221–225.

Smith, T., Groen, A. D., & Wynn, J. W. (2000). Randomized trial of intensive early intervention for children with pervasive developmental disorder. *American Journal of Mental Retardation, 105*(4), 269–285.

Snyder, R., Turgay, A., Aman, M., Binder, C., Fisman, S., Carroll, A., Risperidone Conduct Study Group (2002). Effects of risperidone on conduct and disruptive behavior disorders in children with subaverage IQs. *Journal of the American Academy of Child and Adolescent Psychiatry, 41*, 1026–1036.

Srinath, S., Janardhan Reddy, Y. C., Girimaji, S. R., Seshadri, S. P., & Subbakrishna, D. K. (1998). A prospective study of bipolar disorder in children and adolescents from India. *Acta Psychiatrica Scandinavica, 98*, 437–442.

Srivastava, V. K., Sitholey, P., Dwivedi, C. M., & Tripathi, S. K. (1988). Influence of socio-cultural factors on delusions: A study on children and adolescents. *Child Psychiatry Quarterly, 21*, 121–128.

Swedo, S. E., Rapoport, J. L., Leonard, H. L., Lenane, M., & Cheslow, D. (1989). Obsessive compulsive disorders in children and adolescents: Clinical phenomenology of 70 consecutive cases. *Archives of General Psychiatry, 46*, 335–343.

Thakur, A., Jagadheesan, K., & Sinha, V. K. (2003). Psychopathological dimensions in childhood and adolescent psychoses: A confirmatory factor analytical study. *Psychopathology, 36*, 190–194.

Tharoor, H., Kar, N., & Jagdisha, S. (2002). Profile of childhood depression in a south Indian clinic population. *Indian Journal of Psychiatry, 45*, s9.

Van Karnebeek, C. D. M., Scheper, F. Y., Abeling, N. G., et al. (2002a). Aetiology of mental retardation or borderline cognitive delay in 281 children referred to a tertiary care center: A prospective study. In C. D. M. Van Karnebeek (Ed.), *Mental retardation: Diagnostic studies on aetiology [doctoral thesis]* (pp. 75–108). Amsterdam, Netherlands: Department of Pediatrics/Emma Children's Hospital and Department of Clinical Genetics, Academic Medical Centre, University of Amsterdam.

Van Karnebeek, C. D., Jansweijer, M. C., Leenders, A. G., Offringa, M., & Hennekam, R. C. (2005). Diagnostic investigations in individuals with mental retardation: A systematic literature review of their usefulness. *European Journal of Human Genetics, 13*, 6–25.

Van Karnebeek, C. D., Koevoets, C., Sluijter, S., et al. (2002b). Prospective screening for subtelomeric rearrangements in children with mental retardation of unknown aetiology: The Amsterdam experience. *Journal of Medical Genetics, 39*, 546–553.

Vitiello, B., Severe, J. B., Greenhill, L. L., Arnold, L. E., Abikoff, H. B., Bukstein, O. G., et al. (2001). Methylphenidate dosage for children with ADHD over time under controlled conditions: Lessons from the MTA. *Journal of the American Academy of Child and Adolescent Psychiatry, 40*(2), 188–196.

Walter, G., & Rey, J. M. (1997). An Epidemiological Study of the Use of ECT in Adolescents. *Journal of the American Academy of Child and Adolescent Psychiatry, 36*, 809–815.

Webster-Stratton, C., Reid, M. J., & Hammond, M. (2004). Treating children with early-onset conduct problems: Intervention outcomes for parent, child, and teacher training. *Journal of Clinical Child and Adolescent Psychology, 33*, 105–124.

Weiss, M. J. (1999). Differential rates of skill acquisition and outcomes of early intensive behavioral intervention for autism. *Behavioral Interventions, 14*(1), 3–22.

Yang, P. C., Liu, C. Y., Chiang, S. Q., Chen, J. Y., & Lin, T. S. (1995). Comparison of adult manifestations of schizophrenia with onset before and after 15 years of age. *Acta Psychiatrica Scandinavica, 91*, 209–212.

Zaw, F. K. K., Bates, G. D. L., Murali, V., & Benthan, P. (1999). Catatonia, autism, and ECT. *Developmental Medicine and Child Neurology, 41*, 843–845.

Zito, J. M., Safer, D. J., dosReis, S. et al. (2003). Psychotropic practice patterns for youth: A 10-year perspective. *Archives of Pediatrics & Adolescent Medicine, 157*, 17–25.

Chapter 14
Nosology and Diagnostic Issues in Child and Adolescent Psychiatry

Pravin Dullur

'Diagnosis is not the end but the beginning of practice'.
Martin Fischer—German–American physician and writer

1 Introduction

Diagnosis, classification and nosology are often lumped together as the same entity and the three terms are sometimes used interchangeably. It is important to clarify the difference between these entities. Nosology is the study of classification of disorders. Classification or grouping is an innate part of human development. For example, babies are able to mentally bisect space into left versus right categories (Quinn 2012) and can categorise people (mother vs. others) by the age of 4 months. Classification, therefore, is not necessarily only about classifying disorders. For example, there is a World Health Organisation (WHO) classification of psychosocial circumstances (WHO 1998).

The main systems of classification in psychiatry are the WHO sponsored International Classification of Diseases (ICD) (WHO 1992) and the American Psychiatric Association's (APA) Diagnostic and Statistical Manual of Mental Disorders (DSM) (APA 1994). The DSM was created in 1952 with the specific aim of having a standardised classification system to diagnose psychiatric disorders. Revisions of the DSM have paralleled advances in the field of psychiatry, such as theoretical models, epidemiology, genetics, symptoms groups and treatment. The ICD is a WHO-generated classification of all groups of diseases. Mental illnesses were included as disorders in the 8th edition of the ICD in 1968. Over time, these two systems have

P. Dullur, Staff Specialist

P. Dullur (✉)
University of New South Wales, Sydney, NSW 2052, Australia
e-mail: dullurpravin1@yahoo.com

S. Malhotra and S. Chakrabarti (eds.), *Developments in Psychiatry in India*,
DOI 10.1007/978-81-322-1674-2_14

in parallel, emerged as the main classification systems in psychiatry. Efforts are on for the last few decades to bring these two systems as close to one another as possible, and a "harmonisation committee" is currently attempting this. Other classificatory systems are specific to younger children, e.g. the classification 0–3 (DC: 0–3) in 1994, its revised second version (DC: 0–3R) in 2005, and the Research Diagnostic Criteria-Preschool Age (RDC-PA) in 2002.

The Webster's dictionary defines diagnosis as "the art or act of identifying a disease from its signs and symptoms". This is true for all of medicine. The difficulty, with psychiatry in general and child and adolescent psychiatry in particular, is in defining what these signs and symptoms are, and what they actually mean. Some related terms are syndrome, disorder and disease. All of these are wrongly used interchangeably at times. A syndrome is a set of signs and symptoms, which occur together more frequently than chance alone would dictate. An example is Down's syndrome, in which various clinical signs and symptoms such as low intelligence, characteristic mongoloid face and a simian crease occur together. A syndrome does not necessarily imply either the cause or functional impairment. In Down's syndrome of course, the aetiology is known (for example, trisomy chromosome 21). In other instances (e.g. Asperger's syndrome), the aetiology is less clear. A disease is traditionally defined as a condition with a known aetiology. For example, diabetes is considered to be a disease, since it has multiple sign and symptoms (high blood sugar, polyuria and polydipsia) with a known aetiology (low insulin due to various factors, e.g. loss of the islets of pancreas). Most psychiatric entities are not "diseases" in the traditional sense of the term, since their exact aetiology is not currently known. Therefore, the term "disorder" is favoured. As per the ICD 10 (WHO 1992), a "disorder" implies the existence of a clinically recognisable set of symptoms or behaviour, associated in most cases with distress and with interference with personal functions. Therefore, the two pillars of making a diagnosis are as follows: firstly, the presence of a syndrome, meaning clear and specific signs and symptoms, and secondly, the presence of dysfunction.

2 Diagnosis Versus Formulation

So why is diagnosis important?

This is depicted in the following case vignette:

> Ravi, a 13 year old boy, came to the clinic with his parents who complained that he was persistently disobedient and aggressive. The aggression was noted both at home and school and was often planned. He persistently carried a grudge. He often ran away from home and had been warned twice by the police. He smoked cigarettes and occasionally marijuana. The parents reported that he never accepted responsibility for what he did.

Non-diagnostic labels in such a person could include "a troubled child", a "behaviourally disturbed child" or "too strict parents". The treatment could be very variable. It could include working on the "external circumstances", which led to his outbursts (e.g. counselling his parents or changing his school) to individual sessions with him (e.g. to find out what makes him angry and help him to find new coping strategies). It could also result in incorrect assumptions about the prognosis and outcome (e.g. "he will just grow out of it"). A diagnostic assessment, on the other hand, if done in a careful manner might reveal a diagnosis,in this instance one of conduct disorder. It should be pointed out that the basis for applying the diagnostic label is only the child's behaviour, which must fit a certain pattern (e.g. aggression across multiple settings, deceitfulness and lacking respect for rules). These patterns make up the bulk of the classificatory manuals such as the ICD 10 and the DSM-IV. In modern schemes, the defining criteria for nearly all psychiatric diagnoses are purely descriptive and phenomenological (Dilling 2000). Identifying the criteria, therefore, acts as a clinical assessment tool, so that the presence of aggression and disobedience trigger certain lines of enquiry. For example, the DSM criteria for conduct disorder include aggression to people or animals, destruction of property, deceitfulness or theft and serious violation of rules. Knowing the DSM or ICD criteria would not only lead the clinician to objectively diagnose conduct disorder, but also help the clinician to rule out other diagnoses, such as Attention deficit hyperactivity disorder (ADHD) and specific reading disorders (dyslexia), which are comorbid in about one-third of patients with conduct disorder (Rutter et al. 1998).

If a diagnosis of conduct disorder is made, a considerable knowledge base is accessible in research. Thus, we know that Ravi's long-term outlook without treatment is relatively poor; 40 % of children with conduct disorder go on to be convicted of three offences by the age of 17 (Farrington 1995). So suggesting that "he will grow out of it" would be misleading. The prognosis would be worse if the onset of his conduct disorder was before 4 years of age, if antisocial behaviour was frequent and widespread, if his IQ or reading age was low, if hyperactivity was present and if his parents were hostile towards him (Robins 1978). Having a diagnosis would also impact on the type of treatment chosen. For example, for conduct disorder, treatment options include cognitive problem solving therapy, parent management, functional family therapy and multi-systems therapy (Kazdin 1997).

However, no causal mechanisms are necessarily implied while making a diagnosis. This is significantly different from older theories, which attributed disorders to causes that could not be tested. (For example, suggesting that the boy in the above vignette has "castration anxiety") Those who believe that the phenomenological approach taken in psychiatric classification is inferior or less scientific than that prevalent in physical medicine are mistaken—after all, epilepsy, hypertension and asthma are all diagnosed on the basis of observable phenomena with no assumptions of causality required. That is because the aetiology for the vast majority of psychiatric disorders is simply not known.

Thus systems of classification such as the DSM or the ICD serve multiple functions. Firstly, they define disorders, that is, serve to make diagnoses. Secondly, they serve as systems of classification. For example, the ICD 10 has classified psychiatric disorders into 10 different categories with multiple diagnoses within each category. Thirdly, they serve as means of communication between clinicians, researchers and other stakeholders such as consumers, policy makers, politicians and insurance companies. Finally, they drive research.

In general, child and adolescent psychiatric disorders are classified as internalising disorders, externalising disorders and developmental disorders. This is in addition to all the other traditional "adult" diagnoses such as psychotic or mood disorders. Internalising disorders, as the name suggests, are predominantly problems related to anxiety, fear, shyness, low self-esteem and emotional disturbances.

Traditionally, these are less likely to be disruptive as parents or teachers may not necessarily notice them or consider them worthy of intervention. Internalising disorders include separation anxiety disorder, phobias of childhood and sibling rivalry disorder. Externalising problems, on the other hand, predominantly include behaviours such as hyperactivity, aggression and impulsivity. Diagnoses include ADHD, oppositional defiant disorder (ODD) and conduct disorder. Development colours all aspects of psychiatric disorders in children and adolescents. Independently though, developmental disorders are classified into problems of global impairment (mental retardation) or specific disorders (e.g. speech delay). The separation between these disorders is by no means absolute. Depressive symptoms can occur in conduct disorders, anxiety symptoms can occur in ADHD, and intellectual impairment can occur with any disorder.

3 Multi-axial Framework

Both the ICD 10 and DSM-IV have a multi-axial framework for psychiatric disorders in childhood and adolescence (WHO 1996). The ICD 10 axes are described below.

Axis I: Clinical psychiatric syndromes: Here, criteria for particular diagnoses are applied, as described in the relevant manuals for ICD 10.

Axis II: Specific disorders of development: These include disorders of speech and language, reading, spelling and motor development.

DSM-IV codes Axis I and Axis II of the ICD 10 on Axis I.

Axis III: Intellectual level: Mental retardation is primarily coded on this Axis. In DSM-IV, mental retardation is included in Axis II.

The multi-axial system for diagnosing mental illness does not necessarily convey details about mental retardation itself. Therefore, Dr Satish Girimaji (2008) proposes the following multi-axial system specifically for mental retardation:

Axis I: Presence and degree of mental retardation (e.g. mild mental retardation)

Axis II: Aetiologic or syndromal diagnosis (e.g. fragile X syndrome)

Axis III: Associated medical problems (e.g. epilepsy)

Axis IV: Associated psychiatric problems (e.g. ADHD)

Axis V: Family and psycho-social axis (e.g. poor awareness, high stress levels and over-expectation).

It is notable that words and terminology have a way of evolving over time, especially in the context of stigma. The words “idiot”, “imbecile” and “moron” were scientific ways of describing degree of mental retardation in the early part of the twentieth century before giving way to “mental retardation”. The term “intellectual disability” is preferred in both the DSM-5 and ICD 11 classifications (Luis Salvador-Carull 2011).

Axis IV: Associated medical conditions: All medical conditions are coded on Axis IV. A few have specific associations with psychiatric disorders, for example, tuberosclerosis predisposes to autism and Cornelia de Lange syndrome to self injury. Even when there is no specific disorder, congenital syndromes are often characterised by a particular pattern of behaviour (Flint and Yule 1994). In DSM-IV, medical conditions are included under Axis III.

Axis V: Associated abnormal psychosocial conditions: These include a range of psychosocial hazards, from abnormal intra-familial relationships, e.g. physical or sexual abuse, family history of mental disorders, distorted intra-familial communication patterns, abnormal upbringing (e.g. in an institution), acute life events and chronic interpersonal stress arising from difficulties at school. As the number of psychosocial adversities goes up, the rate of psychiatric disorders increases (Garmezy and Masten 1994). Rutter (1987) found that no single psychosocial adversity was associated with any particular disorder; rather, the total number of adverse situations was important. Those with only one adverse situation had no increase in disorders over those without adversity, whereas those with two adverse situations had a 4-fold increase in disorders. Conduct disorder is particularly associated with a poor immediate psychosocial environment (Steinhausen and Erdin 1992), whereas emotional disorders are associated more with acute life events and school-related chronic stressors (Moselhy et al. 1997). Psychosocial issues are coded on Axis IV in the DSM-IV.

Axis VI: Global social functioning: Here, a judgement is made on a dimensional scale, ranging from superior social functioning to profound and pervasive social disability. Studies based on DSM-IV criteria often use the Children's Global Assessment Scale (CGAS) (Shaffer et al. 1983). DSM-IV includes global functioning on Axis V.

Of importance is that the DSM-5 (APA 2013) has done away with the multi-axial system, specifying that all diagnoses are equally important, and therefore, a multi-axial framework is no longer necessary.

4 Diagnostic Formulations

An important and distinct, yet related concept is that of the diagnostic formulation. The formulation is a statement, which puts the patient in perspective. While a diagnosis is not tailored for an individual patient, a formulation is designed to do precisely that. It answers the question: "Why is this patient here, now?"

This is depicted in the following case vignette:

Sita is a 6 year old girl who presented to the clinic with school refusal. Sita lives in Bangalore, with her parents, both software engineers. She was cared for at her grandparent's house by her grandparents while both parents went to work. The fear of school started when her parents had talked about school in a casual way, discussing the punishments they had been given when they had started school, years ago. This fear was heightened, when on a visit to the school prior to start of the session, a teacher had said jokingly, that '"bad children" were often punished by being locked up in the bathroom with cockroaches. On the first day of school, Sita and her mother went together, but Sita cried so loudly that the school advised her mother to take her back home. This pattern was repeated over the next few days. As a result, she would constantly cling to her mother in the mornings and would cry for long time after her mother left for work. Her grandparents reported that the crying did not settle after her mother left, but would continue for hours together later. Her mother spent increasingly longer times at home trying to settle Sita down, but Sita's clinginess worsened. As a result, the mother found that she could no longer reach work on time. As time passed, Sita started complaining of significant abdominal pain in the morning. This resulted in several trips to specialists to identify the cause of the pain and treat it, to no avail. The pain would often disappear when the family decided they would stop trying to send her to school for that day. All attempts to get her to school resulted in severe screaming and "tantrums". After giving up trying to get her to school, the parents would go to work, leaving Sita at home with the grandparents. She would pass her time by watching TV and playing computer games. However, at home, her clinginess to her mother worsened and she started complaining of repeated dreams of a monster taking away her mother, and could no longer sleep in her own bed. This fear of something happening to mother extended to all situations and the mother found that she could neither work, nor socialise. Her relationship with her husband worsened as her husband would blame her for not managing Sita's anxiety. One professional they visited labelled her as an "anxious child" and said "anxiety is common around getting to school" and advised the parents to "give her time". Another suggested that the parents were being "too soft" on her, and that "tough love" was needed.

In this case, careful assessment and application of proper criteria revealed that she fulfilled several criteria of separation anxiety disorder including: developmentally inappropriate and excessive anxiety concerning separation from a key figure (in this case the mother), excessive distress, school refusal, nightmares around separation, difficulty sleeping and repeated complaints of physical symptoms. Significant dysfunction included loss of education for Sita, loss of work for her mother and marital discord between the parents.

On further assessment, Sita was anxious by temperament. Both her parents had social phobia. The parents described themselves as anxious by nature as well. A related feature was that they tended to have constantly anxious interactions with Sita (e.g. "Don't go to there, an insect might bite you").

Therefore, the diagnosis would be as follows:

Axis I: Separation anxiety disorder
Axis II: Nil
Axis III: Nil
Axis IV: Nil
Axis V: Family history of anxiety, anxious interactions between parents and child, marital discord, loss of education and work opportunities
Axis VI: CGAS score of 60.

Making the diagnosis does not necessarily lead to proper management. A formulation, specific to the case is needed. Formulations are of several types: these include a diagnostic formulation, which incorporates key diagnostic criteria, a psychodynamic formulation, which explains symptoms in a psychodynamic way (Perry et al. 1987) or a clinical formulation which incorporates a biopsychosocial model (RANZCP guidelines 2012). A clinical formulation incorporates vulnerability and precipitating factors and links these to maintaining factors.

Therefore, a useful formulation in Sita's case would be:

"Sita is a 6 year old girl who presented with severe separation anxiety with school refusal. This has significantly impacted the functioning of the family. Sita is vulnerable to anxiety

> disorders due to the following factors: biologically: a family history of anxiety, anxious temperament; and, psychologically, due to anxious interactions resulting in a negative appraisal of normal stimuli. The disorder was precipitated by social factors (being scared by teacher) and seems to be maintained by avoidance behaviours at home (computer games).

Based on the formulation, the following management was done.

> Sita and her family were seen by a child psychiatrist. After the above diagnosis and formulation were made, the psychiatrist spent a long time in educating the parents regarding the illness. Medical illness such as hypothyroidism and anaemia were ruled out. Interventions included forming a good therapeutic relationship with Sita, relaxation exercises and a program of graded exposure coupled with relaxation exercises, which involved both the school situation and separation anxiety. The psychiatrist worked with both parents and through them, with the school. Medication was deferred in view of the age of the child. The parents agreed to seek treatment for their own anxiety disorders. Four months later, Sita was well integrated at school, but continued to be anxious. The mother was able to return to work.

Thus, diagnosis and formulation are the twin pillars on which management should be based.

Several important issues dog the ICD and DSM systems of classification. These include, the use of categorical versus dimensional approaches (Coghill and Sonuga-Barke 2012); the use of multiple axes or a single axis (Taylor and Rutter 2008); the excessive number of diagnostic categories (Rutter 2011), the large number of "Not otherwise specified NOS" diagnoses (Rutter 2011); whether to diagnose comorbid disorders separately (as in the DSM), or to have combined diagnoses (e.g. hyperkinetic conduct disorder or depressive conduct disorder in the ICD 10) (Rutter and Uher 2012); whether functional impairment will need to be made a necessary criterion for making a diagnosis (Rutter 2011); how to integrate the ICD and DSM systems; the issue of homogeneity versus heterogeneity of diagnoses (Scott 2001) and so on. These will not be discussed further in this chapter.

5 Influence of Child and Adolescent Issues on Specific Diagnoses and Their Classification

Given that children are constantly growing, a good knowledge of normal development is necessary to correctly differentiate the normal from the pathological. For example, temper tantrums are normal at the age of two, not at the age of eight years. Imaginary friends are usual for five-year-olds, but not 15-year-olds. A depressed 5-year old child will not be able to articulate suicidal thinking patterns, while a 16-year old would. The ability to identify time patterns is poor in a 5-year old child, average in an 11-year old one and adult like by the age of 15 years. This means that an 8-year old would not be able to describe events in a chronological sequence, whereas a 15-year old adolescent would. Therefore, flexibility is required while attempting to fit particular behaviours into a diagnostic category. An important issue in making a diagnosis is an understanding of the context in which the problem occurs. These contextual factors could be family, school or sociocultural issues. For example, poor attention at school in a child due to an inappropriate school placement would not merit a diagnosis of attention deficit disorder. Understimulation in a child who may have a slow to warm-up temperament may result in quasi-autistic symptoms, which resolve readily when the child is placed in a different environment. Cultural differences may also affect diagnostic concepts and practice. Economic disadvantage, for example, is associated with conduct and attentional problems, but the meanings of such relationships often remain unclear.

Once developmental difficulties are identified, it is helpful to decide if abnormalities are due to delay or to deviance from the usual pattern of development. For example, a child may exhibit a speech problem. If she produces only a handful of words, but in the appropriate context, she may suffer from expressive speech delay. A diagnosis, however, can be made only if the delay is exclusive to speech and not part of a global delay. If global delay exists, a diagnosis of mental retardation (intellectual disability) would be more appropriate. If the delay in the speech is greater than the mental age of an intellectually delayed child, both mental retardation and a speech delay should be diagnosed. On the other hand, if the speech is atypical, e.g. lacking reciprocity or tone and accompanying gestures, a diagnosis of autism might be considered.

6 Psychiatric Disorders Among Children and Adolescents

This section deals with some of the disorders specific to children and adolescents and explores the differences between the two prevalent systems of classification, the DSM and the ICD.

Anxiety disorders: The ICD 10 defines emotional disorders in children as "mainly exaggerations of normal developmental trends rather than phenomena that are qualitatively abnormal in themselves". It also affirms that developmental appropriateness is the key diagnostic feature, which differentiates these disorders from other neurotic disorders. For example, agoraphobia is not part of childhood anxieties and so is abnormal irrespective of the age of the child. On the other hand, separation anxiety is normal at the age of 18 months, but not at age six years. The ICD and DSM systems differ significantly with relation to anxiety disorders in childhood. The ICD 10 includes separation anxiety disorder, phobic anxiety disorder of childhood (abnormal degree of normal childhood fears), social anxiety disorder of childhood (extreme wariness of strangers or new situations) and sibling rivalry disorder (severe emotional disturbance usually following birth of a younger sibling). The DSM, on the other hand, recognises only separation anxiety disorder as a discrete diagnosis among the above. As a result, studies (e.g. Adornetto et al. 2012) have found poor concordance between ICD 10 and DSM-IV diagnoses of childhood anxiety disorders. A PubMed search with the keywords "sibling rivalry disorder" returned no results, while a search with keywords "sibling", "rivalry" and "disorder" revealed a single relevant article (Snowling 2011), which talks of the sibling relationship, but not of "sibling rivalry disorder". In the absence of any research, this disorder could perhaps be eliminated from the ICD 11. This is one of the issues raised by Sir Michael Rutter (2011), who has suggested that the number of diagnostic categories in the ICD 10 is excessive and some are rarely used; therefore, there is a need to eliminate some of the diagnoses in the DSM-5 as well.

Conduct disorder: The ICD 10 and the DSM-IV are quite discordant in the classification of conduct disorders. The ICD 10 category of conduct disorder includes: conduct disorder in the family context, unsocialised conduct disorder, socialised conduct disorder and ODD. The DSM-IV, on the other hand, describes conduct disorder as standalone diagnosis, with onset in childhood or adolescence, and identifies ODD as a separate condition. Clinical experience in India suggests that the "conduct disorder within the family context" is a commonly seen condition. However, researchers suggest that sub-classification of conduct disorder in the ICD-10 has not proved satisfactory and recommend that it be discontinued in the ICD 11 (Ruter 2011). Another issue is that in both DSM-IV and ICD-10, sub-classification differs between childhood and adulthood. For example, conduct disorder in childhood is sub-classified as described above, whereas antisocial personality disorder (ASPD) is not. Psychopathic features are necessary in diagnosing antisocial personality, but not necessary for diagnosing conduct disorder in childhood. Furthermore, conduct disorder is treated as an Axis I clinical disorder in both classificatory systems, whereas ASPD is treated as an Axis II disorder. Given the extensive evidence for continuity over time between the two, that makes little sense. This is particularly so because the diagnosis of ASPD in DSM-IV requires evidence of conduct disorder in childhood. Therefore, a lifespan approach, which brings conduct disorders and ASPD together, is much needed (Moffitt et al. 2008). Yet, it must be noted that in over half the patients with an onset in childhood, the disorder does not persist into adult life (Odgers et al. 2007a).

One of the principles of the ICD 10 is that it encourages clinicians to make a combined diagnosis wherever possible. Therefore, it includes two such categories: depressive conduct disorder (which highlights the fact that a high proportion of children with conduct disorder have depressive features) and hyperactive conduct disorder (comorbid ADHD and conduct disorder). Odgers et al. (2007b) comment on the persistence of conduct disorder into adulthood and propose that ASPD is more likely if it is accompanied by over-activity. Therefore, they recommend that the criteria for conduct disorder should include both components. This is done to an extent in the ICD 10 in the shape of the hyperactive conduct disorder category. However, research is unclear whether this represents separate disorders or not.

Robins and Guze, in a seminal paper in 1970, defined the criteria to label a particular entity as a disorder. These included a clinical description, laboratory studies, delimitation from other disorders, follow-up studies and family studies. In psychiatric nosology, identifying laboratory studies is probably the least helpful to establish the validity of a diagnosis, owing to the lack of such studies. Hence, researchers have attempted to use other indicators. The difficulty in child and adolescent psychiatry is the high rate of comorbidity between disorders. As mentioned, the ICD 10 tends to integrate comorbid conditions into a separate diagnosis, while DSM aims to diagnose them as separate entities. Therefore, some studies have tried to identify these patterns and establish whether these are same or different disorders.

In a retrospective study from India (Malhotra et al. 1999), the clinical and phenomenological correlates of hyperkinetic conduct disorder and conduct disorder, as per the ICD-10 diagnostic criteria were examined. Twenty patients with hyperkinetic conduct disorder and 25 patients with conduct disorder were compared on socio-demographic variables, temperament and specified clinical variables. The two groups differed in terms of the hyperkinetic conduct disorder group having a younger age of onset, a more gradual development of and a longer duration of conduct symptoms as compared to the children with conduct disorder. Children with hyperkinetic conduct disorder had differences in temperament, e.g. distractibility, lower IQ, more perinatal complications and delayed milestones, as compared to the conduct disorder group. The authors proposed that the two disorders followed different pathways of development towards conduct symptomatology, lending some credibility to the separation of these two disorders.

Obsessive-compulsive disorder: A study by Steinberger et al. (2002) aimed to distinguish the criteria for obsessive-compulsive disorder (OCD) across DSM and ICD criteria in children and adolescents suffering from OCD. The sample was of 61 children and adolescents assessed at a specialised outpatient clinic for OCD. They noted that only 45.9 % of patients could be diagnosed by ICD 10 criteria, whereas 95.1 % could be diagnosed using DSM-IV criteria. The patient's age, age at onset and the duration of the illness did not influence the diagnostic stability of DSM-IV criteria. In contrast, in the ICD 10, the majority of subjects diagnosed as full OCD were adolescents. This appeared to be primarily because the ICD 10 includes "presence of insight" as a major criterion to establish obsession as a phenomenon. Naturally, younger children are more inclined to have a poor insight into the absurdity of the symptom. An unusual finding was that there was no significant difference in age and age at onset between the group "with full insight" and that "with poor insight". This suggests that poor insight may be more typical of the disorder than of the developmental phase. The study concluded that the DSM-IV criteria are superior to that of ICD-10 for diagnosing OCD in children and adolescents, because they are age-adapted and provide a more detailed and age-independent description of the obsessive and compulsive symptoms.

In an Indian study on this subject, Jaisoorya et al. (2003) examined the phenotypic characteristics of juvenile OCD (current age less than or equal to 18 years, $n = 39$) and juvenile-onset adult OCD (onset less than or equal to 18 years, current age greater than 18 years, $n = 87$) and adult-onset OCD (onset greater than 18 years, $n = 105$). They noted that the juvenile OCD was associated with male preponderance, elevated rates of certain obsessive-compulsive symptoms, attention deficit hyperactivity disorder, chronic tics, body dysmorphic disorder and major depression. In addition, juvenile-onset adult OCD differed from juvenile OCD in having later age at onset and low rate of ADHD. Juvenile-onset adult OCD was positively associated with social phobia and chronic tics more often than adult-onset OCD. Thus, juvenile OCD appears to be different from both juvenile-onset adult OCD and adult-onset OCD, supporting previous observations that juvenile OCD could be a developmental subtype of the disorder.

Psychosis: Yet another Indian study (Reddy et al. 1993) attempted to study the nosology of psychosis in children and adolescents. Their sample included 50 children aged between 5 and 16 years, meeting criteria for a psychotic illness as per ICD 9 criteria. They applied criteria of ICD 9, ICD 10 and the DSM-III R to these children. They found that concordance rates between the three systems were highest for schizophrenia (90 %) and the least for schizo-affective disorders (72 %).

They concluded that most of the subjects could be classified into one of the major psychosis categories. The study suggested that use of adult criteria for diagnosing psychotic disorders in children and adolescents was justified.

ADHD: ADHD is yet another disorder common in children and adolescents. Community surveys in India suggest a rate of 1.6 %. The three key features of ADHD are inattention, hyperactivity and impulsivity. The ICD 10 term is hyperkinetic disorder (HKD), while the DSM-IV has retained the term ADHD. A longitudinal perspective suggests that symptoms of hyperactivity and impulsivity tend to improve over a period of time, but inattention and social dysfunction do not (Larsson et al. 2011; Faraone et al. 2006). Much debate exists on the ICD versus DSM diagnoses. For example, in a German study, 2,452 children aged 7–17 years were examined through an extensive battery of investigations (Dopfner et al. 2008). A prevalence of 5.0 % as per DSM criteria was reported, but the prevalence rate was only 1.0 % according to ICD 10 criteria. Therefore, it appears that the DSM criteria are far more likely to pick up ADHD, as opposed to the ICD 10 criteria. An Indian study (Sitholey et al. 2012) attempted to compare the usefulness of the two systems of diagnosis in a clinical sample of 62 children (54 boys and 8 girls). Diagnoses were made using the Kiddie Schedule for Affective disorders and Schizophrenia—present and lifetime version, followed by application of DSM-IV or ICD-10 DCR criteria for ADHD or HKD. Global assessment of functioning was estimated on the CGAS. The important clinical finding was that all children could be diagnosed with ADHD. However, only 44 (71 %) could be diagnosed with HKD. The authors suggested that DSM-IV criteria should be used in Indian children, rather than ICD 10 criteria.

7 Changes to the 5th Edition of the DSM (DSM-5)

The DSM-5 (APA 2013) was released in May 2013. Therefore, it would be useful to understand the changes made in the DSM and how it would impact child and adolescent psychiatric disorders. This section reviews a limited number of diagnoses specific to child and adolescent psychiatry.

8 Autism Spectrum Disorder

DSM-IV refers to autism spectrum disorders as pervasive developmental disorders. Diagnoses included are autistic disorder, Asperger's disorder, pervasive developmental disorder-NOS, Rett's disorder and childhood disintegrative disorder. (The ICD 10 has an extra diagnosis called atypical autism). These 5 disorders are considered together since they share a common denominator of having reciprocal social interaction deficits and communication difficulties. Retts syndrome and childhood disintegrative disorder are considered different as they both suppose a period of normal development prior to regression of development resulting in an autistic state.

The following have changed in the DSM-5:

1. A single autism spectrum disorder (ASD) diagnosis now subsumes all the DSM-IV subtypes
2. Both domains (social interaction/communication and restricted, repetitive behaviours) are needed to make the diagnosis
3. The DSM-IV-TR domains of social interaction and communication have merged into one. The criteria have been simplified into 3 primary subcriteria: deficits in socioemotional reciprocity, deficits in non-verbal communicatory behaviours and deficits in relationships
4. For the domain of restricted behaviour, interests and activities, the subcriteria remain comparable with those in DSM-IV-TR, with the addition of hyper- or hyporeactivity to sensory stimuli or unusual interest in sensory aspects of the environment
5. Severity levels (1–3) ranging from "requiring support" to "requiring very substantial support" are described
6. A key point of importance is that abnormalities in only the social communication/interaction domain would result in a diagnosis of social communication disorder being made.

The restructuring of the autism spectrum disorders will have significant repercussions across multiple domains. Commentators (Witwer and Lecavalier 2008) have suggested that discarding labels often viewed as less stigmatizing—such as pervasive developmental disorder-NOS and Asperger's—may deter individuals with milder symptoms from seeking care. Rather than eliminating these subtypes, Ghaziuddin (2010) called for their inclusion in DSM-5 with further refinement of their diagnostic criteria. It is possible that with the restructure, more children previous labelled as "on the autism spectrum" but not necessarily impaired will receive an ASD diagnosis, resulting in over-diagnosis. This then will further impact funding for systems such as schools and disability.

9 Attention Deficit/Hyperactivity Disorder

The DSM-IV and ICD 10 criteria for ADHD have already been described. The DSM-5 retains the same basic structure with 2 primary domains of inattention and hyperactivity/impulsivity (APA 2013) and has retained all the criteria in the DSM-IV. The DSM-5 attempts to provide a life span perspective. Therefore, it includes descriptions of behaviours from different age ranges. For instance, the DSM-IV criterion "is often forgetful in daily activities" now reads "is often forgetful in daily activities, chores and running errands (for older adolescents and adults, returning calls, paying bills, and keeping appointments)."

Other points of importance are described in this paragraph. The age of onset criterion has been relaxed from 7 years in the DSM-IV to 12 years in the DSM-5.

Coding types (combined type, predominantly inattentive type and predominantly hyperactive-impulsive hyperactive type) have been preserved but relabelled as "presentations" instead of "types". Finally, severity specifiers have been added.

The ADHD developmental subgroup (2013) went through a series of proposals which were not included finally. Four new criteria were proposed initially to the hyperactivity/impulsivity domain: tending to act without thinking, often being impatient, being uncomfortable doing things slowly and systematically, and finding it difficult to resist temptations or opportunities. A "restrictive predominantly inattentive presentation" (the number of hyperactive/impulsive symptoms needed to be 2 or less) was proposed. Coghill and Seth (2011) had highlighted the lack of empirical evidence for the restrictive predominantly inattentive subtype and the 4 new impulsivity criteria. The work group acknowledged the limited empirical data for the restrictive subtype. The flip side of the argument was that it satisfies a clinical need and would serve as an impetus for further research. In addition, the work group proposed age-specific variability in the number of criteria required for diagnosis. None of these were adopted.

The DSM-5 work group advised gathering information from parents and teachers for children and young adolescents and from third parties for older adolescents and adults. This is in keeping with the life span approach to ADHD and meets recommendations suggested by the American Academy of Paediatrics (2000).

A concern raised by Francis (2010) is that the higher age of onset criterion could theoretically expand the number of false positives. Other evidence does not support this claim. For example, in a recent prospective cohort study, raising the age of onset criterion to age 12 years increased the ADHD prevalence by only 0.1 % (Polanczyk et al. 2010).

Disruptive mood dysregulation disorder and the paediatric bipolar disorder debate among the most controversial changes in DSM-5 is the inclusion of the diagnosis disruptive mood dysregulation disorder (DMDD), formerly called temper dysregulation disorder with dysphoria. The disorder is characterised by a baseline mood of persistently negative affect (angry or irritability) that is punctuated by severe recurrent temper outbursts occurring 3 or more times per week. Intensity and duration criteria have been described. The key differential diagnosis is bipolar disorder. DMDD excludes those patients who exhibit full symptom hypomanic symptoms for longer than 1 day.

The creation of the DMDD diagnosis is in response to ongoing controversy about the nature of paediatric bipolar disorder. Researchers (Biederman 2006; Mick et al. 2005) have postulated that bipolar disorder in children is a chronic as opposed to episodic illness, characterised by severe irritability and episodic aggressive outbursts. They see it on a continuum of ADHD. We (Jairam et al. 2012) and others (Geller et al. 2008) recommend that it should be considered similar to adult bipolar disorder (episodic illness, acute biphasic disorder: "classic or narrow-spectrum bipolar disorder").

In an Indian study, Jairam et al. (2004) assessed 25 children who were diagnosed with bipolar disorder prior to age 16. They noted that it was possible to diagnose these children using adult criteria. Follow-up of these children over 4–5 years showed that the diagnosis stayed true and was certainly episodic in nature. On the other hand, the children as described in the broad spectrum bipolar certainly present frequently to child and adolescent psychiatry clinics. Liebenluft et al. (2003) labelled this group of disorder as "Severe Mood dysregulation (SMD)". The outlined criteria specify that onset should be between age 7 and 17, and the mood should be abnormal: specifically, anger or sadness should be present for at least half a day on most days. Hyperarousal, e.g. insomnia, agitation, pressured speech or intrusiveness, was required. The key criterion was the presence of marked increased reactivity to negative emotional stimuli such as extended temper tantrums, verbal rages and aggression. Presence of cardinal bipolar symptoms such as elevated mood and grandiosity would exclude the diagnosis.

Recent studies have thrown more light on SMD. ADHD and depression (not bipolar disorder) are more common in follow-up studies of this population (Brotman et al. 2006; Stingaris et al. 2011). Family genetic studies have suggested that kids with SMD have family members with lower psychiatric morbidity rates than those seen in BD, ADHD and ODD/CD (Carlson 2007). This points to SMD possibly being a separate entity and raises more questions about its genetic basis. Proponents argue that the irritability in bipolar disorder is more severe than that found in ADHD or ODD and that these children are, in fact, exhibiting complicated mood cycling (Wozniak et al. 2005).

The DMDD category was created in an effort to provide a diagnostic "home" for the children with severe, non-episodic irritability and, presumably, to lower the rates of assignment of paediatric bipolar diagnosis. The authors of the DSM (DSM-5 Childhood and Adolescent Disorder Work Group 2010) state that they hope that the addition of the diagnosis will increase public awareness of the clinical needs of this patient population, generate new research, and lead to identification of appropriate treatment interventions (DSM-5 Bipolar Disorder Task Force, 2010). This is all the more important, given that treatment for bipolar disorder is shifting towards use of atypical antipsychotics rather than traditional mood stabilisers and there are growing reports of significant metabolic side effects of atypical antipsychotics in adolescents (Correll et al. 2009; Dullur et al. 2012; Eapen et al. 2012).

Anxiety disorders in childhood: The key change in DSM-5 is that the separation anxiety disorder (SAD) has been classified as an anxiety disorder. In the DSM-IV, it was classified under disorders usually first diagnosed in infancy, childhood or adolescence. Specifically, the criterion that age of onset of the disorder must be before the age of 18 years has been removed. The target of separation anxiety fears now includes "major" attachment figures instead of only listing parents. Avoidance behaviours include adult settings such as work, rather than primarily school refusal.

Recent evidence justifies the move. Adult-onset SAD is increasingly being reported (Shear et al. 2006; Pini et al. 2010). On the other hand, Starcevic (2013a) argues that separation anxiety in adults should be seen as a manifestation of associated anxiety disorders such as generalised anxiety or panic. This viewpoint is supported by the high rates of comorbidity observed in adult SAD (Shear et al. 2006).

10 Feeding and Eating Disorders

The eating disorder (ED) category of DSM-IV-TR currently consists of anorexia nervosa, bulimia nervosa and ED NOS. The DSM-5 has expanded the category to include pica, rumination disorder, avoidant/restrictive food intake disorder (formerly called feeding disorder of infancy or early childhood), anorexia nervosa, bulimia nervosa and binge ED (currently classified within the DSM-IV-TR appendix as an area warranting further research).

Anorexia retains the basic structure of DSM-IV. However, the amenorrhoea criterion has been eliminated. The amenorrhoea is irrelevant in pre-menarchial girls, postmenopausal women or women taking oral contraceptives. Binge ED has been formalised. This is especially important given that cognitive behaviour therapy (CBT) approaches have been found useful for this category (Wonderlich et al. 2009).

11 Oppositional Defiant Disorder (ODD)/Conduct Disorder (CD)

Both ODD and CD have been moved into the category of "disruptive, impulse control and conduct disorders", the underlying difficulty being problems in self control of emotions and behaviour.

There is no change to the criteria for diagnosis of ODD. However, the symptoms are classified within 3 categories as follows: (1) angry/irritable mood, (2) defiant/headstrong behaviour; and (3) vindictiveness. A severity index has been added.

Conduct disorder retains the same basic structure and age of onset specifier. A new specifier "with limited prosocial emotions" has been added. To qualify for this specifier, a person would need to display at least two of the following characteristics: lack of remorse or guilt, Callous-lack of empathy, unconcerned about performance and shallow or deficient affect.

Potential new categories to be included:

The DSM-5 suggests the following as proposed disorders that are included in Section III of the DSM-5, meaning they are not recognised as disorders but require more research. The following are especially relevant to child and adolescent psychiatry.

Attenuated Psychosis Syndrome (APS): The DSM-5 describes APS in terms of psychotic symptoms that are attenuated but clinically important. Duration and frequency criteria are specified. Identified risks include that the reliability and validity of the syndrome are still unclear (Yung et al. 2010) and that only a minority progress into Schizophrenia (Ruhrmann et al. 2010). This then would increase the risk of unnecessary treatment with antipsychotics. On the other hand, APS could potentially identify high-risk patients who may be helped by judicious use of medication.

Non-suicidal self injury (NSSI): NSSI refers to intentional, self-inflicted damage to one's body, e.g. cutting or burning with no suicidal intent. The purpose of the behaviour is to either induce a positive feeling state or to obtain relief from a negative state or to resolve an interpersonal difficulty. The DSM-IV only recognises this behaviour within the context of a borderline personality disorder. This category reflects recent research that NSSI behaviour is common in adolescents (Madge et al. 2008) and can occur in a heterogeneous group of conditions (Brausch and Gutierrez 2010).

Internet gaming disorder: The Internet has transformed all aspects of life including education, social networking and gaming. Behavioural addictions have been described by various researchers and incorporate key concepts as related to substance addictions, e.g. tolerance, salience, withdrawal, and loss of control (Kuss and Griffiths 2012). A question often asked is "What exactly is the child addicted to"? The Internet is seen as a medium, not a substance, just as one is addicted to alcohol, not a bar. Therefore, Starcevic (2013b) argues that this term should be dropped. Similarly, gaming may be online or offline, adding to the confusion. Thus, the DSM-5 proposes "Internet gaming disorder".

The criteria strongly reflect drug dependence criteria such as preoccupation with games, withdrawal symptoms and tolerance (increased time spent). Only non-gambling gaming is included. The term Internet gaming was preferred rather than Internet addiction. Finally, use of the Internet for recreational/social/sexual uses is excluded.

Some evidence on the correlates of "Internet addiction" is emerging. Floros and Siomos (2013) conceptualised Internet addiction as being attributed to seeking social comfort, evading feelings of loneliness and/or depression having diminished impulse control and seeking distraction from other problems. Parenting styles, e.g. overprotection, are seen as contributory factors. The addiction in gaming is maintained by a combination of incentives (e.g. more points), disincentives (e.g. loss of points on logging off), social/moral consequences (e.g. logging out would result in the team losing points collectively) and so on (Kuss and Griffiths 2012).

Clinically, while criteria for addiction may be more difficult to establish, harmful use may probably be easier to establish and work with. A sensible clinical approach is to routinely ask about technology use in the patient, just as one would screen for illicit drugs.

12 Conclusion

Classificatory manuals are the backbone of the entire field of psychiatry. They serve as the gold standard for making diagnosis and providing treatment. They form the basis of organising services and driving research. They continue to have far reaching implications across multiple fields including law, education, disability, social welfare services, government policy, insurance and public perceptions of psychiatric disorders. Given this broad impact, the authors of these manuals face incredible pressure from several domains. As such, the enormous work done in putting together and updating classificatory systems needs to be commended. All too often, these manuals are either criticised (often not unreasonably), or ridiculed, or taken to ridiculous lengths. For example, Bentall (1992) argues for the inclusion of happiness as disease state. Given that our knowledge about the aetiology of the diseases we treat remains woefully inadequate, it is understandable that classificatory systems will be constantly evolving, and there are bound to be discrepancies between different editions of the manuals. These discrepancies are likely to continue till the aetiological and genetic underpinnings of psychiatric disorders are understood better. This is all the more relevant in the era of corporate governance, evidence-based medicine and funding models, which often require every patient to fall neatly into a particular category. Meanwhile, clinical skill, logic, compassion and common sense continue to be the psychiatrist's greatest resources. As long we are guided by our patient's needs, as long as we base our interventions on the Hippocratic Oath and the Rogerian principle of unconditional acceptance of our patients, we will do well as a profession.

References

Adornetto, C., Suppiger, A., In-Albon, T., Neuschwander, M., & Schneider, S. (2012). Concordances and discrepancies between ICD-10 and DSM-IV criteria for anxiety disorders in childhood and adolescence. *Child and Adolescent Psychiatry and Mental Health, 6*, 40.

American Psychiatric Association. (1994). *Diagnostic and statistical manual of mental disorders (DSM-IV)* (4th ed.). Washington, DC: American Psychiatric Association.

American Psychiatric Association. (2013). *Diagnostic and statistical manual of mental disorders (DSM-5)* (5th ed.). Washington, DC: American Psychiatric Association.

American Academy of Pediatrics, Committee on Quality Improvement, Subcommittee on Attention-Deficit, Hyperactivity Disorder. (2000). Clinical practice guideline: diagnosis and evaluation of the child with attention-deficit/hyperactivity disorder. *Pediatrics, 105*, 1158–1170.

Bentall, P. (1992). A proposal to classify happiness as a psychiatric disorder. *Journal of Medical Ethics, 18*, 94–98.

Biederman, J. (2006). The evolving face of pediatric mania. *Biological Psychiatry, 60*, 901–902.

Brausch, A., & Gutierrez, P. (2010). Differences in non-suicidal self-injury and suicide attempts in adolescents. *Journal of Youth and Adolescence, 39*, 233–242.

Brotman, M. A., Schmajuk, M., Rich, B. A., Dickstein, D. P., Guyer, A. E., Costello, E. J., et al. (2006). Prevalence, clinical correlates, and longitudinal course of severe mood dysregulation in children. *Biological Psychiatry, 60*, 991–997.

Carlson, G. A. (2007). Who are the children with severe mood dysregulation, a.k.a. "Rages"? *American Journal of Psychiatry, 164*, 1140–1142.

Coghill, D., & Seth, S. (2011). Do the diagnostic criteria for ADHD need to change? Comments on the preliminary proposals of the DSM-5 ADHD and disruptive behavior disorders committee. *European Child and Adolescent Psychiatry, 20*, 75–81.

Coghill, D., & Sonuga-Barke, E. J. (2012). Annual research review: Categories versus dimensions in the classification and conceptualisation of child and adolescent mental disorders—implications of recent empirical study. *Journal of Child Psychology and Psychiatry, 5*, 469–489.

Correll, C. U., Manu, P., Olshanskiy, V., Napolitano, B., Kane, J. M., & Malhotra, A. K. (2009). Cardiometabolic risk of second-generation antipsychotic medications during first-time use in children and adolescents. *JAMA, 302*(16), 1765–1773.

Dilling, H. (2000). Classification. In M. G. Gelder, J. J. Lopez-Ibor Jr., & N. C. Andreasen (Eds.), *New Oxford textbook of psychiatry* (pp. 109–133). Oxford: Oxford University Press.

Döpfner, M., Breuer, D., Wille, N., Erhart, M., & Ravens-Sieberer, (2008). How often do children meet ICD-10/DSM-IV criteria of attention deficit-/hyperactivity disorder and hyperkinetic disorder? Parent-based prevalence rates in a national sample–results of the BELLA study. *European Child and Adolescent Psychiatry, 1*, 59–70.

DSM-5 Childhood and Adolescent Disorders Work Group. (2010). Issues pertinent to a developmental approach to bipolar disorder in DSM-5 [APA DSM-5 Development website]. (2010). Available at: http://www.dsm5.org/Proposed%20Revision%20Attachments/APA%20Developmental%20Approaches%20to%20Bipolar%20Disorder.pdf. Accessed 14 Feb 2013.

DSM-5 Childhood and Adolescent Disorders Work Group. Justification for temper dysregulation disorder with dysphoria [APA DSM-5 Development website]. (2010). Available:http://www.dsm5.org/Proposed%20Revision%20Attachments/Justification%20for%20Temper%20Dysregulation%20Disorder%20with%20Dysphoria.pdf. Accessed 14 Feb 2013.

DSM-5: options being considered for ADHD. Available at: http://www.dsm5.org/Proposed%20Revision%20Attachments/APA%20Options%20for%20ADHD.pdf. Accessed 15 Feb 2013.

Dullur, P., Eapen, V., & Trapolini, T. (2012). Metabolic syndrome in an adolescent psychiatric unit. *Australas Psychiatry., 20*(5), 444–445.

Eapen, V., Brac, GF., Ward, P., Hazell, P., Barton, G., Asghari-Fard, M. et al. (2012). Evaluation of weight gain and metabolic parameters among adolescent psychiatric inpatients: Role of health promotion and life style intervention programs. *Journal of Metabol Syndrome*, 109. doi:10.4172/2167-0943.1000109.

Faraone, S. V., Biederman, J., & Mick, E. (2006). The age dependent decline of attention deficit hyperactivity disorder: A meta-analysis of follow-up studies. *Psychological Medicine, 36*, 159–165.

Farrington, D. (1995). The development of offending and antisocial behaviour from childhood: Key findings from the Cambridge study in delinquent development. *Journal of Child Psychology and Psychiatry, 36*, 929–964.

Flint, J., & Yule, W. (1994). Behavioural phenotypes. In M. Rutter, E. Taylor, & L. Hersov (Eds.), *Child and adolescent psychiatry: Modern approaches* (pp. 666–687). Oxford: Blackwell.

Floros, G., & Siomos, K. (2013). The relationship between optimal parenting, Internet addiction and motives for social networking in adolescence. *Psychiatry research*. doi:10.1016/j.psychres.2013.01.010. pii: S0165-1781(13)00031-0 (Epub ahead of print).

Frances A. DSM5 plans to loosen criteria for adult ADD. Psychology today. April 20, 2010. Available at: http://www.psychologytoday.com/blog/dsm5-in-distress/201004/dsm5-plansloosen-criteria-adult-add?page_2. Accessed 15 Feb 2013.

Garmezy, N., & Masten, A. (1994). Chronic adversities. In M. Rutter, E. Taylor & L. Hersov (Eds.) *Child and adolescent psychiatry: Modern approaches* (pp. 191–208). Oxford: Blackwell.

Geller, B., Tillman, R., Bolhofner, K., & Zimerman, B. (2008). Child bipolar I disorder: Prospective continuity with adult bipolar I disorder; characteristics of second and third episodes; predictors of 8-year outcome. *Archives of General Psychiatry, 65*(10), 1125–1133.

Ghaziuddin, M. (2010). Should the DSM V drop Asperger syndrome? *Journal of Autism and Developmental Disorders, 40*, 1146–1148.

Girimaji, S.C. (2008). Clinical practice guidelines for the diagnosis and management of children with mental retardation. *Indian Journal of Psychiatry.*

Jairam, R., Prabhuswamy, M., & Dullur, P. (2012). Do we really know how to treat a child with bipolar disorder or one with severe mood dysregulation? Is there a magic bullet?. *Depress Research Treatment*. 967302.

Jairam, R., Srinath, S., Girimaji, S. C., & Seshadri, S. P. (2004). A prospective 4–5 year follow-up of juvenile onset bipolar disorder. *Bipolar Disorders, 5*, 386–394.

Jaisoorya, T. S., Janardhan Reddy, Y. C., & Srinath, S. (2003). Is juvenile obsessive-compulsive disorder a developmental subtype of the disorder?—Findings from an Indian study. *European Child and Adolescent Psychiatry, 12*(6), 290–297.

Kazdin, A. E. (1997). Practitioner review: Psychosocial treatments for conduct disorder in children. *Journal of Child Psychology and Psychiatry, 38*(2), 161–178.

Kuss, D. J., & Griffiths, M. D. (2012). Internet gaming addiction: A systematic review of empirical research. *International Journal of Mental Health and Addiction, 10*, 278–296.

Larsson, H., Dilshad, R., Lichtenstein, P., & Barker, E. D. (2011). Developmental trajectories of DSM-IV symptoms of attention deficit/hyperactivity disorder: Genetic effects, family risk and associated psychopathology. *Journal of Child Psychology and Psychiatry, 52*, 954–963.

Leibenluft, E., Charney, D. S., Towbin, K. E., Bhangoo, R. K., & Pine, D. S. (2003). Defining clinical phenotypes of juvenile mania. *American Journal of Psychiatry, 160*, 430–437.

Luis Salvador-Carull, (2011). Intellectual developmental disorders: towards a new name, definition and framework for "mental retardation/ intellectual disability" in ICD-11. *World Psychiatry, 10*, 175–180.

Madge, N., Hewitt, A., Hawton, K., et al. (2008). Deliberate self-harm within an international community sample of young people: comparative findings from the child & adolescent self-harm in Europe (CASE) study. *Journal of Child Psychology and Psychiatry, 49*, 667–677.

Malhotra, S., Aga, M., Balraj, & Gupta, N. (1999). Comparison of conduct disorder and hyperkinetic conduct disorder: A retrospective clinical study from north India. *Indian Journal of Psychiatry, 41*(2), 111–121.

Mick, E., Spencer, T., Wozniak, J., & Biederman, J. (2005). Heterogeneity of irritability in attention-deficit/hyperactivity disorder subjects with and without mood disorders. *Biological Psychiatry, 58*, 576–582.

Moffitt, T. E., Arseneault, L., & Jaffee, S. R. (2008). Research review: DSM-V conduct disorder. research needs for an evidence base. *Journal of Child Psychology and Psychiatry, 49*(1), 3–33.

Moselhy, H., Vostanis, P., & Winkley, L. (1997). Psychosocial abnormalities (ICD–10, Axis V) in child psychiatric outpatients: Relationship with patterns of referral, diagnosis and attendance. *European Journal of Psychiatry, 11*, 27–34.

Odgers, C. L., Caspi, A., Broadbent, J. M., et al. (2007a). Prediction of differential adult health burden by conduct problem subtypes in males. *Archives of General Psychiatry, 64*, 476–484.

Odgers, C. L., Milne, B. J., Caspi, A., et al. (2007b). Predicting prognosis for the conduct problem boy: Can family history help? *Journal of the American Academy of Child and Adolescent Psychiatry, 46*, 1240–1249.

Perry, S., Cooper, A. M., & Michels, R. (1987). The psychodynamic formulation: Its purpose, structure, and clinical application. *American Journal of Psychiatry, 144*(5), 543–550.

Pini, S., Abelli, M., Shear, K. M., et al. (2010). Frequency and clinical correlates of adult separation anxiety in a sample of 508 outpatients with mood and anxiety disorders. *Acta Psychiatrica Scandinavica, 122*, 40–46.

Polanczyk, G., Caspi, A., Houts, R., Kollins, S. H., Rohde, L. A., & Moffitt, T. E. (2010). Implications of extending the ADHD age-of-onset criterion to age 12: Results from a prospectively studied birth cohort. *Journal of the American Academy of Child and Adolescent Psychiatry, 49*, 210–216.

Quinn, P. C. (2012). Evidence for mental subdivision of space by infants: 3–4 month-olds spontaneously bisect a small-scale area into left and right categories. *Psychonomic Bulletin and Review, 19*(3), 449–455.

RANZCP formulation guidelines for candidates OCI/MOCI Examination Page 1 of 8 Approved: Chair OI Subcommittee (2012) Version 5. Accessed 15 Feb 2013.

Reddy, Y. C., Girimaji, S. R., & Srinath, S. (1993). Comparative study of classification of psychosis of childhood and adolescent onset. *Acta Psychiatrica Scandinavica, 87*(3), 188–191.

Research Diagnostic Criteria—Preschool Age (RDC-PA) (2002) www.infantinstitute.org/RDC-PA.htm. Accessed 15 Feb 2013.

Robins, L. N. (1978). Sturdy childhood predictors of adult antisocial behaviour: Replications from longitudinal studies. *Psychological Medicine, 8*, 611–622.

Robins, E., & Guze, S. B. (1970). Establishment of diagnostic validity in psychiatric illness: Its application to schizophrenia. *American Journal of Psychiatry, 126*, 983–987.

Ruhrmann, S., Schultze-Lutter, F., Salokangas, R. K., et al. (2010). Prediction of psychosis in adolescents and young adults at high risk: Results from the prospective European prediction of psychosis study. *Archives of General Psychiatry, 67*, 241–251.

Rutter, M. (1987). Psychosocial resilience and protective mechanisms. *American Journal of Orthopsychiatry, 57*, 316–331.

Rutter, M. (2011). Research Review: Child psychiatric diagnosis and classification: concepts, findings, challenges and potential. *Journal of Child Psychology and Psychiatry, 52*(6), 647–660.

Rutter, M., Giller, H., & Hagell, A. (1998). Antisocial behavior by young people. In J. Tizard & K. Whitmore (Eds.), *Education*. Cambridge: Cambridge University Press.

Rutter, M., & Uher, R. (2012). Classification issues and challenges in child and adolescent psychopathology. *International Review of Psychiatry, 24*(6), 514–529.

Scott, S. (2001). Classification of psychiatric disorders in childhood and adolescence: Building castles in the sand? *Advances in Psychiatric Treatment, 8*, 205–213.

Shaffer, D., Gould, M., Brasic, J., et al. (1983). A children's global assessment scale (CGAS). *Archives of General Psychiatry, 40*, 1228–1231.

Shear, K., Jin, R., Ruscio, A. M., Walters, E. E., & Kessler, R. C. (2006). Prevalence and correlates of estimated DSM-IV child and adult separation anxiety disorder in the National Comorbidity Survey Replication. *American Journal of Psychiatry, 163*, 1074–1083.

Sitholey, P., Agarwal, V., & Bharti, V. (2012). A clinical comparison study of attention deficit/hyperactivity disorder (DSM-IV) and hyperkinetic disorder (ICD-10) in Indian children and Adolescents. *Journal of Indian Association Child Adolescent Mental Health, 8*(1), 6–11.

Snowling, M. J. (2011). Editorial: What's behind sibling rivalry: Checks and balances in the sibling relationship. *Journal of Child Psychology and Psychiatry, 52*(6), 629–630.

Starcevic, V. (2013a). Separation anxiety disorder in adults: Is the neglect real? *Australia and New Zealand Journal of Psychiatry, 47*, 188–189.

Starcevic, C. (2013b). Is Internet addiction a useful concept? *Australia and New Zealand Journal of Psychiatry, 47*, 16–19.

Steinberger, K., & Schuch, B. (2002). Classification of obsessive-compulsive disorder in childhood and adolescence. *Acta Psychiatrica Scandinavica, 106*, 97–102.

Steinhausen, H., & Erdin, A. (1992). Abnormal psychosocial situations and ICD–10 diagnoses in children and adolescents attending a psychiatric service. *Journal of Child Psychology and Psychiatry, 33*, 731–740.

Stringaris, A. (2011). Irritability in children and adolescents: A challenge for DSM-5. *European Child and Adolescent Psychiatry, 20*(2), 61–66.

Taylor, E., & Rutter, M. (2008). Classification. In M. Rutter, D. Bishop, D. Pine, S. Scott, J. Stevenson, E. Taylor, & A. Thapar (Eds.), *Rutter's child and adolescent psychiatry* (5th ed., pp. 18–31). Oxford: Wiley-Blackwell.

WHO. (1996). *Multiaxial classification of child and adolescent psychiatric disorders*. Cambridge: Cambridge University Press.

Witwer, A. N., & Lecavalier, L. (2008). Examining the validity of autism spectrum disorder subtypes. *Journal of Autism and Developmental Disorders, 38*, 1611–1624.

Wonderlich, S. A., Gordon, K. H., Mitchell, J. E., Crosby, R. D., & Engel, S. G. (2009). The validity and clinical utility of binge-eating disorder. *International Journal of Eating Disorders, 42*, 687–705.

World Health Organization. (1992). *The ICD-10 classification of mental and behavioural disorders: Clinical descriptions and diagnostic guidelines*. Geneva: World Health Organization.

World Health Organization. (1998). *Diagnostic and management guidelines for mental disorders in primary care: ICD-10 chapter V primary care version* (2nd ed.). Geneva: World Health Organization.

Wozniak, J., Biederman, J., Kwon, A., et al. (2005). How cardinal are cardinal symptoms in pediatric bipolar disorder? An examination of clinical correlates. *Biological Psychiatry, 58*, 583–588.

Yung, A. R., Nelson, B., Thompson, A. D., & Wood, S. J. (2010). Should a "risk syndrome for psychosis" be included in DSMV? *Schizophrenia Research, 20*, 7–15.

Zero to Three. (1994). *Diagnostic classification of mental health and developmental disorders of infancy and early childhood*. Washington, DC: Zero to Three Press.

Zero to Three. (2005). *Diagnostic classification of mental health and developmental disorders of infancy and early childhood DC:0-3R*. Washington, DC: Zero to Three Press.

Chapter 15
Autism Spectrum Disorder: 70 Years on and the Plot Thickens

U.S. Naik

1 Introduction

Autism spectrum disorder (ASD) is characterised by patterns of delay and deviance in the development of social, communicative and cognitive skills, arising in the first years of life.

In October 2010, Donovam and Zucker published an article in The Atlantic, "Autism's First Child" or "Leo Kanner's Case No. 1, Don T". The authors through painstaking detective work tracked down Donald who will be eighty this year.

In their own words, "*Later chapters in his life remained unwritten, leaving us with no detailed answer to the question: Whatever happened to Donald?*

There is an answer. Some of it we turned up in documents long overlooked in the archives of Johns Hopkins. But most of it we found by tracking down and spending time with Donald himself. His full name is Donald Gray Triplett. He's 77 *years old. And he's still in Forest, Mississippi. Playing golf*' (Donovan and Zucker 2010).

Oliver Triplett, the father, of Case No. 1, sent a preliminary report to Kanner that was 33 pages long. "Oliver's *observations were the first detailed listing of symptoms that are now instantly recognisable to anyone who knows autism.—The child was withdrawn "into his shell," to "live within himself," "perfectly oblivious to everything about him." "No apparent affection" "a mania for spinning blocks and pans and other round objects." "A fascination for numbers, musical notes, letters of the alphabet, which he enjoyed reciting in reverse order,"—he also had intense dislikes: milk, swings, tricycles—"almost a horror of them" "When interfered with, he has temper tantrums, during which he is destructive*".

U.S. Naik, Emeritus Professor

U.S. Naik (✉)
Department of Psychiatry, Osmania Medical College, Hyderabad, India
e-mail: naikusha@gmail.com

S. Malhotra and S. Chakrabarti (eds.), *Developments in Psychiatry in India*,
DOI 10.1007/978-81-322-1674-2_15

By the age of 2, he could recite the 23rd Psalm and knew 25 questions and answers from the Presbyterian catechism by heart.—And the random humming he engaged in while spinning blocks turned out not to be quite so random after all. Rather, he always "picked three notes that, if played simultaneously on a keyboard, would blend into a perfect chord" (Donovan and Zucker 2010).

To this Kanner, America's leading psychiatrist, at that time was to write these most famous words to Donald's mother, Mrs. Triplett:

> Nobody realizes more than I do myself that at no time have you or your husband been given a clear-cut and unequivocal … diagnostic term.";—"If there is any name to be applied to the condition of Don and those other children, I have found it best to speak of it as "autistic disturbance of affective contact" (Donovan and Zucker 2010).

These words were to mark the description of a new childhood condition, *infantile autism*, now called ASD. Kanner's original description still continues to form the core of the diagnosis of autism, a condition which is rapidly being reported across the globe and puzzling scientists, families and therapists. India too has published extensively in several aspects of the condition. This chapter will highlight Indian research while noting current world opinion.

2 Definition and Prevalence

2.1 Definition

Autism is now defined as a disorder characterised by the following:

(a) Deficits in social communication and social interaction manifested by all three of the following:

- Deficits in social–emotional reciprocity
- Deficits in nonverbal communicative behaviours used for social interaction
- Deficits in developing and maintaining appropriate relationships

(b) Restricted repetitive patterns of behaviour, interests or activities manifested by at least two of the following:

- Stereotyped or repetitive speech, movements or use of objects
- Excessive adherence to routines or rituals
- Restricted interests
- Hyper- or hypo-sensitivity to sensory stimuli

  These symptoms should be noticed in early childhood and interfere with function. Three levels of severity are also included (American Psychiatric Association 2013).

2.2 Prevalence

The centre for disease control (CDC) has documented that more children are being diagnosed with an ASD than ever before. A conservative estimate is of 1/500 children. However, the CDC in 2008 reported the overall estimated prevalence of ASDs as 11.3 per 1,000 (one in 88) children aged 8 years. ASD prevalence estimates varied widely across all sites (range: 4.8–21.2 per 1,000 children aged 8 years. The risk is 3–4 times higher in males than in females (CDC 2012).

In an important review commissioned by the WHO, in most studies reported after 2000, the median prevalence is 17/10,000 for AD and 62/10,000 for all pervasive developmental disorders (PDDs) (Elsabbagh et al. 2012).

Most reports from India tend to be from hospital-based samples. Erna Hoch, a Swiss psychiatrist, who worked in Kashmir, reported 2.9 % of cases in a missionary hospital to be infantile autism. Subsequently, patients were reported from tertiary care centres (Hoch 1967). One of the earliest studies was from Bangalore (Narayanan 1978).

The following studies from a tertiary care centre report clinic figures. Four patients were noted to have attended the outpatient clinic between 1981 and 1982 (Malhotra and Chaturvedi 1984). Another study found 16 children diagnosed with autism over a 2-year period (Singhi and Malhi 2001). Five patients with childhood disintegrative disorder were reported from 1980 to 1989 (Narayanan 1978) and three patients with Asperger's syndrome from 1989 to 1999. Between 1989 and 1999, 46 patients with autism spectrum disorder were seen, of which 22 had autism, 12 had childhood disintegrative disorder, 5 had atypical autism, 4 had Asperger's syndrome and 2 children had Rett's syndrome (Malhotra and Chaturvedi 1984; Singhi and Malhi 2001; Malhotra et al. 2003; Malhotra and Vikas 2005). Thirty-one patients were reported between 1981 and 1984 at a tertiary centre in South India (Bharat et al. 1997; Srinath et al. 1989). In another clinic in North India of 641 cases, 121 or 18.9 % had PDDs (Juneja et al. 2012).

Special schools have also yielded clusters of subjects with autism. Out of 500 special school children screened for autistic disorder, 74 were diagnosed with autism (14.8 %) (Subbalakshmi 2012). Through retrospective analysis of records of an early intervention programme (EIP), one study demonstrated that 4 % of children attending an EIP centre had autism (Kaur et al. 2006). In a study in Barwani district, in a total of 262 children with ID evaluated for psychiatric disorders, the following rates were observed: attention deficit hyperactivity disorder (ADHD), 6.5 %; autism and 4.2 % anxiety (Lakhan 2013). In the past, attempts have also been made to create a central registry of cases (Seth and Kalra 2006; Kalra et al. 2005). *However a cohesive picture of the prevalence and incidence of autism spectrum disorder is missing in India. It is imperative that epidemiological studies which are multi-centric, representative and well designed using an instrument with high fidelity be carried out* (Sharan 2006).

3 Aetiology

The quest for the aetiology of autism has generated an astounding amount of research. Different theories abound with genetic, immunological, epigenetic, and environmental effects.

There is a good body of research from India, particularly in the study of genes that have been implicated as relevant.

(i) **Genetic factors**

In a review in the Pediatric Clinics of North America, the genetic and chromosomal disorders associated with autism were categorised as metabolic, mitochondrial, chromosomal and single-gene conditions (Torielo 2012). The metabolic disorders were phenylketonuria, purine metabolism disorders, succinyl semialdehyde dehydrogenase deficiency, disorders of creatine transport metabolism, cerebral folate deficiency and Smith–Lemli–Opitz syndrome. Mitochondrial involvement was suggested by elevated lactate levels and respiratory chain disorders. The chromosomal anomalies were Dup7q11.23, Dup or Del 16p11.2, Del 17q12, Del or dup 15q13, and Del 22q13.

Under the monogenic conditions were listed Rett's, Angelman's, CHARGE and Cornelia de Lange syndromes, neurofibromatosis, tuberous sclerosis, myotonic dystrophy and Fragile X syndrome (Torielo 2012). Whereas in the past, the focus was on a search for a chromosomal cause, chromosomal microarray analysis (CMA) has identified copy number variants in as many as 8 % of children (Tchaconas and Adesman 2013). The interplay of several genes is now considered as aetiologically important. Genome-wide association studies suggest that a propensity to ASD appears to stem from common genetic polymorphisms, which exert substantial additive genetic effects on ASD (Klei et al. 2012).

5HIAA and HVA: Studies from India reflect the quest for aberrant gene transmission in families. In an early Indian study, 5HIAA and HVA was not increased in the CSF of 17 children with autism (Narayan et al. 1993).

Glutamate: In a study of 10 children with ASD and 10 controls, blood glutamate levels were measured using high-performance liquid chromatography technique, and brain glutamate levels were measured using proton magnetic resonance spectroscopy (MRS). The levels of glutamate were significantly raised and correlated with each other (Choudhury et al. 2012).

Tryptophan hydroxylase 2: Based on the premise of serotoninergic pathway involvement as an endophenotype for ASD, the association of tryptophan hydroxylase 2 (*TPH2*), the rate-limiting enzyme in 5-HT biosynthesis, and integrin beta-chain 3(*ITGB3*) a serotonin quantitative trait locus with ASD was investigated in the Indian population. The results indicated the likely involvement of *ITGB3* and *TPH2* in the pathophysiology of ASD in the Indian population (Singh et al. 2013).

Folate pathway: Folate pathways were assessed in 138 children with autism and 138 children without autism and were tested for 5 genetic polymorphisms related to the folate pathway. Of the genes studied using PCR-restriction fragment length polymorphism were methylene tetrahydroflate reductase (MTHFR C677T and MTHFR A1298C). MTHFR C677T was found to be a risk factor with MTHFR A1298C acting additively to increase risk (Mohammad et al. 2009).

Serotonin transporter gene (*SLC6A4*): Hyperserotoninemia, response to SSRIs and linkage to 17q11, has generated interest in studying the serotonin transporter gene SL6A4 (solute carrier family 6). The serotonin transporter gene (SLC6A4) was studied in 93 children with autism, their families and 160 controls. No preferential allelic transfer to the probands was noted (Guhathakurta et al. 2008).

Engrailed 2 (*EN2*): The epigenetic evaluation of *EN-2* a homeobox transcription factor, in the cerebellum of patients with autism indicates a persistent upregulation of a gene that normally undergoes perinatal downregulation to ensure normal Purkinje cell differentiation. *EN-2* has now been verified to be one of several candidate genes that have both genetic and epigenetic associations with autism including brain-derived neurotrophic factor, the reelin gene (RELN), oxytocin, HOXA1, MeCP2 and screening for Fragile X (FXS; Tr Psyr). A study in Assam of Engrailed 2 (EN2) involved in the patterning of the cerebellum in development has been found to map to the 7q36.3 region, which has previously been shown to be associated with ASD and language disorders like childhood dysphasia. Five markers in the promoter, exon 1 and intron region of the EN2 gene were studied. Two intronic markers were transmitted with a significant bias in favour of females, which has not been reported before (James et al. 2013; Sen et al. 2010).

Reelin gene: The RELN is located on chromosome 7q22, an important and critical region for autism, identified through several genome-wide scans. The first of the two studies from Assam was conducted with 73 persons with autism and 129 parents and 80 controls. There was no difference in allelic and genotypic distribution between patients and controls. Though there was a difference in allele repeats between Indian and other populations, there was no difference between patients and controls in the three markers of the RELN (Dutta et al. 2007). A subsequent study investigated six more single nucleotide polymorphisms (SNPs) in 102 patients, 182 parents and 101 healthy controls. No preferential parental transmission of any alleles of the markers to affected offspring, or any biased allelic or genotypic distribution between the cases and controls was noted (Dutta et al. 2008). Thus, this study suggested that SNPs of RELN are unlikely to be associated with ASD in the Indian population.

Glutamate 6 receptor: Glutamate receptor 6 gene (GLu R6 or GRIK2) was studied in 101 cases, 180 parents and 152 controls, but no biased transmission of alleles or haplotypes to the affected offspring was detected (Dutta et al. 2007).

Glutathione S-transferases: Glutathione S-transferases (GST) are antioxidant enzymes that play an important role in the cellular detoxification and have been associated with ASD. Six patients with ASD and 8 controls were assessed for GST activity. Fifty one patients with ASD and 45 controls were recruited for GST mu (GSTM1) and G theta (GSTT1) genotyping. While no significant differences in frequencies of GSTM1 and GSTT1 genotypes was noted, the mean erythrocyte GST activity in ASD was significantly decreased compared with controls (Hermawati et al. 2011).

HOXA1 and HOXB1: Some negative correlations and lack of association of HOXA1 and HOXB1 variants with autism in an Indian study (Gangopadhyay et al. 2007).

Fragile X screening and checklist: The Fragile X syndrome is the most frequent hereditary cause of mental retardation. It has been the focus of several studies. The *FMR1* gene is classified into normal 5–44; gray zone 45–54; premutation 55 to <200; and full mutation ≥200 repeats. About 705 women from Tamil Nadu, South India, were screened for the *FMR1* allelic variation by using radioactive polymerase chain reaction–polyacrylamide gel electrophoresis (PAGE) analysis. One in 353 women carried the premutation. No full mutations were observed. Ms-PCR is more suitable for routine screening and clinical testing compared with rPCR-PAGE analysis. In a study reporting screening for Fragile X (FXS) in 157 individuals with various neurobehavioural problems, only four were confirmed as FXS (3.18 % prevalence among neurobehavioural outpatients). Thirty distinct alleles with 12–49 CGG repeats were detected, by the FRAXA checklist. In a clinically useful study, when clinical features were analysed in 327 males and 41 females, six clinical features were statistically significant in FRAXA individuals, namely hyperactivity, poor eye contact, hyperextensibility of joints, large ears, macro-orchidism and a family history of mental retardation. Using this checklist would improve the reliability of FRAXA testing (Manjunatha et al. 1989; Rai 2011; Indhumathi et al. 2012; Bhowmik et al. 2009; Guruju et al. 2009).

Fragile sites: In 150 subjects selected from 140 families, 132 families had a single child with autism, while in 8 families, multiple sibs were affected. Among the 150 subjects analysed for various fragile sites, 12 individuals were found to be positive for Fragile "X" chromosome (Manjunatha et al. 2001).

Tuberous sclerosis complex: Tuberous sclerosis complex (TSC) is an autosomal dominant disorder with loci on chromosome 9q34.3 (TSC1) and chromosome 16p13.3 (TSC2). In a study, a total of 12 mutations were studied; of these, seven mutations were novel. A single previously known deletion in the TSC1 gene was identified. In addition, three and eight variants/polymorphisms in the TSC1 and TSC2 genes, respectively, were detected. Of these, three were novel SNPs (Ali et al. 2004).

MRNA: A systematic analysis of the CNV-miRNAs based on their interactions with the target genes enabled the identification of top 10 miRNAs as hub molecules. These CNV-miRNAs in turn affected transcription factors and their target genes with a role in neurodevelopment and synapse formation. This was possibly the first report to highlight the significance of CNV-microRNAs and their contribution towards the genetic heterogeneity of autism (Vaishnavi et al. 2013).

Systems biology: Using a systems biology approach, starting with 675 genes for ASD and 713 genes for bipolar disorder and using a consensus path database, networks for 4 pathways were identified: (1) neuroligand receptor interaction pathway, (2) synaptic transmission, (3) circadian rhythm pathway and (4) catecholamine synthesis pathway (Ragunath et al. 2011).

Twin studies and the shared environment: It needed a twin study done in California to highlight the importance of a shared environment in contributing to concordance. Structured diagnostic assessments were completed on 192 twin pairs. For strict autism, concordance for male twins was 0.58 for 40 monozygotic pairs and 0.21 for 31 dizygotic pairs; for female twins, the concordance was 0.60 for 7 monozygotic pairs and 0.27 for 10 dizygotic pairs. The conclusion was that the susceptibility to ASD has moderate heritability and a substantial shared twin environmental component (Surén et al. 2013).

(ii) **Immunological factors**

Immune function alterations have been repeatedly demonstrated in patients with autism and their families. These include neuroinflammation in brain tissue, elevated cytokines in blood and CSF and antibodies directed against neural tissue (Vargas et al. 2005). Infections may also contribute to immune dysfunction. Cytokines implicated in autism are IL-1B, IL-6, IL-4, IFN-γ and TGF-B (Tchaconas and Adesman 2013; Vargas et al. 2005; Onore et al. 2012; Singh 1996).

Nuclear factor kappa B (NF-κB): A clear period of normal development followed by regression and subsequent improvement with treatment suggests a multifactorial aetiology. Viral and bacterial infections, hypoxia or medication could affect both the foetus and the infant. These stressors could upregulate transcription factors like nuclear factor kappa B (NF-κB), a master switch for many genes including some implicated in autism like tumour necrosis factor (TNF). Based on this hypothesis, one Indian study chose to determine NF-κB in children with autism. Peripheral blood samples of 67 children with autism and 29 control children were evaluated for NF-κB using electrophoretic mobility shift assay (EMSA). A significant increase in NF-κB DNA binding activity was noted in peripheral blood samples of children with autism. As NF-κB levels reflect a response to stressors of several kinds, and in turn NF-κB controls many genes, the significance of its role in autism needs further elucidation (Naik et al. 2011).

Allergies: *Ninety-four* serum samples of patients were tested for IgG. Although egg, milk, wheat, peanuts and buckwheat are the most common food allergens, in this study, egg allergy was seen in 5.08 % of patients, milk allergy was seen in 7.62 % and wheat flour allergy was seen in 5.93 % of patients. Peanut allergy was seen in 47.45 % of the subjects (Rao 2010).

(iii) **Environmental factors**

Environmental toxins include heavy metals like lead and mercury; pesticides like organochlorines, organophosphates, and pyrethoids; and two halogenated aromatic hydrocarbons, namely polychlorinated biphenyls (PCBs) and polybrominated diphenyl ethers (PBDEs). Recently, PBDEs have been shown to influence the expression of autism-related genes in the brain of experimental animals and human brain tissue. The role of environmental factors in earlier described mechanisms like cytokine regulation reflects a close interplay of the environment with immune mechanisms (LaSalle et al. 2013; Goines and Ashwood 2013).

Folate intake: In a Norwegian cohort that enrolled 109,000 children born from 2002 to 2008, the mothers were recruited during pregnancy at approximately 18 weeks' gestation. It was found that those mothers who started taking folic acid before getting pregnant were about 40 % less likely to have a child who developed autism. Folic acid supplements were best started 4 weeks before conception. In children whose mothers took folic acid, 0.10 % had autistic disorder, compared with 0.21 % in those unexposed to folic acid. This finding has a simple lesson of supplementation of folic acid before conception as preventive strategy (Hallmayer et al. 2011). Also implicated have been maternal infections in pregnancy, low birthweight, increased paternal age and twin pregnancies (Tchaconas and Adesman 2013).

Trophoblastic inclusions in the placenta: An interesting new study suggests that examining the placenta for trophoblastic inclusions may help predict autism in high-risk infants (Walker et al. 2013).

Toxins (*trace elements percentage and toxic elements*): In 45 children with autism and 5 controls, levels of copper, polybenium and mercury were significantly higher in the hair and nails of children with autism, with direct relation to severity. The trace elements magnesium and selenium were reduced in children with low-functioning autism (Priya and Geetha 2011).

Oxidative stress markers: Urinary levels of oxidative stress markers, namely thiobarbituric acid-reacting substances, lipid hydroperoxides, 4-hydroxynonenal, protein carbonyls, sulfhydryl groups, total antioxidant capacity, total peroxide content, oxidative stress index and also UA/Cr ratio, can be considered as the measure of oxidative stress index in children with autism. The significant correlation between severity of autism and urinary lipid peroxidation products also supports the use of oxidative stress markers and antioxidants as biomarkers of autism (Damodaran and Arumugam 2011). A recent brief report discussed the possibility of vitamin B12 deficiency as a causative mechanism in a patient with childhood disintegrative disorder (Malhotra et al. 2013).

Mouse models: Valproic acid was used as a toxicant in mice with a deletion of glutathione-S-transferase M1 (GSTM1), a gene associated with increased risk of autism that codes for an enzyme involved in the management of toxicant-induced oxidative stress. Valproic acid treatment caused significant increases in apoptosis in granule cells of the hippocampus and cerebellum. Valproic acid treatment resulted in deficits in social behaviours, not found in control mice without the gene deletion (Yochum et al. 2010).

Electromagnetic fields: Electromagnetic fields emitted during the operation of electronic gadgets do not have enough energy to cause DNA alterations directly; however, ample evidence is available from in vitro and in vivo studies to demonstrate their ability to cause DNA alterations indirectly as well as epigenetic modifications (Ahuja et al. 2013).

(iv) **Neuroimaging**

The three methods used for imaging in autism are positron emission tomography (PET), single-photon emission tomography (SPECT) and MRS. Three neurotransmitters have been studied: serotonin, dopamine and amino butyric acid (GABA). PET studies have shown a prolonged period of higher brain levels of serotonin synthesis, and also asymmetries of marker uptake in the thalamus, cerebellum and frontal cortex. SPECT studies have shown increased whole brain dopamine binding. MRS studies have shown decrease in *N-acetyl aspartate* (NAA) levels in children with autism (Chugani 2012). In a SPECT study of 22 children with autism, fifteen children had no perfusion abnormalities on SPECT imaging. Of the remaining seven, decreased perfusion in the left frontoparietal cortex was seen in three children and in the left inferior and medial frontal cortex in two children (Singhi et al. 2008). In another SPECT study, 10 children, with ASD, showed hypoperfusion in frontal prefrontal and subcortical areas (Gupta and Ratnam 2009). In a third study, temporal tubers were found to correlate with symptoms of autism in children with TSC (Kothur et al. 2008).

(v) **Psychological theories and birth-related issues**

Psychological stressors: Pathological changes in the cerebellum in autism are thought to correspond to an event before 30–32 weeks' gestation. Incidence of stressors during each 4-week block of pregnancy was recorded. Incidence of stressors in the blocks prior to and including the predicted time period (21–32 weeks' gestation) in each group of surveys was compared to the other prenatal blocks. A higher incidence of prenatal stressors was found in autism at 21–32 weeks' gestation, with a peak at 25–28 weeks. This does support the possibility of prenatal stressors as a potential contributor to autism (Beversdorf et al. 2005). In an early Indian case series, four cases were reported where children manifested symptoms of autism after severe psychological stress (Kapur 1989).

Cultural issues: Many cultural issues can change the identification, help-seeking behaviour and diagnosis of children with ASD. African Americans were 2.6 times less likely to receive a diagnosis of autism on their first specialty visit but instead were labelled ADHD (Mandell et al. 2007). Some traits of Asian children like avoiding eye contact with elders may be a sign of respect and not ASD. Studying Indians outside India, in a survey of 24 families with children with autism, three groups of families emerged: (i) primarily Western in their beliefs, (ii) primarily Indian and (iii) endorsed a combination of Western and Indian beliefs and practices. The observation was that when working with culturally diverse families, it is best not to assume the group as homogenous (Ravindran and Myers 2012).

Traits: In an interesting cross-cultural study, the expression of autistic traits were compared in students from three cultures the UK, India and Malaysia, using the autism spectrum quotient (AQ). Behaviours associated with autistic traits were greater in the Eastern group. Males scored higher than females, as did science students versus non-science students; Indian students scored higher on the imagination subscale and Malaysian students on the attention switching subscale (Freeth et al. 2013).

(vi) **The gut microbiome**

Newer research avenues have been explored in the past few years. The gut microbiome estimated "that up to a hundred trillion microbial cells have made a home of us". The human microbiome project was started in 2007 at the National Institute of Health (NIH), USA, to establish the nature of these organisms and their genome. The impact of this unrecognised "organ" in neurological and psychiatric disorders, and more particularly autism is under scientific scrutiny (Mulle et al. 2013).

It is obvious that there is no single aetiology for ASD. A complex array of genetic, environmental, epigenetic and psychosocial stressors may function in an untold number of permutations and combinations to lead to a clinical diagnosis.

4 Symptoms and Nomenclature

On 18 May 2013, Jeffery A. Lieberman, Director of the National Institute of Mental Health (NIMH), USA, issued a joint statement, with the President of the American Psychiatric Association (APA).

> This week, my good friend and colleague Tom Insel and I issued a rare joint statement clarifying the National Institute of Mental Health's (NIMH) support of the Diagnostic and Statistical Manual of Mental Disorders (DSM) as the gold standard of care for 2013 and for years to come. We did this because of a blog post on the NIMH Website about our collective frustration with the progress of brain science, the paucity of new treatments for brain diseases to help our patients and the need for future-looking researchers to think outside the box. We were concerned that comments about how to move beyond some of our traditional, symptom-based methods of diagnosis—which are, at the moment, the gold standard of science—were widely misreported as NIMH changing its position on the newly revised DSM-5. This is, of course, a preposterous notion. The NIMH was involved in all phases of the revision of the DSM, including the moments during the 10-year process when we all realized that the science that we hoped by now would have given us laboratory, imaging and electrophysiologic procedures to help diagnose mental illnesses was still coming up short (Jeffrey and Lieberman 2013).

The disappointments of the past 20 years are that we are still a phenomenological group struggling to find our disease markers. Of course, one must not forget that finding clear biochemical or imaging tests will promptly take the condition away to other disciplines! One important study conducted by Daley in India was assuring, as the majority of psychiatrists, paediatricians and psychologists used the ICD-10 or the DSM-IV for diagnosis (Daley and Sigman 2002). In 2010, data from 643 paediatricians in 1998 and 643 paediatricians in 2008 suggested a greater awareness and recognition of cases was reported with appropriate criteria for diagnosis (Daley and Barua 2010). It would be interesting to see the response to the new DSM criteria, while experts in the USA like Volkmar and Reichow (2013) have diametrically opposite views on the changes in the autism category. The main concern is that with greater specificity, some sensitivity will be lost and milder forms of the disorder and high-functioning individuals will not receive a diagnosis and therefore no treatment.

The symptomatology of autism began with Kanner's case notes. While gathering material for this paper, one reference turned up "India" in a Kanner article, called "*The conception of wholes and parts in early infantile autism*". What was the reference to India?

In one of the early cases, Malcolm H. saw a picture in an encyclopaedia. His mother said it was the *Taj Mahal in India—He then went through the whole library for days searching for pictures of India (Taj Mahal)*—"He was disturbed because the next two pictures of the Taj Mahal were different and "*found solace in getting the encyclopaedia and looking at the picture he had seen there first*" (Kanner 1951).

Leo Kanner's amazing attention to detail cannot be matched, and symptom descriptions like these still form the basis of a diagnosis of autism.

In India, Tito, an exceptionally bright but less verbal adolescent, wrote an insider's view of autism through three books written when he was 8, 11 and 17 years of age. Writing in the third person about "the boy," he writes:

> The hand had made a strange relationship with its shadow and he fluttered it and spent his hours contented with the lone company of his shadow. And his worries stopped. He shut away the world and felt secure in the presence of the shadow. If only the world could be a game with the shadow. But the reality was that he was drawing himself away and away into the world of his shadow. Nights were terrible. He searched everywhere for his shadow. He flapped to call it, there was nothing but darkness. He cried for it betrayed by the friend (Tito).

When asked why he flapped, he replied in writing, "*I am calming myself. My senses are so disconnected, I lose my body. So I flap. If I don't do this, I feel scattered and anxious*" (Mukhopadhyay 2000). Sceptical BBC producers documented his story with amazement, and his mother Soma has gone on to describe her treatment strategies based on her care of Tito and his feedback.

Several updates to symptomatology are added regularly to the world literature (Nazeer and Ghaziuddin 2012). The literature on symptomatology in the Indian literature mainly comprises case reports. There is also a wealth of unpublished literature. Clinical observations date back to 1978 (Narayanan 1978). Some of the case reports are on childhood disintegrative disorder, Rett's disorder, CHARGE syndrome and tuberous sclerosis (Malhotra and Singh 1993; Malhotra et al. 2002; Malhotra and Gupta 2002; Kumar et al. 2004; Sitholey et al. 1998). A descriptive hospital-based study was published in 2005 (Pushker et al. 2012). Disorders in speech articulatory function have been reported, which might serve as early indicators (Juneja et al. 2005). In vernacular speech, in Malayalam-speaking children, echolalic ability was observed to be present independent of the general language ability (Sullivan et al. 2013). Fifteen children with ASD were compared with 10 controls for speech abnormalities: exaggerated pitch, pitch range, pitch excursion and pitch contours were observed in autism. These are distinctive characteristics of *motherese,* suggesting a distinct vocal output (Aithal et al. 2011).

Pull to sit and hypotonia: A head lag at 6 months appeared to predict autism and could be evaluated further as an early marker (Sharda et al. 2010).

Log reports of time spent: In one interesting study of 140 preschool children with developmental disability, hourly log reports of time spent demonstrated differences between children with ASD from the rest of the group. Children with ASD spent thrice the time on sedentary or exclusion activities like watching television (21 % of the time) or playing alone (14 %). Conversely, playing with peers was 1.7 % and home schooling 0.3 % of the time (Shah 2012).

Epilepsy and neurological symptoms: The figure for epilepsy in autism varies at approximately 30 % before adolescence—with two peaks, one in early childhood and again in adolescence (Venkatesan 2005). Abnormalities in auditory brain stem responses were described (Silver and Rapin 2012). In a study to compare the developmental profiles of children with autism and children with developmental delay, the children with autism showed lower social skills, whereas children with developmental delays showed poorer motor skills (Shivashankar and Satishchandra 1989).

Intelligence: Data on intellectual ability from seven sites were combined; 38 % of children with ASDs were classified in the range of intellectual disability (ID) (i.e. IQ $\leq$ 70, 24 % in the borderline range (IQ 71–85) and 38 % had IQ scores >85). The proportion of children classified in the range of ID ranged from 13 % in Utah to 54 % in South Carolina (CDC) (CDC 2012). Michael Rutter, the doyen of child psychiatry and authority on autism, discussed the following areas to be evaluated in ASD, namely developmental regression, savant skills and epilepsy and additional psychiatric diagnosis. To these may be added sleep disorders, which are so characteristic of ASD (Jayarama and Bhat 2004).

Regression: Regression is defined as the loss of previously acquired skills. About Kanner's Case No. 3, his parents stated "*It seems that he has gone backward mentally gradually for the last 2 years*". At the current time, as Ozonoff stated in 2010, "Behavioural signs of autism are not present at birth but emerged through diminished social communication behaviours. More children may present with regression than previously thought, but parent reports do not capture this phenomenon". While gaze, smiles and vocalisations were mostly comparable at 6 months, infants who later went on to receive a diagnosis of ASD showed distinct differences by 12 months of age (Rutter 2011). Regression is determined through retrospective parental accounts, prospective laboratory studies and home video recordings which complement parent reports, counts or when a child cannot come into the laboratory to be observed (Ozonoff et al. 2010). According to Ozonoff, 19 of 22 young children who went on to develop autism showed a decline in gaze directed to faces between 6 and 36 months of age. However, only three parents reported any regression in their child's behaviour (Rutter 2011). In our own experience, parents have initially not reported any regression, and later acknowledged regression while participating in parent groups. When asked why, one mother said she did not wanted to be labelled as a mother who had missed the early signs of autism, in her son. In one study, 35 children with ASD and regression were compared with 35 children with ASD without regression. The mean age of regression was 22 months with the majority regressing between 12 and 24 months (Jones 2012). A single patient with regression also responded well to a comprehensive multimodal treatment approach in motor, language and social domains, and also in the activities and skills of daily living (Malhi and Singhi 2005). In a study of 51 children, regression occurred in 68.4 % of the sample; 21.5 % regressed before 12 months, 41.1 % regressed between 12 and 24 months, and 5.8 % regressed between 24 and 36 months (Nizamie et al. 2010). When the milestones of very young children with regressive autism are studied, it becomes likely that regression may have occurred even before the regression with clear-cut behaviour change, for which help is being sought. A child may have normal development for social smile and eye contact, but be delayed in stranger anxiety with the simultaneous onset of sensory issues. The difference between infants who regress and infants who do not may be in terms of change in those who regress and delay in those who do not (Abbagani 2006). This could well lead to the parent reporting that the child had multiple regressions at 15–18 months. Descriptive terms like "shy, stubborn and scared" were more often used in the non-regressive behaviour. In another small study of 31 children with regression and 37 normally developing children, regression was assessed on the following: turning to sound or name, carrying out commands, pointing waving bye-bye, speech, eye contact, self-help skills, indication of toilet needs, quality of play, interests, curiosity and sleep routines. These questions had good discriminatory value as only one normally developing child had regression (in toilet skills for a brief period after joining school). It was found useful in data retrieval to ask parents about each milestone, not only the time of achievement of the milestone but also if the achieved language or social skills had changed in any qualitative way. Our study found the following: turning to sound or voice, eye contact, socialisation, speech or vocalisation and sleep as the most frequently noted indicators of regression. Of these, 1–3 have been used to document regression based on home videos (looks at people, smiles at people, language and joint attention). The consensus is on prospective data collection and development of simple screens to sensitise paediatricians to the earliest behavioural manifestations of autism. This would lead to early identification, referral, evaluation and treatment without necessarily labelling a child (Abbagani et al. 2008). In a recent workshop, the participants also agreed to consider regression in autism as distinct from CDD, which is characterised by a very severe and rapid loss of skills after 2 years of age (Ozonoff et al. 2010).

Sleep disturbances: Children with ASD more prone to sleep disturbance and in an earlier study 40–80 % reported problems of sleep. Problems described have been in all areas of sleep: problems in onset of sleep, sleep maintenance, settling and nocturnal awakening. In children with ASD, nocturnal awakening may be characterised by laughing, vocalisation, screaming and playing alone with toys and objects (Naik et al. 2012). In one study, 51 children between the ages of one-and-a-half and six years with ASD and abnormalities in the development of sleep–wake cycles were seen in 62 % of children with autism. Resistance to sleep and waking were the most frequently reported. Sleep patterns included difficulty falling asleep, having disturbed sleep and waking up at night (Nizamie et al. 2010). In another study, using the Owen's "The Children's Sleep Habits Questionnaire" (CSHQ), 27 children with regressive autism were compared with 37 typically developing children. Significant differences were found in regularity of bedtime, sleep duration, bedtime resistance, latency and night wakening. In addition to the quantitative aspects of sleep disturbance, noteworthy were the following qualitative aspects: complex bedtime routines which included rocking, swinging, and clinging to objects; excessive need for silence and darkness, and long car rides; special objects needed to sleep, e.g. a blanket to chew on, plastic bottles, lids, and toothpaste tubes; night awakening quality like, crying, screaming, playing with non-toys disregarding parent, watching television, and difficulty in returning to sleep; and unusual activities like walking over sleeping parents or siblings. These sleep-related issues contributed greatly to parental stress and coping abilities (Cortesi et al. 2010). The cultural aspects of sleep arrangements, like *Child falling asleep in Parents' bed* (To the Indian Parent this is normal), or *Item 3 Child falls asleep in own bed* (Often, no separate bed is available for a small child even in affluent families), need to be considered. These cultural differences can have international consequences. An Indian family in Norway could not explain their differences in child rearing practices and sleeping arrangements, to child health authorities with serious turmoil all round (Abbagani et al. 2012).

Savant skills: ASD has been associated with special skills often highlighted in films like "Rain Man" and books like "The curious case of the dog in the night time" (The Hindu 2012). In a very well-designed study, savant skills were specified as "an outstanding skill/knowledge clearly above participant's general level of ability *and* above the population norm." Exceptional cognitive skills were defined as applied to Wechsler subtest scores at least 1 standard deviation above general population norms, and 2 standard deviations above the participant's own mean subtest score. Twenty-four out of 93 individuals were identified as having one or more savant skills (total = 26 %). There were 14 calendrical calculators, four others with computational skills and three individuals with superior visuospatial skills. One individual had a musical talent, one had an exceptional memory skill, and one had skills in both memory and art (Greenwell 2004). Understanding strengths may help optimise a child's outcome, if these strengths are properly recognised and channelized (Howlin et al. 2009). In a review of 51 patients, parental report suggested 39 out of 51 children had exceptional skills in some area of cognition, amounting to 75 % of children, but no testing was done to verify the true nature of these abilities (Nizamie et al. 2010).

Differential diagnosis and comorbidity: Comorbidity of other conditions in autism has been well documented. The first step is ascertaining the presence or absence of ID, in which global developmental delay will be present, unlike in autism where abilities and deficits are not uniform. If there is no ID, ADHD, anxiety, mood disorders and psychosis should also be considered high incidences of coexisting ID have been reported in different studies, as high as 95 % (Seth and Kalra 2006; Nazeer and Ghaziuddin 2012; Gupta and Maitra 2002; Kar et al. 1993). The prevalence of comorbidities was found to be high, and it increased with severity of ID, except for ADHD, autism and violent behaviour, which decreased (Purkayastha et al. 1997). In children with ID in the Barwani district, ADHD was diagnosed in 6.5 % of children and autism in 4.2 % (Lakhan 2013).

Differential diagnosis: Differential diagnosis has not been discussed much in the literature. A study discusses the need to keep in mind language and learning disorders (Jauhari et al. 2012).

Bipolar disorder is hard to recognize in children with autism. ADHD, anxiety, depression and OCD are other comorbid conditions (Jayarama and Bhat 2004). In reporting diagnostic overshadowing, the example of study of a 9-year-old female child was cited. In a 5-year follow-up of a patient with an initial diagnosis of separation anxiety disorder during the course of follow-up, the child began to exhibit features of PDD, not otherwise specified (Baird et al. 2001).

The core symptoms still define ASD. However, regression and savant skills make the condition unique and mysterious.

5 Assessment

Reaching care has different routes. Who makes the diagnosis? Fortunately, the medical fraternity in the country appears to be following the ICD 10 or DSM IV with reasonable uniformity over the pattern of diagnosis. Level 1 screening measures are intended to be used by physicians to differentiate children at risk for ASDs from healthy children. Level 2 tools are used in developmental clinics to differentiate those at risk for having ASDs and other developmental disabilities, and as part of a diagnostic evaluation (Meera et al. 2012). These include the Autism Behaviour Checklist (ABC), the Childhood Autism Rating Scale (CARS), Gilliam Autism Rating Scale (GARS-2), the AQ, adolescent version, and the Social Communication Questionnaire (SCQ).

Brief Infant–Toddler Social and Emotional Assessment: The Brief Infant–Toddler Social and Emotional Assessment (BITSEA) subscales were evaluated in detecting risk for 456 toddlers. Results provided support for the BITSEA as a Level I screener for social emotional problems and a Level II screener for ASD symptoms at community sites such as well child clinics (Dyches 2011).

Assessment Kit for Autism (AKA): The action for autism (AFA) has made a new tool kit, and this needs to be used in a standardised manner through training to unify assessment and is intended to ensure that more and more children can be identified early. The AKA has three components:

1. A "quick scan" of child behaviours, completed by asking parent or persons who spend most time with the child a set of five questions.
2. Suggested activities for the professional to conduct, which will provide more information on the child's behaviours.
3. Suggested questions for people who spend the most time with the child to get information about usual patterns of behaviour and activity, since all the relevant information may not be evident in one sitting with the child (Gardner et al. 2013).

Indian Scale for Assessment of Autism (ISAA): The NIMH Hyderabad has developed the ISAA based on the CARS. It has 40 items and six domains: social relationship and reciprocity; emotional responsiveness; speech language and communication; behaviour patterns; sensory aspects; and cognitive component. It has been used with success in clinic settings (Singhal: http://www.autism-india.org).

The Vineland Adaptive Behaviour Scales: The Vineland Adaptive Behaviour Scales-II edition, 2005 (Vineland-II), is useful in assessing abilities in autism spectrum disorder. Difficulties in administration of the scale to Indian children are related to cultural differences in gender roles and in the way some self-care tasks are performed (Patra and Arun 2011).

The CARS: The CARS has been evaluated for use in the Indian population, and with a CARS score of 33, a sensitivity of 81.4 % and a specificity of 78.6 % for diagnosis of autism have been found. There was high concordance with ICD-10. Another expert recommended the scale for use in the Indian context. In a study of 51 children with autism (DSM IV), the mean CARS rating was 44, while when the suggested cut-off of 67 was used, only 40 of 51 children were diagnosed to be autistic. It was suggested by the authors that the cut-off should be lowered to 45 to increase sensitivity in the Indian context (Manohari et al. 2013).

The Aberrant Behaviour Checklist has been validated internationally between a special school in Vishakhapatnam and a Swiss Institute (Russell 2010).

The Autism Behaviour Check list has also been studied in the Indian context (Varisco et al. 2009).

The Parenting Stress Index: The Parenting Stress Index (PSI) is a scale specifically developed to assess the magnitude of parental stress in various disorders. In a study, it was used to quantify stress experienced by 51 mothers of children with autism, before and after psychosocial and other interventions, with a follow-up period of 18 months. Significant improvement was seen in the parental subdomains of competence, attachment, role restriction, depression, isolation and health ratings following intervention, suggesting the usefulness of this tool in measuring change in parental stress (Juneja et al. 2010).

Too many tools: A recent study examined the measurement tools and target symptoms/skills used to assess treatment response during ASD intervention trials from 2001 to 2010. Data from 195 prospective trials were analysed. There were 289 unique measurement tools, of which 61.6 % were used only once, and 20.8 % were investigator designed. Only three tools were used in more than 2 % of the studies, and none were used in more than 7 % of studies (Abbagani et al. 2013). There is an obvious lack of consensus in the area of outcome measurement, which needs to be addressed. These results represent a lack of consistency in outcome measurements in ASD intervention trials. These findings highlight the need to set guidelines for appropriate outcome and assessment measures.

In general, assessment is one area where appropriate tools have been developed, which may need cross-validation in some cases, but some kind of consensus needs to be arrived if comparable research goals are to be met.

6 Investigation

Assessments are vital, necessary and sufficient to make a diagnosis of autism. No testing is needed for a diagnosis. Much to the chagrin of all concerned, we do not have the respectability of a confirmatory biomarker for validation of ASD. So, sadly enough, even in 2013, we do not need tests to confirm a diagnosis. However, if any test aids in treatment, it should be performed whatever the cost and difficulty. For example, the American Association of Paediatrics (AAP) recommendation of chromosomal microarray analysis gives a yield of about 8 % of various genes involved. It is available in very few centres in the country like the CDFD and CCMB, though private laboratories would certainly welcome the recommendation. As research evolves and more specific recommendations become available, it would be useful to investigate along the lines of American recommendations. In a recent review, the recommendations of the AAA have been summarised and brought up to date several tests conducted on children as clinical have only academic relevance. It is better to learn from the experience of wealthier countries. In a recent review, recommendations of the past have been overturned because of the low yield of tests.

Tchacomas and Adesman (2013) have the following suggestions:

> *Genetic testing*: CMA is suggested as the most robust of these tests. The AAP's autism tool kit recommends this test for every child with ASD. In our context, we can wait a while to learn from the experience of better endowed countries. As these tests do not detect Fragile X or Rett's syndrome, our policy should stay with these two tests when indicated by clinical features or family history.
>
> *Neuroimaging*: MRIs are recommended only in acute regression, microcephaly, midline facial abnormalities, neurocutaneous lesions and confirmed neurological signs on clinical examination. Anyone who has witnessed the struggle of parents in sedating a child for diagnostic imaging would find relief in these recommendations.
>
> *Electoencephalograms* are suggested only for those children who have clinical or suspected seizures, sudden regression or unexplained behavioural changes.
>
> *Metabolic testing*: Testing should be conducted in children with failure to thrive, hypotonia, vomiting, lethargy, unusual odours, possibility of storage disorders and movement disorders. When indicated, tests would include renal and liver function, amino acids, pyruvate, lactate carnitine and acylcarnitine.

Blood lead would be indicted in children with pica. In children on antipsychotics, regular monitoring of lipid levels is necessary.

7 Treatment

"*Let me hold your shoulder like I used to when you started pointing and communicating she said trying to find a way. This time it was easy for the boy to write as he could feel the presence of the hand, his own hand linked to his body at the shoulder point where his mother was holding him. I have a concrete proof that to start with any new activity it is important for autistics like the boy, to be held at that part of the body which does the work as the relating ability develops slowly through practice. Then it can be faded out as the person gets the habit of that particular work*" (Mukhopadhyay 2003).

Tito again! Today many forms of therapy use the prompt offered by a gentle touch to help the child with autism master many fine motor skills like writing. The goals of treatment are twofold: to reduce disruptive behaviour and to increase communication and learning Treatment will depend on the age at the time of referral. The different treatment options can be bewildering. Children need to receive a combination of psychoeducational approaches and medical interventions with family support. Assessment forms, checklists for history taking, assessment of regression, symptom checklist, age-based intervention recommendations, early psychosocial interventions and summaries of medication-related studies are included in the Indian Psychiatry Society guidelines for childhood and adolescent problems (Mukhopadhyay 2003). Effective early intervention (EI) programmes for children should provide an autism-specific curriculum content focusing on attention, compliance, imitation, language and social skills in a highly structured and supportive teaching environment with opportunities to generalise skills. The best interventions are the most intensive and focused. The best known behavioural programme is the applied behaviour analysis (ABA), which uses one-on-one interaction between the adult and the child. Another method is TEACCH which is a "whole life" approach aimed at supporting children, adolescents and adults with autism through the provision of "visual information, structure and predictability". Family support is essential and can help relieve the tremendous stress faced by parents of children with autism. The different treatment options can be bewildering. Children need to receive a combination of psychoeducational approaches and medical Interventions. Regarding new medical interventions, a technical expert panel has recommended that a child with ASD should receive comprehensive evaluation within 60 days of diagnosis, family concerns should be specifically addressed and 25 h of intervention per week is necessary (Naik 2007).

Seeking treatment: Help-seeking behaviour and EI have been underresearched.

Different reports exist as to when children comes for medical diagnosis. Reports vary as to the age at which self-referral takes place and diagnosis is made. There is an increased awareness about autism in the Indian Paediatric community, but for the most part, a lack of appropriate services is perceived as the main problem. Daley in 2004 studied the delay in reaching care (Maglione et al. 2012). The age of identification was less than 2 years in 83 % of patients in one centre, and less than 4 years in the remaining (Shivashankar and Satishchandra 1989). Conversely, another study showed a delay of 32 months between parents identifying a problem in the child's development and a diagnosis of autism being given to the child. Deviance or delay in speech was the main concern (Daley 2004). In a survey in Gujarat, 192 paediatricians expressed that barriers to early referral were insufficient time, lack of treatment choices and lack of knowledge regarding referral options (Chakrabarti 2009; Desai and Mohite 2011). This suggests proving more training and resources would help. In an update from the diasporas, a small study of eight South Asian parents, who were currently raising a child diagnosed with an ASD in Canada, barriers to diagnosis and treatment that were reported by parents were examined; 75 % of parents reported that they did not reveal their child's ASD diagnosis to their friends and their own family members, including their parents and siblings. Their most imperative needs were for information regarding services their child might receive in the future. (Grewal 2010). One study suggests that in the diaspora parents of children with ASD, outside the country cannot be considered as a single entity (Ravindran and Myers 2013).

Early Intervention in children with autism: When a child is younger, the brain has much more plasticity or ability to change and so changing or teaching new behaviour is much easier. Earlier studies showed that only half of all children with autism would gain speaking abilities. Recognising and diagnosing autism before preschool age has been uncommon until the last few years. Listening carefully to caregivers as they voice their earliest concerns would facilitate early recognition (Singhi and Malhi 2001; Kishore and Basu 2011). Interesting new work has emphasised the earliest indicators of autism by following up high-risk "baby sibs" (Barbaro and Dissanayake 2013). In future, it is likely that autism will be diagnosed for most children in the toddler age period (18–30 months). Intervention should start as soon as characteristics of ASD are noted and continue for as long as required. When intervention starts early, children experience success and are more likely to engage socially and learn language and communication skills. Children are also less likely to become frustrated with a consequent decrease in challenging behaviours. Commencing working with the parents early in the therapeutic relationship can alleviate the distress. Anecdotal evidence of suicide in parents especially mothers abound. The importance o f psychological support and intervention with parents of ASD cannot be underestimated (Malhotra et al. 2002).

Learning (DEALL): One innovative Indian programme has been started in Bangalore by Karanth. The training for each child is based on the profile of the child and covers several developmental domains such as motor, communication, social and cognitive development. It also addresses other related issues such as eye contact, attention and sitting tolerance, compliance and behaviour. Ideally, enrolment to the DEALL program should take place by the age of 2.5–3 years. There should be a 1:4 staff: student ratio and therapy take place with 12 children per unit, 3 h per day/5 days a week. Training of trainers has also been initiated. Incidentally, Tito and Karanth felt she was a kind therapist from whom the boy benefitted (Karanth et al. 2010).

The Combined psychoeducational and biomedical approach: As part of an interventional programme, a combined psychoeducational and biomedical approach was used as an 18-month prospective, longitudinal, intervention study with 51 children with autism, aged one-and-a-half to six years, who fulfilled the DSM IV diagnostic criteria for autism with a developmental quotient (DQ) above 50 and normal gross motor milestones (walking by 15 months). The families had to be willing to follow a GF CF diet. Activities and intervention programmes were developed and tailor-made for each child depending on the level of functioning and development. The program was implemented on the basis of the TEACCH model. The TEACCH program was developed for children with autism at the University of North Carolina, Chapel Hill, in the 1960s and is popular worldwide. The TEACCH program involves structured teaching to train children and individuals with autism in the areas of social skills, communication skills, independent living skills, vocational skills and leisure skills. The diet was an elimination diet which was gluten-free, casein-free, sugar-free and preservative-free diet. Vitamin and mineral supplements were always provided. GI treatment was provided. Every patient was discussed individually with the child's paediatrician to monitor growth and nutrition. Children had free access to the paediatrician from the National Institute of Nutrition, who attended the hospital daily to discuss any dietary issues. Monitoring on a six-monthly basis on the CARS, PEP-R, REELS expressive, and REELS receptive scales was significant at ($p < 0.001$) on all four scales and on the overall developmental score. Both methods complemented each other. The biomedical approach helped the child pay attention to and benefit from the individualised training programme. Parental stress scores came down considerably during treatment (Abbagani et al. 2011).

The Early Start Denver models (*ESDM*): A recent a clinical trial comparing ESDM with conventional autism therapy services randomly assigned 48 toddlers (aged 18–30 months) to receive either ESDM therapy or the EI services routinely available in their communities (Seattle). Both groups received roughly 20 h of weekly therapy for two years. Overall, those in the ESDM group showed greater increases in IQ, language and adaptive behaviour than children in the community-intervention group. This more typical pattern of brain activity was associated with improved social behaviour including improved eye contact and social communication (Dawson et al. 2012).

The Developmental, Individual, Relationship-based (*DIR*) *model*: The developmental, individual, relationship-based (DIR) model, designed by Stanley Greenspan in 1989, describes 6 milestones as crucial to a child's development. Parents and professionals involved with the child must comprehend how the milestones affect a child's emotional and intellectual growth. The six milestones are the following: self-regulation and interest, intimacy, two-way communication, complex communication, emotional ideas and emotional thinking. The major element of this approach entails that (a) professionals do floor time with the child, (b) parents observe floor time being done with their child and (c) parents change their style of relating to the child with regard to a given milestone. Floor time is a systematic way of working with a child with autism to help him or her. A study was conducted to establish the efficacy of floor time for the development of social behaviour in preschool children with ASD. The children who received intervention showed a qualitative change in their interactive behaviour (Lal and Chhabria 2013).

Social stories: *In a case–control study*, reading such stories and role playing led to significant improvement over controls in the RSSM rating scale for self-management (Lal and Ganesan 2011).

Sensory integration: In a qualitative study of 65 parents on sensory integration perception of mothers, it was found that the children were not averse to sensory integration, and this in turn encouraged participation (Joshi 2008).

Visual strategies: Objects, pictures, symbols and manual signs were used as visual tools with 14 one-on-one sessions; communication skills were considerably improved (Lal and Bali 2007).

Auditory processing methods: Common to both dyslexia and autism have been used to facilitate auditor communication (Sampath et al. 2010).

Coaching: Based on the premise that parents of children with autism have less positive experiences in parent–child interactions, parents were taught to break down tasks into achievable and objective components. This served to enhance a sense of mastery in the parent when goals were achieved (Raj and Kumar 2009).

Milieu therapy: The children who underwent intervention based on milieu approach showed an increased use of target language and functional communication skills across settings and conversational partners (Vishnu et al. 1992).

Parental Involvement Scale: In a pilot study at a Mumbai School using a Parental Involvement–Engagement Scale, it was found that higher parental involvement made for greater progress in emotional, social, language cognitive and motor skill development (Srivastava and Mukhopadhyay 2011).

The Lovaas method: Children below 6 years of age were treated at a Delhi hospital using parents as chief therapists. A mainly behavioural approach based on the Lovaas method was used. Parents were expected to spend at least 60–90 min per day training the child. A significant improvement was seen in DQ, the CARS and the ABC scores at the end of 8–30 months (Juneja et al. 2012).

Music therapy: Music therapy was used in children in an improvised interactive way to improve communication skills (Mukherjee 2008).

Yoga: The use of integrated approach to yoga therapy (IAYT) as a complementary therapy for children in a small study reported improvement in imitation skills and social and non-verbal communication (Radhakrishna 2010).

Several other techniques have been used, but have not been reported adequately in the Indian literature. These include speech therapy, cognitive behaviour therapy and sensory integration. Treatments based on traditional systems of Ayurveda and Yoga have emerged. They too need scientific validation. Music therapy is recommended as "a non-invasive, enjoyable and cost-effective therapy; unique outcomes are possible". Art as an EI tool has been described (Christopher 2011). Drama education and the use of masks have been used to improve social communication (Nelson 2011).

Augmentative Communication (AC): In one Mumbai-based study, 8 children received 12 sessions of language intervention using augmentative communication (AC); significant change was noted both in language and social behaviour (Lal 2010).

Picture Exchange Communication (PEC): The use of PECs in a 7-year-old male child was reported with 60 % improvement on several of the instruments used (Shahzadi Malhotra et al. 2010).

Assistive technology: Studying an emotional hearing aid-assistive technology, which enables children with autism to understand the facial expression of individuals in the social environment improvements, was reported (Nancy 2012).

Special care during other medical problems: A case report of a severe case of bruxism treated by dental intervention under anaesthesia was used to discuss the special patience and care needed in children with autism (Nagendra and Jayachandra 2012; Muthu and Prathibha 2008).

The best elements of many of these measures may be combined in a cost-effective manner and used even where optimum resources are lacking. In the Lovaas method, discrete trial training has gained popularity (Lovaas 2003).

7.1 Innovative and Emerging Treatments

Uncommon sense toys: Uncommon sense toys, being researched in Bangalore, encourage social interaction among children with autism. The toys have audiovisual and tactile feedback, which can be triggered by a child's action movement and voice. The toys help the child to engage in collaborative play through both individual responses and shared responses. Orientation, touch and expression are required to operate the three specifically designed toys (Dsouza et al. 2010).

Robotic technology: Robotic technology, appeals to children with ASD. This fact can be used to provide repeatable, accurate and individualised intervention services. In a study, a humanoid robot had its vision augmented by a network of cameras for real-time head tracking using a distributed architecture. The robot could intelligently adapt itself in an individualised manner to generate prompts and reinforcements, based on the child's head movements to promote skills in social orienting. The system was validated for feasibility, accuracy and performance with six children with ASD, and a control group of six typically developing children (Welch et al. 2010).

Virtual environment: In another study of robotic technology using the same technique in children with ASD, a virtual environment has been designed where children with autism could participate in social activities with the social robots. Gaze and social distance are being studied as an initial step (Bekele et al. 2012).

Personalised learning: The authors propose a smart e-learning tutoring model for patients with ASD, with machine learning capabilities, which help in generating dynamic e-learning sessions and maximise learning opportunities through personalisation of the programme (Vullamparthi et al. 2011).

Ideas from other work New Ideas by Sinha: His first research on people with the disorder, in 2003, focused on the ability of children with ASD to integrate a visual scene. The autism literature is fuzzy on the subject, with some studies showing clear deficits and others showing none. Sinha believes he can help children with autism to achieve greater visual integration (Ostrovsky et al. 2009).

Drug development: Attempts are on to model proteins like Shank3, also known as proline-rich synapse-associated protein 2 (ProSAP2). ProSAP2 is a protein encoded by the SHANK3 gene which could be used for drug designing (Ostrovsky et al. 2009).

Animal studies: The role of green tea extract was studied in reversing behavioural changes induced by valproate and oxidative stress markers in mice. Both behavioural assessments and histopathological studies confirmed the usefulness of green tea extract (Mujawar et al. 2013).

7.2 Family Support and Community Support

Family support is essential and can help relieve the tremendous stress faced by parents of children with autism. Parent groups serve this purpose. Breaking the news can be a difficult procedure as many parents have heard of autism and cannot believe it is happening to them. Parents have a great need to know more about this problem, and nothing can substitute for time spent with the family. In a study in Goa, twenty interviews and nine focus group discussions were carried out with families of children with autism and with teachers and TD families. The key findings were the following: (1) raising a child with ASD places severe stress on the families with initial withdrawal, (2) personal and wider impact with discrimination, (3) parents respond well to supportive measures, (4) health education and religious sectors do not have awareness of these needs and (5) this study serves to identify the unmet needs of families with ASD (Banji et al. 2011).

Parental stress: Barua describes her own experiences of life with her son: the shock of the diagnosis, acceptance, unconditional love and affirmation (Barua 2007).

The Parenting Stress Index and brief psychological interventions: The PSI was used to assess stress among children with disability and autism with three-fourths of the group having significant stress. A qualitative analysis was further undertaken to evaluate the nature of these stresses. Even brief psychological interventions of 3–56 sessions addressing different issues like behavioural, supportive and educational techniques can ameliorate some of the emotional issues of parents of children with autism (John 2012). The importance of acceptance is stressed in the following account.

Community support: Kanner's case No. 1 stayed on in the community where he grew up. The community was proud of his abilities and protective.

"*Donald's neighbours not only shrug off his oddities, but openly admire his strengths—while taking a protective stance, with any outsider whose intentions toward Donald may not have been sufficiently spelled out. On three occasions, while talking with townspeople who know Donald, we were advised, in strikingly similar language each time: "If what you're doing hurts Don, I know where to find you." We took the point: in Forest, Donald is "one of us.*" (Donovan and Zucker 2010)".

Staunch community support can certainly have beneficial effects.

7.3 Psychopharmacology

Medication should be used for targeted symptoms, in the smallest dose for the shortest period of time, keeping the side effects in mind. The question is sometimes asked as to why do not drugs work in autism "*Numerous studies have documented that autism stands out from almost all other psychiatric disorders in showing no marked benefits of psychotropic medication on core symptoms (such as impaired social reciprocity and social communication). Why? One possible implication is that the basic deficit does not involve neurotransmitters; if not, what does it involve? It is important to pose the question, not so much because of the implications for treatment today, but rather because a satisfactory answer could have important implications for the neural basis of autism. For the moment, medication is of some value for associated problems, but the enigma is why that seems to be all.*" (Jayarama and Bhat 2004; Buitelaar 2003).

Risperidone and aripiprazole have FDA approval. Effective for the target symptoms of irritability, they come with side effects which should be carefully monitored (Tchaconas and Adesman 2013). The parameters that need monitoring include blood glucose, lipids, liver function tests, prolactin and thyroid-stimulating hormone. Hyperactivity can be managed by methylphenidate and atomoxetine, though less successfully than in ADHD. Melatonin is effective in sleep issues; two new drugs hold promise, arbaclofen in Fragile X and an enzyme replacement proprietary combination, CM-AT (Tchaconas and Adesman 2013). Supplementation with omega-three fatty acids, nacyl cystiene and l carnosine have all been tested in RCTs and found useful. An Indian study replicated the usefulness of risperidone (Singhi Nagaraj et al. 2006). The use of donpezil in treating autism is reported as case study (Srivastava et al. 2011). However, there is serious concern that the core symptoms of autism seem to respond less readily to psychopharmacology, than in other psychiatric disorders. For a review of pharmacological treatment of ASD, practice guidelines may be useful, as also a more recent review (Mukhopadhyay 2003; Nazeer 2011).

7.4 Complementary and Alternative Therapies

Complementary and alternative therapies are defined as "a group of diverse medical and health care systems, practices and products that are not considered to be part of conventional medicine". They are called complementary when used together with conventional medicine and alternative when used instead of conventional treatment. In an extensive review of the subject, an interesting classification of treatments has been made. SECS stands for safe, easy, cheap and sensible; RUDE stands for risky, unrealistic, difficult and expensive. This method serves to categorise well-tested drugs as recommended, for example melatonin in sleep disorders and acceptable in conditions where costly or difficult or risky treatments do not get similarly categorised. This seems a useful tool for the clinicians as well (Lofthouse et al. 2012).

Complementary and Alternative Interventions as seen by social workers: A Czech student analysed attitudes of social workers to alternative treatment in Kerala. One response was stigma and fear of side effects in traditional medicine. Yoga was approved, but not Ayurveda; spiritual help was not recommended, whereas biological treatments were (Hudec 2012).

A Review of GFCF diets: New evidence suggests that a gluten-free (GF), casein-free (CF), or gluten- and casein-free diets (GFCF) can ameliorate core and peripheral symptoms and improve developmental outcome in some cases of autism spectrum conditions. The majority of published studies indicate statistically significant positive changes to symptom presentation following dietary intervention. Changes in communication, attention and hyperactivity are detailed (Whiteley et al. 2012). Specific characteristics of best and non-responders to intervention are not yet understood.

The Scan Brit RCT: The Scan Brit, randomised, controlled, single-blind study of a gluten- and casein-free dietary intervention for children with ASD assigned 72 Danish children to diet (A) or non-diet (B) groups by stratified randomisation. Data for 26 diet children and 29 controls demonstrated significant improvement in mean diet group scores on subdomains of the ADOS, the GARS and the ADHD-IV measures. Predefined statistical thresholds were surpassed in the GFCF group, so Group B was assigned to GFCF as well. At 24 months, while there was evidence of sustained clinical group improvements, there was a possible plateau effect for intervention in some cases at this point (Pennesi and Klein 2012).

Responders and non-responders to GFCF diets: Attempts have been made to study responders and non-responders to GFCF diets. In one questionnaire-based survey from 387 parents, the presence of GI symptoms, food allergy and sensitivities and strict diet implementation was indicative of greater improvement in ASD behaviours, physiological symptoms and social behaviours compared with children whose parents reported none of these symptoms (Whiteley et al. 2010).

The Chennai GFCF study: In a small study from Chennai of 50 children with autism, children on restricted diets showed improvement over a 2-month period in attention, sleep and reduction in hyperactivity and anxiety (Nazni et al. 2008).

Treatment of ASD has been the subject of intense research activity. While we can learn from the experience of others, consolidating proven useful measures and scaling treatments is urgently needed. Drug treatment has not been as effective as in other psychiatric disorders and must be balanced carefully with monitoring of side effects. Certain complementary and alternative measures which are categorised as safe may be tried with parental consent.

8 Follow-up and Prognosis

> DONALD LIVES ALONE NOW, in the house where his parents raised him. FOR ALL THE PROGRESS that Donald has made in the decades since—the driving, the golfing—conversation is an art that continues to elude him. Except for once a month, that is, when he walks out the front door and leaves town. Perhaps the most remarkable aspect of Donald's life is that he grew up to be an avid traveller. He has been to Germany, Tunisia, Hungary, Dubai, Spain, Portugal, France, Bulgaria, and Colombia—some 36 foreign countries and 28 U.S. states in all, including Egypt three times, Istanbul five times, and Hawaii 17 times. He's notched one African safari, several cruises, and innumerable PGA tournaments.
>
> This is the same man whose favourite pastimes, as a boy, were spinning objects, spinning himself and rolling nonsense words around in his mouth. At the time, he seemed destined for a cramped, barren adulthood—possibly lived out behind the windows of a state institution. Instead, he learnt to golf, to drive, and to circumnavigate the globe—skills he first developed at the respective ages of 23, 27, and 36. In adulthood, Donald continued to branch out (Donovan and Zucker 2010).

Regular follow-up is required. Parents often shop for treatment, so ideally, all services can be offered in one setting, but this has been mostly difficult to achieve. With early and appropriate intervention, long-term outcomes have improved, and some children grow into self-sufficiency in adulthood, while several are able to function with support. The improvement in several children can be so remarkable that we need to adopt a more optimistic attitude. However, caution is needed in children with evidence of motor delay.

"Two factors that have been consistently associated with prognosis are language development and IQ. Very few children who have not developed some useful communicative speech by the age of 5–6 years have a positive outcome and, conversely, individuals who were either cognitively un-testable as children, or who had non-verbal scores below 50 were almost invariably reported as highly dependent. Best outcomes have been found for individuals with an IQ of at least 70 in childhood (Jayarama and Bhat 2004)".

Some years after presentation, older children around the age of 10 years to adolescence develop seizures unrelated to the severity of autism. In adults, affective disorders and obsessive compulsive behaviour are known to develop (Venkatesan 2005; Jayarama and Bhat 2004).

Optimal outcome individuals: In a study by Fein, at the University of Connecticut, several children lost their diagnosis of autism on all scales of assessment. These optimal outcome individuals ($n = 34$) were compared on standardised measures to age-, sex- and IQ-matched individuals with high-functioning autism ($n = 44$) or typical development (TD group, $n = 34$). The optimal outcome (OO) and TD groups' mean scores did not differ on socialisation, communication, face recognition or most language subscales, although three OO individuals showed below-average scores on face recognition. Early in their development, the OO group displayed milder symptoms than the HFA group in the social domain, but had equally severe difficulties with communication and repetitive behaviours. These results substantiate the possibility of OO from autism spectrum disorders and demonstrate an overall level of functioning within normal limits for this group (Fein et al. 2013). In an Indian study, a single adult was followed up and showed inadequate social functioning (Chaudhari et al. 2008). In a small study, 33 of 37 children diagnosed as autistic disorder retained their diagnosis. Only 1 out of 6 children labelled PDD NOS retained the diagnosis. The follow-up was for about a year (Malhi and Singhi 2011).

9 Ethics

The main issue of ethics arise (a) at the patient and family level in using proven methods of treatment and (b) in maintaining confidentiality. As the use of Internet increases and parent groups stay in touch across the globe, it is important to be aware of new developments in the field and explain pros and cons of different remediable approaches, permitting parents to make informed choices. In a broader framework, it is necessary to protect Indian families and children from experimental use of new drugs, whose side effect profile is not yet fully understood. This is more the case when children cannot explain their discomforts. By and large, we have kept ourselves from being targeted for drug trials, but constant vigilance is necessary. Greater attention to ethical issues will enhance the quality of epidemiological, genetic and treatment studies (Daley et al. 2013).

10 Facilities

10.1 The Action for Autism (AFA)

An important development has been the formation of the AFA by Mrs Merry Barua. The AFA was started in 1991 to provide support and services to persons with autism and their families, and to create an environment in India, in which people with autism are able to grow to their full potential. The AFA is now the primary organisation in South Asia specialising in ASDs. The AFA is a non-profit organisation whose mission is to facilitate a barrier-free environment, empower families of individuals with ASD, act as a catalyst for change and build community responsibility for mainstreaming of all persons with ASD.[1] In a review of facilities available for children with autism and mental retardation, the models in use were special schools, inclusive schools, home-based education and units established by parent groups; 46.8 % preferred home-based education, 25.8 % were in special schools, and 19.4 % were in inclusive schools (Karnath Aluri and Karanth 2002). The educational support systems available to children with ASD have been reviewed elsewhere (Narayan et al. 2005).

---

[1] Action for Autism www.autism-india.org/afa.

Architecture: Architects too have shown interest in designing environments. It is possible to design better environments for children with autism by using tools like the researcher environment checklist (REC), teacher performance scale (TPS) and teacher environment rating checklist (TEC). Guidelines could be formulated for building design and landscaping to create the most conducive environment (Khare and Mullick 2008).

Organisations like the AFA can serve as an umbrella organisation to facilitate multicentre epidemiological studies, uniform assessment, early detection, intervention, follow-up and advocacy for children with autism. Already, the AFA has brought autism under the purview of the National Act for Persons with Disabilities and under the National Trust.

10.2 Government Initiatives

Services for persons with autism have been summarised by Bhargava as a report. She has summarised the details of several schemes available to persons with ASD (Bhargava 2010).[2, 3]

The National Trust: Setting up the National Trust for the Welfare of Persons with Autism, Cerebral Palsy, Mental Retardation and Multiple Disabilities Act, 1999, was an important step. The Act facilitates the realisation of equal opportunities, protection of rights and full participation of persons with disabilities and provision for appointment of legal guardian for persons with disabilities.

To promote inclusive school education, the following facilities have been created:

(a) Sarva Shiksha Abhiyan (SSA)

The key objective of SSA is Universalisation of Elementary Education (UEE), three important aspects of which are access, enrolment and retention of all children aged 6–14.

(b) Inclusive education for the disabled at secondary stage (IEDSS)

The IEDSS, launched in April 2009, provides assistance for the inclusive education of children with disabilities of Classes IX–XII including autism. Funds are provided for activities such as identification and assessment, assistive devices, allowance for transport, escorts, readers, uniforms, books and stationary.

(c) Capacity building of special teachers

Course curricula have been developed and standardised by the Rehabilitation Council of India (RCI) for (i) Diploma in Special Education (ASD) and (ii) B.Ed. in Special Education to handle the special needs of students with disabilities according to the National Trust in inclusive classrooms.

---

[2] National Trust for the Welfare of Persons with Autism, Cerebral Palsy, Mental Retardation and Multiple Disabilities Act 44 of 1999. New Delhi.

[3] Persons with Disability Act. Government of India. Persons with disabilities (Equal opportunities, Protection of rights and Full participation), Act, 1995, New Delhi.

(d) Support for children with autism

The Central Board of Secondary Education (CBSE) has made several changes in the examination by-laws in February 2009 to help children with disabilities, including those with autism, giving the board (public) examinations of Class X and XII, which strengthen earlier relaxations.

(e) Other benefits

Health insurance, scholarships, income tax benefits to families, travel concessions, banking simplification and legal support have also been simplified.

10.3 The Role of NGOS

In a recent review, Patel has specifically called for the inclusion of MHNGOs as full partners of the government services in the National Mental Health Programme. Such a partnership could take several forms, including participation in committees to monitor the NMHP in each district, become providers of the DMHP services or provide community-based services like day care centres. NGO placements should become mandatory for psychiatric training, and NGO representation should be sought in all committees, planning at the state and national levels (Thara and Patel 2010).

11 Conclusion

In the past 70 years since the world became aware of autism, a great deal of scientific advance has taken place and information grown exponentially, but we still cannot see the woods for the trees. As a postgraduate student, one of my early seminars was on childhood autism and I believe my abiding interest in autism began in 1975. At that time, the incidence was reported to be 1:10,000–1:40,000 children. In 70 years, we have not improved on the inclusion criteria for diagnosis. Autism continues to be a disorder characterised by patterns of delay and deviance in the development of social and communicative skills with behavioural problems, often associated with exceptional skills, and arising in the first few years of life. Everything else about autism is a controversy. The name we call it by, the prevalence rate, the assessment, the aetiology, the investigation and treatment and of course prognosis. For every little step of progress comes a question. In 2013 comes the contradiction that the theory of a lack of neural connectivity noted on functional MRI may be an artefact caused by movement of the head. Some of these artefacts could be got rid off by "scrubbing", but the neural theories would need a rethinking (Deen and Pelphrey 2012; Wolff et al. 2012). We no longer blame parents for being cold and unemotional, but instead are confronted by an array of causative possibilities. Older fathers and migrant mothers have been implicated. Epigenetics is being given greater recognition in all branches of medicine. The interplay of several genes is now considered as aetiologically relevant. Every day brings new additions to the list of implied causative genes; a gene encoding a sodium proton exchanger is a new entrant. Markers of inflammation are being increasingly identified with elevated levels of cytokines and transcription factors in children with autism. Earlier gold standards like the ADOS will now have to be revised in the light of DSM V. Along the way, we seem to have created and consolidated encapsulated areas in the gestalt of autism best exemplified by Insel's *Kingdoms*.

On 26 February 2013, Thomas R. Insel, Director NIMH, wrote on his blog that there appear to be Four Kingdoms of Autism.[4] He has hypothesised that the current perspectives on autism seem like four well-fortified kingdoms "each with its own truths. And each too often fails to understand or even recognize that their truths may not apply to all kingdoms". Much like Kipling's blind men of Hindostan, each was partly in the right.

(i) The *Illness* kingdom: Here, the search is for disease biomarkers to assist in diagnosis and molecular targets for drug treatments—and—eventually reduce the need for services.
(ii) The *Identity* kingdom: This supports adults who were once on the spectrum and now face problems in the "neurotypical" world rather than seeking to become "neurotypical", they advocate for acceptance or inclusion ("nothing about us without us") as well as recognition that autistic thinking may yield innovative solutions. As Temple Grandin asks rhetorically "Who do you think made the first stone spears?—The Asperger's guy. If you were to get rid of all the autism genetics, there would be no more Silicon Valley.[5]"
(iii) The *Injury* Kingdom: One of the more heated arguments surrounding autism has been on the possible role of vaccination and has led parents to feel betrayed by mainstream medicine who have then "turned to alternative treatments based on detoxification, diet, or oxidative stress. This kingdom advocates for prevention, recognising that identifying the cause is the most direct path to stopping the soaring prevalence of autism".
(iv) The *Insight* kingdom: These scientists use autism as s as an opportunity to study the social brain through procedures like mapping of the brain.

Insel rightly suggests that while all this work is going on, the most important activity would be for all concerned to work towards the goal of "ensuring that every person on the spectrum, irrespective of wealth, geography, or ethnicity, receives the best treatments and services". The best strategy to reunite the kingdoms is though proven efficacy of prevention and intervention. Every delay hurts some child somewhere and keeps some family in distress. This frantic pace of research, the evolving theories and the need for convergence of different disciplines emphasise the need for multicentre studies. In India, the most immediate research need is for epidemiological studies. These should be followed by training therapists in EI and best management practices. A parent body that would supervise and link collaborating agencies in a fund-efficient and cooperative manner seems the need of the hour. Much like

---

[4] Insel T, http://www.nimh.nih.gov/about/2013/the-four-ingdoms-of-autism.shtml. The four kingdoms of Autism Thomas Insel on February 26, 2013.

[5] Tedtalk TEDTalk 2010 Temple Grandin.

protocols are shared in several countries for diseases like cancer, an Indian consortium of interested medical and other professionals including basic scientists, educationists, psychologists, social workers, occupational and physiotherapists, speech and language specialists and dialecticians would save time, enhance the quality of research and prevent duplication. Using tried and tested methods would translate into meaningful patient and family care. To conclude, we are short of time, and we cannot wait another 70 years to solve all the mysteries of autism. Our time starts now.

References

Abbagani, K.L. (2006). *A study of children with autism and effectiveness of psychosocial interventions with them.* The thesis submitted to the Osmania University for the award of Degree of Doctor of Philosophy in social Work June 2006.

Abbagani, K. L., Anandaraj, H., & Naik, U. (2011). *A combined psychoeducational and biomedical approach to autism treatment.* Paper presented at global autism convention, May 19–21, 2011, Bangalore.

Abbagani, K. L, Anandaraj, H., & Naik, U. S. (2013). Use of the parenting stress index (PSI) in mothers of children with Autism. *Indian Journal of Cerebral Palsy Under publication.*

Abbagani, K. L., Naik, U. S., Kommuri, S., & Balakrishna, N. (2012). *Assessment of sleep issues in autism-early assessment in the Indian context.* Paper presented at a Symposium at the 13th World Congress of the World Association for Infant Mental Health Conference held from April 17–21, 2012 at Cape Town, South Africa.

Abbagani, K. L., Naik, U., Niranjan, D., & Srinivas, U. (2008). *A typical development in some children with autism prior to regression.* Paper presented at first national congress of BSCNDD on 'improving quality of life of children with neurodevelopmental disabilities' held in Dhaka, Bangladesh from March 17–18, 2008. Jointly organized by Shishu Bikash Network and DFID.

Ahuja, Y. R., Sharma, S., & Bahadur, B. (2013). Autism: An epigenomic side-effect of excessive exposure to electromagnetic fields. *Medicine and Medical Sciences, 5*(4), 171–177. EMF AHuja.

Aithal, S., Manjunath, Y. N., & Shyamala, K. C. (2011). Language in India.

Ali, M., Markandaya, M., Girimaji, S. C., Shukla, A. K., Sachhidanand, S., & Kumar, A. (2004). Genetic variation in the TSC1 and TSC2 genes in 24 TSC families from India.

American Psychiatric Association (2013) Desk Reference to the Diagnostic Criteria from DSM-5(TM) Paperback, May 27, 2013.

Baird, G., Charman, T., & Santosh, P. J. (2001). Clinical considerations in the diagnosis of autism spectrum disorders. *The Indian Journal of Pediatrics, 68*(5), 439–449. DD Baird.

Banji, D., Banji, O. J., Abbagoni, S., Hayath, M. S., Kambam, S., & Chiluka, V. L. (2011). Amelioration of behavioral aberrations and oxidative markers by green tea extract in valproate induced autism in animals. *Brain Research, 1410*, 141–151.

Barbaro, J., & Dissanayake, C. (2013). Early markers of autism spectrum disorders in infants and toddlers prospectively identified in the social attention and communication study (SACS). *Autism, 17*(1), 64–86.

Barua, M. (2007). Lessons from Neeraj, my son with autism. *Journal of Religion, Disability and Health, 11*(2), 29–40.

Bekele, E., Lahiri, U., Swanson, A., Crittendon, J., Warren, Z., & Sarkar, N. (2012). A Step Towards Developing Adaptive Robot-Mediated Intervention.

Beversdorf, D. Q., Manning, S. E., Hillier, A., Anderson, S. L., Nordgren, R. E., Walters, S. E., et al. (2005). Timing of prenatal stressors and autism. *Journal of Autism and Developmental Disorders, 35*(4), 471–478.

Bharat, S., Srinath, S., Sheshadri, S. P., & Girimaji, S. (1997). Child and adolescent psychiatry—in patient facility. *Indian Journal of Psychiatry, 64*(6), 829–832.

Bhargava, A. (2010). Information of measures and policies on special education and topics on education in each country. *Prefatory Note*, 8.

Bhowmik, D. A., Dutta, A., Chatterjee, A., Sinha, A. K., Chattopadhyay, A., & Mukhopadhyay, K. (2009). Screening for fragile X syndrome among neurobehavioural patients from Kolkata, Eastern India. *Journal of Clinical and Diagnostic Research, 3*, 1266–1273.

Buitelaar, J. K. (2003). Why have drug treatments been so disappointing. *Autism: Neural Basis and Treatment Possibilities, 51*, 235–249.

CDC. (2012). Prevalence of Autism Spectrum Disorders—Autism and Developmental Disabilities Monitoring Network, 14 Sites, United States, 2008. *Surveillance Summaries*, CDC, Home March 30, 2012/61(SS03); 1–19.

Chakrabarti, S. (2009). Early identification of autism. *Indian Pediatrics, 46*, 412–414.

Chaudhari, D., Sitholey, P., Aggrawal, V., Gupta, N., & Kumar, P. (2008). Adult Manifestation of Childhood Autism. One case has been studied.

Choudhury, P. R., Lahiri, S., & Rajamma, U. (2012). Glutamate mediated signaling in the pathophysiology of autism spectrum disorders. *Pharmacology, Biochemistry and Behavior, 100*(4), 841–849.

Christopher, S. (2011). Nicole martin: Art as an early intervention tool for children with autism. *Journal of Autism and Developmental Disorders, 41*(5), 685.

Chugani, D. C. (2012). Neuroimaging and neurochemistry of autism. *Pediatric Clinics of North America, 59*(1), 63–73.

Cortesi, F., Giannotti, F., Ivanenko, A., & Johnson, K. (2010). Sleep in children with autistic spectrum disorder. *Sleep Medicine, 11*(7), 659–664.

Daley, T. C. (2004). From symptom recognition to diagnosis: Children with autism in urban India. *Social Science and Medicine, 58*(7), 1323–1335.

Daley, T. C., & Barua, M. (2010). *Diagnostic practices and awareness of utism among Indian pediatricians: A decade of data*. Paper presented at IMFAR Philadelphia. May 21, 2010.

Daley, T. C., & Sigman, M. D. (2002). Diagnostic conceptualization of autism among Indian psychiatrists, psychologists, and pediatricians. *Journal of Autism and Developmental Disorders, 32*(1), 13–23.

Daley, T. C., Singhal, N., & Krishnamurthy, V. (2013). Ethical considerations in conducting research on autism spectrum disorders in low and middle income countries. *Journal of autism and developmental disorders*, 1–13.

Damodaran, L. P. M., & Arumugam, G. (2011). Urinary oxidative stress markers in children with autism. *Redox Report, 16*(5), 216–222.

Dawson, G., Jones, E. J., Merkle, K., et al. (2012). Early behavioral intervention is associated with normalized brain activity in young children with autism. *Journal of the American Academy of Child and Adolescent Psychiatry, 51*(11), 1150–1159.

Deen, B., & Pelphrey, K. (2012). Perspective: Brain scans need a rethink. *Nature, 491*, S20.

Desai, P. P., & Mohite, P. (2011). An exploratory study of early intervention in Gujarat state, India: Pediatricians' perspectives. *Journal of Developmental and Behavioral Pediatrics, 32*(1), 69–74.

Donovan, J., & Zucker, C. (2010). The Atlantic, August 30, 2010.

Dsouza, A., Barretto, M., & Raman, V. (2010). Uncommon sense: Interactive sensory toys that encourage social interaction among children with autism. In *Workshop paper presented at IDC* (Vol. 12).

Dutta, S., Das, S., Guhathakurta, S., Sen, B., Sinha, S., Chatterjee, A., et al. (2007a). Glutamate receptor 6 gene (GluR6 or GRIK2) polymorphisms in the Indian population: A genetic association study on autism spectrum disorder. *Cellular and Molecular Neurobiology, 27*(8), 1035–1047.

Dutta, S., Guhathakurta, S., Sinha, S., Chatterjee, A., Ahmed, S., Ghosh, S., et al. (2007b). Reelin gene polymorphisms in the Indian population: A possible paternal 5′ UTR-CGG-repeat-allele effect on autism. *American Journal of Medical Genetics Part B: Neuropsychiatric Genetics, 144*(1), 106–112. Reelin.

Dutta, S., Sinha, S., Ghosh, S., Chatterjee, A., Ahmed, S., & Usha, R. (2008). Genetic analysis of reelin gene (RELN) SNPs: No association with autism spectrum disorder in the Indian population. *Neuroscience Letters, 441*(1), 56.

Dyches, T. T. (2011). Assessing diverse students with autism spectrum disorders. *The ASHA Leader, 16*(1), 5–6.

Elsabbagh, M., Divan, G., Koh, Y. J., Kim, Y. S., Kauchali, S., Marcín, C., et al. (2012). Global prevalence of autism and other pervasive developmental disorders. *Autism Research, 5*(3), 160–179.

Fein, D., Barton, M., Eigsti, I. M., Kelley, E., Naigles, L., Schultz, R. T., et al. (2013). Optimal outcome in individuals with a history of autism. *Journal of Child Psychology and Psychiatry, 54*(2), 195–205.

Freeth, M., Sheppard, E., Ramachandran, R., & Milne, E. (2013). A Cross-cultural comparison of autistic traits in the UK, India and Malaysia. *Journal of Autism and Developmental Disorders,* 1–15.

Gangopadhyay, P. K., et al. (2007). Lack of association of HOXA1 and HOXB1 variants with autism in the Indian population. *Psychiatric Genetics, 17*(1), 1.

Gardner, L. M., Murphy, L., Campbell, J. M., Tylavsky, F., Palmer, F. B., & Graff, J. C. (2013). Screening accuracy for risk of autism spectrum disorder using the brief infant-toddler social and emotional assessment (BITSEA). *Research in Autism Spectrum Disorders, 7*(5), 591–600.

Goines, P. E., & Ashwood, P. (2013). Cytokine dysregulation in autism spectrum disorders (ASD): Possible role of the environment neurotoxicity and teratology (pp. 67–81) March–April 2013. (Special issue: Environmental influences and emerging mechanisms in the etiology of autism).

Greenwell, B. (2004). The curious incidence of novels about Asperger's Syndrome. *Children's Literature in Education, 35*(3), 271–284.

Grewal, S. (2010). Diagnosis and Treatment Barriers Faced by South Asian Families in Canada Who Have Children Diagnosed with an Autism Spectrum Disorder.

Guhathakurta, S., Sinha, S., Ghosh, S., Chatterjee, A., Ahmed, S., Gangopadhyay, P. K., et al. (2008). Population-based association study and contrasting linkage disequilibrium pattern reveal genetic association of SLC6A4 with autism in the Indian population from West Bengal. *Brain Research, 1240*, 12–21.

Gupta, S., & Maitra, K. (2002). Exploring ability in disability: A case for children with autism. *Gifted Education International, 16*(3), 278–284. Special talents have been described 4 cases were studied to use strengths to advantage.

Gupta, S. K., & Ratnam, B. (2009). Cerebral perfusion abnormalities in children with autism and mental retardation: A segmental quantitative SPECT study. *Indian Pediatrics, 46*(2), 161–164.

Guruju, M. R., Lavanya, K., Thelma, B. K., Sujatha, M., OmSai, V. R., Nagarathna, V., et al. (2009). Assessment of a clinical checklist in the diagnosis of fragile X syndrome in India. *Journal of Clinical Neuroscience, 16*(10), 1305–1310.

Hallmayer, J., Cleveland, S., Torres, A., Phillips, J., Cohen, B., Torigoe, T., et al. (2011). Genetic heritability and shared environmental factors among twin pairs with autism. *Archives of General Psychiatry, 68*(11), 1095.

Hermawati, D., Then, S. M., Winarni, T. I., Faradz, S. M., & Jamal, R. (2011). Lower erythrocyte GST activity in autism spectrum disorder (ASD) patients compared to normal controls. *Asia-Pacific Journal of Molecular Medicine*, 1–6.

Hoch, E. M. (1967). *Indian children on psychiatrist's playground.* New Delhi: Indian Council of Medical Research.

Howlin, P., Goode, S., Hutton, J., & Rutter, M. (2009). Savant skills in autism: Psychometric approaches and parental reports. *Philosophical Transactions of the Royal Society B: Biological Sciences, 364*(1522), 1359–1367.

Hudec, T. (2012). The attitudes of social workers in Kerala to complementary and alternative interventions for children with autism spectrum disorders.

Indhumathi, N., Singh, D., Chong, S. S., Thelma, B. K., Arabandi, R., & Srisailpathy, C. S. (2012). Fragile X CGG repeat variation in Tamil Nadu, South India: A comparison of radioactive and methylation-specific polymerase chain reaction in CGG repeat sizing. *Genetic Testing and Molecular Biomarkers, 16*(2), 113–122.

James, S. J., Shpyleva, S., Melnyk, S., Pavliv, O., & Pogribny, I. P. (2013). Complex epigenetic regulation of Engrailed-2 (EN-2) homeobox gene in the autism cerebellum. *Translational Psychiatry, 3*(2), e232.

Jauhari, P., Bhargava, R., Bhave, A., Kumar, C., & Kumar, R. (2012). Comorbidities associated with intellectual disability among pediatric outpatients seen at a teaching hospital in northern india. *Journal of Policy and Practice in Intellectual Disabilities, 9*(1), 10–16.

Jayarama, S., & Bhat, J. S. (2004). Epidemiological profile of children with autism in comparison with other communicatively challenged children attending early intervention centre. *Indian Journal of Community Medicine, 29*(3), 145–146.

Jeffrey, A., & Lieberman, M. D. (2013). The American Psychiatric Association's 2013 Annual Meeting, May 18–22, San Francisco, California.

John, A. (2012). Stress among mothers of children with intellectual disabilities in Urban India: Role of gender and maternal coping. *Journal of Applied Research in Intellectual Disabilities, 25*(4), 372–382.

Jones, R. (2012). Workshop report: Regression in autism SFARI Simons Foundation Autism Research Initiative, 17 April 2012.

Joshi, A. (2008). Sensory integrative therapy services in India—A qualitative analysis of parents' perspective. *Indian Journal of Occupational Therapy, 40*(2), 49.

Juneja, M., Jain, R., & Mishra, D. (2012a). Referral profile of a child development clinic in Northern India. *The Indian Journal of Pediatrics, 79*(5), 602–605.

Juneja, M., Mukherjee, S. B., & Sharma, S. (2005). A descriptive hospital based study of children with autism. *Indian Pediatrics, 42*(5), 453.

Juneja, M., Mukherjee, S. B., Sharma, S., Jain, R., Das, B., & Sabu, P. (2012b). Evaluation of a parent-based behavioral intervention program for children with autism in a low-resource setting. *Journal of pediatric neurosciences, 7*(1), 16.

Juneja, M., Sharma, S., & Mukherjee, S. B. (2010). Sensitivity of the autism behavior checklist in Indian autistic children. *Journal of Developmental and Behavioral Pediatrics, 31*(1), 48–49.

Kalra, V., Seth, R., & Sapra, S. (2005). Autism—Experiences in a tertiary care hospital. *The Indian Journal of Pediatrics, 72*(3), 227–230.

Kanner, L. (1951). The conception of wholes and parts in early infantile autism. *American Journal of Psychiatry, 108*(1), 23–26.

Kapur, S. O. (1989). Infantile autism-case studies. *Nimhans Journal, 7*(1), 83–85.

Kar, N., Khanna, R., & Kar, G. C. (1993). Autistic features in children with mental retardation. *Indian Journal of Psychiatry, 39*(4), 304–308.

Karanth, P., Shaista, S., & Srikanth, N. (2010). Efficacy of communication DEALL—An indigenous early intervention program for children with autism spectrum disorders. *Indian Journal of Pediatrics, 77*(9), 957–962.

Karnath Aluri, U., & Karanth, P. (2002). Rehabilitation facilities available for children with autism/PDD in Bangalore city—A survey. *Asia Pacific Disability Rehabilitation Journal, 13*(2), 115–124.

Kaur, P., Chavan, B. S., Lata, S., Kaur, A., Tinku, S., Arora, Y., et al. (2006). Early intervention in developmental delay. *The Indian Journal of Pediatrics, 73*(5), 405–408.

Khare, R., & Mullick, A. (2008). Educational spaces for children with autism: Design development process. *CIB W 084 Proceedings, Building Comfortable and Liveable Environment for All,* pp. 66–75.

Kishore, M. T., & Basu, A. (2011). Early concerns of mothers of children later diagnosed with autism: Implications for early identification. *Research in Autism Spectrum Disorders, 5*(1), 157–163.

Klei, M. A., Klei, L., Sanders, S. J., Murtha, M. T., Hus, V., Lowe, J. K., et al. (2012). Common genetic variants, acting additively, are a major source of risk for autism. *Molecular Autism, 3*(1), 1–13.

Kothur, K., Ray, M., & Malhi, P. (2008). Correlation of autism with temporal tubers in tuberous sclerosis complex. *Neurology India, 56*(1), 74.

Kumar, S., Alexander, M., & Gnanamuthu, C. (2004). Recent experience with Rett syndrome at a tertiary care center. *Neurology India, 52*(4), 494.

Lakhan, R. (2013). The coexistence of psychiatry disorders and intellectual disability in children aged 3–18 years in the Barwani District, India.

Lal, R. (2010). Effect of alternative and augmentative communication on language and social behavior of children with autism. *Educational Research and Reviews, 5*(3), 119–125.

Lal, R., & Bali, M. (2007). Effect of visual strategies on development of communication skills in children with autism. *Asia Pacific Disability Rehabilitation Journal, 18*(2), 120–130.

Lal, R., & Chhabria, R. (2013). Early intervention of autism: A case for floor time approach. Early Intervention of Autism: A Case for Floor Time Approach http://dx.doi.org/10.5772/54378.

Lal, R., & Ganesan, K. (2011). Children with autism spectrum disorders: Social Stories and self management of behaviour. *British Journal of Educational Research, 1*(1), 36–48.

LaSalle, J. M., Vallero, R. O., & Mitchell, M. M. (2013). Epigenetics at the interface of genetics and environmental factors in autism. In *Environmental epigenomics in health and disease* (pp. 97–114). Berlin, Heidelberg: Springer.

Lofthouse, N., Hendren, R., Hurt, E., Arnold, L. E., & Eric Butter, E. (2012). A review of complementary and alternative treatments for autism spectrum disorders. *Autism Research and Treatment, 2012*, 1–21.

Lovaas, O. (2003). *Teaching individuals with developmental delays better intervention techniques*. Austin TX: Pro-Ed.

Maglione, M. A., Gans, D., Das, L., Timbie, J., & Kasari, C. (2012). Nonmedical interventions for children with ASD: Recommended guidelines and further research needs. *Pediatrics, 130*(Supplement 2), S169–S178.

Malhi, P., & Singhi, P. (2005). Patterns of development in young children with autism. *The Indian Journal of Pediatrics, 72*(7), 553–556.

Malhi, P., & Singhi, P. (2011). Follow up of children with autism spectrum disorders: Stability and change in diagnosis. *The Indian Journal of Pediatrics, 78*(8), 941–945.

Malhotra, S., Chakrabarti, S., Gupta, N., Kumar, P., & Gill, S. (2003). Pervasive developmental disorders and its subtypes: Sociodemographic and clinical profile. *German Journal Psychiatry, 6*, 33–39.

Malhotra, S., Chakrabarti, S., & Nehra, A. (2002a). Psychological interventions with parents of autistic children. *Indian Journal of Psychiatry, 44*(2), 108–117.

Malhotra, S., & Chaturvedi, S. K. (1984). Patterns of childhood psychiatric disorders in India. *Indian Journal Paediatrics, 51*, 235–240.

Malhotra, S., & Gupta, N. (2002). Childhood disintegrative disorder—Re examination of the current concept. *European Child and Adolescent Psychiatry, 11*, 108–114.

Malhotra, S., Kumar, D., & Gupta, N. (2002b). Rett's syndrome. A neurodevelopmental disorder: Report of two cases. *Neurology India, 50*, 330–333.

Malhotra, S., & Singh, S. P. (1993). Disintegrative psychosis of childhood: An appraisal and case study. *Acta Paedopsychiatrica, 56*, 37–40.

Malhotra, S., Subodh, B. N., Parakh, P., & Lahariya, S. (2013). Brief report: Childhood disintegrative disorder as a likely manifestation of vitamin B12 deficiency. *Journal of Autism and Developmental Disorders*, 1–4.

Malhotra, S., & Vikas, A. (2005). Pervasive developmental disorders: Indian scene. *Journal of Indian Association for Child and Adolescent Mental Health, 1*(5).

Mandell, D. S., Ittenbach, R. F., Levy, S. E., & Pinto-Martin, J. A. (2007). Disparities in diagnoses received prior to a diagnosis of autism spectrum disorder. *Journal of Autism and Developmental Disorders, 37*(9), 1795–1802.

Manjunatha, K. R., Chetan, G. K., Arathi, R., Padma, S., Venkatesh, H. N., Srinath, S., et al. (2001). Genetics of autism: Association of chromosomal fragile sites. *Indian Journal of Human Genetics, 1*(4), 293–299.

Manjunatha, K. R., Narayanan, H. S., Rao, B. S. S. R., Srinath, S., & Girimaji, S. R. (1989). Cryptogenetic investigations in autistic children: A preliminary study on the detection of fragile X chromosome. *Nimhans Journal, 7*(2), 163–167.

Manohari, S. M., Raman, V., & Ashok, M. V. (2013). Use of vineland adaptive behavior scales-II in children with autism—An Indian experience. *Journal of Indian Association for Child and Adolescent Mental Health, 9*(1), 5–12.

Meera, S. S., Kaipa, R., Thomas, J., & Shivashankar, N. (2012). Brief report: An unusual manifestation of diagnostic overshadowing of pervasive developmental disorder—Not otherwise specified: A five year longitudinal case study. *Journal of Autism and Developmental Disorders*, 1–4.

Mohammad, N. S., Jain, J. M. N., Chintakindi, K. P., Singh, R. P., Naik, U., & Akella, R. R. D. (2009). Aberrations in folate metabolic pathway and altered susceptibility to autism. *Psychiatric Genetics, 19*(4), 171–176.

Mujawar, S., Kandale, V., & Welasly, P. (2013). Sequence analysis and homology modeling of SHANK3 protein involved in Autism. *Indian Streams research Journal, 3*(4).

Mukherjee, B. B. (2008). *Musical interaction with children with autistic spectrum disorder in an Indian context* (Doctoral dissertation, Strathclyde).

Mukhopadhyay, T. R. (2000). *Beyond the silence: My life, the world and autism.* London, UK: National Autistic Society.

Mukhopadhyay, T. R. (2003). *The mind tree: A miraculous child breaks the silence of autism.* New York: Arcade Publishing.

Mulle, J. G., Sharp, W. G., & Cubells, J. F. (2013). The gut microbiome: A new frontier in autism research. *Current Psychiatry Reports, 15*(2), 1–9.

Muthu, M. S., & Prathibha, K. M. (2008). Management of a child with autism and severe bruxism: A case report. *Journal of Indian Society of Pedodontics and Preventive Dentistry, 26*(2), 82.

Nagendra, J., & Jayachandra, S. (2012). Autism spectrum disorders: Dental treatment considerations. *Journal of International Dental and Medical Research, 5*(2), 118–121.

Naik, U. (2007). Practice parameters for childhood autism child and adolescent psychiatry clinical practice guidelines for psychiatrists in India. In S. Gautam, A. Avasthi, S. Malhotra (Eds.), *Task force on clinical practice guidelines for psychiatrists in India* (pp. 210–237). Indian Psychiatry Society.

Naik, U. S., Abbagani, K. L., Amita Shree Balakrishna N. (2012). *Assessment of regression in autism.* Paper Presented at a Symposium at the 13th World Congress of the World Association for Infant Mental Health Conference, Cape Town, South Africa (pp. 17–21), April 2012.

Naik, U. S., Gangadharan, C., Abbagani, K., Nagalla, B., Dasari, N., & Manna, S. K. (2011). A study of nuclear transcription factor-kappa B in childhood autism. *PLoS One, 6*(5), e19488.

Nancy, A. A. (2012). Deployment of assistive technology in the emotional hearing aid for children with autism. *International Journal of Research in Communication Technologies-IJRCT, 1*(1).

Narayan, M., Srinath, S., Anderson, G. M., & Meundi, D. B. (1993). Cerebrospinal fluid levels of homovanillic acid and 5-hydroxyindoleacetic acid in autism. *Biological Psychiatry, 33*(8), 630–635.

Narayan, J., et al. (2005). Analysis of educational support systems for children with mental retardation and autism spectrum disorders. *International Journal of Rehabilitation Research, 28*(4), 365–368.

Narayanan, H. S. (1978). A report of clinical observations and management in 7 cases of childhood autism. *Indian Journal of Psychiatry, 20*, 93–97.

Nazeer, A. (2011). Psychopharmacology of autistic spectrum disorders in children and adolescents. *The Pediatric clinics of North America, 58*(1), 85–97.

Nazeer, A., & Ghaziuddin, M. (2012). Autism spectrum disorders: Clinical features and diagnosis. *The Pediatric Clinics of North America, 59*(1), 19–25.

Nazni, P., Wesely, E. G., & Nishadevi, V. (2008). Impact of casein and gluten free dietary intervention on selected autistic children. *Iranian Journal of Pediatrics, 18*(3), 244. (Persian edition).

Nelson, A. (2011). Drama education for individuals on the autism spectrum. In *Key concepts in theatre/drama education* (pp. 177–181). The Netherlands: Sense Publishers.

Nizamie, A., Sengupta, U., Mishra, B. R., Praharaj, S. K., & Nizam, H. (2010). Multimodal Cse report Role of Early Multimodal Interventions in a Case with Autistic Regression. *Acta Neurolrologica Taiwan, 19*, 51–56.

Onore, C., Careaga, M., & Ashwood, P. (2012). The role of immune dysfunction in the pathophysiology of autism. *Brain, Behavior, and Immunity, 26*(3), 383–392.

Ostrovsky, Y., Meyers, E., Ganesh, S., Mathur, U., & Sinha, P. (2009). Visual parsing after recovery from blindness. *Psychological Science, 20*(12), 1484–1491.

Ozonoff, S., Iosif, A. M., Baguio, F., Cook, I. C., Hill, M. M., Hutman, T., et al. (2010). A prospective study of the emergence of early behavioral signs of autism. *Journal of the American Academy of Child and Adolescent Psychiatry, 49*(3), 256–266.

Patra, S., & Arun, P. (2011). Use of Indian scale for assessment of autism in child guidance clinic: An experience. *Indian Journal of Psychological Medicine, 33*(2), 217. NIMH Scale.

Pennesi, C. M., & Klein, L. C. (2012). Effectiveness of the gluten-free, casein-free diet for children diagnosed with autism spectrum disorder: Based on parental report. *Nutritional Neuroscience, 15*(2), 85–91.

Priya, M. D. L., & Geetha, A. (2011). Level of trace elements (copper, zinc, magnesium and selenium) and toxic elements (lead and mercury) in the hair and nail of children with autism. *Biological Trace Element Research, 142*(2), 148–158.

Purkayastha, M., Girimaji, S., Srinath, S. & Sheshadri, S. P. (1997). Clinical profile in mental retardation. In R. Hegde, S. Malhotra, L. P. Shah (Eds.), *Research endeavours in child and adolescent psychaitry in India* (pp. 48–53).

Pushker, N., Tinwala, S., Khurana, S., & Sen, S. (2012). Bilateral microphthalmos with unilateral superior cyst in a child with autism and CHARGE syndrome. *International ophthalmology,* 1–4.

Radhakrishna, S. (2010). Application of integrated yoga therapy to increase imitation skills in children with autism spectrum disorder. *International Journal of Yoga, 3*(1), 26.

Ragunath, P. K., Chitra, R., Mohammad, S., & Abhinand, P. A. (2011). A systems biological study on the comorbidity of autism spectrum disorders and bipolar disorder. *Bioinformation, 7*(3), 102.

Rai, V. (2011). Autism genetics and cytogenetic abnormalities. *Trends in Molecular Sciences, 3*(1), 1–13.

Raj, A., & Kumar, K. (2009). Optimizing parent coaches' ability to facilitate mastery experiences of parents of children with autism. *International Journal of Psychosocial Rehabilitation, 14*(2), 25–36.

Rao, A. N., et al. (2010). Food Allergy investigations and its significance in autism spectrum disorders. *International Journal of Pharma and Bio Sciences, 1*, 1–8. ([PDF] from www.ijpbs.net).

Ravindran, Neeraja, & Myers, Barbara J. (2012). Cultural influences on perceptions of health, illness, and disability: A review and focus on autism. *Journal of Child and Family Studies, 21*(2), 311–319.

Ravindran, N., & Myers, B. J. (2013). Beliefs and practices regarding autism in indian families now settled abroad an internet survey. *Focus on Autism and Other Developmental Disabilities, 28*(1), 44–53.

Russell, P. S. S., et al. (2010). Diagnostic accuracy, reliability and validity of childhood autism rating scale in India. *World Journal of Pediatrics, 6*(2), 141–147.

Rutter, M. L. (2011). Progress in understanding autism: 2007–2010. *Journal of Autism and Developmental Disorders, 41*, 395–404.

Sampath, H., Sivaswamy, J., & Indurkhya, B. (2010). Assistive systems for children with dyslexia and autism. *ACM SIGACCESS Accessibility and Computing, 96*, 32–36.

Sen, B., et al. (2010). Family-based studies indicate association of Engrailed 2 gene with autism in an Indian population. *Genes, Brain and Behavior, 9*(2), 248–255.

Seth, R., & Kalra, V. (2006). Autism in India. *Indian Pediatrics, 43*(5), 456.

Shah, A. P. (2012) Indian Pediatr, 2012—indianpediatrics.net Weak head and neck control early indicator of autism (*11th Annual Meeting for Autism Research—IMFAR, Abstract 9882.*

Shahzadi Malhotra, G. R., Bhatia, M. S., & Singh, T. B. (2010). Effects of picture exchange communication system on communication and behavioral anomalies in autism. *Indian Journal of Psychological Medicine, 32*(2), 141.

Sharan, P. (2006). Need for epidemiological work on autism in India. *Journal of Indian Association of Child and Adolescent Mental Health, 2*(3), 70–71.

Sharda, M., Subhadra, T. P., Sahay, S., Nagaraja, C., Singh, L., Mishra, R., et al. (2010). Sounds of melody—Pitch patterns of speech in autism. *Neuroscience Letters, 478*(1), 42–45.

Shivashankar, N., & Satishchandra, P. (1989). Auditory brainstem responses in autistic children. *Nimhans Journal, 7*(2), 159–162. Auditory brainstem.

Silver, W. G., Rapin, I. (2012). Neurobiological basis of autism. *Pediatric Clinics of North America, 59*(1), 113–128, 43–61.

Singh, V. K. (1996). Plasma increase of interleukin-12 and interferon-gamma. Pathological significance in autism. *Journal of Neuroimmunology, 66*(1), 143–145.

Singh, A. S., Chandra, R., Guhathakurta, S., Sinha, S., Chatterjee, A., Ahmed, S., & Rajamma, U. (2013). Genetic association and gene–gene interaction analyses suggest likely involvement of *ITGB3* and *TPH2* with autism spectrum disorder (ASD) in the Indian population. *Progress in Neuro-Psychopharmacology and Biological Psychiatry.*

Singhi, P., & Malhi, P. (2001). Clinical and neurodevelopmental profile of young children with autism. *Indian Paediatrics, 38*, 384–390.

Singhi, P., Mittal, B. R., Nagaraj, R., & Malhi, P. (2008). Single photon emission tomography in children with autism. *Journal of Pediatric Neurology, 6*(3), 221–225.

Singhi Nagaraj, R., Singhi, P., & Malhi, P. (2006). Risperidone in children with autism: Randomized, placebo-controlled, double-blind study. *Journal of Child Neurology, 21*(6), 450–455.

Sitholey, P., Aga, V. M., Agarwal, V., & Prasad, M. (1998). Childhood autism in tuberous sclerosis. *The Indian Journal of Pediatrics, 65*(4), 615–617.

Srinath, S., Chowdhury, J., Bhide, A. V., Narayanan, H. S., & Shivaprakash (1989). Descriptive study of infantile autism. *Nimhans Journal, 7*(1), 77–81.

Srivastava, R. K., Agarwal, M., & Pundhir, A. (2011). Role of donepezil in autism: Its conduciveness in psychopharmacotherapy. *Case reports in Psychiatry, 2011.*

Srivastava, Seema, & Mukhopadhyay, Anjana. (2011). Optimism-pessimism and emotional competence measures of parents of children with symptoms of autism. *Indian Journal of Community Psychology, 7*(1), 130–138.

Subbalakshmi, N. K. (2012). Prevalence of autism, autistic features and associated risk factors in subjects attending special schools in our community.

Sullivan, K., Sharda, M., Greenson, J., Dawson, G., & Singh, N. C. (2013). A novel method for assessing the development of speech motor function in toddlers with autism spectrum disorders. *Frontiers in Integrative Neuroscience, 1*, 0.

Surén, P., Roth, C., Bresnahan, M., Haugen, M., Hornig, M., Hirtz, D., et al. (2013). Association between maternal use of folic acid supplements and risk of autism spectrum disorders in children. *JAMA, 309*(6), 570–577. doi:10.1001/jama.2012.155925.

Tchaconas, A., & Adesman, A. (2013). Autism spectrum disorders: A pediatric overview and update. *Current Opinion in Pediatrics, 25*(1), 130–144.

Thara, R., & Patel, V. (2010). Role of non-governmental organizations in mental health in India. *Indian Journal of Psychiatry, 52*(Suppl 1), S389.

The Hindu. (2012, March 23). How the Child Welfare Service got the Bhattacharya Kids.

Torielo, H. V. (2012). Approach to the genetic evaluation of the child with autism. *Pediatric Clinics of North America, 59*(1), 113–128.

Vaishnavi, V., Manikandan, M., Tiwary, B. K., & Munirajan, A. K. (2013). Insights on the functional impact of MicroRNAs present in autism-associated copy number variants. *PLoS One, 8*(2), e56781.

Vargas, D. L., Nascimbene, C., Krishnan, C., Zimmerman, A. W., & Pardo, C. A. (2005). Neuroglial activation and neuroinflammation in the brain of patients with autism. *Annals of Neurology, 57*(1), 67–81.

Varisco, S., Kempf-Constantin, N., Lehotkay, R., Devi, T. S., Raju, M. V. R., Giroud, M., et al. (2009). A comparison of use of the aberrant behaviour checklist at the "Lebenshilfe" (Visakhapatnam, Andhra Pradesh, India) and at "La Castalie"(Monthey, Valais, Switzerland). *Schweizer Archiv für Neurologie und Psychiatrie, 160*(7), 280–283.

Venkatesan, S. (2005). Activity log of preschool children with developmental disabilities and autism spectrum disorders. *Asia Pacific Disability Rehabilitation Journal, 16*, 68–76.

Vishnu, K. K., Leela, M., Rao, T. S., & Chengappa, S. K. (1992). Language in India.
Volkmar, F. R., & Reichow, B. (2013). Autism in DSM-5: Progress and challenges. *Molecular Autism, 4*, 13.
Vullamparthi, A. J., Khargharia, H. S., Bindhumadhava, B. S., & Babu, N. S. C. (2011, July). A smart tutoring aid for the autistic-educational aid for learners on the autism spectrum. In *2011 International Conference on Technology for Education (T4E)*, IEEE (pp. 43–50).
Walker, C. K., Anderson, K. W., Milano, K. M., Ye, S., Tancredi, D. J., Pessah, I. N., et al. (2013). Trophoblast inclusions are significantly increased in the placentas of children in families at risk for autism. *Biological Psychiatry*.
Welch, K. C., Lahiri, U., Warren, Z., & Sarkar, N. (2010). An approach to the design of socially acceptable robots for children with autism spectrum disorders. *International Journal of Social Robotics, 2*(4), 391–403.
Whiteley, P., Haracopos, D., Knivsberg, A. M., Reichelt, K. L., Parlar, S., Jacobsen, J., et al. (2010). The scan brit randomised, controlled, single-blind study of a gluten-and casein-free dietary intervention for children with autism spectrum disorders. *Nutritional Neuroscience, 13*(2), 87–100.
Whiteley, P., Shattock, P., Knivsberg, A. M., Seim, A., Reichelt, K. L., Todd, L. et al. (2012). Gluten-and casein-free dietary intervention for autism spectrum conditions. *Frontiers in Human Neuroscience, 6*.
Wolff, J. J., Gu, H., Gerig, G., et al. (2012). Differences in white matter fiber tract development present from 6 to 24 months in infants with autism. *American Journal of Psychiatry, 169*, 589–600.
Singhal, N. (2013). The Assessment Kit (AK) for Autism, AFA Email: actionforautism@gmail.com URL: http://www.autism-india.org.
Yochum, C. L., Bhattacharya, P., Patti, L., Mirochnitchenko, O., & Wagner, G. C. (2010). Animal model of autism using GSTM1 knockout mice and early post-natal sodium valproate treatment. *Behavioural Brain Research, 210*(2), 202–210. Mouse Model VPA.

Chapter 16
Adolescent Psychiatry: An Overview of the Indian Research

M. Mehta, R.D. Pattanayak and R. Sagar

1 Introduction

Adolescence is a period of transition from childhood to adulthood, which is marked by several biological, cognitive and psychosocial changes. It is a unique developmental phase in one's life and is often shaped by the prevalent socio-economic and cultural context. The World Population day, 2003 declared it as the year of 'one billion adolescents' with a call for action towards health, information and services for adolescents (UNFPA 2003). Nearly, one-fourth of the world's adolescents reside in India (Census of India 2001). With over 15 % of adolescents meeting the criteria for *caseness* internationally, it translates into huge absolute numbers for India (Roberts et al. 1998). The mental health needs of this population group are distinct from both children and adults. Adolescent health has recently gained some prominence in national health policies, but the focus has largely been on sexual or reproductive health, while the mental health continues to be low in priority.

This chapter reviews and summarises the available Indian research on psychological health and psychiatric disorders among adolescents, highlighting the gaps in the evidence and provides future directions for adolescent mental health in India. Child psychiatry has been covered elsewhere as a separate chapter in this book. While WHO defines adolescence as spanning between 10 and 19 years, however, it has been more variable in Indian studies. As 18 years is the legal age for adulthood, most clinical services in India consider those between 12 and 18 years as adolescents.

M. Mehta, Professor of Clinical Psychology; R.D. Pattanayak, Assistant Professor; R. Sagar, Additional Professor

---

M. Mehta (✉) · R.D. Pattanayak · R. Sagar
Department of Psychiatry, All India Institute of Medical Sciences, New Delhi, India
e-mail: drmanju.mehta@gmail.com

S. Malhotra and S. Chakrabarti (eds.), *Developments in Psychiatry in India*,
DOI 10.1007/978-81-322-1674-2_16

2 Profile of Indian Adolescents

There are nearly 240 million adolescents in India, who form more than 22 % of the population. The sex ratio for adolescents is 882 females per 1,000 males (Census of India 2001; UNICEF 2011).[1] The social and cultural profile of adolescents in India is briefly summarised here.

In India, the onset of adolescence is often marked by religious or ritualistic ceremonies and adolescent boys and girls are expected to follow a code of conduct. Certain restrictions are imposed on girls' behaviour after the onset of puberty, while boys begin to exercise greater freedom to move about and seek educational and vocational pursuits more freely. Adolescent lifestyles often vary as a result of factors such as residence, ethnicity and socio-economic status of their families. Adolescent boys in rural families often engage in learning vocation or family craft, while adolescent girls are engaged in household responsibilities (cooking, cleaning, taking care of younger siblings, sewing, etc.) in preparation of an early marriage. In contrast, urban adolescents from higher socio-economic status have access to resources for educational and other pursuits and may lead a more westernized lifestyle. Adolescents from urban lower class or urban slums are least privileged in several respects and are quite vulnerable to malnutrition, poor health, sexual exploitation and drug use.

As per the findings of the National Family Health Survey-3, 2005–2006 (NFHS-3), 27 % of girls are married and 50 % of boys between 15 and 19 years are employed (National Family Health Survey-3 2007). Nearly 25 % in rural areas and 10 % in urban areas are illiterate. Gender disparities persist in the education sector, with enrolment rates being lower for girls at all stages of school. Boys and girls (15–19 years) reported relatively more high-risk sexual activity and lower use of condoms compared to 20–24 years age group (National Family Health Survey-3 2007).

The recent socio-cultural changes, weakening of social support from kinship, ambiguity of societal values and increasing gap between aspirations and possible achievements have contributed to inter-generational conflicts. Nonetheless, family as an institution continues to play a large role in influencing adolescents across all sections of the society in India.

3 Adolescent Psychiatry: Need for a Separate Emphasis?

George Patton argued for the need to view adolescent mental health as a unique subspecialty on its own, distinct from the child mental health (Patton 1996). While it was met with considerable debate (Birleson and Luk 1997), nonetheless, it raises an important issue of placing a special, *if not separate*, emphasis on adolescent mental health.

In the Indian context, the available mental health studies on younger population have either not included, or only partially included the adolescent group (with a cut-off of 14 or 16 years for child samples) and more often than not, the

[1] Planning commission. Report of the working group on adolescents for 10th five year plan. Government of India. Available at: http://www.planningcommission.nic.in/aboutus/committee/wrkgrp/wg_adolcnts.pdf. Accessed on May 19, 2013.

sub-analysis for adolescent age groups is often not found in the study findings. The studies exclusively focussing on mental health of adolescents are far few between and have emerged only in recent years. The need for a special emphasis on adolescent mental health is highlighted below.

(1) Adolescence is remarkably different from childhood in psychological development, with a potential bearing on the approach, assessment and interview styles (Pataki 2009). The unique characteristics which emerge during adolescence involve:
    (a) a tendency to experiment and seek novel experiences
    (b) a heightened sense of invulnerability, invincibility or a low risk perception
    (c) an intense desire for independence, rebelliousness
    (d) an inner search for self-identity
    (e) high influence of role models
    (f) need for peer approval, peer opinions valued higher than authority figures
    (g) higher cognitive/prefrontal cortex functions not yet mature (decision making, reasoning, impulse control).
(2) Several psychological issues and concerns are unique to adolescent years. There may be dissatisfaction with one's body image or there may be confusion over one's identity as an individual. At times, the academic expectations may be set high for self and the constant reinforcement by parents may lead to unrealistic demands or goals, posing an increased stress during board examinations. The experimentation with 'gateway' drugs such as tobacco, alcohol and inhalants may lead to indulgence in high-risk behaviours, such as driving under influence. The issues of intimacy and initiation of romantic relationships are another common source of conflict with parents, especially as the adolescent is still a minor. All these behaviours are likely to lead to psychological ill health and affect the functioning at home or school.
(3) The prevalence and pattern of mental and behavioural disorders show a discernible change during adolescence. Depressive disorders become more prevalent, different manifestations of anxiety emerge. Behavioural disturbances, such as suicidality, eating disorders and substance abuse, which are uncommon during childhood, may begin to emerge in these years. Schizophrenia and psychotic disorders typically mark their onset by end of adolescence or youth years. Pre-existing psychiatric disorders may often extend from childhood to adolescence interfering with psychosocial adjustment or may be precursors for another mental disorder. There is a considerable burden of illness associated with adolescent mental disorders and there is also a potential scope for primary or secondary preventive interventions at this age (Patton 1996, 1998).

4 Prevalence of Adolescent Mental Health Problems in India

Worldwide, mental and behavioural disorders pose the highest disease burden among the adolescent age group. Problems related to mental health and behaviour account for 24.7 % of total disability adjusted life years (DALYs) among the 10 to 19 year olds across the world (with mental illness contributing 18.6 %, self afflicted injury to 3.2 % and alcohol use disorders 2.9 % of total DALYs, Mathers 2009).

5 Community Surveys

Some of the earliest epidemiological surveys on general population in India had included individuals across all age groups, including those aged between 10 and 20 years (Sethi et al. 1967; Pillai et al. 2008). The prevalence rates for mental disorders in this younger sub-sample varied between 1.8 and 9.6 % across the surveys, as summarised in Table 1. It is to be noted, however, that these surveys were not specifically geared towards detecting morbidity in adolescents. Most of earlier surveys had used same instruments or interviews for adult as well as younger population groups, which could have lead to under-detection of mental morbidity.

While some recent surveys are now available for prevalence of psychiatric disorders in child population, but there are hardly any surveys focusing on adolescent age groups. A methodologically robust study by Srinath et al. (2005) reported a prevalence rate of 12 % among children aged 4–16 years. In such surveys with upper cut-off of 14 or 16 years, the adolescent rates have not been provided separately. It is, therefore, clear that there has been a lack of separate emphasis on adolescent mental health in the psychiatric epidemiological surveys from India.

A recent population-based survey by Pilli et al. (2008) attempted to assess current mental morbidity among 2,048 adolescents (aged 12–16 years) from urban and rural areas of Goa. The current prevalence of any DSM–IV diagnosis was 1.81 % [95 % CI 1.27–2.48]. The most common diagnoses were anxiety disorders (1.0 %), depressive disorder (0.5 %), behavioural disorder (0.4 %) and attention-deficit hyperactivity disorder (0.2 %).

In a prospective study for incidence of psychiatric disorders, school children (aged 4–11 years) were followed after 6 years, at which time the sample was aged between 10 and 17 years (Malhotra et al. 2009). The incidence for child and adolescent psychiatric disorders was 18 per thousand per year (95 % CI: 0–37), of which half had neurotic, stress-related and affective disorders; and 10 % had personality and behavioural disorders. Overall, about 40 % children presented with disorders that had onset specific to childhood, while rest of conditions were early onset psychiatric disorders which are usually seen in adults. Separate findings for adolescent sample were, however, not available.

5.1 School Surveys

Recent surveys have attempted to assess the prevalence of mental health problems in school-going adolescents (Rao 1978), Nair et al. (2012). In addition, these also provide some insight into the academic, family or personal problems affecting the mental health of students in secondary or higher secondary classes (Table 2).

Bhasin et al. (2010) assessed all students from standard 9–12 for presence of depression, anxiety and stress in a purposively selected school sample, with adolescents mostly from affluent backgrounds. A significant proportion of the students had a high level of depression, stress and anxiety scores, which were correlated with each other, and inversely related to academic performance. Depression and stress was significantly

Table 1 Community-based surveys: findings for adolescent sample

Study reference	Survey methods	Adolescent sub-sample	Prevalence	Profile
Sethi et al. (1967) (Lucknow-urban)	Head of household/ housewife interview	$n = 388$ 11–20 years	20 patients (5.1 %)	Psychoneurosis (anxiety, conversion) was common in entire sample Age-wise distribution of morbidity not provided
Sethi et al. (1972) (Lucknow-rural)	Head of Household interview	$n = 509$ 10–20 years (19 % of total sample)	10 patients (1.9 %)	Mental subnormality ($n = 7$) and psychoneurosis ($n = 3$) Rates same as in adult sample
Premrajan et al. (1993) (Pondicherry-urban)	House to house survey	$n = 209$ 13–20 years	6 patients (2.9 %)	All six patients were females Rates lower than adult sample
Nandi et al. (2000) (West Bengal –rural)	Door to door survey (in 1972 and 1992)	$n = 488$ (in 1972) $n = 851$ (in 1992) 12–23 years (22–24 % of total sample)	1972: 9.6 % 1992: 4.0 %	Age specific distribution of mental morbidity not provided for this age group Rates lower than adult sample
Srinath et al. (2005) (Bangalore and Lucknow; urban/rural)	Screening f/u by Diagnostic interview schedule for children–parent version DISC-P and parent interview (12-16 yrs)	Bangalore: 2064 Lucknow: 2325 (0–16 years) Figure for adolescent sub-sample not known	Bangalore: 12 % (in 4–16 yrs group) Lucknow: 11.8 % & 3.6 % in adolescent boys and girls, respectively	Mood and anxiety disorders found in only 0.1–0.2 % of sample Boys more psychopathology than girls, especially during adolescent years at the Lucknow centre
Pillai et al. (2008) (Goa- urban/rural)	DSM IV diagnosis (Development and well-being assessment)	$n = 2,048$ 12–16 years	Current prevalence 1.81 %	Anxiety/depression: 1 % each Behavioural disorders: 0.4 % ADHD: 0.2 % Association with urban residence, non-traditional lifestyles, lack of safety and history of abuse

Table 2 School surveys of adolescent mental health problems

Study reference	Instruments	Sample	Findings
Rao (1978)	General health questionnaire-60; clinical interview	$n = 428$ urban 13–16 years	Total prevalence: 19.6 % Girls slightly higher prevalence than boys One of the initial school studies in India; part of a thesis
Mehta et al. (1991) ICMR funded	Child behaviour questionnaire	$n = 2055$ rural school 6–12 years	Prevalence found to be 13.28 % (total)
Ahmad et al. (2007)	Screening f/u by ICD-10	$n = 390$ 10–19 years	Prevalence: 17.9 % in overall sample; and highest in 14–15 years old (25 %) Educational problems, substance abuse, conduct disorder, anxiety, common problems
Arun and Chavan (2009)	General health questionnaire; Mooney problem checklist	$n = 2402$ Standard 7–12th	45.8 % reported psychological problems 50 % perceived problems with role as students 45 % experienced academic decline 9 % reported life as a burden and 6 % had suicidal ideation
Bhasin et al. (2010) (NCR-Greater Noida)	DASS-1 (Depression anxiety stress scale)	$n = 242$ students Standard 9–12th	Median scores for depression (0–42), anxiety (0–42), stress (0–42) sub-scales were 10, 8 and 14, respectively (population norms not available for DASS) More in females More in board classes (10th/12th)

(continued)

Table 2 (continued)

Study reference	Instruments	Sample	Findings
Reddy et al. (2011)	Strength and difficulties score (SDQ)	$n = 354$ 11–16 years Standard 10th	10.4 % had an abnormal SDQ score Scores on hyperactivity (12 %), conduct problems (16.7 %), emotional problems (12.4 %) and peer (6.2 %) subscales were abnormal in significant percentage Emotional sub-scale score particularly high in female adolescents 19 % had definite difficulties, of which 1/4th were for over a year, which affected functioning in various areas
Samanta et al. (2012) (Bangalore)	Self report questionnaire	$n = 199$ Males only Standard 8–10th	Mental health problems such as loneliness (10–17 %), worrying (11–17 %) and suicidal thoughts (14–19 %) were common, with higher figures in urban students Physical violence/bullying was more prevalent for urban students in various settings at home/school
Singh and Mishra (2012) (Delhi, Lucknow-urban/rural)	Adolescent lifestyle survey	$n = 1{,}500$ Standard 6–11th	Suicidal attempts reported by 18 % of sample. Several lifestyle concerns (related to eating, sleeping, risk behaviours) commonly seen in the sample
Nair et al. (2012) (Kerala)	Teenage Screening Questionnaire-Trivandrum (TSQ-T)	$n = 11{,}501$ Standard 11th	15.2 % reported adjustment problems; 65.8 % body image-related problems; 61.2 % scholastic problems; 22.1 % family-related problems; and 31.9 % personal problems

Table 3 Hospital-based studies: pattern of psychiatric disorders in adolescent patients

Study reference	Instruments	Adolescent patients	Findings
Nagaraja et al. (1981–1983) (ICMR multi-site study) (Bangalore, Delhi, Lucknow, Waltair, AP)	Semi-structured interview; Rutter' classification and ICD-9 diagnosis used	$n = 1{,}015$ 12–16 years	Psychosis (41 %), hysterical neurosis (27 %) and conduct disorder (7 %) were common; 10–20 % sample had associated abnormal psychosocial factors
Bharath et al. (1997) (Bangalore)	Chart review for admitted patients over one-year period	152 adolescent in-patients	Hysterical neurosis (31 %) Psychosis (25 %), conduct disorder (10 %), hyperkinetic syndrome (9.8 %) Average stay: 4–12 weeks
Malhotra et al. (2007) (Chandigarh)	Retrospective chart review (1980–2005) of patients ($\leq$15 years)	Average 100–144 adolescents per year—largest sub-group	Among entire sample ($\leq$15 years), common diagnoses were mental retardation, neurotic and stress-related disorders and childhood disorders (separate analysis not provided for adolescents)
Sidhu (2012) (Patiala, Punjab)	Semi-structured proforma ICD-10 diagnosis	$n = 500$ 10–19 years	Mood disorders (24.8 %), neurotic, stress-related and somatoform disorders (23.6 %)-common diagnosis 13.2 % had positive family history Prevalence more in nuclear families

associated with the number of adverse events in the student's life over past one year. Anxiety and stress was particularly high in board classes (standards 10th and 12th).

Reddy et al. (2011) assessed urban school adolescents for mental and behavioural problems and found that 28 % had either abnormal or borderline abnormal score on the Strengths and Difficulties Questionnaire (SDQ). Nearly, one in ten had an abnormal SDQ score, and one in five had a difficulty. While male adolescents had higher scores on conduct problems, female adolescents scored particularly high on the emotional symptoms subscale.

In another large-scale school-based study, 61.2 % adolescents reported scholastic problems, 22.1 % family-related problems, 31.9 % personal problems and 15.2 % adjustment problems, with boys reporting a higher percentage. Body image disturbances were present in two-thirds of adolescents (Nair et al. 2012).

5.2 *Hospital-based Studies*

Several researchers have described the profile and pattern of psychiatric disorders among the treatment seeking adolescent patients, Nagaraja et al. 2005, Sidhu (2012) as summarised in Table 3. Psychosis, mood disorders, neurotic and stress-related, and somatoform disorders were the most common reasons for consultation. Conduct disorder was also a common reason for consultation in the clinic-based sample. This profile of adolescent disorders is quite different from that in children visiting psychiatry clinics.

6 Factors Affecting the Psychological Health of Indian Adolescents

There is often a complex socio-ecological framework of risk factors operating in various contexts, which are central to the lives of adolescents (self, home, school, peer group and neighbourhood). There is sufficient evidence, including evidence from low- and middle-income countries that factors such as dysfunctional family structure and relationships, poverty, urbanisation, academic failure, substance use, and physical and sexual abuse are associated with impaired emotional functioning in adolescents (Patel et al. 2008). There is a significant role of genetic factors as seen in many international studies, and a few hospital-based studies from India. For example, a family history of psychiatric illness was seen in about 40 % of child and adolescent sample with mood disorders (Sagar et al. 2012).

There is a dearth of large-scale systematic studies exploring population-based risk factors for adolescent psychiatric disorders. In a large community-based sample from Goa, the following emerged as significant risk factors associated with adolescent mental disorders (Pillai et al. 2008):

- residence in urban areas
- an outgoing 'non-traditional' lifestyle (frequent partying, going to the cinema, shopping for fun and having a boyfriend or girlfriend)

- difficulties with studies
- lack of safety in the neighbourhood
- gender discrimination
- a history of physical or verbal abuse
- tobacco use.

Among higher secondary school-going adolescents ($n = 811$; average age of 16 years), nearly one-third reported experiencing some form of sexual abuse over past 12 months and 6 % reported experiencing forced sex. Both boys and girls reported experiencing sexual abuse. These adolescents had significantly poorer academic performance, poorer mental and physical health, greater substance abuse, poorer parental relationships and higher rates of consensual sexual behaviours (Patel and Andrew 2001).

Runaway adolescents were found to have high hopelessness, depression, suicidal attempts, and history of physical and sexual abuse, substance use and behavioural problems. Such vulnerable groups of adolescents are at risk of suffering from a wide array of mental health problems (Khurana et al. 2004).

Some of the psychosocial factors which are especially relevant in context of psychological health of Indian adolescents have been discussed below:

6.1 Family Factors

Having one's family as the primary source of social support is associated with lower prevalence of mental disorders (Pillai et al. 2008). In traditional societies, the joint family system ensures a strong role of extended family members in the upbringing of children. In the past few decades, several socio-economic changes such as urbanisation, migration and consumerism have contributed to an increase in nuclear families, and if sufficient parental attention is not paid to them, adolescents may face loneliness and isolation. In general, the emotional unavailability of parents is likely to have long-term psychological consequences in the form of low self-esteem and vulnerability to depression.

In a large school-based sample (13–15 years), high levels of parental involvement (indicated by regular homework checking, parental understanding of their child's problems, and parental knowledge of their child's free-time activities) was significantly associated with better mental health. Adolescents with more parental involvement were less likely to have loneliness, insomnia due to anxiety, sadness and hopelessness (Hasumi et al. 2012).

6.2 School/Academic Factors

Overall, the education in India is a tremendously competitive field, though recently some measures have been taken to change the educational system. A high level of stress is frequently seen among students, and even parents, as a result of unrealistically high academic targets set for students. The parental pressure to over-perform, or enormous expectations from an adolescent in secondary or higher secondary classes, is a frequently seen stressor in clinical practice. The term 'examination' was found to be a fairly common life event predating the onset of depression in school-going adolescents visiting the child and adolescent clinic at the All India Institute of Medical Sciences (AIIMS), New Delhi especially in the months of February and March when the semester ends in most schools (Garg 2004). Headache was observed to a common presentation among adolescents who are high achievers in school, with rigid and perfectionistic traits in another study from the same institute (Kayal 2006). At times, adolescents may struggle hard to be a topper in order to seek parental approval. Constant comparison between siblings and parental affection conditional on the adolescent's achievement promotes an unhealthy competition between the siblings and acts as a stressor.

6.3 Life Events and Stressors

Adolescents with psychopathology report significantly more stressful life events compared to healthy counterparts (Patel et al. 2008). An identifiable stressor or life event was reported by 50 % of the younger sample (mean age: 13.68 ± 2.53 years) with mood disorders presenting to the child and adolescent clinic of the AIIMS (Sagar et al. 2012). These were as follows (in decreasing order of frequency): illness or death of a family member, interpersonal conflicts, academic stressors like failure in examination, and change of residence or school. Parental divorce is a common stressor seen in clinics in urban settings, which may translate to peer rejection, low self-esteem, and change of school or residence, all of which may pose additional stress. The gender atypical behaviour in adolescence may lead to inner conflicts and parental or societal disapproval. The adolescent coming to terms with homosexual orientation may feel rejected and lonely and may be at a greater risk for substance use, depression and suicide (Russell and Joyner 2001). The socio-economic stressors faced by adolescents in India such as parental unemployment or poverty may lead to chronic stress among adolescents.

6.4 Lifestyle Issues and Concerns

Several lifestyle-related issues (eating behaviours, sexual behaviours and substance use) may have the potential to impact the physical as well as mental health of adolescents. In a large sample of 1,500 adolescents, inappropriate dietary practices (fast food consumption, cold drinks, low fruit and vegetable intake), sedentary activities, irregular sleeping habits, less religiosity, milder activity pattern, unhealthy daily routine and pursuance of different forms of risk behaviours were commonly seen (Singh and Mishra 2012). Between 10 and 30 % of school-going adolescents in India are overweight and nearly 5 % have obesity. It is especially more among adolescents from parts of Punjab, Maharashtra, Delhi, and south India, and among affluent urban adolescents. (National Family Health Survey-3 2007; Srihari et al. 2007; Singhal et al. 2010; Mehta et al. 2007). The prevalence of some form of sexual activity or contact varies between 8 and 30 % among adolescent boys and 6–15 % of adolescent girls

(Shashikumar Ramadugu et al. 2011; Lakshmi et al. 2007). Four per cent of males and 1 % of females reported sexual intercourse (Lakshmi et al. 2007). Adolescents having unfriendly relationship with parents had higher likelihood of sex initiation, and those who reported sexual abuse, sexually transmitted disease symptoms, smoking and those who had not read scientific literature on reproductive and sexual health were more likely to have initiated sex from an early age (Sahay et al. 2013). A number of health problems may arise from risky behaviours, such as sexual activity and substance abuse initiated from an early age. Irregular dietary practices, being overweight and early initiation of sex or substance use, may influence the psychological health of the adolescent population in addition to increasing the likelihood of physical disorders.

It is also important to keep in mind that some of the abnormal adolescent behaviours or lifestyles might represent just the extreme end of normal distribution, and there may be difficulty in labelling them as pathological. It is better to take into account the normative peer behaviours, and the familial and socio-cultural context to seek a better understanding of mental health problems of adolescents.

7 Adolescent Psychiatric Disorders: Indian Studies

7.1 Behavioural Disorders with Onset in Childhood (Attention Deficit Disorders, Conduct Disorder)

Some disorders with onset during childhood may extend into adolescence and beyond. Such disorders may interfere with the normal psychological development, social skills acquisition, academic performance and adjustment at school.

Attention-deficit/hyperactivity disorder (ADHD) is a common and chronic condition requiring long-term management. While hyperactivity often subsides during early adolescence, but inattention may continue to persist. Most Indian studies on ADHD have, however, focussed only on samples of children. Few adolescents, even if included, were not described separately in terms of phenomenology, co-morbidity or management. A comparative study of DSM IV and ICD-10 criteria for diagnosing attention deficit disorders found that while there was a significant overlap between the two, the ICD-10 criteria could diagnose only 70 % of the children and adolescents in contrast to 100 % in case of DSM IV (Sitholey and Agarwal 2012). In another study on comorbidity, 13.5 % children and adolescents with ADHD also had comorbid bipolar disorder (Sivakumar et al. 2013). There is also an increased likelihood of progression to substance use disorders beginning from an early age among those with ADHD (Sringeri 2008). A 6-month outcome of children and adolescents with ADHD on treatment was assessed in a prospective study. The SDQ revealed significant reduction in total difficulty score, the conduct problem sub-scale and peer relationship problem score. Significant improvement in severity of ADHD and academic and psychosocial functioning is possible in ADHD (Deb et al. 2011).

The prevalence of the conduct disorder varies from 7 to 11 % during childhood in most studies and is more common in boys. The ratio of male to female conduct disorders is lower for the adolescent-onset type than for the childhood-onset type (Shastri et al. 2010).

Children and adolescents with conduct disorder are at increased risk of developing antisocial personality disorder and psychopathy later in life. A biological study from India sought to investigate whether any developmental abnormalities are present in the uncinate fasciculus of younger individuals (27 adolescents and 16 healthy controls) with conduct disorder using DT-MRI tractography (Sarkar et al. 2013). Participants in the conduct disorder group had a history of serious aggressive and violent behaviour, including robbery, burglary, grievous bodily harm and sexual assault. Adolescents with conduct disorder had a significantly increased fractional anisotropy and reduced perpendicular diffusivity, in the left uncinate fasciculus. The study concluded that the adolescents with conduct disorder have significant differences in the 'connectivity' and maturation of uncinate fasciculus.

7.2 Mood Disorders Adolescents with Depression

7.2.1 Depression

Adolescent depression shows discernible changes from childhood depression in terms of prevalence, gender differences and phenomenology (Pattanayak et al. 2012; Das 2003). The prevalence rates of depression show an increase from childhood (1–2 %) to adolescence with a cumulative probability of 10–20 % by late adolescence, which is same as adult rates. The rates of depression which are similar across both genders in children are almost twice in adolescent females compared to adolescent males. Certain depressive symptoms, e.g. subjectively depressed mood, hopelessness, guilt, atypical and melancholic symptoms are typically reported by adolescents with depression, rather than depressed children. There is a higher risk of suicidal attempts or completion among adolescents compared to children with depression. Approximately, 40–90 % adolescents with depression have a comorbid psychiatric disorder, which includes anxiety disorders, conduct disorders, substance abuse and personality disorders in case of adolescents and hyperactive and conduct disorders in childhood (Pattanayak et al. 2012; Das 2003). The issue of aetiological continuity versus discontinuity in childhood, adolescent and adult depression remains debatable. Depression and stress are prevalent in school-going adolescents, especially among girls. Further, it was found to be associated with a number of significant life events over past one year of the adolescent's life (Bhasin et al. 2010). Few studies have attempted to assess depression in adolescents who are school dropouts. About 11 % of school dropouts had severe and extreme grades of depression on Beck's Depression Inventory (BDI) in contrast to 3 % among school-going adolescents (Nair et al. 2004). Depression during the formative adolescent years may lead to several adverse long-term consequences. The levels of depression, stress and anxiety were inversely related to academic performance (Bhasin et al. 2010). Proper identification of depression is crucial to early management and prevention of suicidal risk. The psychometric properties of the BDI and Children Depression Rating Scale-Revised (CDRS-R) were found to be satisfactory for use among Indian adolescent subjects visiting primary-care and paediatric settings. Basker et al. (2007a, b) and Russell et al. (2012) compared the diagnostic accuracy of a self-rated (BDI) and a clinician-rated (CDRS-R) measure of depression in Indian adolescents across three schools. While BDI was found to have a better sensitivity, CDRS-R had a better specificity. It might be prudent to use both these instrument simultaneously to improve the identification of depression in primary-care settings, including school or college health clinics. Not much research is available on course or outcome of adolescent depression in India.

7.2.2 Bipolar Disorder/Mania

Few available studies have assessed the profile, comorbidity and course of adolescent bipolar disorder. Reddy et al. (1997) sought to examine the clinical profile of mania in bipolar disorder in a sample of 21 children and adolescents. The most common symptoms were pressure of speech, irritability, elation, distractibility, increased self-esteem, expansive mood, flight of ideas and grandiose delusions, which appeared to be more or less similar to adult mania. Additionally, 61 % had delusions and/or hallucinations. No subject had comorbid attention-deficit hyperactivity disorder (ADHD) in this study, but as many as 25 % of child and adolescent subjects with bipolar disorder had comorbid ADHD in another study from north India (Sivakumar et al. 2013). Anxiety disorders are another common comorbidity in early onset bipolar disorder. Among the 46 adolescent subjects with remitted bipolar disorder, the prevalence of current and lifetime anxiety disorders was 28 and 41 %, respectively. Compared with others, adolescents with anxiety had more lifetime suicidal ideation, more number of episodes, lower physical, psychosocial, and total subjective quality of life, and lower global functioning. Anxiety disorders were associated with a poorer course and low functioning in bipolar disorder. Prompt recognition and treatment of anxiety disorders in mood disorders are important for comprehensive management. Ratheesh et al. (2011), Srinath (1998) conducted a study to assess the course and predictors in early onset bipolar disorder. A total of 30 subjects in childhood and adolescence were assessed systematically at baseline and 4–5 years later. All subjects had recovered from their index episodes and none exhibited chronicity, however, two-thirds had relapsed, mostly within 2 years of recovery from index episodes. No specific predictors of recovery and relapse could be identified. The study implied that in view of the high rates of relapse in the crucial developmental phase of a young individual, long-term maintenance medication should be considered in juvenile bipolar patients, even if it is a first episode (Srinath 1998). Family stressors such as parental substance use, marital discord and lower socio-economic status are associated with poor treatment response (Kayal 2006).

7.3 Suicide and Self Harm

Suicide is a leading cause of death among young people in India. One of the earliest papers on suicidal attempts among student population was by Venkoba Rao (1972) who described 35 young people with attempted suicide, of which seven attempts proved fatal. In a study evaluating the cause of death among those aged 10–19 years in a rural population of 108,000 in south India, suicide accounted for about a quarter of all deaths in boys and between 50 and 75 % of all deaths in girls. The average suicide rate for girls was 148 per 100,000 and for boys, 58 per 100,000 (Aaron et al. 2004). These rates are one of the highest for young population across the world.

Most studies from India have found that about 4–16 % of adolescents have suicidal ideation and nearly 0.4–5 % have attempted suicide (Arun 2009; Pillai et al. 2009; Sharma et al. 2008). Females had higher prevalence of suicidal thoughts and attempts compared to male adolescents. A retrospective analysis of 222 cases of suicidal deaths in age group 10–18 found that the commonest age group was 15–18 years in both the sexes and most common method was hanging (57 % in girls, 49.5 % in boys) followed by poisoning (Lalwani et al. 2004). Adolescent suicidal behaviour is associated with female gender, premarital sex, physical abuse at home, lifetime experience of sexual abuse, probable common mental disorders, psychological distress, academic incompetence, mother's working status and peer relationship problems (Pillai et al. 2009; Sharma et al. 2008).

Adolescent who attempted suicide had significantly higher levels of depression, hopelessness, lethality of event and stressful life events compared to adults (Sudhirkumar 2000). Poor impulse control, childhood trauma and life events are also commonly seen in association with adolescent suicide behaviours. The common life events preceding suicidal attempts are mostly failure in examinations, anticipated punishment and impending loss of love or romantic relationship, among others (Jena and Siddhartha 2004). A recent study by Nair et al. (2013) sought to characterise the need and identify the predictive factors for preventive consultation or hospitalisation for adolescent suicide in a rural community setting. Of the 500 adolescents, 2 and 0.6 % required emergency consultation and hospitalisation, respectively. Males needed more preventive action. Age, gender, and presence of anxiety or depressive disorder independently predicted a need for protective action and, together contributed to a parsimonious predictive model. More such studies assessing the preventive strategies implemented at a community level and identifying vulnerable individuals are needed.

7.4 Neurotic, Stress Related and Somatoform Disorders

7.4.1 Anxiety Disorders

Anxiety disorders are commonly encountered among adolescent population. Deb and Walsh (2010) assessed anxiety among a group of 460 adolescents (aged 13–17 years) from Kolkata using the State-trait Anxiety Inventory. Results show that anxiety was highly prevalent in the sample with 20 % of boys and 18 % of girls having high anxiety levels. Anxiety was significantly associated with following being a boy, studying in Bengali medium schools, belonging to middle socio-economic class (middle socio-economic group) and having working mothers. Results also show that a substantial proportion of the adolescents perceived they did not receive quality time from fathers (32.1 %) and mothers (21.3 %) and did not feel comfortable sharing their personal issues with their parents. Social withdrawal in adolescents is also thought to emanate from fear or social anxiety, though recent study by Bower and Raja (2011) observed that it is best conceptualized as a multifaceted construct.

7.4.2 Chronic Headache

Chronic headache is a frequent cause of distress for adolescents, often prompting them to seek medical or paediatric consultations. Many a times, the chronic headache is associated with psychological or psychiatric, rather than medical reasons. Chronic headaches of all kinds and not just due to somatoform pain disorder are discussed here. In a clinic-based study on phenomenology of chronic daily headache in Indian children and adolescents, majority had a more or less specified time of onset of regular headache spells. In all patients, phenomenology of headache included a significant vascular component. Heightened level of anxiety mostly related to academic stress and achievement was noted in the majority (Chakravarty 2005). Presence of high ambitions, perfectionist traits and need to succeed were observed in the adolescents with migrainous headaches (70 %) and tension type headaches (47 %). Parents also had high expectations of academic achievement from these adolescents (Mehta 2002).

In a large-scale study of 2,235 adolescents, 58 % reported having recurrent headaches in past one year (Gupta et al. 2009). Migraine was the most prevalent type of headache (17.2 %), followed by unspecified type of headache (15 %), and tension type of headache (11 %). Average age of onset of headache was 11.33 years, and it was progressive in 37 % since its onset. Family history of headache was common in adolescents with headache. Headache was more prevalent in higher grades and among girls. In another study from Delhi, headache types seen in adolescents were migraine, tension-type headache and unspecified headache, in that order. Stress was seen to be a major precipitant in 40 % of headaches irrespective of type. Majority had been suffering for 1–2 years before taking a formal consultation (Mishra 2013). Stress management techniques may help in effective prevention and control of triggers for headache.

7.4.3 Post-traumatic Stress Disorder

Psychological responses to disasters in adolescents vary widely across cultures. A study of adolescents ($n = 447$) after the Orissa super-cyclone found that a majority had psychological symptoms. Post-traumatic stress disorder (PTSD) was present in 30.6 %, and an additional 13.6 % had sub-syndromal PTSD. Parents and teachers reported mental health concerns in only 7 %. The study demonstrated that PTSD is a valid clinical construct among adolescents in an Indian set-up and, though highly prevalent, may be missed without clinical screening (Kar et al. 2007). About a year after a super-cyclone, psychiatric presentations in adolescents were a conglomeration of PTSD (27 %), depression (17.6 %) and anxiety symptoms (12 %). The proportion of adolescents with any diagnosis was 37.9 %, and comorbidity was seen in 39.0 % of them. Prolonged periods of helplessness and lack of adequate post-disaster psychological support were perceived as probable influencing factors, as well as the severity of the disaster (Kar and Bastia 2006). In a post-tsunami study of adolescents from the Andaman and Nicobar Islands, Math et al. assessed adolescent survivors using the MINI International Neuropsychiatric Interview (MINI). The most common psychiatric morbidities observed among the primary and secondary survivors were adjustment disorder, depression, panic disorder and PTSD, among other disorders (Math et al. 2008). Available research highlights the need for identification and intervention for post-disaster psychiatric morbidities in adolescent survivors. Low cost, community-based culture-sensitive models should be developed for use in disaster affected areas.

7.4.4 Obsessive Compulsive Disorders (OCD)

There is very little research on phenomenology, course or treatment of adolescents with OCD. In a study of 54 adolescents with OCD, comorbidity was found in 69 % of the sample: 22 % were diagnosed with disruptive disorders; 20 % met criteria for mood disorders; 19 % had anxiety disorders; and 17 % had tic disorders (Reddy et al. 2000).

7.4.5 Eating Disorders

Eating disorders have not been captured in any of the community or school surveys and are uncommon in clinical settings in India. There is a perception that eating disorders are more likely to be prevalent in Western cultures and may not be as common in Asian cultures. It is also possible that the disorder differs somewhat in its clinical manifestation among Non-Western cultures. Few case reports or series have described symptoms or management of patients with eating disorders from India (Mendhekar et al. 2009; Khandelwal et al. 1995; Basker et al. 2013). A recent study a tertiary-care clinic in north India has described the period prevalence (2001–2006) of eating disorders as 1.25 % among clinic population less than 18 years of age (Basker et al. 2013). Psychogenic vomiting (85.4 %) was fairly common in these patients, and only six patients (14.6 %) with anorexia nervosa were noted.

In a descriptive series of seven adolescent patients with eating disorders, there were three boys and four girls. Diagnosis could be made in all of them using standard criteria. Five of them were managed in in-patient setting with nutritional rehabilitation and family-based therapy. Four patients who had strong family support recovered (Mammen et al. 2007). A multidisciplinary approach to treatment appears to be essential for a good outcome.

7.5 Schizophrenia and Psychotic Disorders

Schizophrenia has been considered to be a neurodevelopmental disorder and typically has an onset in late adolescence or among youth. Adolescent psychosis is rare in community surveys, though it is relatively more common in clinic populations. The clinic prevalence of schizophrenia and psychotic disorders among those visiting child and adolescent clinic, AIIMS over a two-year period was 2.5 % (mean age: 14.17 ± 1.07 years) (Mammen et al. 2007). Acute transient psychoses was commonest diagnosis followed by schizophrenia, other and unspecified psychotic disorders

The clinical presentation of psychosis is likely to be age, development and possibly culture specific and merits a further research attention. Hallucinations were commonest symptoms (auditory 56.5 %; visual 17.4 %) followed by persecutory delusions

(26.1 %) in the clinic sample of early onset psychosis. One-third had long-standing academic difficulties and one-third had comorbid psychiatric disorder. Family history of psychiatric illness was present in 30 % of sample (Pattanayak et al. 2010). In the first ever SPECT study of early onset schizophrenia from India, a sample with onset at or before 14 years of age was examined (mean age of onset: 12.4 ± 1.4 years) and compared with healthy controls. Patients had perfusion anomalies in the left temporal, frontal and parietal areas and also showed impaired executive functioning on neuropsychological assessments (Malhotra et al. 2006). There is a minimal data on the use of electroconvulsive therapy (ECT) in adolescents from India. But available data show safety and efficacy of its use. This is especially important in the context of recent Mental Health Care Bill in India which prohibits use of ECT in population below 18 years of age. In a sample of 25 adolescents (aged 13–18 years) who received ECT treatment at a tertiary care-centre, catatonic symptoms (68 %) were the most common. An average of 10 ECTs was administered per patient (range: 2–21). Response rates varied between 77 % and 92 % according to diagnosis, indicating that ECT is effective in the treatment of severe psychiatric disorders in adolescents (Grover et al. 2013).

7.6 Substance Abuse

Community surveys suggest that tobacco and alcohol are prevalent substances of abuse among Indian adolescents. The Global Youth Tobacco Survey (Global Youth Tobacco Survey: India 2009) was conducted on a large sample of school-going adolescents ($n = 10{,}112$) aged between 13 and 15 years found that 14.6 % of adolescents were currently using any tobacco product. The finding from a systematic review of studies published in India between 1991 and 2007 also indicate that the median prevalence of tobacco ever use among school-going adolescents in India is quite high (18 %) (Pal and Tsering 2009). In the National Household Survey, 21 % of the subsample was between 12 and 18 years of age ($n = 8{,}587$). (Ray 2004) Of total adolescent sample, 3.4 % were current alcohol users, 0.6 % cannabis users and 0.1 % opioid users. Adolescents constitute only a small percentage of treatment seekers in drug dependence treatment settings ($\leq$ 15 years: 0.4 % and 16–20 years: 4.6 %). Among the adolescents who were in contact with *Nehru Yuva Kendras* across the country, use of heroin was seen in 3.3 % of the adolescents using drugs. Potentially serious complications such as sexual risks, violence and other high-risk behaviours were reported in association with adolescent substance use, which may pose a significant public health problem (Ray 2004). In a 25 year chart review from a tertiary-care clinic settings, the commonest substance of abuse was opioids (76.2 %), of which heroin was reported by 36 % of patients (Saluja et al. 2007). Mean age at first use of the primary substance was 14.8 years and mean age at first presentation was 17 years. About one-fifth (21.2 %) of the subjects indulged in high-risk behaviours such as having sexual intercourse with multiple sexual partners. Nearly half of the subjects had positive family history of either drug dependence (40.2 %) or psychiatric disorder (5.5 %). Few studies or reports are available on the drug use among street children in India (Ray et al. 2009; Benegal et al. 2013) and those admitted to juvenile observation homes

(Pagare et al. 2004). Substance use was a common phenomenon in this vulnerable population and at times and was reported to be necessary for survival on streets. Inhalant use is especially common in a large majority as it is cheap and easily accessible. An intervention based on life skills money management and building self-esteem delivered on streets by means of various activities in six sessions was developed, tested and found effective in improving some of the aspects (Ray et al. 2010). Inhalant use has also been reported by children or adolescents who are out of school but living with their families, and also among those who are school-going students (Ningombam et al. 2011). Some studies have described the clinical profile of users of inhalants seeking treatment at tertiary-care settings (Kumar et al. 2008; Verma et al. 2011a, b). Although biochemical and haematological abnormalities have been described in literature, but these were not seen in treatment seeking users of inhalants from India (Quraishi et al. 2014). Comorbid psychiatric disorders are common especially with early onset substance use. More externalising problems were present, and internalising problems were also present, though to a lesser extent. A substantial percentage of adolescents using substances had conduct disorder (48–73.3 %), ADHD (16.6–17.4 %) and learning disorders in some of them. Further, high-risk behaviours were seen in over 10 %, while cognitive impairments were noticed in inhalants users. Low self-esteem and inadequate coping skills, poor social and family functioning and impaired communication skills were frequently noticed, which showed some improvement after administration of the treatment module developed as part of the study.

8 Adolescent Service Delivery Models and Interventions: Indian Research

Few researchers have attempted to develop and test various models for service delivery aimed at adolescent health, including mental health. Schools are important places for prevention, promotion and early identification of common mental health problems or stressors. Prof. Malvika Kapur has worked extensively towards the development of school mental health programmes using only limited resources and trained personnel. A descriptive and experiential account has been provided on various issues, e.g. process of designing a programme, identification of teachers as counsellors, specific strategies of counselling and training of teachers (Kapur 1997). A model of health promotion among adolescents using life skills approach in secondary schools has been described by Bharath and Kumar (2010). The model uses experiential learning with peers using participatory methods, thereby enabling the adolescent with psychosocial skills. The school infrastructure and teachers are involved for its implementation as a co-curricular activity for maximum effect. It covers nearly 55,000 adolescents in secondary schools across four districts in Karnataka. The adolescents in the programme had significantly better self-esteem, perceived adequate coping and better adjustment in general, and specifically with teachers, in school, and pro-social behaviour. Compared to dispensary-based adolescent health clinics, utilisation was significantly higher in a school-based clinics, particularly for psychosocial problems (which were fairly common) relative to medical problems (Kumar et al. 2008). It may be worthwhile to explore the service delivery models described in context of adolescent reproductive and sexual health. Psychological and behavioural issues figured prominently in these settings. A school-based intervention on 'health education' covered basic issues pertaining to adolescent health, sexual education, pubertal changes and psychological problems usually encountered during adolescence led to an improvement in knowledge among adolescent girls (Das et al. 2010). A significant improvement in positive attitudes was also observed with regard to substance abuse in the adolescent period.

Naik et al. (2013) described the development of a community (*taluk* hospital)-based approach for adolescent care and counselling services, as a part of the initiatives for adolescent health and sexual health. These clinics were well utilised with 1,588 adolescents visiting them over a two-year period. Apart from medical and reproductive problems, psychosocial problems ranged from minor anxieties, sadness and adjustment problems to psychiatric disorders. In another study by same researchers, (Nair et al. 2012) an intervention in the form of 'family life and life skills education package' was delivered across 103 higher secondary schools in a district. Consistent improvement in knowledge was seen six months after intervention. Many randomised-controlled trials from low- and middle-income countries have found a host of treatment approaches to show some efficacy among adolescents with mental health problems (Nair et al. 2012). These include culture-specific coping mechanisms, mind–body skills (including meditation and breathing techniques), cognitive behaviour therapy delivered by lay counsellors in low-resource environments. Some of them have described working with the family members as part of intervention and some others have used an eclectic mix of narrative, creative, social and cognitive approaches. While some or all of the above may be useful in Indian settings, there is a need to conduct the research to examine their efficacy and feasibility in Indian settings.

Some of the research pertaining to development of psychological interventions for adolescents has been done at Department of Psychiatry, AIIMS. A cognitive behaviour therapy (CBT)-based treatment module was developed by Sharma et al. (unpublished) to treat adolescents with substance use with behaviour problems. Another CBT module, currently being developed as part of a department thesis, focuses on anger management among school-going adolescents (Pandey et al. unpublished). A coping skills module based on principles of CBT was developed by Chugh et al. (unpublished) and found to be effective in decreasing scores of internalising and externalising problems in school-going adolescents. Results also showed an increase in competencies of adolescents, e.g. positive expression to cope with anger, problem solving, self-efficacy and social skills. Novel interventions such as computer-assisted interventions may be employed especially for urban adolescents. One such computer-assisted cognitive behaviour therapy (CBT) for adolescents with depression is being developed at Department of Psychiatry, AIIMS (Srivastava et al. 2013).

9 Adolescent Mental Health Care: Current Status and Future Directions

Mental health problems affect 10–20 % of adolescents worldwide. Despite their relevance, adolescent mental health needs have been neglected in policies, especially in low- and middle-income countries. In India, adolescent mental health clinics are limited to only a handful of academic centres and tertiary-care hospitals in India. The sub-optimal functioning of the primary-care system and inadequate inter-sectoral linkages add up to the treatment gap. There is a tremendous scarcity of human resources for mental health (0.2 psychiatrists, 0.05 psychiatric nurses as well as 0.03 psychologists and social workers per 100,000 population), (Thirunavukarasu and Thirunavukarasu 2010) leading to a slow pace of growth for most psychiatric sub-specialties. In order to strengthen child and adolescent mental health care in a country, it should be supported by the necessary policies, programmes, legislations, therapeutic drug policy, substance abuse policy, budget, primary-care system, training programmes and service delivery system (Russell et al. 2012). However, most of this is currently lacking in Indian context, even though a few positive initiatives have been taken recently. Some issues discussed in the context of child psychiatry and child mental health services hold true for adolescent mental health as well, and those shall not be discussed in detail here. Following are some of the steps needed to promote adolescent mental health in the clinical services, research and policies of the country:

9.1 General

- Lack of uniformity or consensus in the age parameter for defining the group of adolescents is a major impediment in gathering homogenous data from various studies (which have used variable cut-offs of 14, 16, 18 or 19 years). Adolescents are most often subsumed with either children (0–14 years of age) or youth (15–24 years of age). Different policies and programmes define the adolescents' age group differently. For example, the Constitution of India and labour laws consider people up to the age of 14 as children, whereas the Reproductive and Child Health Programme mentions adolescents as being between 10 and 19 years of age, while psychiatric services consider 12–18 years as adolescents. Internationally, the age group of 10–19 years is considered to be the age of adolescence as per the WHO definition. Such heterogeneity hinders the generation of prevalence data and information on various aspects of mental health in adolescents.

9.2 Research

- Studies exclusively focusing on adolescent mental health problems are a recent phenomenon in India. Adolescents are distinct from children as well as adults in terms of psychological, emotional, development and social issues. A separate emphasis on different aspects of adolescent mental health should be reflected while designing a particular study or presenting the findings.

- In terms of the volume of literature, adolescent mental health studies few and far between. Most of the information on phenomenology, comorbidity or management is available from only a few studies. There is a need to fuel the research on adolescents in the Indian context, especially focusing on areas which are culturally more relevant.
- Course and outcome studies are universally lacking in Indian adolescent research. There is a need to plan larger, multi-site longitudinal studies across the country to know the culture-specific prognostic factors, if any, and outcome in Indian adolescents.
- There is a dearth of tools and instruments in adolescent mental health which are suitably translated and validated for use in Indian settings. There is also a need to develop culture-specific instruments of assessment, incorporating the *emic* items.
- There is a need to develop low-cost models of intervention, which can be delivered by teachers, school counsellors or health workers across various settings. These interventions should focus on development of life skills, coping resources, stress management and relaxation and early detection and referral for mental disorders.
- Cost effectiveness of various school or community-based approaches needs to be assessed, which is important to guide decisions related to large-scale implementation.
- Families and parents have an important role to play in the care of adolescents. Unlike many Western countries, Indian culture promotes the dependence and reliance on family members throughout adolescence and early youth. So far, the research on adolescent mental health has not taken the family member's perspective into account. There is a need to examine the ways in which family support can be utilised as a resource for promotion of mental health of adolescents. Many adolescents with psychological distress report stress as a result of conflict with parents, and effective communication strategies can be targeted as part of family interventions in such adolescents.

9.3 Service Development

- Strengthening of the primary-care system through the District Mental Health Programme shall go a long way to improve the current mental health situation. The upcoming Five Year Plan aims to upscale the District Mental Health Programme to include every single district in the country. In the future, it shall eventually lead to a more available, accessible and affordable system of mental health care for all, including the adolescent population.
- Integration and linkage of child and adolescent mental health with paediatric practice: There is a need to develop more effective linkages with paediatricians and paediatric services across the country, which can focus on the effective screening and management of priority mental health disorders in children and adolescents. The two-tier diagnostic approach of using a screening measure (e.g. the Child Behaviour Checklist), followed by confirmation using reference standard clinical criterion may be used in paediatric settings.
- School and college mental health promotion can be done using the available resources (teachers. Counsellors and school infrastructure) and some of the

components, e.g. life skills education can be an integral component of the curriculum from early years. While many such initiatives have been taken in various states, but there is a need to provide support and increase the coverage of the schools and districts in the country.

- Capacity building and training of manpower: Various categories of professionals such as school counsellors, teachers, educators, physicians, paediatricians and nurses can be trained in relevant aspects. The 'training-of-trainers' can facilitate regular training programmes for building manpower resources for adolescent mental health promotion and preventive activities.
- Inter-sectoral linkages: As adolescent mental health problems occur in a wider psychosocial context, there is a need to develop effective inter-sectoral linkages with the educational system, the legal and juvenile justice system, social welfare and voluntary organisations and non-governmental organisations. There is a need for more effective linkage of adolescent mental health with the National Rural Health Mission and the Reproductive and Child Health Programme.
- Adolescents are generally considered to be a relatively disease-free group; however, some of the lifestyles and patterns of risky behaviours (e.g. substance use or unsafe sex) which are initiated during adolescence have implications on their present and future health. In this regard, there is a need to have a countrywide initiative to reduce or delay the onset of substance use. There is an important role for brief interventions in adolescents engaged in risky behaviours such as driving under influence. There is also a need to have multi-modal interventions, including promotion of awareness and effective law enforcement.

9.4 Policy

- Only recently, steps have been taken to develop a mental health policy in the country. There is no child and adolescent mental health policy so far. A mental health policy specifically for younger population is crucial in order to provide a developmental framework to enhance mental health resources and guide adequate development of services, advocacy, and proper access to care, prevention, promotion and appropriate budget allocation.

10 Conclusions

Adolescents comprise 22 % of Indian population, yet very little attention has been paid to the mental health issues in this age group. Between 20 and 45 % of school-going adolescents appear to have psychological problems, and 1.8–9.6 % of the adolescents appear to have a diagnosable mental disorder as per the available surveys. The major psychiatric disorders continue to be under-researched in adolescents. There are several deficits in services, manpower and no country—specific policy to address child and adolescent mental health. There is a need to develop more research evidence on psychiatric or psychological problems of adolescents and to focus on the development of low-cost interventions to promote adolescent mental health. Effective integration and linkages across various sectors will go a long way to promote adolescent mental health. There is an urgent need for a child and adolescent mental health policy, which can act as a developmental framework to enhance mental health resources for adolescents.

References

Aaron, R., Joseph, A., Abraham, S., Muliyil, J., George, K., Prasad, J., et al. (2004). Suicides in young people in rural southern India. *The Lancet, 363*, 1117–1118.

Ahmad, A., Khalique, N., Khan, Z., & Amir, A. (2007). Prevalence of psychosocial problems among school going male adolescents. *Indian Journal of Community Medicine, 32*, 219–221.

Arun, Priti, & Chavan, B. S. (2009). Stress and suicidal ideas in adolescent students in Chandigarh. *Indian Journal of Medical Sciences, 63*, 281–287.

Basker, M. M., Mathai, S., Korula, S., & Mammen, P. M. (2013). Eating disorders among adolescents in a tertiary care centre in India. *Indian Journal of Pediatrics, 80*, 211–214.

Basker, M., Moses, P. D., Russell, S., Swamidhas, P., & Russell, P. S. S. (2007a). The psychometric properties of beck depression inventory for adolescent depression in a primary-care paediatric setting in India. *Child and Adolescent Psychiatry and Mental Health, 1*, 8. doi:10.1186/1753-2000-1-8.

Basker, M., Russell, P. S. S., Russell, S., & Moses, P. D. (2007b). Validation of child depression rating scale- revised for adolescents in a primary-care paediatric use in India. *Child and Adolescent Psychiatry and Mental Health, 1*, 8. doi:10.1186/1753-2000-1-8.

Benegal, V., Sheshadri, S. P., Chand, P. K., Lakshmana, G., Subodh, B. N. (2013). Inhalant use among street children in Bangalore (Part of WHO Biennium activity), NIMHANS, Bangalore. Available at: http://www.nimhans.kar.nic.in/cam/CAM/Drug_abuse_among_street_children.pdf. Accessed on May 17, 2013.

Bharath, S., & Kumar, K. K. (2010). Empowering adolescents with life skills education in schools—School mental health program: Does it work? *Indian Journal of Psychiatry, 52*, 344–349.

Bharath, S., Srinath, S., Seshadri, S., & Girimji, S. (1997). Child and adolescent psychiatry in-patient facility. *Indian Journal of Pediatrics, 64*, 829–832.

Bhasin, S. K., Sharma, R., & Saini, N. K. (2010). Depression, anxiety and stress among adolescent students belonging to affluent families: A School-based Study. *Indian Journal of Pediatrics, 77*, 161–165.

Birleson, P., & Luk, E. S. (1997). Continuing the debate on a separate adolescent psychiatry. *Australian and New Zealand Journal of Psychiatry, 31*, 447–451.

Bower, J. C., & Raja, R. (2011). Social withdrawal subtypes during early adolescence in India. *Journal of Abnormal Child Psychology, 39*, 201–212.

Census of India. (2001). *Office of registrar general and census Commissioner of India*. New Delhi: Ministry of Home Affairs. Government of India.

Chakravarty, A. (2005). Chronic daily headache in children and adolescents: A clinic based study from India. *Cephalalgia, 25*, 795–800.

Das, P., Pal, R., & Pal, S. (2010). Awareness on psychosomatic health among adolescent girls of three schools in north Kolkata. *Indian Journal of Psychiatry, 52*, 355–359.

Deb, K. S., Mittal, A., Sagar, R., Mehta, M. (2011). Effectiveness of treatment on psychosocial adjustment and academic outcome in children with Attention Deficit Hyperactivity Disorder (ADHD): A six month follow-up study. XIth Biennial Conference Indian Association for Child & Adolescent Mental Health. Nov 17–19, 2011.

Deb, S., & Walsh, K. (2010). Anxiety among high school students in India: Comparisons across gender, school type, social strata and perceptions of quality time with parents. *Australian Journal of Educational and Developmental Psychology, 10*, 18–31.

Global Youth Tobacco Survey: India 2009 Fact Sheet. Available at: http://www.who.int/fctc/reporting/Annexoneindia.pdf. Accessed on May 19, 2013.

Grover, S., Malhotra, S., Varma, S., Chakrabarti, S., Avasthi, A., & Mattoo, S. K. (2013). Electroconvulsive therapy in adolescents: A retrospective study from North India. *The Journal of ECT, 29*, 122–126.

Gupta, R., Bhatia, M. S., Dahiya, D., Sharma, S., Sapra, R., Semalti, K., et al. (2009). Recurrent headache in Indian adolescents. *Indian Journal of Pediatrics, 76*, 733–737.

Hasumi, T., Ahsan, F., Couper, C. M., Aguayo, J. L., & Jacobsen, K. H. (2012). Parental involvement and mental well-being of indian adolescents. *Indian Pediatrics, 49*, 915–918.

Jena, S., & Siddhartha, T. (2004). Non-fatal suicidal behaviors in adolescents. *Indian Journal of Psychiatry, 46*, 310–318.

Kapur, M. (1997). *Mental health in Indian schools*. New Delhi: Sage Publications.

Kar, N., & Bastia, B. K. (2006). Post-traumatic stress disorder, depression and generalised anxiety disorder in adolescents after a natural disaster: A study of comorbidity. *Clinical Practice Epidemiology in Mental Health, 26*(2), 17.

Kar, N., Mohapatra, P. K., Nayak, K. C., Pattanaik, P., Swain, S. P., & Kar, H. C. (2007). Post-traumatic stress disorder in children and adolescents one year after a super-cyclone in Orissa, India: Exploring cross-cultural validity and vulnerability factors. *BMC Psychiatry, 14*(7), 8.

Khandelwal, S. K., Sharan, P., & Saxena, S. (1995). Eating disorders: An Indian perspective. *International Journal of Social Psychiatry, 41*, 132–146.

Khurana, S., Sharma, N., Jena, S., Saha, R., & Ingle, G. K. (2004). Mental health status of runaway adolescents. *Indian Journal of Pediatrics, 71*, 405–409.

Klasen, H., & Crombag, A. C. (2013). What works where? A systematic review of child and adolescent mental health interventions for low and middle income countries. *Social Psychiatry and Psychiatric Epidemiology, 48*, 595–611.

Kumar, S., Grover, S., Kulhara, P., Mattoo, S. K., Basu, D., Biswas, P., et al. (2008a). Inhalant abuse: A clinic-based study. *Indian Journal of Psychiatry, 50*, 117–120.

Kumar, R., Prinja, S., & Lakshmi, P. V. M. (2008b). Health care seeking behavior of adolescents: Comparative study of two service delivery models. *Indian Journal of Pediatrics, 75*, 895–899.

Lakshmi, P. V. N., Gupta, N., & Kumar, R. (2007). Psychosocial predictors of adolescent sexual behavior. *Indian Journal of Pediatrics, 74*, 923–926.

Lalwani, S., Sharma, G. A. S. K., Kabra, S. K., Girdhar, S., & Dogra, T. D. (2004). Suicide among children and adolescents in South Delhi (1991–2000). *Indian Journal of Pediatrics, 71*, 701–703.

Malhotra, S., Biswas, P., Sharan, P., & Grover, S. (2007). Characteristics of patients visiting the child and adolescent psychiatric clinic: A 26-year study from North India. *Journal of Indian Association Child Adolescence and Mental Health, 3*, 53–60.

Malhotra, S., Gupta, N., Bhattacharya, A., & Kapoor, M. (2006). Study of childhood onset schizophrenia (COS) using SPECT and neuropsychological assessment. *Indian Journal of Psychiatry, 48*, 215–222.

Malhotra, S., Kohli, A., Kapoor, M., & Pradhan, B. (2009). Incidence of childhood psychiatric disorders in India. *Indian Journal of Psychiatry, 51*, 101–107.

Mammen, P., Russell, S., & Russell, P. S. (2007). Prevalence of eating disorders and psychiatric co-morbidity among children and adolescents. *Indian Pediatrics, 44*, 357–359.

Math, S. B., Tandon, S., & Nagaraja, D. (2008). Psychological impact of the tsunami on children and adolescents from the Andaman and Nicobar Islands. *Primary Care Companion to the Journal of Clinical Psychiatry, 10*, 31–37.

Mathers, C. (2009). Global burden of disease for women, children and adolescents. In J. E. Ehiri & M. M. Meremikwu (Eds.), *Global perspectives on maternal and child health*. New York: Springer.

Mehta, M., Bhasin, S. K., Agrawal, K., & Dwivedi, S. (2007). Obesity amongst affluent adolescent girls. *Indian Journal of Pediatrics, 74*, 619–622.

Mehta, M., Mukhim, E., & Sagar, R. (2002). Achievement motivation in adolescents with headache. *Abstracted in 10th World Congress on Pain* (p. 521). IASP Press.

Mehta, M., Pandav, C. S., & Pandey, P. (1991). Mental health problems in rural school children. *Indian Journal of Society Psychiatry, 7*, 32–39.

Mendhekar, D. N., Arora, K., Lohia, D., Aggarwal, A., & Jiloha, R. C. (2009). Anorexia nervosa: An Indian perspective. *National Medical Journal of India, 22*, 181–182.

Mishra, D., Sharma, A., Juneja, M., Singh, K. (2013). Profile of recurrent headache in pediatric outpatients at a public hospital in Delhi. *Indian Pediatrics*, E-pub ahead of print Apr 5, 2013; PII: S097475591200602.

Nagaraja, J., Parkash, S., & Sitholey, P. (2005). A study of pattern of child and adolescent psychiatric disorders (1981–1983). In Mental Health Research in India. Division of non-communicable diseases, Indian Council of Medical Research (ICMR). Available at: www.icmr.nic.in/publ/Mental%20Helth%20.pdf. Accessed on May 31, 2013.

Nair, M. K., Chacko, D. S., Indira, M. S., Siju, K. E., George, B., & Russell, P. S. (2012a). A primary care approach for adolescent care and counseling services. *Indian Journal of Pediatrics, 79*(Suppl 1), S79–S83.

Nair, M. K., Leena, M. L., George, B., Kasthuri, N., Chandramohan, K., & Russell, P. S. (2012b). School based adolescent care services: A district model. *Indian Journal of Pediatrics, 79*(Suppl 1), S11–S18.

Nair, M. K., Paul, M. K., & John, R. (2004). Prevalence of depression among adolescents. *Indian Journal of Pediatrics, 71*, 523–524.

Nair, M. K. C., Russell, P. S. S., Shankar, S. R., Subramaniam, V. S., Nazeema, S., Mammen, P., et al. (2013). Adolescent suicide: Characterizing the need and identifying the predictive factors for preventive consultation or hospitalization in a rural community setting. *International Journal of Adolescent Medicine and Health, 25*, 81–86.

Nandi, D. N., Banerjee, G., Mukherjee, S. P., Ghosh, A., Nandi, P. S., & Nandi, S. (2000). Psychiatry morbidity of a rural Indian community: Changes over a 20 year period. *The British Journal of Psychiatry, 176*, 351–356.

National Family Health Survey-3. (2007). International Institute for Population Sciences (IIPS) and Macro International. National Family Health Survey (NFHS-3), 2005–2006, India: Key Findings. Mumbai: IIPS.

Ningombam, S., Hutin, Y., & Murhekar, M. V. (2011). Prevalence and pattern of substance use among the higher secondary school students of Imphal, Manipur, India. *National Medical Journal of India, 24*, 11–15.

Pagare, D., Meena, G. S., Singh, M. M., & Saha, R. (2004). Risk factors of substance use among street children from Delhi, New Delhi. *Indian Pediatrics, 41*, 221–225.

Pal, R., & Tsering, D. (2009). Tobacco use in Indian high-school students. *International Journal of Green Pharmacy, 3*, 319–323.

Pataki, C. S. (2009). Adolescent development. In B. J. Sadock, V. A. Sadock, & P. Ruiz (Eds.), *Kaplan and Sadock's comprehensive textbook of psychiatry* (9th ed., pp. 3356–3365). Lippincott Williams and Wilkins: Philadephia.

Patel, V., & Andrew, G. (2001). Gender, sexual abuse and risk behaviours: A cross-sectional survey in schools in Goa. *National Medical Journal of India, 14*, 263–267.

Patel, V., Flisher, A. J., Nikapota, A., & Malhotra, S. (2008). Promoting child and adolescent mental health in low and middle income countries. *Journal of Child Psychology and Psychiatry, 49*, 313–334.

Pattanayak, R. D., & Mehta, M. (2012). Childhood and adolescent depression. In U. Nayar (Ed.), *International handbook on mental health of children & adolescents: Culture, Policy & Practices* (pp. 21–38), New Delhi: Sage Publications.

Pattanayak, R. D., Sagar, & R., Mehta, M. (2010). Clinical profile of early onset non affective psychosis patients (≤16 years) presenting at a tertiary care centre (abstract). In Proceedings of the international conference on schizophrenia, ICONS, SCARF, Oct 22–24, 2010.

Patton, G. (1996). An epidemiological case for a separate adolescent psychiatry? *Australian and New Zealand Journal of Psychiatry, 30*, 563–566.

Patton, G. (1998). Adolescent psychiatry: Its potential to reduce the burden of mental disorder. *European Archives of Psychiatry and Clinical Neuroscience, 248*, 1–3.

Pillai, A., Andrews, T., & Patel, V. (2009). Violence, psychological distress and the risk of suicidal behaviour in young people in India. *International Journal of Epidemiology, 38*, 459–469.

Pillai, A., Patel, V., Cardozo, P., Good man, R., Weiss, H. A., & Andrew, G. (2008). Non-traditional lifestyles and prevalence of mental disorders in adolescents in Goa, India. *The British Journal of Psychiatry, 192*, 45–51.

Premarajan, K. C., Danabalan, M., Chandrasekar, R., & Srinivasa, (1993). Prevalence of psychiatry morbidity in an urban community of Pondicherry. *Indian Journal of Psychiatry, 35*, 99–102.

Quraishi, R., Pattanayak, R. D., Dhawan, A., & Jain R. (2014). A descriptive study of clinical, hematological and biochemical parameters of inhalant users seeking treatment at a tertiary care centre in India. *Indian Journal of Psychological Medicine, 35*(2), 174–179.

Ramadugu, S., Ryali, V. Srivastava, K., Bhat P. S., & Prakash, J. (2011). Understanding sexuality among Indian urban school adolescents. *Industrial Psychiatry Journal, 20*, 49–55.

Rao, V. A. (1972). Attempted suicide and suicide among students in Madurai. *Indian Journal of Psychiatry, 14*, 389–397.

Ratheesh, A., Srinath, S., Reddy, Y. C., Girimaji, S. C., Seshadri, S. P., Thennarasu, K., et al. (2011). Are anxiety disorders associated with a more severe form of bipolar disorder in adolescents? *Indian Journal of Psychiatry, 53*, 312–318.

Ray, R. (2004). National survey on extent, pattern and trends of drug abuse in India. Ministry of social justice and empowerment and United Nations office on drug and crime regional office for South Asia.

Ray, R., Dhawan, A., Ambekar, A., Yadav, D., & Chopra, A. (2009). Inhalant use among street children in Delhi—A situation assessment. Developed under the Ministry of Health, Government of India and WHO Collaborative Programme. Report submitted to WHO, India.

Ray, R., Dhawan, A., Ambekar, A., Yadav, D., & Chopra, A. (2011). Co-ordination and convergence of Delhi district health services programmes and drug use intervention for the out of school child 2010–2011. National drug dependence treatment centre, All India Institute of Medical Sciences. Under Government of India and World Health Organization Collaborative Program (Biennium 2010–2011).

Reddy, B. S., Biswas, A., & Rao, H. (2011). Assessment of mental health of Indian adolescents studying in urban schools. *Malaysian Journal of Paediatrics and Child Health Online Early, 17*. Available from: http://mjpch.com/index.php/mjpch/article/view/276. Accessed on May 31, 2013.

Reddy, Y. C., Girimaji, S., & Srinath, S. (1997). Clinical profile of mania in children and adolescents from the Indian subcontinent. *Canadian Journal of Psychiatry, 42*, 841–846.

Reddy, Y. C., Reddy, P. S., Srinath, S., Khanna, S., Sheshadri, S. P., & Girimaji, S. C. (2000). Comorbidity in juvenile obsessive-compulsive disorder: A report from India. *Canadian Journal of Psychiatry, 45*, 274–278.

Roberts, R. E., Attkisson, C. C., & Rosenblatt, A. (1998). Prevalence of psychopathology among children and adolescents. *American Journal of Psychiatry, 155*, 715–725.

Russell, P. S., Basker, M., Russell, S., Moses, P. D., Nair, M. K. C., & Minju, K. A. (2012a). Comparison of a self-rated and a clinician-rated measure for identifying depression among adolescents in a primary-care setting. *Indian Journal of Pediatrics, 79*(Suppl 1), S45–S51.

Russell, S. T., & Joyner, K. (2001). Adolescent sexual orientation and suicide risk: Evidence from a national study. *American Journal of Public Health, 91*, 1276–1281.

Russell, P. S., Mammen, P., Nair, M. K., Russell, S., & Shankar, S. R. (2012b). Priority mental health disorders of children and adolescents in primary-care pediatric setting in India 1: Developing a child and adolescent mental health policy, program, and service model. *Indian Journal of Pediatrics, 79*(Suppl 1), S19–S26.

Sagar, R., Pattanayak, R. D., & Mehta, M. (2012). Clinical profile of pediatric mood disorders at a tertiary care centre. *Indian Pediatrics, 49*, 21–23.

Sahay, S., Nirmalkar, A., Sane, S., Verma, A., Reddy, S., & Mehendale, S. (2013). Correlates of sex initiation among school going adolescents in Pune, India. *Indian Journal of Pediatrics*. Published online Apr 19, 2013. doi:10.1007/s12098-013-1025-8.

Saluja, B. S., Grover, S., Irpati, A. S., Mattoo, S. K., & Basu, D. (2007). Drug Dependence in adolescents 1978–2003: A clinic-based observation from North India. *Indian Journal of Pediatrics, 74*, 455–458.

Samanta, A., Mukherjee, S., Ghosh, S., & Dasgupta, A. (2012). Mental health, protective factors and violence among male adolescents: A comparison between rural and urban schools of West Bengal. *Indian Journal of Public Health, 56*, 155–158.

Sarkar, S., Craig, M. C., Catani, M., Dell'acqua, F., Fahy, T., Deeley, Q., et al. (2013). Frontotemporal white-matter microstructural abnormalities in adolescents with conduct disorder: A diffusion tensor imaging study. *Psychological Medicine, 43*, 401–411.

Sethi, B., Gupta, S., & Kumar, R. (1967). 300 urban families: A psychiatric survey. *Indian Journal of Psychiatry, 9*, 280–302.

Sethi, B., Gupta, C., Kumar, R., & Kumar, P. (1972). A psychiatric survey of 500 rural families. *Indian Journal of Psychiatry, 14*, 183–196.

Sharma, R., Vijay, L., & Chaturvedi, S. (2008). Suicidal behavior amongst adolescent students in South Delhi. *Indian Journal of Psychiatry, 50*, 30–33.

Shastri, P. C., Shastri, J. P., & Shastri, D. (2010). Research in child and adolescent psychiatry in India. *Indian Journal of Psychiatry, 52*(Suppl1), S219–S223.

Sidhu, T. K. (2012). Evaluation of psychiatric morbidity in adolescents in Patiala district Punjab. *Indian Journal of Community Health, 24*, 63–66.

Singh, A. P., & Mishra, G. (2012). Adolescent lifestyle in india: Prevalence of risk and promotive factors of health. *Psychology and Developing Societies, 24*, 145–160.

Singhal, N., Misra, A., Shah, P., Rastogi, K., & Vikram, N. K. (2010). Secular trends in obesity, regional adiposity and metabolic parameters among Asian Indian adolescents in north India: A comparative data analysis of two selective samples 5 years apart (2003, 2008). *Annals of Nutrition and Metabolism, 56*, 176–181.

Sitholey, P., Agarwal, V., & Bharti, V. A. (2012). Clinical comparison study of attention deficit/hyperactivity disorder (DSM-IV) and hyperkinetic disorder (ICD-10) in Indian children and adolescents. *Journal of Indian Association for Child and Adolescent Mental Health, 8*, 6–11.

Sivakumar, T., Agarwal, V., & Sitholey, P. (2013). Comorbidity of attention-deficit/hyperactivity disorder and bipolar disorder in North Indian clinic children and adolescents. *Asian Journal of Psychiatry, 6*, 235–242.

Srihari, G., Eilander, A., Muthayya, S., Kurpad, A. V., & Seshadri, S. (2007). Nutritional status of affluent Indian school children: What and how much do we know? *Indian Pediatrics, 44*, 204–213.

Srinath, S., Girimaji, S. C., Gururaj, G., Seshadri, S., Subbakrishna, D. K., Bhola, P., et al. (2005). Epidemiological study of child and adolescent psychiatric disorders in urban and rural areas of Bangalore, India. *Indian Journal of Medical Research, 122*, 67–79.

Srinath, S., Janardhan, Y. C., Girimaji, S. R., Seshadri, S. P., & Subbakrishna, D. K. (1998). A prospective study of bipolar disorder in children and adolescents from India. *Acta Psychiatrica Scandinavica, 98*, 437–442.

Sringeri, R. (2008). The association between attention-deficit hyperactivity disorder and early-onset alcohol dependence—A retrospective study. *Indian Journal of Psychiatry, 50*, 262–265.

Sudhirkumar, C. T. (2000). A study of psychosocial and clinical factors associated with adolescent suicide attempts. *Indian Journal of Psychiatry, 42*, 231–242.

Thirunavukarasu, M., & Thirunavukarasu, P. (2010). Training and national deficit of psychiatrists in India—A critical analysis. *Indian Journal of Psychiatry, 52*, 83–88.

UNICEF The State of the World's Children 2011 India: Risk and opportunities for the world's largest national cohort of adolescents. Adolescence: An age of opportunity, p 1 Available at http://www.unicef.org/sowc2011/pdfs/India.pdf. Accessed on May 19, 2013.

United Nations Fund for Population Activities (UNFPA). (2003). *The state of world population 2003: Making 1 Billion count—Investing in adolescents' health and rights*. New York: United Nations Fund for Population Activities.

Verma, R., Balhara, Y. P., & Deshpande, S. N. (2011a). Inhalant abuse: A study from a tertiary care de-addiction clinic. *East Asian Arch Psychiatry, 21*, 157–163.

Verma, R., Balhara, Y. P., & Dhawan, A. (2011b). Inhalant use: An exploratory study. *Industrial Journal of Psychiatry, 20*, 103–116.

Pandey, V., Mehta, M., & Sagar, R. Anger in adolescents: Psychopathology and management. Department of Psychiatry, A.I.I.M.S., New Delhi. (ongoing Ph D thesis; unpublished).

Srivastava, P., Mehta, M., Sagar, R., Ambekar A. (2013). Conceptualizations guiding a computerized cognitive behavior therapy for adolescents with depression. In *Proceedings of 41st International Conference of British Association of Cognitive and Behavior Therapists*, 32–33.

Rao, P. N. (1978) Psychiatric morbidity in adolescence: An epidemiological survey of prevalence in high school adolescents. Unpublished M.D. thesis. Bangalore University, Bangalore, India.

Garg, R. (2004) Clinical study of psychosocial factors and comorbidity in major depressive disorder in adolescents, Unpublished M.D. thesis, All India Institute of Medical Sciences, New Delhi.

Kayal, M. (2006) Familial predictors of treatment outcome in adolescents with depression. Unpublished M.D. thesis, All India Institute of Medical Sciences, New Delhi

Das, N. (2003) Clinical study of phenomenology of major depressive disorder in adolescents. Unpublished M.D. thesis, All India Institute of Medical Sciences, New Delhi.

Sharma, R., Mehta, M., Dhawan, A. & Jain R. Psychological aspects and family factors among adolescents with substance use disorders and development of a treatment module, Department of Psychiatry, A.I.I.M.S., New Delhi. (unpublished M.D. thesis).

Bhad, R., Jain, R., Dhawan, A. & Mehta, M. Clinical assessment and biochemical validation of adolescent inhalant users in treatment settings, Department of Psychiatry, A.I.I.M.S., New Delhi. (unpublished M.D. thesis).

Bhattarai, R., Dhawan, A., Mehta, M. & Sagar, R. Clinical assessment of psychiatric co morbidity in adolescent inhalant users. Department of Psychiatry, A.I.I.M.S., New Delhi. (unpublished M.D. thesis).

Chugh, G., Mehta, M., Sagar, R. & Dhawan, A. Development and assessment of effectiveness of strategies for coping skills in adolescents. Department of Psychiatry, A.I.I.M.S., New Delhi. (unpublished Ph D thesis).

Chapter 17
Intellectual Disability in India—An Update

S.C. Girimaji

1 Introduction

Intellectual Disability (ID) can be viewed from a number of perspectives—as an extreme variation of the Gaussian distribution of intelligence, a trait, a biomedical condition as a consequence of underlying brain disease, or as a disability arising out of complex interaction between cognitive impairments and the living environment. However, the best way to understand ID is from a bio-psychosocial perspective. ID belongs to a class of neurodevelopmental disorders, which have onset in childhood and lead to impaired development of one or more human capacities. The core concept of ID—namely onset in childhood, significant impairments in global cognitive or intellectual functions, and concurrent deficits in adaptive behaviours—has remained the same over the centuries, though the condition has carried different names in different epochs in history. The most recent approach likely to be adapted by ICD-11 and by DSM 5 is to classify ID under the 'parent category' of neurodevelopment disorders with a new name of "intellectual developmental disorders" (Salvador-Carulla et al. 2011).

The approach of society towards people with ID has varied across ages and societies. For instance, there was widespread institutionalisation of these people in industrialised societies in the nineteenth and the early twentieth century. It was only later that these societies realised that it was a costly and unfortunate error. Since then they have been advocating family and community-based care. Institutionalisation has never occurred in a big way in India, and families have always looked after these individuals with a sense of duty and compassion. The reasons are not far to seek—the closely-knit

S.C. Girimaji, Professor

S.C. Girimaji (✉)
Department of Child and Adolescent Psychiatry, National Institute of Mental Health and Neurosciences, Bengaluru, India
e-mail: girimaji.nimhans@nic.in

S. Malhotra and S. Chakrabarti (eds.), *Developments in Psychiatry in India*,
DOI 10.1007/978-81-322-1674-2_17

family and kinship systems in India have always kept their member in their fold, despite their disabilities and hardships that they have had to face in the process. However, the scenario is changing in the last 2 or 3 decades, because of the rapid social changes that we are undergoing, with major implications for the individuals with ID and their families. A lot of discussion, debate and development of approaches have been happening on how do we face these new challenges, and organise services for individuals and their families. There is no doubt that more widespread, more efficient, and more comprehensive services and support systems from a life-span perspective have to be developed to ensure adequate quality of life for individuals with ID and their families.

The beginnings of organised services in this area can be traced to establishment of special schools in many cities in the 1950s and the 1960s by Non Governmental Organizations (NGOs) and by the voluntary sector. A number of child guidance clinics (CGCs) and mental retardation clinics were also set up in hospitals, sometimes by departments of psychology or child development in university set-ups. These schools and CGCs became the hub of activity for providing services, imparting training, and also for spreading awareness. They also developed many innovations, for instance group parental counselling, parent training, and home-based interventions. Tools to assess intelligence and social development such as Binet-Kamat test and the Indian version of Vineland Social Maturity Scale were developed, which are still in use today. Professional enthusiasm reached such great proportions in the late 1960s and early 1970s that a new journal devoted to ID—the Indian Journal of Mental Retardation was started in 1968, though it was discontinued after a few years. There was a sustained interest in the epidemiology of ID in the 1970s, either as a part of general psychiatric surveys, or specifically on ID; these brought out the magnitude of the problem and ID was no longer a hidden reality (Srinath and Girimaji 1999). The number special schools have seen a phenomenal growth in the past decade and there are now more than 1,200 such schools all over India now.

In this chapter, some of the most significant developments in the last 3 decades are reviewed and a roadmap is offered for future. Many of these developments have been reviewed elsewhere (Girimaji and Srinath 2010) and readers could also refer to clinical practice guidelines for ID prepared for the Indian Psychiatric Society for further information (Girimaji 2008).

2 Family Issues and Family-Focussed Interventions

Studying the implications and consequences for families caring for an individual with ID has been recurring theme of research. These include parental attitudes, family stress, burden, coping, and family needs. (Seshadri 1983; Wig et al. 1985; Narayan et al. 1993; Dhar 2009). The popularity of behaviour modification and training parents in behaviour modification skills for home-based training received considerable attention in 1980s. Varma and Seshadri (1989) developed an outpatient model for children with mild ID that involved individualised family intervention with components of parent education and counselling, parent-child relationship, and imparting training skills to parents. One of the earliest efforts was by Mehta and Ochaney (1984) who reported that it was possible to train parents in behaviour modification skills. Group parental counselling approach in centres that saw a large number of children with ID was another novel development (Girimaji et al. 1990; Peshwawaria et al. 1991), with the aim of parent education, orientation, providing emotional support, and to encourage and equip them for home-based training. Several variations of this approach, such as parental workshops, caregiver training workshops, self-help group workshops, have developed over the years and are being practiced widely all over India. Brief centre-based family-focussed intervention is another innovation where children are admitted along with their families for a comprehensive intervention by a multi-disciplinary team. At the National Institute of Mental Health and Neurosciences (NIMHANS) such intervention has been going on almost 3 decades (Narayanan et al. 1988). An evaluation of efficacy of this model was carried out through a ICMR funded project with very encouraging results; social adaptive skills improved, behaviour problems decreased, family stress came down and family coping was better (Girimaji 1996), a new semi-structured instrument to evaluate stress and coping in these families was developed (Girimaji et al. 1999), and a manual for counsellors was prepared. Similarly, the Vellore model at the *Nambikai Nilayam* has been quite popular, where the family-focussed intervention is done along with other interventions by a multi-disciplinary team (Russel et al. 1999). Adaptation of similar interventions has happened all over India.

High-risk intervention, early detection and intervention is another area, which has seen some development over the years. One positive development has been the increasing interest of paediatricians in developmental disorders in general and early intervention in particular. There have been several reports of early intervention in India, with some of them indicating positive results (APAWMR 1992; Pandit et al. 1992; Thomas 1992; Kaur et al. 2006; de Souza et al. 2006; Nair et al. 2009).

3 Parent Associations

The idea of parents coming together and forming associations for mutual support, service development, advocacy, and brining about positive changes in policies and legislation, and implementation of these caught up in 1980s, especially after a WHO-NIMHANS workshop in Bangalore in 1981. Several parent associations were formed in different parts of India, especially after receiving a strong push for the movement by the National Institute for the Mentally Handicapped, Secunderabad. There are now more than 180 such associations spread over 28 states, and they have come together to form an umbrella organization called *Parivar*—National Confederation of Parent Organisations (*Parivar*-NFPO). This positive development in the recent years has definitely contributed to empowerment of individuals and their families, and ensuring that their rights are not neglected.

4 Comorbid Problem Behaviours and Psychiatric Disorders

Mental health problems are quite common in ID, whether in the form of comorbid psychiatric disorders or problem behaviours. Psychiatric disorders are at least 2 to 3 times more common people with ID, compared to general population (Einfeld et al. 2011). Presence of these comorbid problems in people with ID has major negative consequences for them and their families—for instance exclusion from educational settings, and increased family stress. These conditions are often under-diagnosed and under-treated because of a number of reasons, for example, misattribution of symptoms to ID itself—diagnostic overshadowing (Reiss 1982), or masking of symptoms because of presence of ID. There are a number of studies from India that have documented high rates of comorbid psychiatric disorders in this population (Chaturvedi and Malhotra 1983; Kishore et al. 2004; Shivakumar et al. 2008). It is a primary task of the psychiatrist to recognise, evaluate and carry out multi-modal management of these mental health issues.

5 Legislation and Policies

India, in keeping with the trends all over the world, has been moving from a charity-based to welfare-based to rights-based approach to develop services for people with disabilities. The 2 important legislations—the Persons with Disabilities Act of 1995 and the National Trust Act of 1999 have been, in many ways, landmark legislations. The latter legislation especially has made significant contributions. The National Trust set up under this act has been quite active and introduced a number schemes such as health insurance, caregiver training programmes, group homes and respite and residential care services. Both these Acts are in the process of undergoing revision to bring them in line with United Nations Convention for Rights of Persons with Disabilities (UNCRPD), to which India is a signatory. Another major development in the education sector has been the *Sarva Shiksha Abhiyan* (SSA), which promotes inclusion education for 6–14 year old children, with a zero rejection policy. Implementation of the SSA, though uneven across India, has offered some hope for inclusion of children with ID into the mainstream school system. The recent Right to Education Act has now mandated this approach.

6 Community-Based Rehabilitation (CBR)

CBR programs emerged in India in the 1980s. These were initially initiated by NGOs, and later funded by governmental agencies. CBR programmes began with outreach services, satellite clinics and camps run by centres that were already providing some support to this population, but which felt the need to extend their involvement, driven by the philosophy of 'reaching the unreached'. These centres were also engaged in the training of workers at the grassroots level. To start with, CBR programmes included only physical disabilities. Soon, NGOs running these programmes realised that they were seeing a large number of individuals with ID, and were interested in including this as an agenda. Basic activities under the CBR programmes are survey and enumeration of individuals with ID, conducting community awareness programmes, providing services in the form of enrolment in schools, providing training, parental counselling and parent training, and ensuring access to various governmental facilities and benefits such as disability pension. Evaluation of these programmes are far and few, and the sustainability of the programs once the funding is withdrawn, is often a cause for concern.

7 Human Resource Development

The National Institute for Mentally Handicapped (NIMH), an apex body for ID under ministry of Social Justice and Empowerment was set up in 1984. Within a short time of its inception, the NIMH started a flurry of courses to train professionals at various levels, such as special education, undergraduate and postgraduate courses in ID, and rehabilitation. The NIMH has also been conducting short-term training programmes and refresher courses. A number of useful manuals, handouts, and multi-media materials on early stimulation, education, training, and rehabilitation have been published. Another popular publication is the all India Directory of services. The NIMH has also been involved in development and implementation of innovative care models suited for India. Other notable activities include the Annual National Seminar on Mental Retardation, the Annual Meet of Parent Organisations, the Special Olympics, and the National Meet of Special Employees. The institute has many regional centres all over India, mainly to provide services and run training courses for manpower development. Currently, there are numerous training centres in both public and NGO sectors, who train professionals in ID all over India.

8 Biomedical Research

One notable development in research has been on the description of syndromes and investigation into neurobiological and molecular genetic basis of ID. Genetic disorders that have been investigated include neurometabolic disorders, Down's syndrome, fragile X syndrome, primary microcephaly, copy number variations, and the Rett's syndrome. A collaborative study between the NIMHANS and the Indian Institute of Science on autosomal recessive primary microcephaly has reported a new gene mutation in this condition (Kumar et al. 2009), and has also found mutations in genes already reported earlier (Kumar et al. 2004; Bhat et al. 2011). Recently, the NIMH has brought out a very useful compilation on research in ID in India (Reddy and Narayan 2007).

9 A Roadmap for the Future

As is evident from this update, there is no doubt there have many significant positive developments in a number fronts concerning ID. But, we have long way to go. Large sections of this population continue to under-served, and whatever facilities that are there are under-utilised. There is an urgent need to build comprehensive models to address all the needs of individuals with ID and their families and caregivers. Specific intervention packages at different stages in the life span of individuals with ID have to be developed, especially during adolescence and adulthood. Coordinated action of all stakeholders, and inter-sectoral integration will ensure that services are not fragmented and smoothly flow into one another. Research focusing on biomedical and psycho-social aspects of ID has to continue, focussing on issues relevant to India. Development and evaluation of replicable models of service delivery, whether it is early intervention, family empowerment, health needs, education, training or CBR is a priority. Legislation, policy, and programme development will ensure that systems are built and sustained to respond to the rights of persons with ID and their families.

References

APAWMR Project Report. (1992). *Early intervention with infants at risk for developmental delays*. Hyderabad: UNICEF.

Bhat, V., Girimaji, S. C., Mohan, G., Arvinda, H. R., Singhmar, P., Duvvari, M. R., et al. (2011). Mutations in WDR62, encoding a centrosomal and nuclear protein, in Indian primary microcephaly families with cortical malformations. *Clinical Genetics, 80*(6), 532–540.

Chaturvedi, S. K., & Malhotra, S. (1983). Psychiatric problems in mental retardation. *Child Psychiatry Quarterly, 16*(3), 96.

de Souza, N., Sardessai, V., Joshi, K., Joshi, V., & Hughes, M. (2006). The determinants of compliance with an early intervention programme for high-risk babies in India. *Child: Care, Health and Development, 32*(1), 63–72.

Dhar, R. L. (2009). Living with a developmentally disabled child: Attitude of family members in India. *The Social Science Journal, 46*, 738–755.

Einfeld, S. L., Ellis, L. A., & Emerson, E. (2011). Comorbidity of intellectual disability and mental disorder in children and adolescents: A systematic review. *Journal of Intellectual and Development Disability, 36*(2), 137–143.

Girimaji, S. C. (2008). Clinical practice guidelines for the diagnosis and management of children with mental retardation. Retrieved from www.indianjpsychiatry.org/cpg/cpg2008/CPG-CAP_05.pdf.

Girimaji, S. R., Srinath, S., Seshadri, S. P., Madhu, P. R., & Nardev, (1990). Pattern of utilisation of outpatient group counselling services for parents of mentally retarded persons. *Indian Journal of Psychological Medicine, 13*(2), 153–157.

Girimaji, S. R. (1996). *Final Report of the project evaluation of the effectiveness of brief inpatient family intervention versus outpatient intervention for mentally retarded children*. New Delhi: ICMR.

Girimaji, S. C., & Srinath, S. (2010). Perspectives of intellectual disability in India: Epidemiology, policy, services for children and adults. *Current Opinion in Psychiatry, 23*, 441–446.

Girimaji, S. C., Srinath, S., Seshadri, S. P., et al. (1999). Family Interview for Stress and Coping in Mental Retardation (FISC-MR): A tool to study stress and coping in families of children with mental retardation. *Indian Journal of Psychiatry, 41*, 341–349.

Kaur, P., Chavan, B. S., Lata, S., Kaur, A., Tinku, S., Arora, Y., et al. (2006). Early intervention in developmental delay. *Indian Journal of Pediatrics, 73*(5), 405–408.

Kishore, M. T., Nizamie, A., Nizamie, S. H., & Jahan, M. (2004). Psychiatric diagnosis in persons with intellectual disability in India. *Journal of Intellectual Disability Research, 48*(1), 19–24.

Kumar, A., Blanton, S. H., Babu, M., Markandaya, M., & Girimaji, S. C. (2004). Genetic analysis of primary microcephaly in Indian families: Novel ASPM mutations. *Clinical Genetics, 66*(4), 341–348.

Kumar, A., Girimaji, S. C., Duvvari, M. R., & Blanton, S. H. (2009). Mutations in STIL, encoding a pericentriolar and centrosomal protein, cause primary microcephaly. *American Journal of Human Genetics, 84*(2), 286–290.

Mehta, M., & Ochaney, M. (1984). Training mental retardates: Involving mothers in operant conditioning program. *Indian Journal of Clinical Psychology, 11*, 45–49.

Nair, M. K. C., Philip, E., Jeyaseelan, L., George, B., Mathews, S. & Padma, K. (2009). Effect of child development centre model early stimulation among at risk babies—A randomized controlled trial, *Indian Pediatrics,* 46, s20–s26.

Narayan, J., Madhavan, T., & Prakasham, B. B. (1993). Factors influencing the expectations of parents for their mentally retarded children. *Journal of Intellectual Disability Research, 37*, 161–168.

Narayanan, H. S., Girimaji, S. R., Gandhi, D. H., Raju, K. M., Rao, P. M., & Nardev, G. (1988). Brief in-patient family intervention in mental retardation. *Indian Journal of Psychiatry, 30*(3), 275–281.

Pandit, A., Chaudhari, S., Bhave, S., & Kulkarni, S. (1992). Early intervention programme through the high risk clinic—Pune experience. *Indian Journal of Pediatrics, 59*(6), 675–680.

Peshwawaria, R., Reddi, V. S., Subba, T. A. R., Persha, A. J., & Mohapatra, B. (1991). Group parent training programmes at NIMH: An overview. *Journal of Personality and Clinical Studies, 7*, 169–184.

Reddy, S. H. K., & Narayan, J. (2007). *Research in mental retardation in India*. Secunderabad: National Institute for the Mentally Handicapped.

Reiss, S., Levitan, G. W., & Szyszko, J. (1982). Emotional disturbance and mental retardation: Diagnostic overshadowing. *American Journal of Mental Deficiency, 86*(6), 567–574.

Russell, P. S., John, J. K., & Lakshmanan, J. L. (1999). Family intervention for intellectually disabled children. Randomised controlled trial. *The British Journal of Psychiatry, 174*, 254–258.

Salvador-Carulla, L., Reed, G. M., Vaez-Azizi, L. M., Cooper, S., Martinez-Leal, R., Bertelli, M., et al. (2011). Intellectual developmental disorders: Towards a new name, definition and framework for "mental retardation/intellectual disability" in ICD-11. *World Psychiatry, 10*(3), 175–180.

Seshadri, M. (1983). Impact of the mentally handicapped child on the family. *Indian Journal of Clinical Psychology, 10*, 473–478.

Shivakumar, P. T., Girimaji, S. C., Srinath, S. and Shekar, S. P. (2008). Psychiatric comorbidity in mental retardation. *Indian Journal of Psychiatry*, 542.

Srinath, S., & Girimaji, S. R. (1999). Epidemiology of child and adolescent mental health problems and mental retardation. *NIMHANS Journal, 17*, 355–366.

Thomas, M. (1992). The Action Aid disability programmes: Experiences in early identification and early intervention. *Indian Journal of Pediatrics, 59*(6), 697–700.

Varma, V. K., & Seshadri, M. (1989). Intervention programmes for parents of mentally retarded children. *Annals of National Academics and Medicinal Science (India), 25*, 309–328.

Wig, N. N., Mehta, M., & Sahasi, G. (1985). A study of time utilization and perceived burden of mentally handicapped child in joint and nuclear families. *Indian Journal of Social Psychiatry, 1*, 251–261.

Chapter 18
Perspectives on Interventions in Child Psychiatry in India

B.K. Pradhan

1 Background

The current chapter looks at the child mental health scene in India with respect to interventions, both historical and contemporary. The chapter will broadly review the interventions and developments with regard to common child psychiatric conditions in India, such as depression, anxiety disorders, learning disorders, attention deficit hyperactivity disorder (ADHD), autism spectrum disorders, and intellectual disability. In addition to the various 'Western' treatment options, and indigenous 'home-based interventions', the Indian family's great tenacity in caring for the mentally ill, and their role as an invaluable resource in treatment and rehabilitation will be highlighted. The concluding section will present the challenges and opportunities for future in the field of child psychiatric interventions in India.

2 Child Psychiatric Disorders: Extent of Burden and Importance

2.1 Global Scenario

Children and adolescents constitute almost a third (2.2 billion individuals) of the world's population of these, almost 90 % live in low-income and middle-income countries, where they form up to 50 % of the population (UNICEF 2008). Almost 20 % of all children and adolescents are affected by mental health problems and at

B.K. Pradhan, Assistant Professor

B.K. Pradhan (✉)
Child, Adolescent and Adult Psychiatry, Cooper University Hospital
and Cooper Medical School of Rowan University, Camden, NJ, USA
e-mail: pradhan-basant@cooperhealth.edu

S. Malhotra and S. Chakrabarti (eds.), *Developments in Psychiatry in India*,
DOI 10.1007/978-81-322-1674-2_18

least half of these show impaired schooling and social development (Sawyer et al. 2000). Among children and adolescents, problems such as child abuse and neglect, conduct disorder, alcohol and drug abuse, depression, ADHD, and suicide are all becoming more common than they were initially thought to be (Rutter and Smith 1995; Costello 1998). Furthermore, mental disorders (notably depression) are appearing at a younger age, and they also seem to be increasing in severity (Mrazek and Haggerty 1994). Children and adolescents with mental health problems are twice as likely to report feeling 'very stressed', three times more likely to have poor or fair physical health, three times more likely to perform below grade level at school, three times more likely to use alcohol and other drugs, and six times more likely to think about killing themselves (Zubrick 1995; Costello 1989).

Although most of child and adolescent psychiatry is practiced in industrialized countries, the vast majority of the world's children live in the developing world. The mental health of children in developing countries is important, but a relatively under-explored area. Methodological problems of epidemiological studies in this field include, in addition to other factors, the use of case definitions and disability criteria developed in the West and the assumption that dimensions of disorder and thresholds for reporting problems are similar to European and North American populations.

Psychiatric epidemiological studies from high-income countries indicate that more than a quarter of children and adolescents meet lifetime criteria for a mental disorder (Srinath et al. 2005); about 10 % have distress or impairment that is severe enough to warrant intervention (Brauner and Stephens 2006). Children and adolescents in low- and middle-income countries (LAMIC) constitute 35–50 % of the population. Although many studies report that the burden of child and adolescent mental health poses a significant public health burden, the major challenges are meager resources and manpower, low recognition, lack of much needed policy making, low priority for fund allocation, as well as limited research. For example, mental health research in child and adolescent mental health contributes barely 3–6 % of all published mental health research in the world (Patel and Sumathipala 2001; Saxena et al. 2006, 2007).

2.2 Indian Scenario: Some Recent Epidemiological Data

India is a developing country with a population of more than 1 billion (which is 16 % of the world population), and children below 16 years of age constitute more than 40 % of its population. India presents a unique case, not only in terms of this big volume of child and adolescent population, but also in terms of its immense diversity in the languages spoken, levels of literacy, and social and cultural practices, including the child-rearing practices. Despite our strengths in terms of great tradition and culture and above all abundance of family support, on downside, we have low budgetary resources, interference from competing and conflicting healing systems, scarcity of mental health personnel, 'brain drain', and the stigma against seeking help for problems related to the mental illnesses. In the developed world application of methodological developments such as structured and semistructured diagnostic interviews, statistical methods for estimating prevalence and correlates of mental disorders have established the prevalence of mental disorders, patterns of co-morbidity, correlates and risk factors for mental disorders, and service patterns. In contrast, Indian studies have not as yet definitively and consistently established epidemiological data on mental disorders in children and adolescents. Some notable studies are outlined below:

Attempts at estimating the burden of child and adolescent psychiatric disorders in India have only consisted of a few methodologically sound studies among community samples. These have reported overall point prevalence rates of 9.4 % in children aged 8–12 years (Hackett et al. 1999), 12.5 % in children aged 0–16 years (Srinath et al. 2005), and 1.81 % in adolescents aged 12–16 years (Pillai et al. 2008). In a study from North India (Malhotra et al. 2002a), the prevalence rate of psychiatric disorders in the age group of 4–11 years was found out to be 6.33%; in this sample, enuresis was the most common disorder. In the first ever study on the incidence of child psychiatric disorders in India (Malhotra et al. 2009), which followed up children after 6 years, the research team that included this author reported that the incidence of psychiatric disorders in a representative sample of school children from Chandigarh was 18 per 1,000 per year.

2.3 Specific Disorders: India in Comparison with Global Scenario

Prospective studies tracking the natural course of specific childhood and adolescent mental disorders have not been conducted in Indian community samples. In a recent review (Malhotra and Pradhan 2013), the authors concluded that the prevalence and incidence rates found in the Indian studies are lower than those reported in developed countries; however, further studies clarifying the reasons for these lower rates are needed. The epidemiological data described below are taken from an editorial specifically addressing this issue (Sharan and Sagar 2008).

Mood disorders: The median prevalence estimate of major depression in children and adolescents in studies conducted in developed countries is 4.0 % (range: 0.2–17 %), which is in contrast to much lower rates found in limited studies available from Indian subcontinent.

Anxiety disorders: The median prevalence rate of all anxiety disorders in children and adolescents was reported to be 8 % (range: 2–24 %) based on studies conducted in developed countries; much lower rates have been found in limited studies, which are available from Indian subcontinent. Though school-based samples from India report a higher prevalence of internalizing disorders in girls, the gender difference in the prevalence of anxiety disorders in children and adolescents has not been established in community samples.

Externalizing disorders: The median prevalence rate of ADHD in studies conducted in the developed countries is reported to be 4 % (range: 1.7–17.8 %). However, in some Indian studies, the point prevalence estimate for hyperkinetic disorder is 1.6 %. In one such two-stage study, which specifically assessed ADHD, a prevalence of 12.2 % in preschoolers selected from kindergartens was reported. The median 12-month prevalence rate of disruptive behavior disorders (i.e., conduct disorder or oppositional defiant disorder) is 6 % (range: 5–14 %) in studies conducted in developed countries, whereas one Indian study has reported a point prevalence for conduct and oppositional defiant disorder to be 1.3 %. A school-based study from India (Shenoy et al. 1998) showed that the prevalence of externalizing disorders is higher among boys; however, a definitive statement regarding gender distribution of externalizing disorders awaits replication in community samples.

Substance abuse and dependence: The median estimate of alcohol or drug abuse or dependence in community surveys of adolescents in developed countries is 5 % (range: 1–24 %). The complete absence of substance abuse in a sample from Bangalore, India (Srinath et al. 2005) was linked to the low response rate for the diagnostic interview, youths' unwillingness to reveal such information, and parents' ignorance about the abuse.

Learning disorders: A study in rural India found that more than 80 % of the 172 children in a group of dropouts suffered from learning disability, as diagnosed by a psychological screening test (Pratinidhi et al. 1999). A survey of 1,535 primary school children drawn from schools in Bangalore city found that 15 % suffered from learning disability. Learning problems were associated with a low quality of academic work, poor concentration, not carrying out tasks, low motivation, and under-achievement (Shenoy et al. 1998).

Disorders in very young children: With the exception of pervasive developmental disorders, there has been considerable controversy about the validity of diagnosis of mental disorders in very young children (age < 5 years). Egger and Angold (2006) summarized the rates of childhood mental disorders as follows: ADHD (2–5.7 %), oppositional defiant disorder (4–16.8 %), conduct disorder (0–4.6 %), depression (0–2.1 %), and anxiety disorders (0.3–9.4 %). There was a high degree of co-morbidity in young children with mental disorders; of those with one disorder, approximately 25 % had a second disorder. The proportion of children with co-morbidity increases about 1.6 times for each additional year from age 2 (18.2 %) to 5 (49.7 %) years. In contrast, Srinath et al. (2005) reported that the most common diagnoses in the 0–3 year age group were pica (2 %), behavior disorder NOS (1.8 %), expressive speech disorder (1.4 %), and mental retardation (now called 'intellectual disability', 1.4 %).

Childhood sexual abuse: There are very few reports on child sexual abuse, from developing countries. In a study of school-based adolescents in India, 6 % reported a lifetime experience of coercive sexual intercourse; other types of sexual harassment and abuse were commonly experienced, and sexual abuse was strongly associated with educational failure, poor physical health, and mental health (Patel and Andrew 2001).

In summary, it is evident that the overall rate of psychiatric disorders may be lower in India compared to developed countries. Moreover, the range of disorders may be different in the two settings. In particular, Indian children and adolescents seem to have markedly lower rates of depression, substance use disorders and disruptive behavior disorders, and a greater rate of sub-syndromal disorders (e.g., behavior disorder NOS) and mono-symptomatic conditions such as enuresis and stuttering. It is difficult to disentangle whether the difference in rates and pattern of disorders are due to real differences or due to methodological issues.

3 Interventions from Historical Perspectives: Global and Indian

3.1 Across the Globe

3.1.1 Recognition of Child Psychiatry as a Distinct Discipline

An important antecedent to the specialty of child psychiatry was the social recognition of childhood as a special phase of life with its own developmental stages, starting with the neonate and eventually extending through adolescence. Kraepelin's psychiatric taxonomy, published in 1883, ignored disorders in children (Kanner 1960). It was Sigmund Freud who made initial major contributions about establishing a conceptual framework about childhood as a significant phase of life. Later on, several other intellectuals such as Anna Freud, Eric Erikson, Melanie Klein, Donald Winnicot, Margaret Mahler, and Peter Bloss added developmental dimensions to psychoanalysis, making it applicable to assessment and treatment of disorders among children and adolescents. The term 'child psychiatry' was in use in French as early as 1899, (Manheimer 1900). However, the Swiss psychiatrist Moritz Tramer (1882–1963) was probably the first to define the parameters of child psychiatry in terms of diagnosis, treatment, and prognosis within the discipline of medicine, in 1933 (Eliasberg 1964). The first academic child psychiatry department in the world was founded in 1930 by Leo Kanner (1894–1981), under the direction of Adolf Meyer at the Johns Hopkins Hospital, Baltimore, USA. In 1936, Kanner established the first formal elective course in child psychiatry at the John Hopkins Hospital.

Psychopharmacology: The use of medication in the treatment of children also began in the 1930s, when Charles Bradley opened a neuropsychiatric unit and was the first to use amphetamine for brain damaged and hyperactive children· But it was not until the 1960s that the first National Institute of Health (NIH) grant to study pediatric psychopharmacology was awarded. The era since the 1980s flourished, in large part, because of contributions made in the 1970s, a decade during which child psychiatry witnessed a major evolution as a result of the work carried out by Michael Rutter and colleagues in their first comprehensive population survey of 9- to 11-year-olds, carried out in London and the Isle of Wight. In this influential work, the investigators demonstrated specific continuities of psychopathology over time and the influence of social and contextual factors in children's mental health. They determined the prevalence of ADHD, identified the onset and prevalence of depression in mid-adolescence and the frequent co-morbidity with conduct disorder, and also explored the relationship between various mental disorders and scholastic achievement (Rutter 1990).

3.2 Ancient India: Child Care Guidelines Formulated by the Sage Teachers

To treat a child from a developmental perspective was known even to people of ancient India as evidenced by the clear writings in the *Kashyapa Samhita* (an ancient treatise of *Ayurveda,* meaning 'collections of the sage teacher *Kashyapa*'), the entire writings of which are devoted to childcare. *Kashyapa Samhita* describes 46 disorders out of which 12 are described as disorders of children (*bala roga*). Quite in tune with the modern models of 'integrated maternal and child mental health', in ancient India, the mother and infant were seen as a single unit. The central themes in the *Kashyapa Samhita* are not only the concept of mother–child unit, but also the 'developmental stage model,' which describes the various stages of physical as well as psychological stages of development of the child from conception till adulthood. In addition, this system of child care was in perfect accordance with Mother Nature. For example, a baby was taken out to see the moon in the 3rd month and the sun in the 4th month after its birth; the molding of the front portion of the head (*Chuda karana*) was done around the 6th month to ensure proper fontanel closure; ear piercing was done around the 1st year of the child, the thread ceremony (*Upanayana*, meaning child is cognitively developed enough (a similar ceremony in Christian culture in the West is called *Communion*) is performed around the age of 7 years (which is amazingly in accordance with the modern studies in cognitive development by theorists such as Piaget and others that at age of 7 years, a child achieves preliminary logical thinking). Devoted readers can refer to the story of *Jivaka* (*Vriddha Jivaka Tantra*, i.e., the doctrines of old *Jivaka* Srikrishnamurthy 2002) for further details.

3.3 Modern India: From the First Child Guidance Clinic (1937) to 12th Five-year Plan (2012)

The first Child Guidance Clinic (CGC) was established in India in 1937. By 2003 in India, 164 CGCs were running. However, these were mostly in urban areas, and the rate of about two-and-a-half new CGCs every year is hugely insufficient to cater to the huge burden mental health needs of Indian children. Of note, is the fact that 74 % of Indian children live in rural areas. The National Policy for Children was formulated in 1974. This provided some impetus for further work in policy making and implementation. The National Plan of Action for Children was formulated in 2005, which contributed subsequently to the inclusion of a child-centered focus in the 11th five-year plan in 2007. One of the major advances in epidemiology during the past decade has been the increasing focus on the impact and burden of mental disorders. These data will be very crucial for planning interventions.

The11th five-year plan: This was definitely a child-centered plan. This plan started in 2007 and was completed in March 2012 (Planning Commission 2012). In this plan, the focus rightly shifted to child mental health policy, school mental health policy, including school-based mental health programs, as well as mental health policy for the disabled. This has sparked a renewed interest in the research on interventions in child and adolescent mental health, as well as increased involvement of the non-governmental organizations (NGOs) into the research and service delivery aspects in this field. Despite the recent progress in India in this area, there is still a wide gap between identifying needs, planning, developing policies and effective implementation to bring a difference. Child psychiatry in India indeed has a long way to go.

The 12th five-year plan: This is ongoing as we speak. Independent India has taken fairly good steps in addressing issues such as child literacy and child health, but program implementation in organized manner is not a success story at all. There is neither an independent, nor an integrated child mental health policy in India.

4 Community Needs Versus Service Utilization in India

Ten percent of the child population is in need of special care and treatment, whereas only 1 % gets some care and treatment. Children with borderline intellectual functioning and various learning, speech, and visual and hearing difficulties are conservatively estimated to be 20 % of the total child population (Shastri et al. 2010). Factors associated with service utilization include impairment, co-morbidity, suicide attempts, parental recognition, help-seeking attitude, and family burden. Studies on utilization of services are clearly needed in India. In contrast to adult mental disorders, the economic impact of childhood mental disorders has not been widely studied, and the burden of childhood and adolescent mental disorders is not acknowledged in the global burden of disease estimates. Unlike in the developed nations, a very small number of preventive and promotional interventions have been evaluated in developing countries such as India. For example, in a systematic review (Flament 2007), out of 47 separate programs reviewed, only one had been implemented in the low- and middle-income countries.

5 Specific Interventions in Child Psychiatry in India

More so since 2007, after the implementation of the 11th five-year plan, some more progress in various aspects of child psychiatry including service delivery and research is almost palpable. This is reflected by the fact that in the last few years, accredited fellowship programs in child psychiatry have been made available in two national centers, i.e., the National Institute of Mental Health and Neurosciences (NIMHANS), Bangalore, and recently the Postgraduate Institute of Medical Education and Research (PGIMER), Chandigarh. Despite these very welcoming developments, child psychiatry, more so the intervention aspects of it, has a long way to go. For understandable reasons (some of which have been outlined under the next section: ‘Barriers to effective interventions’), research literature on outcome of child psychiatric intervention is quite meager. Searching the database, one does not come across randomized controlled trials on interventions in this subcontinent but rather sparse case reports and some proposals addressing the felt needs or conceptualizing various desirable service delivery methods that should be implemented.

There have been some published studies about child psychiatric interventions in India, as will be described below:

About interventions on autism, apart from national centers such as NIMHANS, PGIMER, and All India Institute of Medical Sciences (AIIMS), autism interventions are available in India through organizations such as Action For Autism (AFA). These interventions involve elements of Treatment and Education of Autistic and related Communication-handicapped Children (TEACCH), applied behavior analysis (ABA), verbal behavior analysis (VBA), and various forms of assistive and augmentative communication (AAC) including picture exchange communication systems (PECS). Many Indian families try ayurvedic and homeopathic treatments, and a number of centers and doctors in India have begun to advertise their services specifically as it relates to autism. Some descriptions of these can be found in the website www.autism-india.org and other web resources.

In a study (Juneja 2012) examining the efficacy of a parent-based intensive behavioral intervention program in Indian autistic children, 16 children with autistic disorder undergoing the intervention for at least 6 months were enrolled. The mean development, social, expressive, and receptive language quotients, and the Childhood Autism Rating Scale (CARS) and Autism Behavior Checklist (ABC) scores were compared before and after the intervention. The average duration of therapy was 19.5 ± 11.78 months. There was a significant improvement in the development quotient ($P = 0.015$), social quotient ($P = 0.004$), expressive language quotient ($P = 0.03$), CARS ($P = 0.001$), and ABC ($P = 0.014$) scores. The authors concluded that parent-based behavioral intervention programs have a promising role in the management of children with autism in resource-constraint settings.

In another study (Malhotra et al. 2002b) involving parent-based interventions for autism, psychological intervention was carried out with parents of 5 children with autism. The treatment package included a mix of behavioral, supportive, and educational techniques, delivered in 3–6 sessions of 45–60 min each, in the setting of a child psychiatric clinic of the PGIMER. Results showed that on the whole, parents found this brief contact helpful. They rated emotional aspects of the support offered to be the most helpful.

In a study (Malhotra 2006) examining effects of early interventions on primary prevention in child psychiatric disorders, simple intervention consisting of parental counseling, focusing on recognition of the child's temperamental and cognitive individuality, the use of appropriate parenting strategies, and understanding of normal developmental changes were able to contribute to lowering the incidence of mental disorders in children. This intervention contributed to lowering the incidence of mental disorder to 10 per 1,000 per year, in contrast to children in a control group (18 per 1,000 per year) who did not receive any intervention.

In an empirical study (Pradhan, BK, 2005, unpublished data) involving an open trial of yoga and meditation (concentrative type) in symptomatic management of a group of 10 children with attention deficit hyperactivity disorder (ADHD), it was found out that culturally accepted indigenous interventions such as yoga and concentrative-type meditation were able to decrease impulsivity and improved concentration and focus in children with ADHD.

In another controlled study (Goyal 2006), with 122 normal and 117 emotionally disturbed adolescents, a standard package of training in life skills and psychosocial competence benefitted all adolescents, and resulted in symptomatic improvement in about 80 % of adolescents with internalizing disorders.

Despite these preliminary studies, it cannot be overemphasized about huge need of randomized controlled trials on specific child psychiatric interventions examining efficacy of these interventions in Indian setting in treatment of attention deficit and hyperactive disorder (ADHD), depression, bipolar disorder, anxiety disorder, learning disorders, mental retardation, as well as research on preventive interventions in child psychiatry.

6 Importance of Utilizing Indigenous Interventions

As mentioned before, our major strengths have been extended family system, indigenous 'home-based interventions', Indian family's great tenacity in caring for mentally ill population, and their role as great resource in treatment and rehabilitation. In India, the extended family system has provided extremely good family support over the centuries, which has provided an effective buffer against stress and mental illness. Even today grandmothers living in the homes of Indian families help a great deal in child care. However, there are very few studies regarding the role of grandparents and their impact of these aspects of family structure and parenting styles, and on overall growth and the development of the child. These must be evaluated in the appropriate sociocultural context. There is a strong need to study and evaluate the role traditional beliefs and practices play in child development, and how these can be used for promotional or preventive interventions.

Developing a service structure that mimics those used in more developed countries is not feasible in developing countries. Developing widely based community and primary health care is the only feasible, acceptable, and affordable approach for catering to the mental health needs of Indian children (Saxena et al. 2006, 2007). Similarly, there is considerable scope for using culturally sensitive and feasible psychotherapeutic approaches such as yoga and meditation in care and stress management among children and adolescents with psychiatric disorders.

7 Barriers to Effective Interventions

1. Poverty: Evidence thus far suggests that the greatest vulnerability to disorder arises when poverty is associated with food scarcity leading to under-nutrition, or when other factors such as family dysfunction, family violence, criminality, and high levels of neighborhood danger coexist. These factors may be more common among urban as compared to the rural poor.
2. Stigma about mental health and lack of education and awareness: Beliefs about mental illnesses influence help-seeking attitudes and patterns in people. In a study from Bangalore (Srinath et al. 2005), only 37.5 % of the families of children and adolescents with mental disorders perceived that their children had any problem. Another qualitative study from Goa, India found that even parents of children with ADHD attending a child guidance center rarely used biopsychosocial models to explain their child's behavioral problems (Wilcox et al. 2007).
3. Methodological limitations in the studies leading to lack of clear data for planning effective interventions: When research is so meager, planning for intervention as well as effective implementation is difficult. Perhaps the most problematic of all methodological issues has been validity of screening

instruments and the inclusion of specific learning disorders (Merikangas et al. 2009). There is no consensus in India on the inclusion of learning disorders in prevalence estimates of mental disorders in children and adolescents, despite their substantial presence.

4. Another major problem is evaluating the efficacy of interventions. A particular challenge for promotional interventions is to operationalize and quantitatively assess mental well-being in a manner that defines well-being in a positive way, is culturally valid, and goes beyond establishing the presence or absence of disorders.
5. Large gaps exists in the area of prevention, mental health promotion, and early intervention programs. There are limited child and adolescent mental health services in India. Mostly such services are restricted to urban areas. Access to mental health services for children with a mental, emotional, or behavioral disorder is substandard, not provided early enough, not in sufficient supply, and accessible only to a fraction of children and adolescents.
6. Problems with policy making, resource allocations, as well as service delivery system: There is a great need for more training as well as integration with primary care to increase access to interventions.

8 Some Proposed Solutions

8.1 For Improving Data

Clearly, culture-specific assessment instruments must be developed to aid the identification of certain psychiatric disorders. A more rigorous and systematic approach to addressing the challenges of cross-cultural research is needed, through strategies such as using detailed interview-based measures in addition to questionnaires; examining the internal consistency of questionnaire subscales; comparing inter-informant agreement; and including a qualitative component to research projects.

Important role of non-governmental organizations (NGO): Many NGOs are seeking to integrate child psychiatry interventions within a broader child health agenda. This needs to happen at a larger scale to cater to the huge mental healthcare needs of children and adolescents.

Better policy making: Mental health policies need to be child friendly. These should be geared toward effective legislation, better resource allocation, as well as should be encouraging for mental health promotion and effective early intervention.

8.2 Implementation—The Need for Effective Service Delivery Methods

Despite some research, the fact remains that there is virtually no evidence at all specifically for child and adolescent psychiatry outcomes in India. In order to achieve desired outcomes, one should embrace all the services in a multidisciplinary model, which contribute to the mental health care of children and adolescents, whether provided by health, education, social services, or other agencies. It is also crucial to develop partnerships with services whose primary function is not mental health care, such as general practitioners (GPs) and schools. They can always contribute by offering general advice and treatment for less severe problems, contribute toward mental health promotion, identify problems early in their development, and refer to more specialist services. This would explicitly acknowledge that supporting children and adolescents with mental health problems is not the responsibility of specialist services alone. The plan should include primary mental health workers, psychologists, and counselors working in GP practices, pediatric clinics, schools, and youth services. They can offer consultation to families and other practitioners, outreach to identify severe or complex needs, which require more specialist interventions, assessment, treatment, and training where needed.

9 Conclusions

Children are a supremely important asset for any nation. Their nurture and care are our responsibility. Children's programs should find a prominent part in our national plans. There are very few evaluated child and adolescent psychiatry interventions in India. The highest priority in this area must be given to increased resources to develop, implement, and evaluate intervention in child and adolescent psychiatry in India. The key findings of the limited numbers of studies in the developing countries about the effective interventions are that parenting, nutritional, and educational interventions improve psychosocial development in disadvantaged populations and that interventions which combine both nutritional and psychosocial components (such as promoting mother–infant interaction), and those which are implemented as early as possible and for the longest duration have the greatest impact, This positive impact is evident for many years after the intervention. Child mental health is a shared responsibility, and for any intervention to be effective, there should be a synergy between efforts being made by different stakeholders to address the issues. There is a need to create a mechanism that will make such a synergy possible. All children and adolescents, from birth to their 18th birthday, who have mental health problems and disorders, need to have access to timely, integrated, high-quality, multi-disciplinary mental health services to ensure effective assessment, treatment, and support. There has been noticeable progress in addressing the various lacunae related to the interventions in the field of child and adolescent psychiatry. However, there is still a long way to go in terms of developing a locally and nationally relevant and reliable database, effective implementation of legislation and policies, and the development of effective, accessible, and affordable interventions.

References

Brauner, C. B., & Stephens, C. B. (2006). Estimating the prevalence of early childhood serious emotional/behavioural disorders: Challenges and recommendations. *Public Health Reports, 121*, 303–310.

Costello, E. J. (1989). Development in child psychiatric epidemiology. *Journal of the American Academy of Child and Adolescent Psychiatry, 28*, 836–840.

Costello, E. J. (1998). Child psychiatric disorders and their correlates: A primary care pediatric sample. *Journal of the American Academy of Child and Adolescent Psychiatry, 34*, 570–578.

Egger, H. L., & Angold, A. (2006). Common emotional and behavioral disorders in preschool children: presentation, nosology, and epidemiology. *Journal of Child Psychology and Psychiatry, 47*, 313–337.

Eliasberg, W. G. (1964). In memoriam: Moritz Tramer M.D. (1882–1963). *American Journal of Psychiatry, 121*, 103–104.

Flament, M. F., et al. (2007). Evidence-based primary prevention programs for the promotion of mental health in children and adolescents: A systematic worldwide review. In H. Remschmidt, B. Nurcombe, M. Belfer, N. Sartorius, & A. Okasha (Eds.), *The mental health of adolescents. An area of global neglect* (pp. 65–136). Chichester: Wiley.

Goyal, V. (2006). *Impact of life skills training on psychosocial competence of early and middle adolescents*. Chandigarh, India: Study done at the PGIMER.

Hackett, R., et al. (1999). The prevalence and associations of psychiatric disorder in children in Kerala, South India. *Journal of Child Psychology and Psychiatry, 40*, 801–807.

Juneja, M., et al. (2012). Evaluation of a parent-based behavioral intervention program for children with autism in a low-resource setting. *Journal of Pediatric Neurosciences, 7*(1), 16–18.

Kanner, L. (1960). Child psychiatry: Retrospect and prospect. *American Journal of Psychiatry, 117*(1), 15–22.

Malhotra, S. (2006). Community based follow up and treatment of children identified to have psychiatric disorders. An Indian Council of Medical Research (ICMR) project. New Delhi: ICMR.

Malhotra, S., & Pradhan, B. K. (2013). Childhood psychiatric disorders in north-India: Prevalence, incidence and implications. *Adolescent Psychiatry, 3*, 87–89.

Malhotra, S., et al. (2002a). Prevalence of psychiatric disorders in school children in Chandigarh, India. *Indian Journal of Medical Research, 116*, 21–28.

Malhotra, S., et al. (2002b). Psychological intervention with parents of autistic children. *Indian Journal of Psychiatry, 44*(2), 108–117.

Malhotra, S., et al. (2009). Incidence of childhood psychiatric disorders in India. *Indian Journal of Psychiatry, 51*, 101–107.

Manheimer, M. (1900). Les troubles mentaux de l'enfance (review). *Journal of Mental Science, 46*(193), 342–343.

Merikangas, K. R., et al. (2009). Epidemiology of mental disorders in children and adolescents. *Dialogues in Clinical Neuroscience, 11*, 7–20.

Mrazek, P. J., & Haggerty, R. J. (1994). *Reducing risks for mental disorders: Frontiers for preventive intervention research*. Washington, DC: National Academy Press.

Patel, V., & Andrew, G. (2001). Gender, sexual abuse and risk behaviours: A cross-sectional survey in schools in Goa. *National Medical Journal of India, 14*, 263–267.

Patel, V., & Sumathipala, A. (2001). International representation in psychiatric journals: A survey of 6 leading journals. *The British Journal of Psychiatry, 178*, 406–409.

Patel, V., et al. (2007). Treating and preventing mental disorders in low and middle income countries—Is there evidence to scale up? *Lancet, 370*, 990–1005.

Pillai, A., et al. (2008). Non-traditional lifestyles and prevalence of mental disorders in adolescents in Goa, India. *The British Journal of Psychiatry, 192*, 45–51.

Planning Commission, (2012). Government of India: Five Year Plans. Retrieved on 17 Mar 2012 from www.planningcommission.nic.in.

Pratinidhi, A. K., et al. (1999). Epidemiological aspects of school dropouts in children between 7–15 years in rural Maharashtra. *Indian Journal of Paediatrics, 59*, 423–427.

Rutter, M. (1990). Isle of Wight Revisited, Twenty-five years of child psychiatric epidemiology. In S. Chess, & M. Herzig (Eds.), *Annual Progress in Child Psychiatry and Child Development* (Chap. 7). Psychology Press. ISBN 978-0-87630-602-4.

Rutter, M. & Smith, D. J. (1995). *Psychosocial disorders in young people: Time trends and their causes*. Chichester, UK: Wiley.

Sawyer, M., et al. (2000). *Child and adolescent component of the national survey of mental health and well-being*. Canberra: Publication and Production Unit.

Saxena, S., Paraje, G., Sharan, P., Karam, G., & Sadana, R. (2006). The 10/90 divide in mental health research: Trends over a 10-year period. *British Journal of Psychiatry, 188*, 81–82.

Saxena, S., Thornicroft, G., Knapp, M., & Whiteford, H. (2007). Global mental health 2: Resources for mental health: Scarcity, inequity, and inefficiency. *Lancet, 370*, 878–889.

Sharan, P., & Sagar, R. (2008). Editorial: The need for national data on epidemiology of child and adolescent mental disorders. *Journal of Indian Association for Child and Adolescent Mental Health, 4*(2), 22–27.

Shastri, P. C., et al. (2010). Research in child and adolescent psychiatry in India. *Indian Journal of Psychiatry, 52*(1), S219–S223.

Shenoy, J., et al. (1998). Psychological disturbance among 5–8 year-old school children: A study from India. *Social Psychiatry and Psychiatric Epidemiology, 33*, 66–73.

Srikrishnamurthy, K. R. (2002). Kashyapa Samhita (also known as Briddha Jeevakiya Tantra). English translation.

Srinath, S., et al. (2005). Epidemiological study of child and adolescent psychiatric disorders in urban and rural areas of Bangalore, India. *Indian Journal of Medical Research, 122*, 67–79.

UNICEF, (2008). Statistics and monitoring. http://www.unicef.org/statistics.

Wilcox, C. E., et al. (2007). Seeking help for attention deficit hyperactivity disorder in developing countries: A study of parental explanatory models in Goa, India. *Social Science and Medicine, 64*, 1600–1610.

Zubrick, S. R. et al. (1995) Western Australian child health survey. Developing health and well-being in the Nineties. Institute for Child Health Research.

Part V
Developments in Substance Use Psychiatry

Chapter 19
Addiction Research in India

D. Basu, A. Ghosh, B. Patra and B.N. Subodh

1 Introduction

India is a large country, and the Indian culture, often labelled as an amalgamation of several cultures across centuries, spans across the Indian subcontinent and includes traditions that are several millennia old. The dimensions and the diversity of this country have created an overwhelming opportunity for research. However, this potential has been challenged by the lack of resources, motivation and different priorities in medical practice. Addiction as a phenomenon is known in Indian literature from time immemorial. But apart from a few scattered studies, this area remained unexplored till about 50 years ago. This inertia was disappeared with the commencement of regional-level, followed by national-level, epidemiological research. Over the years, more research in clinical, psychosocial and biological areas has been undertaken. Though the volume of published studies might not be enormous, nevertheless, it has reached to a level in which an honest and comprehensive appraisal of the present and the past is highly warranted and worthwhile.

After important but sporadic reports in the earlier parts of the last century, research in various aspects of substance use and addiction has increased voluminously over the past 40 years. This chapter summarises the major trends in research in this area. This

---

D. Basu, Professor; A. Ghosh, Senior Resident; B. Patra, Senior Resident; B.N. Subodh, Assistant Professor

---

D. Basu (✉) · B.N. Subodh
Drug de-Addiction and Treatment Centre, Department of Psychiatry,
Postgraduate Institute of Medical Education and Research (PGIMER), Chandigarh, India
e-mail: db_sm2002@yahoo.com

A. Ghosh · B. Patra
Department of Psychiatry, Postgraduate Institute of Medical Education
and Research (PGIMER), Chandigarh, India

S. Malhotra and S. Chakrabarti (eds.), *Developments in Psychiatry in India*,
DOI 10.1007/978-81-322-1674-2_19

chapter is divided into two major sections. The first section deals with epidemiology. It is subdivided into studies in general population (national as well as regional or local), treatment-seeking populations and special populations (women, children, elderly, medical profession and other workers and the prison population). The second major section covers the research regarding individual categories of substances predominantly used in India (alcohol, opioids, tobacco, cannabis and inhalants) and emerging newer concerns (newer drugs such as 'club drugs' and non-substance ('behavioural') addictions.

2 Epidemiology

Epidemiology is the scientific study of extent, determinant and distribution of disease in a defined geographic area. The knowledge of which is essential to document, understand, control and prevent such conditions, of which substance addiction is an important one. Epidemiological studies in relation to substance abuse can be grouped into two broad categories: studies among general and studies among special populations. In both these subgroups, there may be community-based and clinic-based research studies. In India, there is an overall paucity of epidemiological research especially of community-based studies. In a review by Basu and Mattoo (1999), this is noted to be 'all the more surprising', because of the clinical evidence for a rapidly increasing and changing trend of substance dependence over the last few decades.

3 Studies Among General Population

3.1 Findings from the National-Level Community-Based Studies

3.1.1 Prevalence of Substance Use in the Community

The National Household Survey (NHS) studied the prevalence of substance use in the general population. It reflects the overall level of drug use and lists commonly abused substances among general population in the country as a whole. It covers 40,697 males in the age group of 12–60 years (Table 1).

Among current opiate users, the largest proportions were opium users, followed by heroin, cough syrup and other opiate users. A small number of subjects reported the use of volatile substance, hallucinogens and stimulants. Only 0.1 % individuals reported 'ever'-injecting drugs, and the category is referred to as injectable drug users (IDUs).

As per the National Family Health Survey-2 (NFHS-2),[1] 17 % of the men drank alcohol, 29 % males aged 15 years or more and smoked tobacco and 28 % chewed tobacco. Two percent of the women drank alcohol, 3 % smoked tobacco and more than 10 % used smokeless tobacco. Rani et al. (2003) studied prevalence of tobacco consumption from samples of NFHS-2 and found it to be 30 % among

[1] National Family Health Survey India-2. Available from http://www.nfhsindia.org/nfhs2.html.

Table 1 Prevalence of drug use among males ($N = 40{,}697$)[a]

Substances	Ever use (lifetime) in %	Current use (last 1 month) in %	Dependent user as per ICD-10 criteria (in %)
Tobacco	57.9	55.8	
Alcohol	25.9	21.4	3.6
Cannabis	4.1	3	0.77
Opiates	1	0.7	0.15
Sedative and hypnotics	0.1	0.1	

aData from the National Household Survey (NHS)

individuals 15 years or older. The NFHS-3[2] showed that 11 % of the women and 57 % of the men used tobacco in any form. Only 2 % of the women and one-third of the men drank alcohol.

3.1.2 Prevalence Among Treatment-Seeking Population

The drug abuse monitoring system (DAMS) component of the National Survey obtained data on personvs taking treatment for the substance use disorder. As reported by the treatment-seeking population, alcohol was the commonest drug of abuse (43.9 %). This was followed by opiates (26 %) and cannabis (11.6 %). Other drugs of abuse such as barbiturates and amphetamines and cocaine were reported by 0.2 and 1.7 % of patients, respectively. Use of tobacco and its products was reported by 10.9 % of the respondents.

3.1.3 Prevalence in Hidden Substance Using Population Not Seeking Treatment

The multicentric rapid assessment surveys (RAS) attempted to obtain data from hidden and inaccessible drug users in the community. The RAS was carried out in 14 towns of India (Sethi 2001). The highest proportion of subjects was currently (last one month) abusing heroin, followed by other opiates (propoxyphene, opium, buprenorphine and pentazocine) at 28.6 %.

4 Findings from the Regional-Level Community-Based Studies

In India, many investigators have studied the prevalence of various psychiatric disorders, including the substance use disorders over period of time. Following are the studies, which have investigated the prevalence of substance use disorders (with or without studying the prevalence of other psychiatric disorders) in the community (Table 2).

[2] National Family Health Survey India-3. Available from http://www.nfhsindia.org/nfhs3.html.

Table 2 Regional-level epidemiological studies of alcohol and drug use

Author (year)	State/city	Population	Prevalence (per 1,000)	Outcome studied
Elnager et al. (1971)	West Bengal	1,383	13	Alcohol and drug addiction
Dube and Handa (1971)	Uttar Pradesh	16,725	22.8	Alcohol and drug abuse
Varghese et al. (1973)	Tamil Nadu	2,904	4.8	Chronic alcoholism
Thacore (1972)	Uttar Pradesh	2,696	18.55	Habitual excessive use (A, C)
Nandi et al. (1975)	West Bengal	1,060	0.94	
Lal and Singh (1979)	Punjab	6,699	203.9	Six-month period prevalence for current users (alcohol and drugs)
Sethi and Trivedi (1979)	Uttar Pradesh	2,415	214	Drug abusers A 43.5 %; C 39.2 %; O 1.4 %
Mohan et al. (1979)	Punjab	3,600	57.6	Opium use
Varma et al. (1980)	Punjab	1,031	237	Current alcohol users
Sundaram et al. (1984)	Rajasthan	4,670	247-alcohol abuse; 30-dependence	Alcohol abuse and dependence
Ponnudorai et al. (1991)	Tamil Nadu	2,334	167	Alcoholism (MAST score ≥5)
Premranjan et al. (1993)	Pondicherry	1,115	34.5	Alcohol dependence syndrome
Jena et al. (1996)	Bihar	1,157	A-288, C-251	Alcohol/drug use
Ghulam et al. (1996)	Madhya Pradesh	5,326	386	Current drug use
Singh et al. (1998)	Uttar Pradesh	1,806	104	Alcohol users
Chaturvedi et al. (1998)	Mizoram	375	M-566, F-457	Tobacco use
Hazarika et al. (2000)	Assam	312	T-40 %; A-36.5 %; IDU-1.28 %; Petrol inhalation-0.64 %	Drug users
Sharma and Singh (2001)	Goa	4,022	1	Alcohol dependence
Mohan and Ray (2001)	Delhi	6,004 and 5,599 households in two surveys	T-276, A-126, C-3, O-4	Dependent drug users

(continued)

Table 2 (continued)

Author (year)	State/city	Population	Prevalence (per 1,000)	Outcome studied
Mohan et al. (2002a, b)	Delhi	10,312	M-59/year/1,000 F-12/year/1,000	Incidence of substance use disorders
Mohan et al. (2002a, b)	Delhi	10,312	only T-181, only A-33, A + T-96	Substance use disorder
Meena et al. (2002)	Haryana	4,691	198	Alcohol and substance abuse
Silva et al. (2003)	Goa	1,013	213	Hazardous drinking of alcohol
Gupta et al. (2003)	Maharashtra	50,220	188	Current alcohol users
Benegal et al. (2003)	Karnataka	21,276	153	Alcohol use
Chaturvedi et al. (2003)	Meghalaya	1,831	29.4 %-T, 12.5 %-A, 4.9 %-O	Substance use
Chaturvedi et al. (2004)	Arunachal Pradesh	5,135	30.9 %-T, 30 %-A, 4.8 %- O	Substance use
Gururaj et al. (2004)	Bangalore	10,168	90	Alcohol users
Gururaj et al. (2006)	Bangalore	28,507	320	Alcohol users
Medhi et al. (2006)	Assam	2,264	A-592; A+T-547	Alcohol and tobacco users
Chavan et al. (2007)	Chandigarh	59,470	68.8	Alcohol and drug dependence
John et al. (2009)	Tamil Nadu	345	Lifetime use 467, use in the past year 348 and hazardous use of alcohol was 142	Hazardous use of alcohol (AUDIT scores >8)
Reddy and Chandrasekhar (1998) meta-analysis	All India	33,684	6.9	Alcohol/drug addiction
Joshi et al. (2010)	Gujarat	2,513	329	Current chewable tobacco users

5 Findings from Treatment-Seeking Populations

A recent retrospective chart review by Basu et al. (2012) studied the profile of subjects attending a drug de-addiction and treatment centre in North India over a period of three decades. This study reported an increase in the number of registered patients with a decrease in the age of presentation. The use of synthetic opioids demonstrated a rising trend. Alcohol, benzodiazepines and use of multiple substances have also been increased over the last few decades. Venkatesan and Suresh (2008), Munjal and Jiloha (1986) and Sachdeva et al. (2002) echoed the same changing pattern. A study from Delhi showed a higher prevalence of heroin use, along with other substances (Sharma and Sahai 1990). A gradually increasing trend was also noticed with respect to heroine use (Saxena and Mohan 1984; Adityanjee et al. 1984). Not only the traditional substances, Basu et al. (2014a) reported 5 patients with cocaine dependence and Sarkar et al. (2012) reported 7 patients with tramadol dependence who presented to a de-addiction centre for treatment.

There were a few studies from the general medico-surgical or emergency settings. A study on substance abusers using emergency services showed that majority of them were alcohol abusers, followed by opioid abuse. Importantly, a substantial proportion of opioid users are intravenous drug users (IVDUs) (Bhalla et al. 2006). Babu and Sengupta (1997) studied more than 300 new admissions in the wards of medicine, general surgery and orthopaedics in a general hospital. They found that problem drinking was present in about 15 % of the inpatients. Sri et al. (1997), who had assessed problem drinking with CAGE questionnaire, found a relatively higher prevalence. Similarly, Sampath et al. (2007) observed around 10 % subjects with alcohol dependence in consecutive hospital admissions.

Among studies from psychiatry outpatient settings, Gupta et al. (1987) found 10 % heroin dependence in a tertiary care hospital. Lavania et al. (2012) studied deliberate self-harm in non-depressed patients with substance dependence; their study demonstrated that opioid dependence predisposed to deliberate self-harm.

There is one study from a self-help organisation. Shastri and Kolhatkar (1989) conducted this study in three Narcotics Anonymous Meeting Centres and two drug addiction rehabilitation centres situated in different areas of Mumbai and its suburbs. It was found that all the subjects were taking either cannabis or heroin. Psychosocial issues in the family seemed to predispose to substance abuse.

6 Substance Use in Special Populations

The social stigma and the legal restriction attached to substance addiction make epidemiological studies challenging and difficult. To circumvent such problems, innovative and specialised research has been undertaken throughout the globe to trace the hidden, but important subset of substance-dependent population. Though in India, the extent of studying such 'special' populations is not too comprehensive, the amount of research is reasonably good and gradually expanding.

6.1 Epidemiological Studies in Women

The use of the substance in women outside religious, cultural or medicinal contexts has been seen in India for centuries. The use of substance outside these contexts has not been recognised until recently in India. Even the large national-level study of substance use in India did not include females in their study. Instances of women using substances have emerged in literature in India from around the 1980s. Recently, there are several studies done on female substance use at the national level; regional studies and the hospital-level data on the use of substances by women have also become available. The available studies have some methodological limitations, but the broad findings, which have emerged, have been described below.

The National Family Household Survey-3, which screened a representative sample of 124,385 for use of alcohol and tobacco throughout India, showed that 2 % women aged 15–49 years use alcohol and 11 % of them use tobacco. Among those who use alcohol, 15 % drink alcohol daily and 84 % once a week, or less than once a week. Among those who smoke, 1 % use smoking forms of tobacco and 8 % use smokeless forms. Around one-fourth of smokers report they smoke 10 or more cigarettes or *bidis*. Tobacco use was more prevalent than alcohol use in almost every state. All forms of substance use were more prevalent in rural, than in urban areas. Substance use decreased with increased level of education and income (NFHS-3). There was a change in the trend in the form of increased use of tobacco in National Family Health Survey-3, compared to National Family Health Survey-2, but the use of alcohol remained same. The National-level House to House Survey of 6,266 women in 25 states in India revealed that predominant substances used were alcohol (91.7 %), opioids (87.9 %) and tobacco (85.6 %) (Murthy et al. 2009). Another national-level survey of 1,865 women users by 110 NGOs showed that women who used substances were in their 20s or 30s, and married. The common substances used were alcohol, tobacco, opioids, sedatives and cannabis. Among users, 25 % had lifetime history and 24 % had been injecting in the previous month. The reasons for initiation of the substance use were due to childhood difficulty, peer influence, partner influence and stress (Murthy 2008).

A survey of 4,648 users in 14 cities found that 8 % of the users were women. These users were single, educated, employed and started using before 20 years of age. The common substances were opioid, alcohol, cannabis and minor tranquilisers. The reasons for initiation of the substance were influence of friends, spouse or partner, and stress and 'tension'. Among them, 40 % were IDUs and were involved in unsafe practices, unprotected sex and drug peddling (Kumar 2002). The Gender, Alcohol and Culture: An International Study (GENACIS) assessed alcohol and other substance use across 5 districts of Karnataka among 1,464 females. Most females were middle aged, poorly educated (<6 years), married and earning less. Around one-third of the women users had hazardous drinking, more than a third had husbands who used alcohol and a tenth drank exclusively. Only about 6 % of female drank less than once in the last 12 months (Benegal et al. 2005). A study of 7,445 adult men and 6,919 adult women from South India found that the average consumption on typical drinking occasions, in both men and women, was five standard drinks (12 g of ethanol per drink) (Benegal et al. 2003). Another study in South India found that one-fifth of the people who frequented pubs on weekends were girls aged between 13 and 19 years in Bangalore city (Kumar and Sharma 2008).

6.1.1 Hospital-Based Studies

These data are derived from the people visiting the hospital for substance-related problems. According to the drug abuse monitoring survey (DAMS) of treatment-seeking people in government-sponsored de-addiction centres, 1 % ($N = 117$) of treatment seekers were female during period of September 2006–August 2007. The treatment seekers were middle aged, illiterate, married and doing household activities. The predominant substances used were tobacco, alcohol, opioids, sedatives and cannabis. Majority (87.2 %) of them were first-time treatment seekers. The reason for visiting the hospital was due to physical complications (33.3 %) of substance use (Ray 2004). There are few hospital-based data about the female substance users. The main findings of these studies were that females were middle aged (in their late 30s), married, housewives and poorly educated. They were using alcohol, opioids, tobacco, benzodiazepines and cannabis. They had high physical (34–69 %) and medical comorbidity (23–70 %) (Murthy et al. 1992; Grover et al. 2005).

6.2 Substance Use in Children

There are very few national-level studies, particularly about substance use in children. Though majority of the studies on children have been done on inhalant use, literature is also available for other substance use. Majority of the data have been obtained from the regional studies from the metropolitan cities and from the hospital-based studies. The regional studies are mostly on substance use in street children.

The National Household Survey on Drug Abuse surveyed 40,697 males of whom 8,587 were children (aged 12–18 years). Of these, 3.8 % were using alcohol, 0.6 % were cannabis, and 0.2 % were using opiates (Ray et al. 2004).

In a study of 300 street child labourers in slums of Surat, it was observed that 135 (45 %) used substances. The substances used were smoking tobacco, followed by chewing tobacco, snuff, cannabis and opioids (Bansal and Banerjee 1993). A study of inhalant use in street children in Bangalore showed that tobacco was the predominant substance, followed by inhalants, alcohol, cannabis and opioids (Benegal et al. 1999). Nearly a decade later, in another study of street children from Bangalore, it was observed that inhalants are the commonest substance of abuse, followed by tobacco, alcohol, heroin, cannabis and pharmaceutical preparations. Substance use in street children helps them cope with the rigours of living in the streets (Benegal et al. 2008). A study in the Andamans demonstrated that onset of regular use of alcohol in late childhood and early adolescence is associated with the highest rates of consumption in adult life, compared to later onset of drinking (Benegal et al. 2008). Another study among street children found that among 163 street boys, 132 (80.98 %) were substance abusers. The common substances used were nicotine by 104 (63.8 %), inhalants by 78 (48 %), alcohol by 60 (37 %), sedatives and stimulants by 42 (26 %) and cannabis and opioids by 31 (19 %). A significant portion of the street children had been sexually abused 52 (31.9 %), and 87 (53.3 %) had been physically abused (Gaidhane et al. 2008).

6.2.1 Hospital-Based Studies

There are several case reports of use of the substances in children (Basu et al. 2004a, b; Kumar et al. 2008). A chart review of 85 child and adolescent patients from Chandigarh found that the primary substance of use was opioids, nicotine, alcohol, cannabis, sedatives and inhalants. The reason for use of the substance was curiosity and peer pressure (Saluja et al. 2007).

6.3 Other Populations

A clinic-based study on elderly population has demonstrated a slow but increasing trend of registered elderly patients suffering from substance dependence. There is a preponderance of alcohol dependence, which is followed by opioid dependence (Grover et al. 2008).

A study of the substance use in the 250 auto-rickshaw pullers in New Delhi shows that majority of them used tobacco (79.2 %), followed by alcohol (54.4 %), cannabis (8.0) and opioid (0.8 %). The substance used helped them to remain awake at night while working (Gupta et al. 1986a, b). A study in industrial population about psychiatric prevalence has shown that harmful substance use or substance dependence (42.83 %) is the most common psychiatric condition (Dutta et al. 2007). Another study among industrial workers from Goa estimated a prevalence of 211/1,000 with hazardous drinking using the Alcohol Use Disorder Identification Test (AUDIT) (Silva et al. 2003).

Substance use among medical students has also been examined in several studies (Kumar and Basu 2000; Seshadri 2008). As early as 1977, a drug abuse survey in Lucknow among medical students revealed that 25.1 % abused a drug at least once in a month. Commonly abused drugs included minor tranquilisers, alcohol, amphetamines, *bhang* (cannabis) and non-barbiturate sedatives. In a study of internees on the basis of a youth survey developed by the WHO in 1982, 22.7 % of males 'indulged in alcohol abuse' at least once in a month and 9.3 % abused cannabis, followed by tranquilisers. Common reasons cited were social reasons, enjoyment, curiosity and relief from psychological stress. Most reported that it was easy to obtain drugs such as marijuana and amphetamines (Ponnudurai et al. 1984). Another study in New Delhi of 2,135 medical students showed that current alcohol, tobacco (chewable or smoked) and illicit substance use reported by 7.1, 6.1 and 6.7 % of the respondents, respectively. Use of illicit substances was strongly associated with use of tobacco, alcohol and non-prescription drugs (Rai et al. 2008). A monograph on substance use in the prison population revealed that among the inmates, nearly 80 % had diagnosable psychiatric disorders, and a substantial proportion of them were dependent on substances.

The majority of Indian studies on the special populations have tried to establish the extent of substance use in these populations. Not much work has been done on the treatment-related aspects of substance use in special populations, except among street children using substances.

7 Individual Substance-Related Areas

An attempt has been made to describe the available literature from India on different substances of abuse. To ensure that this section is comprehensive, inclusive and lucid, each of the substance-related sections is further stratified into several subsections based on clinical, biological or treatment-focused research. But, due to paucity of available research in some of these subsections, they are not of uniform length. Studies on comorbid psychiatric disorders, commonly referred as the 'dual diagnosis', are not always substance specific. Hence, there has been some inevitable overlap in this area. This brief summary is based only on original studies and not on reviews of the subject. As expected, most of the published studies are on alcohol problems, followed by opioid dependence. Overall, clinical and psychosocial research substantially outnumbers biological research. Moreover, the majority of these studies have been carried out only in a few centres. Nevertheless, it is encouraging to note that the volume of Indian research is this area is increasing with time.

8 Research on Alcohol-Related Areas

Though the constitution of India has asked for a prohibition for the use of all 'intoxicants' including alcohol, it still remains as one of the most commonly used substances of addiction, as reported by different epidemiological studies. India's reputation as a country with a culture of abstinence especially in matters regarding alcohol is underserved. The country, which has seen a rapid proliferation of city bars and nightclubs in recent years, is fast shedding its inhibitions about alcohol as a lifestyle choice (Prasad 2009).

8.1 Studies on Harmful Effects Incurred by Alcohol Use

Hospital admission rates due to the adverse effects of alcohol consumption are disproportionately high. Several studies indicate that nearly 20–30 % of admissions or consultations are due to alcohol-related problems (direct or indirect) in different healthcare settings but are under-recognised by primary-care physicians (Sri et al. 1997; Benegal et al. 2001). Alcohol misuse has been implicated in over 20 % of traumatic brain injuries (Gururaj 2002; Sabheshan and Natarajan 1987) and 60 % of all injuries reporting to emergency rooms (Benegal et al. 2002). It has a disproportionately high association with deliberate self-harm (Gururaj and Isaac 2001), high-risk sexual behaviour (Chandra et al. 2003), HIV infection, tuberculosis (Rajeswari et al. 2002), oesophageal cancer (Chitra et al. 2008), liver disease (Sarin et al. 1988) and duodenal ulcer (Jain et al. 1999). Association between alcohol dependence and seizures is well recognised. Seizure prevalence of 8–16 % among patients with alcohol dependence has been reported (Matto et al. 2009b). Importantly, a confident diagnosis of withdrawal seizure could be made only in minority of instances (Murthy et al. 2007; Mattoo et al. 2009a, b). A recent estimate from surveillance of major non-communicable diseases in India placed the burden due to alcohol use as most important among all non-communicable disorders (Anand 2000). Hence, huge healthcare expenditure is being incurred due to alcohol use. Using their findings in the Bangalore study, researchers from NIMHANS calculated that the direct and indirect costs are attributable to alcohol addiction to be more than three times the profits of alcohol taxation and several times more than the annual health budget of Karnataka. Extrapolating their findings to the whole of India, they estimated that the total alcohol revenue for the period of 2003–2004 was 216 billion rupees, which fell 28 billion rupees short of the total cost of managing the effects of alcohol addiction (Benegal et al. 2000; Gururaj et al. 2006). Alcohol abuse also causes social dysfunction. In a study from India focusing on the distress of the family members of patients with alcoholism, it was found that relatives of all patients reported behaviours such as excessive spending and disturbance of peace at home to be distressful (Chand and Chaturvedi 2010).

The other side of the coin, the alcohol industry, promotes and nurtures a concept called 'responsible drinking'. The concept, though lucrative for the global trade and excise, should be critically viewed from a health perspective. In a review, it was concluded that currently, there is not enough evidence to promote drinking of alcoholic beverages, even at so-called responsible levels, from a public health and policy perspective (Banerjee et al. 2006).

8.2 Studies on Comorbidity or 'Dual Diagnosis'

Research on 'dual diagnosis' can be well classified into two broad categories based on the locus of the study. Research has been done primarily either in the psychiatry or in the de-addiction clinics, looking for the presence of either of these groups of disorders. Trivedi et al. screened 1,000 consecutive patients presenting to a psychiatric hospital and found that about 8 % of them abused alcohol. The figure indicates that almost half of the all substance abusers were using alcohol. Alcohol was observed to be more commonly used by patients with bipolar and neurotic disorders, rather than patients suffering from schizophrenia (Trivedi and Sethi 1978). Among the second group of studies, Basu and Gupta (2000) noted that the prevalence of drug use among people with mental illness was twice that found in the general population. The prevalence was 16 % in bipolar disorder, 14 % in schizophrenia, 5 % in organic psychosis and 2 % in non-psychotic disorders. Kishore et al. assessed the lifetime prevalence of comorbidity in 43 patients with substance dependence and the chronology of such comorbidity from the de-addiction centre of a tertiary hospital at Lucknow. The substance most commonly used was alcohol. A study was conducted in the Regional Institute of Medical Sciences (RIMS), Manipur, also replicated the findings of higher psychiatric comorbidity among patients with alcohol dependence, compared to controls (Singh et al. 2005). A relatively older clinic-based study from North India, which compared the prevalence of both axis I and axis II psychiatric disorders in patients with alcohol and opioid dependence, found no difference between these patients. The overall prevalence figure for alcohol and opioid dependence was about 60 % (Vohra et al. 2003). In a recent retrospective chart-based review of consecutive patients from the same centre, 13 % patients were found to have any psychiatric disorders. Mood disorders were the commonest comorbidity in both of these studies. A study on 'dual diagnosis' schizophrenia found that patients ascribed hedonistic pursuit as the principal reason for substance use, but reduction in symptoms and distress were also cited as reasons. A trend was discovered for alcohol to be used more for self-medication purposes, compared to opioids and cannabis (Goswami et al. 2003). Another clinic-based study has shown that there is a high frequency of psychiatric comorbidity, predominantly affective disorders, in patients with alcoholic liver disease (ALD) when compared with alcohol dependence alone (Kakunjee 2012). The same group of researchers also found out a substantial and equal occurrence of personality disorders in both ALD and non-ALD groups (Kakunji et al. 2012). Another study, which attempted to assess the prevalence of sexual dysfunction in a clinical sample with alcohol dependence, demonstrated that 72 % had one or more sexual dysfunctions, the most common being premature ejaculation, low sexual desire and erectile dysfunction. The amount of alcohol consumed appeared to be the most significant predictor of developing sexual dysfunction (Arackal and Benegal 2007). Externalising disorders in childhood and adolescence have been found to predate alcohol dependence. Childhood attention-deficit hyperkinetic disorder, which is a member of this group of disorders, was found to be significantly associated with the early-onset subtype of alcohol dependence (Sringeri et al. 2008). In a study from Chandigarh, with a larger sample and better methodology, the same finding was replicated and extended to other childhood disruptive disorders (conduct disorder and oppositional defiant disorder) and adult attention-deficit hyperkinetic disorder (Ghosh 2013). Substance abuse not only predisposes subjects to psychiatric disorders, but also complicates the course of the same. This fact has been substantiated in both patients with alcohol and opioid dependence, where an increase in substance abuse preceded schizophrenic exacerbation in one-third of the patients with 'dual-diagnosis' disorders (Goswami et al. 2003).

8.3 Studies on Other Clinical Issues

Not only psychiatric disorders, but also alcohol dependence is also associated with certain personality traits. In a study to evaluate their personality traits, patients with alcohol dependence obtained significantly higher scores on a variety of traits (Chaudhury et al. 2006). Experience and expression of anger and subsequent lower quality of life were found more commonly among patients with alcohol dependence (Sharma et al. 2011). Individuals with alcohol dependence had significantly lower self-esteem compared with control subjects, and significantly, more of the patients were identified as alexithymic. The same study has also commented on the limited value of MAST and CAGE in the diagnosis of alcohol dependence (Ray and Chandrasekhar 1982). Cross-system diagnostic concordance is contradicted by results from two different studies (Basu et al. 2000a, b; Ray and Neeliyara 1989). Typology of alcohol dependence, which has been studied extensively elsewhere, has not attracted much research attention in India. In a study, multivariate cluster analytic approach to classify alcohol dependence was found to be superior as compared to the univariate one, both in terms of concurrent validity and in terms of predictive validity (Basu et al. 2004a, b). Another study was aimed at finding out clinical, personality and behavioural correlates of age at onset of alcohol dependence. Results showed that early-onset patients with alcohol dependence were higher sensation seekers, higher on the Psychopathic Deviate Scale of the multidimensional personality questionnaire (MPQ) and tended to display aggression, violence and general disinhibition when drinking. On the contrary, late-onset patients with alcohol dependence (age at onset of alcohol dependence more than 25 years) were anxiety prone and guilt ridden and had less alcohol-related problems (Varma et al. 1994). Individuals with chronic alcohol abuse show impairments in several cognitive functions. A study of frontal lobe functions and their association with alcohol consumption variables found that chronic alcohol dependence affects visual scanning, set-shifting and response inhibition abilities. Patients with a fewer number of days of alcohol intake during the past 1 year performed relatively better (SriGowri et al. 2008).

8.4 Studies on Initiation and Course of Alcohol Use

Consumption of alcohol has been attributed to different reasons by consumers. Attitude and knowledge about the substance and addiction can be influenced by the cultural background of the individual. In an effort to develop an instrument to assess the attitude towards drinking, four factors have emerged to the forth, namely 'acceptance', 'avoidance', 'rejection' and 'social dimension' (Basu et al. 1998). A recent study examining the reasons for alcohol intake and the belief about addiction in people with different ethnic backgrounds has found that societal acceptance and pressure, as well as emotional problems, appear to be the major aetiology, leading to higher prevalence of substance dependence in the tribal community (Sreeraj et al. 2012). Another study on information technology professionals has implicated higher rates of professional stress and risk for developing depression in the development of harmful alcohol use (Darshan et al. 2013). Three phases have been defined and characterised in the downhill progression of alcohol dependence (Mattoo and Basu 1997). The early phase is characterised by the absence of any problems; the middle phase, beginning with daily drinking and ending with the use of a bottle of spirits a day, is characterised mainly by social problems; the late phase begins with the onset of morning drinking and is characterised by the onset of physical problems. In a recent effort, the chronology of criteria of dependence in alcohol dependence syndrome was examined (Mattoo and Basu 1997). In order-wise chronology, either craving or tolerance was present as the first criterion and the presence of craving, tolerance or loss of control was observed as the first criterion in more than half of the subjects. Relapse of alcoholism is a rule rather than exception in dependent patients. Lack of cognitive vigilance was observed to be the most common precipitant of relapse. Family and patients' perceptions about the precipitants of relapse were found to be concordant (Malhotra et al. 1999).

8.5 Studies on Biology of Alcohol Dependence

Alcohol abuse disorders result from the interaction between an individual's genetic and environmental susceptibility and repeated intake of alcohol over time. It is not possible to become dependent on alcohol without repeatedly consuming alcohol, but only a small percentage of all drinkers develop alcohol dependence. Although the prevalence of alcohol dependence in the Asian population is low, a sizable number of people in India suffer from alcohol use disorders. Genetic polymorphisms, particularly those of the alcohol-metabolising enzymes alcohol dehydrogenase (ADH) and aldehyde dehydrogenase (ALDH), have been largely implicated in the development of alcohol dependence. Though India represents about one-sixth of the world's population, there are limited data on genes or polymorphisms that confer susceptibility to alcohol dependence in this population. In a study, aldehyde dehydrogenase (ALDH) levels in patients with alcohol dependence and their first degree non-dependent relatives and controls were compared (Murthy et al. 1996). Findings indicated that low erythrocyte ALDH may be considered as a biochemical trait marker associated with alcoholism. Another study from the northern part of India highlighted the uniquely high frequency of the *ALDH2*2/*2* genotype (among subjects with alcohol dependence) being a risk-conferring factor for alcohol dependence. Recently, males with alcohol dependence belonging to six ethnic populations, from four linguistic groups of India, were studied for a single nucleotide polymorphism (SNP) of ALDH2 gene. The small number of haplotypes coding for low-level enzyme activity in this region suggests the strong linkage disequilibrium across the region and confirms the global long-range linkage disequilibrium around the ALDH2 locus (Vaswani et al. 2009). In addition to ALDH polymorphism, it is well established that the central dopaminergic reward pathway is likely involved in alcohol intake and the progression of alcohol dependence. Dopamine transporter (DAT1) mediates the active re-uptake of dopamine from the synapse and is a principal regulator of dopaminergic neurotransmission. A study from the southern part of our country demonstrated a population-specific DAT1 polymorphism determining the vulnerability to alcohol dependence (Bhaskar et al. 2012). Another study provided preliminary insight into genetic risk of alcohol dependence in Indian men (Prasad et al. 2010). It demonstrated two polymorphisms in the *DRD2* gene, which may have clinical implications among Indian men with alcohol dependence.

In addition to the molecular genetic studies, neurobiological and neurophysiological investigations have been undertaken in India. These studies have looked into the high-risk population for alcohol dependence, consisting of either person with family history of alcohol dependence or person having externalising disorders. A study aimed to evaluate corpus callosum morphometry in subjects at high risk for alcoholism found that smaller callosal areas had a negative association with externalising behaviours and might represent yet another marker of susceptibility to alcoholism in high-risk subject (Benegal et al. 2006; Venkatasubramaniam et al. 2007). On similar lines, an electrophysiological study on high-risk subjects showed lower P300 amplitudes over frontal brain areas (Benegal et al. 1995; Murlidharan 2008). Differences were greater in the young, tending to converge with increasing age. There was a strong association between this reduced brain activation and an excess of externalising behaviours in high-risk individuals. Another study in this area concluded that P300 amplitudes varied inversely with the presumed continuum (children with high family loading of alcohol dependence, early-onset alcohol dependence and late-onset alcohol dependence) of risk in those at high risk for developing alcoholism (Silva et al. 2007).

8.6 Studies on Treatment of Alcohol Dependence

Among studies on interventions related to withdrawal and relapse prevention, drug trials outnumber studies on psychosocial interventions. In substance abuse treatment, it is always essential to determine the treatment setting prior to the initiation of actual treatment. Unfortunately, there is no published literature from India on the relative efficacy or indication of inpatient or outpatient treatment. The only retrospective review of inpatient treatment to determine the long-term outcome of both alcohol dependence and opioid dependence revealed that those who were following up at the time of evaluation had significantly longer duration to relapse. Hence, putting emphasis on the follow-up could result in a better long-term outcome (Singh et al. 2008). To ensure an optimal follow-up of patients, it is quite essential to have a multidisciplinary approach.

Lorazepam and chlordiazepoxide are both popular treatments for alcohol-withdrawal syndrome all over the world and so also in India. In a double-blind randomised control trial that was done to compare their efficacy, lorazepam and chlordiazepoxide showed similar efficacy in reducing symptoms of alcohol withdrawal as assessed using the revised Clinical Institute Withdrawal Assessment (CIWA) for Alcohol Scale (Kumar et al. 2009). No difficulties in drug discontinuation or differences in impairing adverse events were observed with either drug. Then again, another study has highlighted the problem with mega doses of lorazepam (Chand and Murthy 2003). Another study demonstrated an increase in the low activity of aldehyde dehydrogenase (ALDH) following administration of either diazepam or chlordiazepoxide in alcohol withdrawal, explaining their efficacy (Murthy 1992).

In India, disulfiram is still the most commonly used agent for relapse prevention, as it is cheap and easily available. Disulfiram in alcohol use disorders in the Indian context is a useful treatment, particularly when compliance with the drug regimen is overseen by family members (Grover and Basu 2004; Grover et al. 2007a, b). An open-label randomised control trial compared the efficacy of disulfiram (DSF) and topiramate (TPM) for preventing alcoholic relapse in routine clinical practice in India (Sousa 2008). Though DSF proved to be more efficacious in terms of time spent in abstinence, TPM-treated patients did show less craving than DSF-treated patients. Another study with similar methodology comparing the efficacy of disulfiram and naltrexone (NTX) demonstrated superior efficacy of DSF in terms of time to relapse (Sousa and Sousa 2004). The third study concluded that DSF is superior to acamprosate (ACP) for preventing relapse in men with alcohol dependence with good family support (Sousa 2005). Comparison of efficacy with DSF and NTX in adolescent population has demonstrated superiority of the former in terms of reducing relapse rate (Sousa 2008). These findings were also replicated in the elderly population (Sousa and Jagtap 2009). All these studies were from same centre and were done by the same research team. Moreover, they had recruited patients with good family support and also provided psychosocial interventions. Hence, the findings of these studies should be interpreted within these limitations. Further comparisons between these drugs in different treatment settings and populations are, thus, warranted. In a retrospective chart review, patients with alcohol dependence who received treatment from an addiction centre were studied to compare those on ACP or NTX versus those on no prophylactic drugs with regard to their demographic and clinical background and short-term outcome after treatment (Basu et al. 2005). Results showed a superiority of ACP over NTX, or no drugs, both in the short term and during follow-up. Despite the popular notion of DSF's potential dangerousness, it has rarely been implicated in serious adverse events. A study was conducted to evaluate the short-term safety of DSF in patients with alcohol dependence with chronic smoking (Galgali et al. 2002). Finding suggested that disulfiram does not significantly alter forced expiratory volume in the first minute (FEV1) values and airway reactivity during the treatment period, thus, could be used safely. Though there is no systemic study on the adverse reactions of these prophylactic medications, there is one case report of possible DSF-induced delirium after 6 weeks of initiation of the medication (Basu 2010).

There are only a handful of studies on psychosocial interventions for alcohol dependence. A five-year follow-up study of 150 patients treated for alcohol dependence using a primarily Alcoholics Anonymous approach reported a modest improvement in outcome, both in short term and in long term (Kuruvilla and Jacob 2007). In a recent study conducted in South India, it was found that individuals randomly assigned to dyadic relapse prevention (i.e. involvement of both patient and family members in the intervention) consistently performed better than those assigned to treatment as usual (Nattala et al. 2010). Intervention was more effective for relapse prevention in terms of reduction in quantity of alcohol, drinking days and number of days with dysfunction in family, occupational and financial dimensions. Another study demonstrated the effectiveness of training community volunteers in imparting knowledge and skills to identify and motivate persons with alcohol and drug dependence to seek treatment (Manickam 1997). Keeping patients with alcohol dependence in the treatment net is one of the most difficult yet a crucial task. Tracing techniques such as home visits were found to be effective in increasing follow-up rates in patients with alcohol dependence (Mahadevappa et al. 1987). Along the same lines, follow-up support and continued care appeared to significantly improve longer-term recovery in this group of patients (Murthy et al. 2009).

Study on the predictors of outcome following alcohol de-addiction treatment has mentioned younger age, higher psychosocial problem index, family history of alcoholism and delayed follow-up after relapse among the few negative predictors (Kar et al. 2003).

9 Research on Opioid-Related Areas

Opium poppy has been cultivated in India since the tenth century. The first Indian text to mention the use of opioids was possibly the '*Dhanvanatari Nighantu*', an ancient Indian medical treatise of the tenth century, which lists opium as a remedy for a variety of ailments. There has been a long-standing history of not only opioid addiction in India, but also managing this addiction through providing access to opioids in a regulated fashion, akin to the agonist maintenance treatment of today. Apart from the epidemiological studies, which have been already mentioned elsewhere, there are only a few biological, clinical and treatment-related studies on opioid dependence from India.

9.1 Studies on Harmful Effects Incurred by Opioid Use

Injecting drug use (IDU) has been strongly associated with HIV. In India too, among all risk groups, prevalence of HIV is highest among IDUs. High prevalence of hepatitis C has also been described among Indian IDU populations. In a review, hepatitis C virus infection is found to co-occur in 30–50 % of IDUs in general and 60–90 % in some high-risk pockets. Hence, the figure indicates an appreciable magnitude of problem that may turn into an epidemic. This review also points towards glaring lacunae of studies on risk behaviours associated with acquiring hepatitis C virus infection in IDUs (Basu 2010). Taking cue from the same, the author has tried to address this issue in a recent study. It was found that seroprevalence of anti-HCV antibody is high in IVDUs compared to non-IVDUs and is primarily related to injecting risk behaviour (Basu et al. 2012, 2013). In a study of consecutive patients, 12.5 % was found to have seizures and most of these were associated with substance use (Mattoo et al. 2009a). Dextropropoxyphene (DPP), a weak opioid, is often abused as a psychoactive substance in India. A retrospective chart review from PGIMER, Chandigarh, has demonstrated that DPP-induced epileptic seizures are common (one in five) and much more frequent than seizures in patients using other opioids. Those with seizures had significantly greater duration of DPP use and higher rates of medical comorbidity compared to patients without seizure (Basu et al. 2009a). Metabolic syndrome (MS) is an emerging condition in present psychiatric literature. A study from India, conducted in Chandigarh, has demonstrated that almost one in three of opioid-dependent patients has metabolic syndrome, and the figure is more than the prevalence of MS in alcohol dependence in the same study. Moreover, the prevalence of MS in both disorders is in turn greater than the general population prevalence (Mattoo et al. 2011).

Studies on comorbidity or 'dual diagnosis': No research till date has exclusively looked into prevalence of psychiatric disorders among patients with opioid dependence. Rather opioid dependence has been studied as a subset of the entire spectrum of substance dependence. In Trivedi et al.'s previously mentioned study, opium was the least sought-after substance among patients with psychiatric illnesses. But, in another study from a de-addiction clinic of Lucknow, opioids were found to be the second most common substances of abuse in patients with dual diagnosis (Kishore et al. 1994). Possibly, the locus of research can explain the discrepancy.

9.2 Studies on Other Clinical Issues

Though subtypes of alcohol dependence have been studied extensively, there are only a few studies on subtyping or profiling of opioid dependence. A study from Chandigarh has shown that the early-onset group was characterised by a significantly younger current age, more urban and unemployed subjects, a higher severity of opioid use, higher sensation seeking and higher global psychopathology in terms of MPQ. These results indicate that the age-at-onset typology in opioid dependence is a feasible way of classifying patients with opioid dependence, and this subtyping has some similarities to age-at-onset typology in alcoholism (De et al. 2003). A recent study from the same centre has sparked renewed the interest in the area of opioid typology. This has compared early- and late-onset opioid patients with opioid dependence on five explanatory domains including clinical (severity), genetic (family history), psychological (sensation seeking and impulsivity), neuropsychological (attention concentration and executive functions) and neurophysiological (P300 evoked response potential). Taking a cue from the classic categorical versus dimensional debate in clinical psychiatry, this research has emphasised that age of onset of opioid dependence is meaningful when the diagnosis of dependence is used as dimension rather than a category (Basu et al. 2014b).

9.3 Studies on Initiation and Course of Opioid Use

Initiation of substance abuse is undoubtedly affected by psychosocial factors. In one study, peer influence was found to have a significant role in initiation of heroin use (Chowdhury and Sen 1992). Sometimes medical prescriptions can initiate opioid use. In a case series of tramadol dependence, prescription of the same medication as an analgesic was found to precede its regular use (Sarkar et al. 2012). Likewise, psychological traits have also been implicated. High sensation seeking combined with alienation, leading to an inability to meet the demands through a socially sanctioned channels, has been hypothesised to foster opioid dependence (Basu et al. 1995). Relapse is a common and distressing aspect of substance dependence mediated by several biological and psychosocial factors (Mattoo et al. 1997, 2009a). A study examined the association between demographic variables, clinical parameters and certain psychosocial factors and relapse among patients with either alcohol or opioid dependence. Patients who had relapsed were significantly more likely to have a positive family history, to have a higher number of previous relapses, to be using maladaptive coping strategies and to have been exposed to a higher total number of 'high-risk' situations and undesirable life events. Conversely, those who had remained abstinent tended to use significantly more number of coping strategies, principally adaptive ones, and scored significantly higher on all measures of self-efficacy. Another study has highlighted on the role of craving in relapse of heroin dependence (Dhawan et al. 2002). Craving was found to be inversely proportional to the duration of abstinence and was not influenced by socio-cultural factors. In a clinic-based study on patients with buprenorphine addiction, a chronic but slowly improving course was ascertained. Substance substitution was found to complicate the overall course and outcome (Basu et al. 2000a, b).

9.4 Studies on Biology of Opioid Dependence

The opioid receptor mu1 (OPRM1) mediates the action of morphine. A study demonstrated the role of OPRM1 receptor polymorphism in the development of opioid addiction (Deb et al. 2010). The same group of researchers also found out the contribution of c-AMP receptor-binding element (CREB) polymorphism to opioid dependence (Kumar et al. 2011). Investigating endophenotypes is an emerging concept, especially for opioid dependence (Singh and Basu 2009). A study has demonstrated maximum abnormality in P300 latency and amplitude, and executive function, in patients with opioid dependence, followed by their healthy relatives, with least abnormalities in the control group (Singh et al. 2009).

9.5 Studies on Treatment of Opioid Dependence

The treatment of opioid dependence syndrome constitutes of treatment for intoxication, withdrawal and relapse prevention. No studies on the treatment of opioid intoxication have been undertaken in India. Buprenorphine has been found to be an effective agent for management of opioid withdrawal symptoms. When compared to clonidine, buprenorphine was found to be efficacious both in terms of less subjective symptoms and in terms of no change in the 'liking' for opioids (Ray et al. 2011). Another study has been conducted to correlate the effect of clonidine in opioid withdrawal with the opiate receptor activity. Clonidine seems to mitigate kappa receptor effects earlier than the mu receptor effects and does not have much effect on delta receptor effects (Chaturvedi 1994).

For long-term management of opioid dependence, one approach is opioid substitution or agonist therapy. Methadone, which has been extensively studied in the West, has been launched only recently in India and is being implemented as a pilot project at five sites in India. The initial clinical experience is encouraging; however, the adequate dose for Indian patients is yet to be determined. Early observations indicate that most Indian patients would require doses ranging between 40 and 80 mg/day. But, there are quite a few studies on the efficacy of another agonist, buprenorphine. A study has demonstrated the low abuse liability of buprenorphine in higher doses (Singhal et al. 2007). De et al. (2001) in a double-blind randomised controlled trial compared different doses of sublingual buprenorphine (2 and 4 mg/day) in an inpatient setting for long-term pharmacotherapy among opiate-dependent subjects. The results indicated that both 2 and 4 mg doses of buprenorphine were effective in pharmacotherapy of opioid dependence without significant difference. Mohan and Ray (1997) did a quasi-experimental study of community-based treatment with buprenorphine for heroin dependence in an urban slum of Delhi. It was seen that 70 % subjects improved with no use or very little use of heroin. Dhawan and Sunder (2008), in a brief overview of buprenorphine substitution in India, have concluded that buprenorphine substitution programmes have been successful in decreasing the harm associated with drug use, as well as decreasing the drug use per se and improving the quality of life. In another study carried out by the All India Institute of Medical Sciences (AIIMS) in Nagaland, 54 patients with opioid dependence on buprenorphine maintenance were followed up for 6 months. There was significant improvement in 'Drug and family domain' of the Addiction Severity Index (ASI), and the subjective well-being scale. Similarly, the treatment centre of TT Ranganathan Clinical Research Foundation, Chennai, found improvement in patients maintained on buprenorphine in their drug use pattern, life functioning, general health, high-risk behaviour, crime rate and arrests. In a multisite study on buprenorphine, Dhawan et al. (2010) reported that the mean dose required was 6 mg/day. Results showed significant abstinence and reduction in addiction severity with buprenorphine at this dose. A recent study found out that buprenorphine and naloxone combination had a higher adherence rate, compared to buprenorphine when used for opioid substitution therapy (Balhara and Jain 2012). In another study, buprenorphine maintenance was found to be helpful not only in terms of diminished use, but also in improving the quality of life (QoL) of patients with opioid dependence (Dhawan and Chopra 2013). Slow-release oral morphine (SROM), a natural derivative of opium and a mu receptor agonist, is relatively cheap with a long duration of action. In India too, SROM has been tried for patients with opioid dependence as a maintenance agent at the Nation Drug De-addiction and Treatment Center (NDDTC), AIIMS, New Delhi. It has been found to be a safe drug with minimal side effects and can be administered in once-daily dosage. Patients showed definite improvement, with a decrease in heroin consumption, improved functioning and a decrease in illegal activities (Rao et al. 2005, 2012). Though opioid substitution therapy has been researched reasonably well, opioid antagonist treatment has been studied rarely. In an open-label study, opioid antagonist naltrexone was found to be efficacious with an overall abstinence rate up to 50 %. It also proved to be acceptable to the patients (Malhotra et al. 2003).

A study, which evaluated sexual dysfunction among men with opioid dependence receiving buprenorphine and naltrexone maintenance therapy, showed a high and equal prevalence of sexual dysfunction in both groups (Ramdurg et al. 2012).

There is an emerging interest of addictive potential of narcotics in pain management, especially in palliative care. A study to determine the extent to which nurses are able to correctly identify drugs as narcotics and to ascertain their perception of the addiction potential of opiates when used for pain management, has shown a lack of appropriate knowledge both in identification and in perception of addictive potential (Desai and Chaturvedi 2003).

10 Research on Tobacco-Related Areas

Tobacco is a unique substance in a sense; it has been studied more by other health professionals rather than the psychiatrists, owing to its wide range of health-related effects, thus culminating in a huge database, which is beyond the scope of this current chapter. Hence, only aspects relevant to psychiatric practice will be discussed here.

10.1 Studies on Harmful Effects Incurred by Tobacco Use

Tobacco-related mortality in India is very high. It increases the number of premature deaths. In a nationally representative sample among both men and women, smoking was associated with twice the mortality when compared to the general population. Smoking was associated with reduction of median survival rate by 6–8 years. Excess deaths among smokers, as compared with non-smokers, were chiefly from tuberculosis and from respiratory, vascular or neoplastic diseases (Jha and Chaloupka 1999). The association of smokeless tobacco with oral cancer is very high. The use of chewable tobacco is associated with coronary vasoconstriction and significant hemodynamic alterations. Although there is no systemic study, it is estimated that 8.3 million cases of coronary artery disease and chronic obstructive airway diseases are also attributable to tobacco each year (Murthy and Saddichha 2010). The economic costs of tobacco use are equally devastating. In addition to the high public health costs of treating tobacco-caused diseases, tobacco kills people at the height of their productivity, depriving families of breadwinners and nations of a healthy workforce (Jiloha 2012).

10.2 Studies on Comorbidity or 'Dual Diagnosis'

For tobacco, primary study samples are almost always the patients with psychiatric illnesses. In a group of 70 patients with schizophrenia, Aich et al. (2004) found that 54.3 % had comorbid substance abuse. Tobacco was one of the commonly abused drugs along with cannabis.

10.3 Studies on Other Clinical Issues

Spontaneous quit attempts in the Indian population are very low, and it has been suggested that only 2 % of users have quit on their own (Jha and Chaloupka 1999). However, one-third of tobacco users had made a quit attempt in the previous year. Among persons who sought a health consultation, less than 50 % have been asked or advised to quit tobacco and less than 10 % provided any form of counselling or pharmacotherapy. Misconceptions among physicians could also influence intervention. In a recent study from South India, about one-third of the doctors believed that smoking only becomes harmful when the number of cigarettes per day was six or more (Thankappan et al. 2009). Smokeless tobacco users are even less likely to have received any intervention. A recent study has demonstrated a differential pattern of cue-controlled craving for the smoked and smokeless form of tobacco (Sarkar et al. 2013).

10.4 Studies on Treatment of Tobacco Dependence

Unfortunately, it appears that patients with tobacco dependence who are unable to stop by themselves are not even advised to stop, let alone not assisted with pharmacotherapy. This possibly explains the alarming paucity of research related to treatment of tobacco dependence. Studies have been carried out either in clinic-based or in community-based settings. Overall, providing simple counselling with proper use of pharmacotherapy is more cost-effective in Indian settings, rather than specialised and more intensive counselling (Murthy and Saddichha 2010; Murthy and Subodh 2010; Thirthalli and Chand 2009).

In a large tobacco cessation clinic-based study from India, use of nicotine replacement therapy (NRT) (along with behavioural counselling) was reported among 10 % of the clients (Varghese et al. 2012). Bupropion was found to be the most commonly used medication. But, studies from India have not consistently found the effectiveness of bupropion among patients with tobacco dependence. Two clinic-based studies among treatment seekers for chest aliments (one open-label study and the other a small randomised controlled trial) demonstrated the effectiveness of bupropion for patients with tobacco dependence, compared to that of counselling. Another open-label non-randomised clinic-based trial also found higher abstinence rates with bupropion (Kumar et al. 2007). But, a small randomised placebo-controlled trial failed to replicate the efficacy of bupropion (Singh and Kumar 2010).

In a multicentre, naturalistic study from tobacco cessation clinics, the efficacy of combined psychosocial and pharmacological intervention was examined among a large number of patients from India, who were receiving some form of behavioural counselling. The use of nicotine gum as well as bupropion was low. At the end of six-week follow-up, 36 % either had quit tobacco or reduced its use by half. Less than 20 % received pharmacotherapy. Among men, use of smokeless tobacco and younger age were associated with good outcome. Behavioural counselling combined with pharmacotherapy was more useful. Having longer-term contact has been associated with better outcome and increasing motivation to quit tobacco in Indian settings (Murthy and Subodh 2010; Varghese et al. 2012). Encouraging results have been published from the Tobacco Cessation Centre at Delhi, the combined group fared better than the counselling only group (Kumar et al. 2007).

Community-based approaches have also been evaluated for their efficacy in tobacco cessation and eventual health benefits (Anantha et al. 1995). In a study from Karnataka, health education was given to the community in the form of screening of films, exhibits and personal contact. In the experimental area, there was a significant decline in tobacco usage both in males and in females. Education using personal and mass media communication in Kerala showed 5-year quit rates of 9.4 % among the experimental group compared with 3.2 % in the control group (Gupta et al. 1986). Annual age-adjusted rates of leukoplakia also decreased in the experimental group at 8–10 years of follow-up (Gupta et al. 1992). Other community interventions have compared minimal and more intensive community-based approaches. A study carried out in the Vaishali district of Bihar used potential volunteer groups and individuals in the community, trained to provide cessation activities. The intervention led to a 4 % quit rate, 3 % dose reduction rate and 2 % reduction in multiple habits (Sinha et al. 2006). The study concluded that community-centred mass approaches with minimal sustained intervention were more effective than a clinic-centred, intensive, individual approach.

11 Research on Inhalant-Related Areas

Published research on inhalants is mainly on socio-demographic and clinical profiles of subjects with inhalant use.

Shah et al. (1999) reported a series of 9 children and adolescents with gasoline abuse. Most of the subjects used gasoline daily, and all subjects reported alcohol abuse in their fathers. All subjects also reported a withdrawal syndrome consisting of irritability, psychomotor retardation, anhedonia, dry mouth, sleep disturbances, craving and increased lacrimation. Waraich et al. (2003) studied 10 children with inhalant abuse. Three of them presented to the clinic in a city in North India; the remaining children were contacted by the community team. Most of the children were from a low socioeconomic background and had dropped out of school. All the children were abusing correction fluid and its thinner, containing toluene. Petrol and nail polish remover were the other solvents used by these children. Other commonly used substances in this group were tobacco, cannabis and alcohol (in descending order). The children reported using the correction fluid because of its easy accessibility, cheap price, the small size of the container (making it easy to conceal), its fast onset of action and the regular ‘high’ that it provided. Basu et al. (2004a, b) reported a series of 5 patients with inhalant abuse coming for treatment. They found that most of the patients had started inhalant abuse during adolescence. All patients, except one, abused typewriter erasing fluid and thinner which contains toluene. All the patients reported using inhalants as addictive substance because of their easy accessibility, cheap price, their faster onset of action and the regular 'high' that they provided.

Praharaj et al. (2008) also described 9 street children with inhalant abuse; these were boys 10–17 years of age, school dropouts and had run away from their homes. In two-thirds of these children, there was a history of domestic violence and conflict in their family, along with physical abuse by family members; in one-third, it was due to alcoholic fathers. The most common method of use was huffing. Kumar et al. (2008) studied the profiles of 21 subjects with inhalant use attending a tertiary care de-addiction centre. These young men were single (100 %), with a mean age of 19 years, unemployed (43 %) or students (38 %), middle socio-economic status (76 %) and poor social support (62 %). They were dependent on inhalants (81 %), inhalants being the only substance of abuse (33 %) and of first or second preference (76 %). Duration of inhalant use ranged 6–60 (mean 16) months. All subjects abused typewriter erasing fluid by sniffing (67 %), huffing (19 %) or bagging (14 %). Initiation was out of curiosity (62 %), under peer pressure (24 %) or as a substitute (14 %). Almost half of the patients (48 %) had a family history of substance dependence. Seth et al. (2005) studied the misuse of toluene among street and working children of Delhi and found emotional deprivation and frustrations, socio-cultural aspects such as work-driven need, others' attitudinal response towards them and their work and lack of parental support as the important determinants of misuse. Verma et al. (2011a) retrospectively reviewed the records of 36 subjects with inhalant abuse or dependence presenting to a drug de-addiction clinic over a period of 2 years. They found that 86 % were adolescents with a mean age of initiation of 14 years. The commonest cause of first use reported by the subjects was experimentation (94 %), and 97 % of them came to know of inhalant use from their inhalant using friends. They also reviewed the records of 25 adolescents with inhalant use presenting to a tertiary care de-addiction centre over a period of one year. The mean age of the initiation of inhalant use was 11.6 years. Experimentation was reported as the reason of the first use by all the adolescents, and all were introduced to inhalants by friends. Sixteen per cent met the DSM-IV criteria for inhalant dependence, and the rest met the criteria for abuse. Concurrently used substances included tobacco (84 %), cannabis (36 %), alcohol (24 %), opioids (16 %) and benzodiazepines (12 %) (Verma et al. 2011b). Narayanaswamy et al. (2013) reviewed the case record of subjects with inhalant use who had utilised psychiatric services over a 10-year period and reported a similar profile. Ray et al. (2009) undertook a national study of misused toluene products among street children in India. A total of 100 inhalant users and 30 non-users were assessed. The mean age of users was 12.8 years with age of first use being 9.3 years (standard deviation 2.8 years). Only four of the users were girls. All the users were working, whereas 16 % of the non-users were students. Most users lived alone on footpaths, streets or railway platforms. The most commonly misused product containing toluene was eraser fluid (83 %), followed by glues (34 %) and petroleum products (3 %). Although toluene was the primary substance of misuse, most children used other drugs concurrently, most frequently tobacco, followed by alcohol, cannabis, raw opium, heroin, sleeping tablets and cough syrups. Sinha et al. (2009) found that the majority of street children who misused volatile substances did not attend school and were employed as unskilled labour and that the nature of their occupation was a significant contributor to their substance misuse. A study on inhalant use among street children in Bangalore found that many inhalant users reported using a variety of drugs, in the preceding two weeks and in the last 24 h. Very few of them knew that inhalant was harmful (22.2 %) and were aware of the harm due to substance use (25.0 %). Majority of them reported that it was difficult to survive in the streets without inhalants (83.3 %). Majority of the inhalant users used inhalants in groups of 1–5 people (75 %) and never felt that using the substance was a problem (81 %). Benefits felt by the inhalant use were that it drove away hunger (36 %), drove away pain (28 %), produced emotional blunting (19 %), reduced pain (11 %) and made then bold (6 %) (http://www.nimhans.kar.nic.in/deaddiction/CAM/Drug_abuse_among_street_children.pdf).

Praharaj and Kongasseri (2012), Srivastava and Nair (2012), Verma et al. (2011c), Das et al. (1995), Pahwa et al. (1998), Mahal and Nair (1978), Gupta et al. (2009), Sood and Sood (2009) and Patra et al. (2011) have all reported several patients of inhalant abuse in the form of naphthalene balls, typewriter correction fluids, kerosene, petrol and glue inhalation.

11.1 Studies on Treatment of Inhalant Dependence or Abuse

There are only a few studies till date addressing this emerging problem. Following a brief intervention consisting of a single viewing of an animated video film and 2 or 3 workbook sessions, a large number of the street children (78 %) had stopped or reduced use of solvent drugs (Benegal et al. 1998). An intervention package using a cognitive behaviour model for street children from streets in Bangalore using inhalant and other substances was devised (Benegal et al. 2008). The sessions were delivered in a group of 5–10 people over 2–3 days. Results showed a significant reduction in the use of substances by street children, increase in the awareness about substance use and increase in help seeking for substance use after 48 h of intervention. Among pharmacological research, only one study from India has examined the effects of baclofen on 3 patients with inhalant dependence; baclofen was found to be effective in reducing the withdrawal (non-specific) symptoms experienced by them (Muralidharan et al. 2008a, b).

12 Research on Cannabis-Related Areas

In India, cannabis has been used for thousands of years in the worship of the Lord Shiva. It is used in an orally administered form called *bhang*, which can be either the wet resinous leaves of the cannabis plant formed into pills, or added to a drink made of milk, cannabis and various other spices, or by smoking the flowering buds of the cannabis plant. This practice is codified in the ancient Vedas as well (Godlaski 2012). A substantive amount of research has been done in India on cannabis abuse.

12.1 Studies on Dual Diagnosis

Chopra and Smith (1974) studied psychotic reactions following cannabis use in 200 patients. Of these patients, 45 % had no previous psychopathology. Most patients recovered fully. Among those with the most severe pre-existing pathology, some patients had a less favourable course; drug psychoses in this group were occasionally dominated by schizophrenic and paranoid symptoms. Potency and dosage schedule of cannabis, as well as a younger age, were generally related to occurrence of a toxic psychosis. Grossman (1969) reported 6 patients with emotional disorders associated with the use *of ganja, bhang* and hashish, products prepared from the plant *Cannabis sativa var. indica*, by Westerners in India. The major psychiatric problems seen were anxiety reactions of moderate-to-severe intensity and psychotic reactions of schizophrenic and schizoaffective types. Basu et al. (1999) carried out a case-control study using a retrospective chart review. The subjects with cannabis psychosis, in contrast to the acute schizophrenic group, had a psychosis of shorter duration characterised by reactive and congruent affect, relative absence of schizophrenic formal thought disorder and a predominantly polymorphic clinical picture. Relapse was always preceded by cannabis use. In an older study, patients with cannabis psychosis of the paranoid type and patients with paranoid schizophrenia were compared (Thacore and Shukla 1976). Most of the patients with cannabis psychosis were violent and panicky and demonstrated bizarre behaviour, but they possessed some insight into the nature of their illness. Patients with schizophrenia manifested these disturbances and characteristics less frequently. Subjects with cannabis psychosis showed rapid ideation and flight of ideas, whereas the characteristic schizophrenic thought disorder was found mostly in schizophrenic patients. Kulhalli et al. (2007) observed patients with cannabis-related psychosis for 7 days in a drug-free protected environment. At the time of presentation, they had unusual thought content, excitement, grandiosity, hallucinatory behaviour and uncooperativeness. Almost half of them presented with cognitive dysfunction. Affective psychosis was the predominant diagnosis. At the end of 1 week of abstinence from cannabis, there was a significant improvement in psychopathology. A recent retrospective file review has implicated cannabis as the commonest substance (20 %) responsible for substance-induced psychotic disorders (Aggarwal et al. 2012a).

12.2 Studies on Other Clinical Issues

The psychological correlates of users of cannabis demonstrated that they reacted slowly, had poor concentration and time estimation and had higher neuroticism and greater perceptuo-motor disturbance, than controls (Menhiratta et al. 1978). *Charas* smokers showed poor memory, lowered psychomotor activity and poor size estimation. Another study also found that users of cannabis were found to react slowly in perceptuo-motor tasks, but not to differ in intelligence or memory tests. The users suffered disability in personal, social and vocational areas and had higher psychoticism and neuroticism scores (Varma et al. 1988). Other studies have revealed that compared to non-users, cannabis users had significantly lower intelligence and memory quotients (Wig and Varma 1977). The users also had significantly lower scores on the speed marking test and made greater errors in correctly perceiving time. However, Ray et al. (1978) did not find any difference in psychosocial factors among chronic users of cannabis, compared to the non-user control group. Physical health and nutrition were relatively poor in users of cannabis, and there were more respiratory complaints. In the social sphere, users of cannabis had a history of poor work record, family maladjustment and episodes of violent behaviour, more often (Mehndiratta and Wig 1975). Chaturvedi et al. (1991) studied the profiles of 100 users of cannabis and found that one-third of them were in the age group 21–30 years and around 37 % of them use 4–6 g/day. The most common cause of starting the use of *bhang* reported was 'pleasure'.

12.3 Studies on Biology of Cannabis Dependence

A PET scan study found that the mean regional glucose metabolisms were higher in bilateral lateral temporal regions in the cannabis-dependent group, as compared to non-drug using controls. The higher metabolism in the left lateral temporal region was statistically significant (Parkar et al. 2010). In another similar study, the same authors found that the cannabis dependence group differed significantly from the schizophrenia group and normal volunteers in their temporal uptakes of cerebral glucose. There was also significant difference in glucose uptake in the medial and lateral temporal regions and the left parietal region between the cannabis dependence group and the schizophrenia group (Parkar et al. 2011).

12.4 Studies on Treatment Related to Cannabis

Detection of cannabis use is complicated by unreliability and inadequacy of information. In these cases, objective evidence could be proven as gold standard. Sharma et al. (2012) found that the high-performance thin-layer chromatographic analysis of urine was sensitive, reproducible and cost-effective, compared to commercial kits.

The sole published research in this area is on cannabis withdrawal. Nanjayya et al. (2010) have investigated and found out the efficacy of Baclofen in a treatment-seeking population of South India. Unfortunately, though widely abused, treatment of cannabis dependence is the least researched area.

13 Research on Non-substance ('Behavioural') Addiction

Growing evidence indicates that people indulge in certain behaviours to the extent that these could be labelled as addictive behaviours. The term 'behavioural addiction' is used to depict non-substance-related pattern of excessive behaviour, which includes pathological gambling, Internet addiction, hypersexual behaviour, compulsive shopping and many other related problems. Research on behavioural addiction in India is still in infancy. There are a few epidemiological studies though; the majority of these are on Internet addiction. The importance of the diagnostic instrument in influencing the prevalence figures for behavioural addictions is underscored by an online survey, which showed a prevalence of Internet addiction as 3.8 and 52 % as per Young's Internet Addiction Diagnostic Questionnaire and ICD-10 diagnosis respectively (Grover et al. 2010).

In a study on the resident doctors from India evaluating their pattern of mobile phone use, nearly 40 % of the participants fulfilled the ICD-10 substance dependence criteria, while 27.1 % of the subjects scored two or more on the CAGE questionnaire. Finally, 23.4 % of the subjects self-rated themselves to be 'addicted' to mobile phones. The authors concluded that among those with excessive use of mobile phones, some may be addicted to their use (Aggarwal et al. 2012a, b). This may impact their work performance and may have health consequences for them. Another study from India, which evaluated young college students, reported that about one-third of the participants met three or more of the ICD-10 diagnostic criteria for substance dependence and more than half (57.1 %) fulfilled two or more items on the CAGE questionnaire (Nehra et al. 2012). Those who fulfilled the dependence criteria spent more time each day on the mobile phone, and this had harmful consequences on various aspects of their life. A recent study seeks to provide a historical overview of gambling and contemporary anti-gambling legislation in India. A surprising lack of contemporary curiosity and scholarly literature on pathological gambling from the region has been underscored in the study (Benegal 2012).

14 Conclusions

Overall, there is substantive amount of research on substance abuse and dependence in India, but with some notable exceptions, the research appears to be sporadic, uncoordinated and conducted from limited centres. Further, some of the major epidemiological and other related data are already old. Substance use and addictions, as well as their clinical features and management, are not static—they change patterns over the years and across places. There is an urgent need to conduct large-scale, multicentre collaborative projects in addiction research in India.

References

Adityanjee, M. D., & Saxena, S. (1984). Heroin dependence: Experience of a de-addiction unit in a general hospital. *Indian Journal of Psychiatry, 28*, 87–88.

Aggarwal, M., Banerjee, A., Singh, S. M., et al. (2012a). Substance-induced psychotic disorders: 13-year data from a de-addiction centre and their clinical implications. *Asian Journal of Psychiatry, 5*, 220–224.

Aggarwal, M., Grover, S., & Basu, D. (2012b). Mobile phone use by resident doctors: Tendency to addiction-like behaviour. *German Journal of Psychiatry, 15*, 50–55.

Aich, T. K., Sinha, V. K., Khess, C. R., et al. (2004). Demographic and clinical correlates of substance abuse comorbidity in schizophrenia. *Indian Journal of Psychiatry, 46*, 135–139.

Anand, K. (2000). Assessment of burden and surveillance of major non-communicable diseases in India. World Health Organization (WHO), South East Asia Regional Office, Workshop Document, New Delhi.

Anantha, N., Nandakumar, A., Vishwanath, N., et al. (1995). Efficacy of an anti-tobacco community education program in India. *Cancer Causes and Control, 6*, 119–129.

Arackal, B. S., & Benegal, V. (2007). Prevalence of sexual dysfunction in male subjects with alcohol dependence. *Indian Journal of Psychiatry, 49*, 109–112.

Babu, R. S., & Sengupta, S. N. (1997). A study of problem drinkers in a general hospital. *Indian Journal of Psychiatry, 39*, 13–17.

Balhara, Y. P. S., & Jain, R. (2012). A urinalysis-based comparative study of treatment adherence on buprenorphine and buprenorphine/naloxone combination used as opioid substitution therapy. *Innovative Clinical Neuroscience, 9*, 24–29.

Banerjee, A., Basu, D., & Malhotra, A. (2006). How responsible is responsible drinking: An evidence based review. *Journal of Mental Health and Human Behaviour, 11*, 23–33.

Bansal, R. K., & Banerjee, S. (1993). Substance use by child labourers. *Indian Journal of Psychiatry, 35*, 159–161.

Basu, D. (2010). Overview of substance abuse and hepatitis C virus infection and co-infections in India. *Journal of Neuroimmune Pharmacology, 5*, 406–496.

Basu, D., Aggarwal, M., Das, P. P., et al. (2012). Changing pattern of substance abuse in patients attending a de-addiction centre in north India (1978–2008). *Indian Journal of Medical Research, 135*, 830–836.

Basu, D., Ball, S. A., Feinn, R., et al. (2004a). Typologies of drug dependence: Comparative validity of a multivariate and four univariate models. *Drug and Alcohol Dependence, 73*(3), 289–300.

Basu, D., Banerjee, A., Harish, T., et al. (2009a). Disproportionately high rate of epileptic seizure in patients abusing dextropropoxyphene. *American Journal of Addiction, 18*(5), 417–421.

Basu, D., Gupta, S., Nebhinani, N., et al. (2014a). Cocaine dependence: First case series from India. *The National Medical Journal of India, 27*, 12–14.

Basu, D., Ghormode, D., Madan, R., et al. (2014b). Age-of-onset of dependence: Does it help our understanding of opioid dependence by generating meaningful categories or by acting as a useful dimension? A critical examination of the classic debate in psychiatry. *Indian Journal of Psychiatry, 56*, 228–237.

Basu, D., & Gupta, N. (2000). Management of dual diagnosis patients: Consensus, controversies and considerations. *Indian Journal of Psychiatry, 42*, 34–47.

Basu, D., Jhirwal, O. P., & Mattoo, S. K. (2005). Clinical characterization of use of acamprosate and naltrexone: Data from an addiction center in India. *American Journal of Addiction, 14*, 381–395.

Basu, D., Jhirwal, O. P., Singh, J., et al. (2004b). Inhalant abuse by adolescents: A new challenge for Indian physicians. *Indian Journal of Medical Science, 58*, 245–249.

Basu, D., Kumar, V., Sharma, A. K., et al. (2013). Seroprevalence of anti-hepatitis C virus (anti-HCV) antibody and HCV-related risk in injecting drug users in northern India: Comparison with non-injecting drug users. *Asian Journal of Psychiatry, 6*, 52–55.

Basu, D., Malhotra, A., Bhagat, A., et al. (1999). Cannabis psychosis and acute schizophrenia. A case Control study from India. *Addiction and Mental Health, 5*, 71–73.

Basu, D., & Mattoo, S. K. (1999). Epidemiology of substance abuse in India: Methodological issues and future perspectives. *Indian Journal of Psychiatry, 41*, 145–153.

Basu, D., Mattoo, S. K., Malhotra, A., et al. (2000a). A longitudinal study of male buprenorphine addicts attending an addiction clinic in India. *Addiction, 95*, 1363–1372.

Basu, D., Gupta, N., Mattoo, S. K., et al. (2000b). Endorsement and concordance of ICD-10 versus DSM-IV criteria for substance dependence: Indian perspective. *Indian Journal of Psychiatry, 42*, 378–386.

Basu, D., Sharma, A., & Nebhinani, N. (2009b). Disulfiram induced delirium: Diagnostic dilemma. *Journal of Mental Health and Human Behaviour, 14*, 105–107.

Basu, D., Varma, V. K., Malhotra, S., et al. (1995). The sensation seeker who is also alienated: Towards a new hypothesis for the genesis of alcohol dependence. *Indian Journal of Psychiatry, 37*, 17–22.

Basu, D., Varma, V. K., Malhotra, A., et al. (1998). Development of a scale to assess attitudes towards drinking and alcoholism. *Indian Journal of Psychiatry, 40*, 158–164.

Benegal, V. (2012). Gambling experiences, problems and policy in India: A historical analysis. *Addiction, 15*, 34–41.

Benegal, V., Gururaj, G., & Murthy, P. (2003). *Report on a WHO collaborative project on unrecorded consumption of alcohol in Karnataka, India*. National Institute of Mental Health and Neurosciences Bangalore, India.

Benegal, V., Jain, S., Subbukrishna, D. K., et al. (1995). P300 amplitudes vary inversely with continuum of risk in first degree male relatives of alcoholics. *Psychiatric Genetics, 5*, 149–156.

Benegal, V., Gururaj. G., & Murthy, P. (2002). Project Report on a WHO Multi Centre Collaborative Project on Establishing and Monitoring Alcohol's Involvement in Casualties. (Monograph on the Internet). Accessed from http://wwwnimhans.kar.nic.in/deaddiction/lit/alcohol%20and%20%20injuries_who%20collab.pdf.

Benegal, V., Nayak, M., Murthy, P., et al. (2005). Women and alcohol in India. In I. S. Obot & R. Room (Eds.), *Alcohol, gender and drinking problems: Perspectives from low and middle income Countries*. Geneva: World Health Organisation.

Benegal, V., Sathyaprakash, M., & Nagaraja, D. (2008). Alcohol misuse in the Andaman and Nicobar Islands. *Report on project commissioned by the Indian Council of Medical Research and funded by Action Aid*, India.

Benegal, V., Velayudhan, A., & Jain, S. (2000). Social costs of alcoholism: A Karnataka perspective. *NIMHANS Journal, 18*, 6–7.

Benegal, V., Venkatasubramanian, G. V., Antony, G., et al. (2006). Differences in brain morphology between subjects at high and low risk for alcoholism. *Addiction Biology, 12*, 122–138.

Bhalla, A., Dutta, S., & Chakrabarti, A. (2006). A profile of substance abusers using the emergency services in a tertiary care hospital in Sikkim. *Indian Journal of Psychiatry, 48*, 243–247.

Bhaskar, L. V., Thangaraj, K., Wasnik, S., et al. (2012). Dopamine transporter (DAT1) VNTR polymorphism and alcoholism in two culturally different populations of south India. *American Journal of Addiction, 21*, 343–347.

Bhateja, G., Nanjayya, S., Grover, S., et al. (2006). Cutaneous complication of parental pentazocine dependence. *German Journal of Psychiatry, 9*, 53–56.

Chand, P., & Chaturvedi, S. K. (2010). Distressing behaviors of alcohol dependence patients: A study from India. *Asian Journal of Psychiatry, 3*, 12–15.

Chand, P. K., & Murthy, P. (2003). Megadose lorazepam dependence. *Addiction, 98*, 1635–1636.

Chandra, P. S., Krishna, V. A., Benegal, V., et al. (2003). High-risk sexual behaviour and sensation seeking among heavy alcohol users. *Indian Journal of Medical Research, 117*, 88–92.

Chaturvedi, S. K. (1994). Amelioration of narcotic withdrawal features with clonidine and opiate receptors activity. *Regulatory Peptides, 22*, 291–292.

Chaturvedi, H. K., Phukan, R. K., & Mahanta, J. (2003). The association of selected sociodemographic factors and differences in patterns of substance use: A pilot study in selected areas of Northeast India. *Substance Use and Misuse, 38*, 1305–1322.

Chaturvedi, H. K., Phukan, R. K., & Mahanta, J. (2004). Sociocultural diversity and substance use pattern in Arunachal Pradesh, India. *Drug and Alcohol Dependence, 74*, 97–104.

Chaturvedi, H. K., Phukan, R. K., Zoramtharga, K., et al. (1998). Tobacco use in Mizoram, India: Sociodemographic differences in pattern. *Southeast Asian Journal of Tropical Medicine and Public Health, 29*, 66–70.

Chaturvedi, G. N., Rai, N. P., Pandey, U. S., et al. (1991). Clinical survey of cannabis users in Varanasi. *Ancient Science of Life, 10*, 194–198.

Chaudhury, S., Das, S. K., & Ukil, B. (2006). Psychological assessment of alcoholism in males. *Indian Journal of Psychiatry, 48*, 114–117.

Chavan, B., Arun, P., Bhargava, R., et al. (2007). Prevalence of alcohol and drug dependence in rural and slum population of Chandigarh: A community survey. *Indian Journal of Psychiatry, 49*, 44–48.

Chitra, S., Ashok, L., Anand, L., et al. (2008). Risk factors for esophageal cancer in Coimbatore, southern India: A hospital-based case-control study. *Indian Journal of Gastroenterology, 23*, 117–118.
Chopra, G. S., & Smith, J. W. (1974). Psychotic reactions following cannabis use in East Indians. *Archives of General Psychiatry, 30*, 24–27.
Chowdhury, A. N., & Sen, P. (1992). Initiation of heroin abuse: The role of peers. *Indian Journal of Psychiatry, 34*, 34–35.
Darshan, M. S., Raman, R., Rao, T. S. S., et al. (2013). A study on professional stress, depression and alcohol use among Indian IT professionals. *Indian Journal of Psychiatry, 55*, 63–69.
Das, P. S., Sharan, P., & Saxena, S. (1995). Kerosene abuse by inhalation and ingestion. *American Journal of Psychiatry, 149*, 7–10.
De, S., Jain, R., Ray, R., et al. (2001). Assessment of differential doses of buprenorphine for long term pharmacotherapy (among opiate dependent subjects). Departmental thesis, Department of Psychiatry, All India Institute of Medical Sciences, New Delhi.
De, B., Mattoo, S. K., & Basu, D. (2003). Age at onset typology in opioid-dependent men: An exploratory study from India. *American Journal of Addiction, 12*, 336–345.
De Sousa, A. A., De Sousa, J., & Kapoor, H. (2008). An open randomized trial comparing disulfiram and topiramate in the treatment of alcohol dependence. *Journal of Substance Abuse Treatment, 34*, 460–463.
Deb, I., Chakraborty, J., Gangopadhyay, P. K., et al. (2010). Single-nucleotide polymorphism (A118G) in exon 1 of OPRM1 gene causes alteration in downstream signaling by mu-opioid receptor and may contribute to the genetic risk for addiction. *Journal of Neurochemistry, 112*, 486–496.
Desai, G., & Chaturvedi, S. K. (2003). Perception and knowledge about narcotics among nurses. *Indian Journal of Palliative Care, 9*, 78–83.
Dhawan, A., & Chopra, A. (2013). Does buprenorphine maintenance improve the quality of life of opioid users? *Indian Journal of Medical Research, 137*, 130–135.
Dhawan, A., Jain, R., & Chopra, A. (2010). Opioid Substitution—Buprenorphine in India: A study report. New Delhi: United Nations Office on Drugs and Crime. Accessed from http://www.unodc.org/documents/southasia/reports/OSB_Report-India.pdf.
Dhawan, A., Kumar, R., Yadav, S., et al. (2002). The enigma of craving. *Indian Journal of Psychiatry, 44*, 138–143.
Dhawan, A., & Sunder, S. (2008). Opioid substitution therapy: The Indian experience. In A. Ambekar & B. M. Tripathi (Eds.), *Drug abuse: News-n-views (Harm reduction: Prevention of HIV among drug users)* (pp. 8–10). New Delhi: National Drug Dependence Treatment Centre, All India Institute of Medical Sciences.
Dube, K. C., & Handa, S. K. (1971). Drug use in health and mental illness in an Indian population. *British Journal of Psychiatry, 118*, 345–356.
Dutta, S., Kar, N., Thirthalli, J., et al. (2007). Prevalence and risk factors of psychiatric disorders in an industrial population in India. *Indian Journal of Psychiatry, 49*, 103–108.
Elnager, M. N., Maitra, P., & Rao, N. N. (1971). Mental health in an Indian rural community. *British Journal of Psychiatry, 118*, 499–503.
Gaidhane, A. M., Zahiruddin, Q. S., Waghmare, L., et al. (2008). Substance abuse among street children in Mumbai. *Vulnerable Children and Youth Studies, 3*, 42–51.
Galgali, R. B., Srinivasan, K., & Souza, G. D. (2002). Study of spirometry and airway reactivity in patients on disulfiram for treatment of alcoholism. *Indian Journal of Psychiatry, 44*, 273–275.
Ghosh, A. (2013). Are childhood externalizing disorders the harbinger of early alcohol dependence? *Bhagwat award Indian Psychiatric Society*.
Ghulam, R., Rahman, I., Naqi, S., et al. (1996). An epidemiological study of drug abuse in urban population of Madhya Pradesh. *Indian Journal of Psychiatry, 38*, 160–165.
Godlaski, T. M. (2012). Shiva, Lord of Bhang. *Substance Use and Misuse, 47*, 1067–1072.
Goswami, S., Singh, G., Mattoo, S. K., et al. (2003). Courses of substance use and schizophrenia in the dual-diagnosis patients: Is there a relationship? *Indian Journal of Medical Science, 57*, 338–346.

Grossman, W. (1969). Adverse reactions associated with Cannabis products in India. *Annals of Internal Medicine, 70*, 529–533.
Grover, S., Basu, D., & Bhateja, G. (2007a). Pharmacoprophylaxis of alcohol dependence: Review and update Part II: Efficacy. *Indian Journal of Psychiatry, 49*, 26–33.
Grover, S., Bhateja, G., & Basu, D. (2007b). Pharmacoprophylaxis of alcohol dependence: Review and update Part I: Pharmacology. *Indian Journal of Psychiatry, 49*, 19–25.
Grover, S., Irpati, A. S., Saluja, B. S., et al. (2005). Substance-dependent women attending a de-addiction center in North India: Socio-demographic and clinical profile. *Indian Journal of Medical Science, 59*, 283–291.
Grover, S., Chakraborty, K., Basu, D. (2010). Pattern of Internet use among professionals in India: critical look at a surprising survey result. *Industrial Psychiatry Journal, 19*, 94–100.
Grover, S., Irpati, A. S., Saluja, B. S., et al. (2008). Drug dependence in geriatric age group: a clinic based study. *German Journal of Psychiatry, 11*, 10–15.
Gupta, P. C., Aghi, M. B., Bhonsle, R. B., et al. (1986a). An intervention study of tobacco chewing and smoking habits for primary prevention of oral cancer among 12 212 Indian Villagers. *IARC Science Publication, 74*, 307–318.
Gupta, S. K., Bali, S., & Jiloha, R. C. (2009). Inhalant use: An over-looked problem. *Indian Journal of Psychiatry, 51*, 160–161.
Gupta, A. K., Jha, B. K., & Devi, S. (1987). Heroin addiction: Experiences from general psychiatry out-patients departments. *Indian Journal of Psychiatry, 29*, 81–83.
Gupta, P. C., Mehta, F. S., Pindborg, J. J., et al. (1992). Primary prevention trial of oral cancer in India: A 10-year follow-up study. *Journal of Oral Pathology and Medicine, 21*, 433–437.
Gupta, R., Narang, R. L., Gupta, K. R., et al. (1986b). Drug abuse among rickshaw pullers in industrial town of Ludhiana. *Indian Journal of Psychiatry, 28*, 145–149.
Gupta, P. C., Saxena, S., & Pednekar, M. (2003). Alcohol consumption among middle-aged and elderly men: A community study from Western India. *Alcohol Alcoholism, 38*, 327–331.
Gururaj, G. (2002). Epidemiology of traumatic brain injuries: Indian scenario. *Neurology Research, 24*, 24–28.
Gururaj, G., Girish, N., Benegal, V., et al. (2006). Burden and socioeconomic impact of alcohol, The Bangalore Study. World Health Organization, South East Asia Regional office, New Delhi.
Gururaj, G., & Isaac, M. (2001). Epidemiology of suicides in Bangalore city. In G. Gururaj & M. Isaac (Eds.), *Epidemiology of suicides in Bangalore city* (1st ed., pp. 34–43). Bangalore: NIMHANS Publication.
Gururaj, G., Isaac, M. K., & Girish, N. (2004). Final report of the pilot study establishing health behaviour surveillance in respect of mental health. *Report submitted to Ministry of Health and Family Welfare,* Government of India and WHO India Country Office, New Delhi.
Hazarika, N. C., Biswas, D., Phukan, R. K., et al. (2000). Prevalence and pattern of substance abuse at Bandardewa, a border area of Assam and Arunachal Pradesh. *Indian Journal of Psychiatry, 42*, 262–266.
Jain, A., Buddhiraja, S., Khurana, B., et al. (1999). Risk factors for duodenal ulcer in north India. *Tropical Gastroenterology, 20*, 36–39.
Jena, R., Shukla, T. R., & Pal, H. (1996). Drug abuse in a rural community in Bihar: Some psychosocial correlates. *Indian Journal of Psychiatry, 38*, 43–46.
Jha, P., & Chaloupka, F. J. (1999). *Curbing the Epidemic: Governments and the economics of tobacco control* (pp. 21–28). Washington, DC: The World Bank.
Jiloha, R. C. (2012). Tobacco smoking: How far do the legislative control measures address the problem? *Indian Journal of Psychiatry, 54*, 64–68.
John, A., Barman, A., Bal, D., et al. (2009). Hazardous alcohol use in rural southern India: Nature, prevalence and risk factors. *National Medical Journal of India, 22*, 123–125.
Joshi, U., Modi, B., & Yadav, S. (2010). A Study on prevalence of chewing form of tobacco and existing quitting patterns in urban population of Jamnagar, Gujarat. *Indian Journal of Community Medicine, 35*, 105–108.

Kakunjee, A. (2012). Psychiatric comorbidity in alcohol dependence with or without cirrhosis—A hospital based comparative study. *Journal of Pakistan Psychiatric Society, 9*, 15–18.

Kakunji, A., Haridas, K., Prabat, C., et al. (2012). Personality profile of persons with alcohol dependence with or without cirrhosis: A hospital based comparative study. *International Journal of Health and Rehabilitation Sciences, 2*, 94–98.

Kar, N., Sengupta, S., Sharma, P., et al. (2003). Predictors of outcome following alcohol de-addiction treatment: A prospective longitudinal study for one year. *Indian Journal of Psychiatry, 45*, 174–177.

Kisore, P., Lal, N., Trivedi, J. K., et al. (1994). A study of comorbidity in psychoactive substance dependence patients. *Indian Journal of Psychiatry, 36*, 133–137.

Kulhalli, V., Isaac, M., & Murthy, P. (2007). Cannabis-related psychosis: Presentation and effect of abstinence. *Indian Journal of Psychiatry, 49*, 256–261.

Kumar, M.S. (2002). Rapid Assessment Survey of Drug Abuse in India. United Nations Office on Drugs and Crime Regional Office for South Asia and Ministry of Social Justice and Empowerment, Government of India. New Delhi, India. Accessed from http://www.unodc.org/india/ras.html.

Kumar, C. N., Andrade, C., & Murthy, P. (2009). A randomized, double-blind comparison of lorazepam and chlordiazepoxide in patients with uncomplicated alcohol withdrawal. *Journal of Studies of Alcohol and Drugs, 70*, 467–474.

Kumar, P., & Basu, D. (2000). Substance abuse by medical students and doctors. *Journal of Indian Medical Association, 98*, 447–452.

Kumar, S., Grover, S., Kulhara, P., et al. (2008). Inhalant abuse: A clinic-based study. *Indian Journal of Psychiatry, 50*, 117–120.

Kumar, R., Kushwah, A. S., Mahakud, G. C., et al. (2007). Smoking cessation interventions and continuous abstinence rate at one year. *Indian Journal of Chest Disease and Allied Sciences, 49*, 201–207.

Kumar, M. S., & Sharma, M. (2008). Women and substance use in India and Bangladesh. *Substance Use and Misuse, 43*, 1062–1077.

Kumar, D., Deb, I., Chakraborty, J., et al. (2011). Polymorphism of CREB binding protein (CREBBP) is a risk factor for addiction. *Brain Research, 1406*, 59–64.

Kuruvilla, P. K., & Jacob, K. S. (2007). Five-year follow up for sobriety in a cohort of men who had attended an alcoholics Anonymous programme in India. *National Medical Journal of India, 20*, 234–236.

Lal, B., & Singh, G. (1979). Drug abuse in Punjab. *British Journal of Addiction, 74*, 411–419.

Lavania, S., Ram, D., Praharaj, S. K., et al. (2012). Deliberate self-harm in nondepressed substance-dependent patients. *Journal of Addiction Medicine, 6*, 247–252.

Mahadevappa, H., Murthy, P., Desai, N. G., et al. (1987). Tracing techniques in the follow up of alcoholics. *Indian Journal of Psychiatry, 29*(4), 377–379.

Mahal, A. S., & Nair, M. C. (1978). Dependence on petrol: A clinical study. *Indian Journal of Psychiatry, 20*, 15–19.

Malhotra, A., Basu, D., Mattoo, S. K., et al. (2003). Acceptability of Naltrexone by patients with opioid dependence. *Hong Kong Journal of Psychiatry, 13*, 6–13.

Malhotra, S., Malhotra, S., & Basu, D. (1999). A comparison of the beliefs of the Indian alcohol dependent patients and their close family members on their reasons for relapse. *Addiction, 94*, 709–713.

Manickam, L. S. (1997). Training community volunteers in preventing alcoholism and drug addiction: A basic programme and its impact on certain variables. *Indian Journal of Psychiatry, 39*, 220–225.

Mattoo, S. K., & Basu, D. (1997). Clinical course of alcohol dependence. *Indian Journal of Psychiatry, 39*, 294–299.

Mattoo, S. K., Basu, D., Sharma, A., et al. (1997). Abuse of codeine-containing cough syrups: A report from India. *Addiction, 92*, 1783–1787.

Mattoo, S. K., Chakrabarti, S., & Anjaiah, M. (2009a). Psychosocial factors associated with relapse in men with alcohol or opioid dependence. *Indian Journal of Medical Research, 130*, 702–708.

Mattoo, S. K., Chakraborty, K., Basu, D., et al. (2011). Prevalence & correlates of metabolic syndrome in alcohol & opioid dependent inpatients. *Indian Journal of Medical Research, 134*, 341–348.

Mattoo, S. K., Singh, S. M., Bhardwaj, R., et al. (2009b). Prevalence and correlates of epileptic seizure in substance-abusing subjects. *Psychiatry and Clinical Neurosciences, 63*, 580–582.

Meena, Khanna P., Vohra, A. K., et al. (2002). Prevalence and pattern of alcohol and substance abuse in urban areas of Rohtak city. *Indian Journal of Psychiatry, 44*, 348–352.

Mehndiratta, S. S., & Wig, N. N. (1975). Psychosocial effects of long term cannabis use in India. A study of fifty heavy users and controls. *Drug and Alcohol Dependence, 1*, 71–81.

Menhiratta, S. S., Wig, N. N., & Verma, S. K. (1978). Some psychological correlates of long-term heavy cannabis users. *British Journal of Psychiatry, 132*, 482–486.

Mohan, D., Chopra, A., & Sethi, H. (2002a). The co-occurrence of tobacco & alcohol in general population of metropolis Delhi. *Indian Journal of Medical Research, 116*, 150–154.

Mohan, D., Mohan, D., Chopra, A., et al. (2002b). Incidence estimates of substance use disorders in a cohort from Delhi, India. *Indian Journal of Medical Research, 115*, 128–135.

Mohan, D., & Ray, R. (1997). Community based treatment for heroin dependence in an urban slum of Delhi (India)—Report submitted to WHO, Searo, New Delhi, India.

Mohan, D., Sharma, N. K., & Sundaram, K. R. (1979). Patterns and prevalence of opium use in rural Punjab (India). Available from https://www.unodc.org/unodc/en/data-and-analysis/bulletin/bulletin_1979-01-01_2_page003.html.

Munjal, G. C., & Jiloha, R. C. (1986). Drug abuse in Delhi: Experiences of a de-addiction unit in a general hospital. *Indian Journal of Psychiatry, 28*, 87–88.

Muralidharan, K., Rajkumar, R. P., Mulla, U., et al. (2008a). Baclofen in the management of inhalant withdrawal: A case series. *Prim Care Companion Journal of Clinical Psychiatry, 10*, 48–51.

Muralidharan, K., Venkatasubramanian, G., Pal, P., et al. (2008b). Transcallosal conduction abnormalities in alcohol-naïve male offspring of alcoholics. *Addiction Biology, 13*, 373–379.

Murthy, P. (2008). Women and drug use in India. Substance, women and high risk assessment study. United Nations Office on Drugs and Crime, Ministry of Social Justice and Empowerment, Government of India and United Nations Development Fund for Women.

Murthy, P., Chand, P. K., Harish, M. G., et al. (2009). Outcome of alcohol dependence: The role of continued care. *Indian Journal of Community Medicine, 34*, 148–151.

Murthy, P., Guru, S. C., Channabasavanna, S. M., et al. (1996). Erythrocyte aldehyde dehydrogenase—a potential marker for alcohol dependence. *Indian Journal of Psychiatry, 38*, 38–42.

Murthy, P., Guru, S. C., Shetty, K. T., et al. (1992). Diazepam and chlordiazepoxide mediated increase in erythrocyte aldehyde activity and its possible implications. *Alcohol, 9*, 199–202.

Murthy, P., & Saddichha, S. (2010). Tobacco cessation services in India: Recent developments and the need for expansion. *Indian Journal of Cancer, 47*, 69–74.

Murthy, P., & Subodh, B. N. (2010). Current developments in behavioral interventions for tobacco cessation. *Current Opinion in Psychiatry, 23*, 151–156.

Murthy, P., Taly, A. B., & Jayakumar, P. N. (2007). Seizures in alcohol dependence. *German Journal of Psychiatry, 10*, 54–57.

Nandi, D. N., Ajmany, S., Ganguli, H., et al. (1975). Psychiatric disorders in a rural community in West Bengal an epidemiological study. *Indian Journal of Psychiatry, 17*, 87–99.

Nanjayya, S. B., Shivappa, M., Chand, P. K., et al. (2010). Baclofen in cannabis dependence syndrome. *Biological Psychiatry, 68*, 9–10.

Narang, R. L., Gupta, R., Mishra, B. P., & Mahajan, R. (1997). Temperamental characteristics and psychopathology among children of alcoholics. *Indian Journal of Psychiatry, 39*, 226–231.

Narayanaswamy, J. C., Viswanath, B., Ravi, M., et al. (2013). Inhalant dependence: Data from a tertiary care center in South India. *Indian Journal of Psychological Medicine, 34*, 136–232.

Nattala, P., Leung, K. S., & Murthy, P. (2010). Family member involvement in relapse prevention improves alcohol dependence outcomes: A prospective study at an addiction treatment facility in India. *Journal of Studies on Alcohol and Drugs, 71*, 234–238.

Nayak, R. B., & Murthy, P. (2008). Fetal alcohol spectrum disorder. *Indian Pediatrics, 45*, 977–983.

Nayak, R., Murthy, P., Girimaji, S., & Navaneetham, J. (2012). Fetal alcohol spectrum disorders—A case-control study from India. *Journal of Tropical Pediatrics, 58*, 19–24.

Nebhinani, N., Aggarwal, M., Mattoo, S. K., et al. (2013). Carisoprodol: An underrecognized drug of abuse in north India. *General Hospital Psychiatry, 35*, 89–92.

Nehra, R., Kate, N., Grover, S., Khehra, N., et al. (2012). Does the excessive use of mobile phones in young adults reflect an emerging behavioural addiction? *journal of Post Graduate Medical Education and Research, 46*, 177–182.

Pahwa, M., Baweja, A., Gupta, V., et al. (1998). Petrol inhalation dependence: A case report. *Indian Journal of Psychiatry, 40*, 92–94.

Parkar, S. R., Ramanathan, S., Nair, N., Batra, S. A., et al. (2011). Are the effects of cannabis dependence on glucose metabolism similar to schizophrenia? An FDG PET understanding. *Indian Journal of Psychiatry, 53*, 13–20.

Parkar, S. R., Ramanathan, S., Nair, N., et al. (2010). Cannabis dependence: Effects of cannabis consumption on inter-regional cerebral metabolic relationships in an Indian population. *Indian Journal of Psychiatry, 52*, 236–242.

Patra, S., Mishra, A., & Shukla, R. (2011). Inhalant abuse: A cause for concern. *Indian Journal of Psychiatry, 20*, 61–63.

Ponnudorai, R., Jayakar, J., Raju, B., et al. (1991). An epidemiological study of alcoholism. *Indian Journal of Psychiatry, 33*, 176–179.

Ponnudurai, R., Somasundaram, O., Indira, T. P., et al. (1984). Alcohol and drug abuse among internees. *Indian Journal of Psychiatry, 26*, 128–132.

Praharaj, S. K., & Kongasseri, S. (2012). Naphthalene addiction. *Substance Abuse, 33*, 189–190.

Praharaj, S. K., Verma, P., & Arora, M. (2008). Inhalant abuse (typewriter correction fluid) in street children. *Journal of Addiction Medicine, 2*, 175–177.

Prasad, R. (2009). Alcohol use on the rise in India. *Lancet, 373*, 17–18.

Prasad, P., Ambekar, A., & Vaswani, M. (2010). Dopamine D2 receptor polymorphisms and susceptibility to alcohol dependence in Indian males: A preliminary study. *BMC Medical Genetics, 11*, 24–28.

Premranjan, K. C., Danabalan, M., Chandrasekhar, R., et al. (1993). Prevalence of psychiatric morbidity in an urban community of Pondicherry. *Indian Journal of Psychiatry, 35*, 99–102.

Rai, D., Gaete, J., Girotra, S., et al. (2008). Substance use among medical students: Time to reignite the debate? *National Medical Journal of India, 21*, 75–78.

Rajeswari, R., Chandrasekaran, V., Suhadev, M., et al. (2002). Factors associated with patient and health system delays in the diagnosis of tuberculosis in South India. *International Journal of Tuberculosis and Lung Disorders, 6*, 789–795.

Ramdurg, S., Ambekar, A., & Lal, R. (2012). Sexual dysfunction among male patients receiving buprenorphine and naltrexone maintenance therapy for opioid dependence. *Journal of Sexual Medicine, 9*, 3198–3204.

Rani, M., Bonu, S., Jha, P., et al. (2003). Tobacco use in India: Prevalence and predictors of smoking and chewing in a national cross sectional household survey. *Tobacco Control, 12*, 34–37.

Rao, R., Dhawan, A., Ambekar, A., et al. (2012). Slow release oral morphine as a maintenance agent in opioid dependence syndrome: An exploratory study from India. *Journal of Substance Use, 17*, 294–298.

Rao, R. V., Dhawan, A., & Sapra, N. (2005). Opioid maintenance therapy with slow release oral morphine: Experience from India. *Journal of Substance Use, 10*, 259–261.

Ray, R. (2004). The Extent, Pattern and Trends Of Drug Abuse In India, National Survey, Ministry of Social Justice and Empowerment, Government of India and United Nations Office on Drugs and Crime, Regional Office for South Asia.

Ray, R., & Chandrasekhar, K. (1982). Detection of alcoholism among psychiatric inpatients. *Indian Journal of Psychiatry, 24*, 389–393.

Ray, R., Dhawan, A., Ambekar, A., et al. (2009). Inhalant use among street children in Delhi: A situation assessment (Report no. SE/08/094199). National Drug Dependence Treatment Centre, All India Institute of Medical Sciences, New Delhi.

Ray, R., Kattimani, S., & Sharma ,H. K. (2011). Opium abuse and its management: Global scenario. Background paper for the Technical Guidelines Development Group (TDG) on Psycho-socially Assisted Pharmacotherapy of Opioid Dependence, WHO (Geneva). UNODC2011 World drug report 2011 Austria, Vienna.

Ray, R., Mohan, D., Prabhu, G. G., et al. (1978). Psychosocial correlates of chronic cannabis use. *Drug and Alcohol Dependence, 3*, 235–241.

Ray, R., & Neeliyara, T. (1989). Alcoholism-diagnostic criteria and variability. *Indian Journal of Psychiatry, 31*, 247–249.

Ray, R., Pal, H., Kumar, R., et al. (2004). Post-marketing surveillance of buprenorphine. *Pharmacoepidemiology and Drug Safety, 6*, 615–619.

Reddy, M. V., & Chandrashekhar, C. R. (1998). Prevalence of mental and behavioural disorders in India: A meta-analysis. *Indian Journal of Psychiatry, 40*, 149–157.

Sabhesan, S., & Natarajan, M. (1987). Alcohol abuse and recovery after head injury. *Indian Journal of Psychiatry, 29*, 143–148.

Sachadev, J. S., Yakhmi, R. S., & Sharma, A. K. (2002). Changing pattern of drug abuse among patients attending de-addiction center at Faridkot. *Indian Journal of Psychiatry, 44*, 353–355.

Saluja, B. S., Grover, S., Irpati, A. S., et al. (2007). Drug dependence in adolescents 1978–2003: A clinical-based observation from North India. *Indian Journal of Pedatrics, 74*, 455–458.

Sampath, S. K., Chand, P. K., & Murthy, P. (2007). Problem drinking among male inpatients in a rural general hospital. *Indian Journal of Community Med, 32*, 93–97.

Sarin, S. K., Bhatt, A., Malhotra, V., et al. (1988). Pattern of alcohol-related liver disease in dependent alcoholics: The Indian dimension. *British Journal of Addiction, 83*, 279–284.

Sarkar, S., Nebhinani, N., Singh, S. M., et al. (2012). Tramadol dependence: A case series from India. *Indian Journal of Psychological Medicine, 34*, 283–285.

Sarkar, S., Sharma, A., & Basu, D. (2013). Comparison of craving between smoked and smokeless tobacco across a variety of cue exposures. *Substance Use and Misuse, 48*, 233–238.

Saxena, S., & Mohan, D. (1984). Rapid increase of heroin dependence in Delhi: Some initial observations. *Indian Journal of Psychiatry, 26*, 41–45.

Seshadri, S. (2008). Substance abuse among medical students and doctors: A call for action. *National Medical Journal of India, 21*, 57–59.

Seth, R., Kotwal, A., & Ganguly, K. K. (2005). Street and working children in Delhi, India, misusing toluene: An ethnographic exploration. *Substance Use and Misuse, 40*, 1659–1663.

Sethi, H. (2001). A rapid assessment study on prevalence of substance abuse disorders in metropolis Delhi. *Indian Journal of Medical Research, 114*, 107–114.

Sethi, B. B., & Trivedi, J. K. (1979). Drug abuse in rural population. *Indian Journal of Psychiatry, 21*, 211–216.

Shah, R., Vankar, G. K., & Upadhyaya, H. P. (1999). Phenomenology of gasoline intoxication and withdrawal symptoms among adolescents in India: A case series. *American Journal of Addiction, 8*, 254–257.

Sharma, P., Murthy, P., & Bharath, M. M. (2012). Chemistry, metabolism, and toxicology of cannabis: Clinical implications. *Iran Journal of Psychiatry, 7*, 149–156.

Sharma, A. K., & Sahai, M. (1990). Pattern of drug use in Indian heroin addicts. *Indian Journal of Psychiatry, 32*, 341–344

Sharma, S., & Singh, M. M. (2001). Prevalence of mental disorders: An epidemiological study In Goa. *Indian Journal of Psychiatry, 43*, 118–126.

Sharma, M. K., Suman, L. N., & Marimuthu, P. (2011). State-trait anger and quality of life among alcohol users. *German Journal of Psychiatry, 14*, 60–65.

Shastri, S. S., & Kolhatkar, K. P. (1989). Socio-demographic features of cannabis and heroin abuse in Bombay. *Journal of Postgraduate Medicine, 35*, 196–198.

Silva, M. C., Benegal, V., Devi, M., et al. (2007). Cognitive deficits in children of alcoholics: At risk before the first sip! *Indian Journal of Psychiatry, 49*, 182–188.

Silva, M. C., Gaunekar, G., Patel, V., et al. (2003). The prevalence and correlates of hazardous drinking in industrial workers: A community study from Goa India. *Alcohol Alcoholism, 38*, 79–83.

Singh, S. M., & Basu, D. (2009). The P300 event-related potential and its possible role as an endophenotype for studying substance use disorders: A review. *Addiction Biology, 14*, 209–298.

Singh, S. M., Basu, D., Kohli, A., et al. (2009). Auditory P300 event-related potentials and neurocognitive functions in opioid dependent men and their brothers. *American Journal of Addiction, 18*, 198–205.

Singh, R. B., Ghosh, S., Niaz, M. A., et al. (1998). Validation of tobacco and alcohol intake questionnaire in relation to food intakes for the five city study and proposed classification for Indians. *Journal of the Association of Physicians of India, 46*, 587–591.

Singh, P., & Kumar, R. (2010). Assessment of the effectiveness of sustained release bupropion and intensive physician advice in smoking cessation. *Lung India, 27*, 11–18.

Singh, S. M., Mattoo, S. K., Dutt, A., et al. (2008). Long-term outcome of in-patients with substance use disorders: A study from North India. *Indian Journal of Psychiatry, 50*, 269–273.

Singh, N. H., Sharma, S. G., & Pasweth, A. M. (2005). Psychiatric co-morbidity among alcohol dependants. *Indian Journal of Psychiatry, 47*, 222–224.

Singhal, A., Tripathi, B. M., Pal, H. R., et al. (2007). Subjective effects of additional doses of buprenorphine in patients on buprenorphine maintenance. *Addictive Behavior, 32*, 320–331.

Sinha, D. K., Ambekar, A., & Tripathi, B. M. (2009). Street children and substance use. In B. M. Tripathi & A. Ambekar (Eds.), *Drug abuse news-n-views* (pp. 3–7). New Delhi: National Drug Dependence Treatment Centre, All India Institute of Medical Sciences.

Sinha, D. N., & Dobe, M. (2004). Effectiveness of tobacco cessation intervention programs. *Indian Journal of Public Health, 41*, 138–143.

Sinha, D. N., Reddy, K. S., Rahman, K., et al. (2006). Linking Global Youth Tobacco Survey (GYTS) data to the WHO framework convention on tobacco control: The case for India. *Indian Journal of Public Health, 50*, 76–89.

Sood, M., & Sood, A. (2009). Glue sniffing intoxication. *Current Pediatric Research, 13*, 59–61.

Sousa, A. D., & Jagtap, J. (2009). An open level trial of naltrexone versus disulfiram in elderly patients with alcohol dependence. *Journal of Pharmacy and Pharmaceutical Sciences, 6*, 85–89.

Sousa, A. D., & Sousa, A. D. (2004). A one-year pragmatic trial of naltrexone vs disulfiram in the treatment of alcohol dependence. *Alcohol Alcoholism, 39*, 528–531.

Sousa, A. D., & Sousa, A. D. (2005). An open randomized study comparing disulfiram and acamprosate in the treatment of alcohol dependence. *Alcohol Alcoholism, 40*, 545–548.

Sreeraj, V. S., Prasad, S., Khess, C. R. J., et al. (2012). Reasons for substance use- a comparative study of alcohol use in tribals and non-tribals. *Indian Journal of Psychological Medicine, 34*, 242–246.

Sri, E. V., Raguram, R., & Srivastava, M. (1997). Alcohol problems in a general hospital—A prevalence study. *Journal of Indian Medical Association, 95*, 505–506.

SriGowri, D. R., Suman, L. N., Rao, S. L., et al. (2008). A study of executive functions in alcohol dependent individuals: Association of age, education and duration of drinking. *Indian Journal of Clinical Psychology, 35*, 14–23.

Sringeri, S. K., Rajkumar, R. P., Muralidharan, K., et al. (2008). The association between attention-deficit/hyperactivity disorder and early-onset alcohol dependence: A retrospective study. *Indian Journal of Psychiatry, 50*, 262–265.

Srivastava, M., & Nair, A. (2012). Spreading tentacles of solvent abuse—A case series study. *National Journal of Medical Research, 2*, 395–398.

Sundaram, K. R., Mohan, D., Advani, G. B., et al. (1984). Alcohol abuse in a rural community in India. Part I: Epidemiological study. *Drug and Alcohol Dependence, 14*, 27–36.

Thacore, V. R. (1972). Drug-abuse in India with special reference to Lucknow. *Indian Journal of Psychiatry, 14*, 257–261.

Thacore, V. R., & Shukla, S. R. (1976). Cannabis psychosis and paranoid schizophrenia. *Archives of General Psychiatry, 33*, 383–386.

Thankappan, K. R., Pradeepkumar, A. S., & Nichter, M. (2009). Doctors' behaviour & skills for tobacco cessation in Kerala. *Indian Journal of Medical Research, 129*, 249–255.

Thirthalli, J., & Chand, P. K. (2009). The implications of medication development in the treatment of substance use disorders in developing countries. *Current Opinion in Psychiatry, 22*(3), 274–280.

Trivedi, J. K., & Sethi, B. B. (1978). Drug abuse in psychiatric patients. *Indian Journal of Psychiatry, 21*, 345–348.

Varghese, A., Beig, A., Senseman, L. A., Rao, S. S., et al. (1973). Social and psychiatric study of a representative group of families in Vellore Town. *Indian Journal of Medical Research, 61*, 608–620.

Varghese, C., Kaur, J., Desai, N. G., et al. (2012). Initiating tobacco cessation services in India: challenges and opportunities. *WHO South-East Asia Journal of Public Health, 1*, 159–168.

Varma, V. K., Basu, D., Malhotra, A., et al. (1994). Correlates of early- and late-onset alcohol dependence. *Addictive Behavior, 19*, 609–619.

Varma, V. K., Malhotra, A. K., Dang, R., et al. (1988). Cannabis and cognitive functions: A prospective study. *Drug and Alcohol Dependence, 21*, 147–152.

Varma, V. K., Singh, A., Singh, S., et al. (1980). Extent and pattern of alcohol use in North India. *Indian Journal of Psychiatry, 22*, 331–337.

Vaswani, M., Prasad, P., & Kapur, S. (2009). Association of ADH1B and ALDH2 gene polymorphisms with alcohol dependence: a pilot study from India. *Human Genomics, 3*, 213–220.

Venkatasubramanian, G., Anthony, G., Reddy, U. S., et al. (2007). Corpus callosum abnormalities associated with greater externalizing behaviors in subjects at high risk for alcohol dependence. *Psychiatry Research, 156*, 209–215.

Venkatesan, J., & Suresh, S. S. (2008). Substance dependence: Decades apart in a teaching hospital. *Indian Journal of Psychiatry, 50*, 100–105.

Verma, R., Balhara, Y. P., & Deshpande, S. N. (2011a). Inhalant abuse: a study from a tertiary care de-addiction clinic. *East Asian Archives of Psychiatry, 21*, 157–163.

Verma, R., Balhara, Y. P., & Deshpande, S. N. (2011b). Workplace inhalant abuse in adult female: Brief report. *Case Reports in Psychiatry, 2*, 102–105.

Verma, R., Balhara, Y. P., & Dhawan, A. (2011c). Inhalant abuse: An exploratory study. *Indian Journal of Psychiatry, 20*, 103–106.

Vohra, A. K., Yadav, B. S., & Khurana, H. (2003). A study of psychiatric comorbidity in alcohol dependence. *Indian Journal of Psychiatry, 45*, 247–250.

Waraich, B. K., Chavan, B. S., & Raj, L. (2003). Inhalant abuse: A growing public health concern in India. *Addiction, 98*, 1169–1172.

Wig, N. N., & Varma, V. K. (1977). Patterns of long-term heavy cannabis use in north India and its effects on cognitive functions: A preliminary report. *Drug and Alcohol Dependence, 2*, 211–219.

Chapter 20
De-addiction Services in India

S.K. Mattoo, S.M. Singh and S. Sarkar

1 Introduction

Mankind has been using substances since time immemorial. India is no exception to this universal historical trend. While the ancient Indian mythological texts mention the consumption of alcohol by demons (*Asuras*) as well as gods (*Devas*), others document recreational and medicinal use of alcohol, opium and cannabis throughout history (Chopra and Chopra 1965). The Mughal period saw the curtailment of the use of alcohol due to the influence of the Islamic traditions; however, it is recorded that the emperors made recreational use of opioids and encouraged the cultivation of opium (Ganguly 2008). When the British took over from the Mughals, they used the opium farming and trade to increase the state revenue. Opium trade to China led to the British China Opium War of 1839–1842 (Cherry et al. 2002). Much later, the British in India tried to kerb and control the use of opium, distributing it through the opium registries of traders and users. District Medical Officers issued licenses to the users to purchase from the traders. Since independence, while this medicalised use of opium has receded, the use of licit and illicit alcohol and drugs has increased gradually.

While the rise in the use and abuse of alcohol is attributed to the globalisation or westernisation, the rise in the abuse of drugs in India, especially in the recent times, has been attributed to a variety of geopolitical circumstances (Charles and Britto 2002). India is located between the two major opium growing regions of the world: the Golden Triangle (Laos, Myanmar and Thailand) and the Golden

S.K. Mattoo, Professor; S.M. Singh, Assistant Professor; S. Sarkar, Senior Resident

S.K. Mattoo (✉) · S.M. Singh · S. Sarkar
Department of Psychiatry, Postgraduate Institute of Medical Education and Research, Chandigarh, India
e-mail: skmattoo@ymail.com

S. Malhotra and S. Chakrabarti (eds.), *Developments in Psychiatry in India*,
DOI 10.1007/978-81-322-1674-2_20

Crescent (Afghanistan, Pakistan and Iran). Large quantities of opioids have been traditionally smuggled into India and trafficked ahead. The geopolitical situation since the late 70s (the Russian invasion followed by US intervention in Afghanistan, the Indo-Pak conflict, the Khalistan movement and terrorism in Punjab and the LTTE movement in Sri Lanka), led to the use of opioids as a currency in the arms trade. Moreover, the problem was accentuated with raw opium being gradually replaced by heroin, which is easily transported, less bulky, more potent and gives a greater rush when injected. This is not to undermine the fact that India is the largest producer of licit opioids being utilised for medicinal purposes (United Nations Office on Drugs and Crime 2012).

Substance use disorders pose a significant problem in India. As a large and diverse country, based on the cultural context and availability of substances, it has a different profile of substance use in different geographical regions. The survey, 'Extent, Pattern and Trends of Drug Abuse in India' revealed that the country has approximately 62.5 million alcohol users, 8.7 million cannabis users and 3 million opioid users (Ray 2004). A meta-analysis concluded that the prevalence of substance use in India is 6.9/1,000 population (Murthy et al. 2010). Such a large quantum of substance using population makes adequate de-addiction services a basic necessity. De-addiction services refer here to the provision of care to reduce or stop substance-taking behaviour and to decrease the harms associated with the use of substances.

Even though the use of different substances varies across different time periods, it is nonetheless associated with a considerable morbidity and mortality and poses a significant healthcare burden (Rehm et al. 2003, 2006). There are also related increases in social problems and criminality, translating into indirect costs to the society (Thavorncharoensap et al. 2009). Hence, to manage the issue of substance use and to reduce the medical and psycho-social problems associated with it, effective de-addiction services are required. This chapter deals with the de-addiction services in India, in a historical perspective. It discusses the service delivery pathways, the models how services are provided, followed by the components of the service delivery. The existing infrastructure and legal framework are discussed, followed by the future outlays and programmes. The needs of special populations are also touched upon.

2 Framework for the Evolution of De-addiction Services in India

Various approaches have been tried to curtail substance use disorders and the consequent harms. Substances had been categorised into licit and illicit substances with initial thrust on implementing legislative measures to control drug-taking behaviours. By bringing possession and consumption of wide range substances under probationary control, it was attempted to regulate the drug abuse problem in the country. However, despite enforcing such punitive measures, a marked decrement in drug-taking behaviours had not been observed, suggesting that deterrence may not work in isolation, and a need for expansion of treatment facilities was felt.

Thus, treatment services were organised, both through the governmental (primary health care, secondary health care, medical colleges and special de-addiction units) and outside of governmental facilities (non-governmental organisations (NGO) and private de-addiction centres). In therapeutic service too, the focus has been initially on abstinence-oriented treatment. Abstinence from any drug-taking behaviour was the aim and was effectuated through detoxification and maintenance on deterrent/antagonist treatment. With time it has been seen that abstinence-based treatment does not necessarily work, and elements of harm reduction were considered. Harm reduction strategy dwells on reducing the harms associated with substance use. Opioid substitution therapies and needle exchange programs are some of the harm reduction measures, which have received attention and have been found to be beneficial in patients with substance use disorders who otherwise have not been able to achieve abstinence.

3 Service Delivery Pathways

De-addiction services can be provided through various pathways and agencies which include the government facilities, the private practitioners, the NGOs or the self-help groups (Abou-Saleh 2006). Government de-addiction services are provided through the government hospitals, primary healthcare clinics and specialised de-addition centres. The funding is provided by the central and/or the state governments. The services are varied in terms of the intensity, expertise and funding. The common feature is that these services are provided for free or at a minimal cost. More intensive de-addiction services are provided mainly at specialised centres at the larger teaching hospitals, though efforts are being made to provide services at the primary care setting, by training the medical officers at the primary health centres. Less intensive detoxification, or mere counselling, may be provided by the less specialised general medical officers. The government service quite often suffers from issues of inadequacy of funding, poor staff motivation and large patient loads. Nonetheless, they provide the backbone of the de-addiction services to the masses.

The private sector de-addiction services are provided through the clinics and rehabilitation centres of private physicians and de-addiction specialists. These operate on fee-for-service basis, and the patients or the families pay for the treatment costs. The profit motive ensures some degree of efficiency and modulation of services according to the demand of the population. However, the services may not be accessible to the poor and downtrodden, who constitute the majority of the population, and whose social and financial spiral is accentuated due to substance use.

The NGO sector comprises of various providers who are not under direct government control and generally work on not-for-profit basis. They often get grants from the government or other benefactors, but work on their particular agenda towards relieving problems affecting the community. Their services can include drug awareness programmes, needle–syringe exchange programmes and rehabilitation shelter programmes. These programmes are useful adjuncts to the existing services and often promote proper utilisation of the services by the substance users (Patel and Thara 2003). However, due to the vast multitude of NGOs with differing interests and inadequate communication with each other, their efforts may not be directed in an efficient manner. For example, many different NGOs may be working in one urban locality on needle–syringe exchange, but with different motives of AIDS control, hepatitis prevention, as a component of opioid substitution, as an intermittent outreach or follow-up or awareness programmes, leading to duplication of efforts in one particular area, while other geographical areas lack in services.

Self-help groups provide yet another pathway of services. Organisations like Narcotic Anonymous, Alcoholic Anonymous, Al-Anon (for friends and family of alcoholics) and Alateen (for teenage or younger family members of alcoholics) provide good support to the substance users and their family members who are also affected due to the patient's substance use problem. Through their weekly or more frequent meetings, these organisations provide inspiration from other's successes at abstinence and foster bonds that promote abstinence from the substance using or substance use promoting behaviours. These are particularly useful in helping in maintaining sobriety and directing to other services when need arises. However, such self-help groups are concentrated in cities and towns and are not available everywhere.

The different service pathways do not necessarily operate exclusive of each other. Patients often shuffle from one service delivery system to another. Also, many a times, these service pathways provide complementary and concurrent services. Apart from the above mentioned modes, patients also take consult from the faith healers and religious institutions, who may help in cessation of substance use through prescription of rituals (e.g. 40 days *jamaat*) and proscription of certain behaviours.

4 De-addiction Treatment Components

De-addiction psychiatry is being increasingly recognised as a specialised branch with requires some degree of training for managing the patient with substance abuse problems. The management of patients with substance use disorders begins with the in-depth assessment of the pattern of substance use, physical harms due to substance abuse and associated psychiatric conditions. The treatment per se involves multiple components of pharmacotherapy, psychotherapy and counselling and rehabilitation measures. All of these are important in improving the outcomes of the patient.

4.1 Pharmacotherapy

Pharmacotherapy for substance use disorders includes medications for either detoxification, or for maintenance. Medications for detoxification vary with the type of substances consumed. Detoxification for alcohol is carried out using long-acting benzodiazepines (diazepam or chlordiazepoxide) or hepatic safe benzodiazepines in cases of liver dysfunction (lorazepam or oxazepam). Detoxification from opioids is carried out using either opioid agonists (like buprenorphine) or other drugs for symptomatic control of withdrawal signs and symptoms (like a combination of clonidine, ibuprofen and nitrazepam). Pharmacoprophylaxis intends at prevention of resumption of substance use or a relapse. This is accomplished by the use of deterrent agents (disulfiram), anti-craving drugs (baclofen or acamprosate) and antagonists (naltrexone). Another approach is to prevent the use of illicit substances by providing through a legalised medical channel the licit medications like agonist agents (buprenorphine or methadone). Many of these agents have been shown to be efficacious in systematic reviews and meta-analyses (Fareed et al. 2012; Minozzi et al. 2011; Rösner et al. 2010). Compliance to these agents is important to maintain abstinence and prevent relapses.

4.2 Counselling and Psychotherapy

It has been seen that pharmacotherapy alone does not work effectively in treatment of substance use disorders. Hence, de-addiction services usually employ some form of 'talk' therapy elements, in varying degrees. These are delivered knowingly or unknowingly and formally or informally while developing rapport with the patient and working with the patient long term in the quest for maintaining abstinence. The formal structured psychotherapies include psychoanalytic, cognitive-behavioural, mindfulness-based, marital and family therapies, eclectic and dialectical therapies among others. In relation to de-addiction services, motivation enhancement therapy and relapse prevention counselling has been found to be of considerable usefulness and effective for treatment of substance use disorders (Dutra et al. 2008).

4.3 Rehabilitation

Apart from pharmacotherapy and psychotherapeutic measures, rehabilitation services are also of relevance to substance users. As substance use disorder progresses, the process of procuring the substance, its use and enjoyment of the effects become the predominant occupation of the patient. As substance use ceases, the patients may have a lot of free time on their hands, which they may find difficult to fill, resulting in re-association with substance using peers and descending again into the loop of substance use and consequent harms. Hence, vocational rehabilitation and engagement can help these patients to remain abstinent. The family, friends or other social supports can play a crucial role in occupational rehabilitation. Social re-integration can also act as a safety net for preventing the person going back to substance use.

4.4 Managing Comorbid Illnesses

De-addiction services need to pay attention not only to the problem of substance use, but also to the issue of other co-morbid medical and psychiatric illnesses. Respiratory disorders, gastrointestinal problems, cardiac problems and poor nutrition are fairly common with substance use disorders. Among other psychiatric illnesses, personality disorders, affective disorders, anxiety disorders and psychotic disorders are frequently encountered. Treatment of these additional disorders can be carried out by the trained physician or psychiatrist dealing with the substance use problem or can be referred to suitable facilities/specialists where these can be addressed.

5 Service Delivery Models

De-addiction services can be delivered through various models of care: outpatient, inpatient, therapeutic communities and through camps and community outreach programmes to schools, colleges and religious institutions (Bruckner et al. 2011). Service delivery is modified when delivering de-addiction services to special populations like prison inmates, women, street children and patients with dual diagnosis.

The majority of the patients with substance use disorders can be dealt on the outpatient basis. The outpatient services involve patients seeking consultation for substance use disorder and prescription of initial detoxification regimen followed by maintenance pharmacoprophylaxis. Counselling and psychotherapeutic interventions are invariably incorporated into the outpatient treatment programmes, and motivation enhancement is attempted. The outpatient facility requires minimal infrastructure and is able to cater to a large number of patients per therapist.

For patients who have multiple substance dependencies, poor health condition, comorbid psychiatric conditions, multiple failed detoxification attempts or lack of supervision, inpatient treatment is better. The inpatient treatment is usually of short stay and involves stabilisation of the medical or psychiatric condition, detoxification, initiation of pharmacoprophylaxis or agonist agent and relevant counselling inputs. The inpatient services provide round-the-clock observation and monitoring, and medical assistance close at hand. Longer inpatient stays are recommended in certain situations when additional psychiatric disorders are present, which require time to remit. Night hospitalisations can be considered in situations where patient engages in productive work in the daytime and rests in the substance-free environment of the inpatient facility in the night.

Therapeutic communities are residential set-ups, which are geared towards making de-addiction services available for a relatively longer duration. The patients are typically voluntarily admitted to the therapeutic community, where they stay and interact with other patients with substance use disorders and try to mend ways of behaving. The focus is on reinforcing abstinent behaviour. There is a hierarchy of residents in the therapeutic community and patients who have recovered guide others towards recovery. There is lesser emphasis on medical management and greater emphasis on changing the psyche to attain recovery. The original model of therapeutic community has been modified in many ways including relaxation of rules, changes in structure and hierarchy, and effective use of adjunct medications.

Another approach that has been utilised has been the camp approach and community outreach. This involves holding ‘camps’, in which awareness is generated in the community, and preliminary treatment is provided to the identified substance users (Chavan et al. 2003; Purohit and Razdan 1988). The aim of such programmes is to generate awareness about the harms of substance use and the treatment modalities available. Since many substance users are unwilling to seek treatment in formal settings due to stigma or other inhibiting factors, this approach attempts to bridge the service gap by bringing the initial treatment to the community at the doorstep of the substance user. However, since treatment of substance use disorders usually requires prolonged contact, the patients are referred to relevant services for further ongoing management. Awareness programs are also conducted in high-risk/vulnerable populations/groups such as schools, colleges, factories, industries and others with information about the services and referral to appropriate centres.

6 Existing Policies and Programmes in India

Supply reduction and demand reduction are the two ways through which the problem of substance use is being tackled in the country. Supply reduction activities aim at reducing the availability of substances (Ray 2009). These are taken care of by the Ministry of Home Affairs, Ministry of Finance and the Department of Revenue and are executed by various enforcement agencies. These measures involve pricing and taxation of the substances, such as alcohol and tobacco, regulation of sale (for example, prohibition of sale to minors) and curtailment of public consumption. Prohibition of sale and consumption of substances is another measure through which supply reduction can be achieved. This has been achieved through legal enforcement of bans against illicit substances, but also has been tried for alcohol in specific states.

Demand reduction focuses upon awareness generation, treatment and rehabilitation services, which are looked after by the Ministry of Health and Family Welfare (MOHFW) and Ministry of Social Justice and Empowerment (MSJE).

The Drug De-addiction Programme (DDAP) was started by the MOHFW in the year 1987–1988 and was later modified in 1992–1993. The programme was initiated as a scheme with funding from the central government and implementation through the states. A one-time grant in aid of Rs. 8 lakhs was given for construction of each drug de-addiction centre, and a recurring grant of Rs. 2 lakhs was given to those established in North Eastern states. Under this programme, a national nodal centre was established in Ghaziabad and two centres have been upgraded, one at PGIMER, Chandigarh and the other at NIMHANS, Bangalore. The nodal centre at Ghaziabad, the National Drug Dependence Treatment Centre (NDDTC) is a 50-bedded facility and provides outpatient and inpatient care. The centre runs specialised clinics: tobacco cession clinic, dual diagnosis clinic and adolescent substance use clinic. It is also actively involved in community programmes, training of the primary healthcare doctors and other trainers. The centre is actively involved with provision of services and research regarding opioid substitution therapy. The centre oversees other de-addiction centres and provides resource personnel for formulation of policies and support services. The de-addiction centre in NIMHANS which has been rechristened as Centre for Addiction Medicine is recognised as the Regional Centre for the Southern India. The centre runs a specialised tobacco cessation clinic and is actively involved in research and planning pertaining to substance use disorders.

The centre at PGIMER Chandigarh is a 20-bedded facility and provides services to a wide range of substance users. The centre provides inpatient and outpatient care and rehabilitative services. The centre runs a tobacco cessation clinic and a dual diagnosis clinic. Integrated management of medical conditions is provided by the attached personnel from internal medicine. With an efficient record keeping, the centre is able to assess the long-term outcome with well documented follow-ups. The centre actively partakes in community de-addiction services by organising awareness camps in the community and in the schools and colleges. The centre is also actively involved in providing guidance to the states of Punjab and Haryana pertaining to matters regarding substance use disorders.

Presently there are about 120 de-addiction centres in India, many of which have been placed at the district hospitals and medical colleges. A considerable proportion of the de-addiction centres are in the North East due to the high prevalence of injectable drug use. The centres in the North East have been functioning better than some other centres due to recurrence of grants to the North East. In some centres, the places marked for de-addiction services is being utilized for a variety of purposes, some of them not directly related to treatment of substance use disorders.

Parallel to the above services, the MSJE has been implementing the Scheme for Prohibition and Drug Abuse Prevention since the year 1985–1986. The scheme aims to provide financial assistance to organisations involved in awareness and preventive education, establishing drug awareness and counselling centres, treatment and rehabilitation centres, and workplace prevention programs and de-addiction camps. Under the scheme, the major portion of the cost of services is borne by the government, and NGOs provide actual services through various means. The MSJE has set up a National Centre for Drug Abuse Prevention (NCDAP) in the National Institute of Social Defence (NISD) for capacity building and training of NGOs running counselling and de-addiction centres. The MSJE has also formed a National Consultative Committee on De-addiction and Rehabilitation (NCCDR), as a consultative mechanism at the national level to advise Central and State Governments on issues connected with drug demand reduction, especially education/awareness building, de-addiction and rehabilitation. Under the umbrella of the MSJE, the Federation for Indian NGOs in Drug Abuse Prevention (FINGODAP) has been created to facilitate networking amongst member NGOs (essentially those funded by the Government of India), so as to gain from each other's experience and also to ensure self-restraint towards implementation of minimum standard of services.

The National Mental Health Programme (NMPH) is the guiding force for the development of mental health services in India (Murthy 2004). Though the initial years of the NMHP did not yield phenomenal strides, the District Mental Health Programme (DMHP) has emerged as a consequence of the NMHP. It aims to decentralise decision-making to the districts and strengthening of the services at the district level at the same time. The other important thrust has been manpower development and emphasis on information–education–communication services. Substance use disorders being common mental disorders have received attention, both in the NMHP as well as the DMHP.

The high prevalence of substance abuse in northern India coupled with the inadequate services resulted in mushrooming of de-addiction centres run by ex-patients. Some of these centres indulged in objectionable activities such as forced detention of the patients, and physical and emotional abuse in the name of treatment or therapeutic community, and no, or inadequate medical care leading to deaths of the inmates, resulted in legal intervention by the Punjab and Haryana High Court. A court established committee of experts, officials and NGO representatives made some recommendations for the checks and balances for operationalising the non-governmental de-addiction centres. Guided by these recommendations, the states of Punjab and Haryana and the Union Territory of Chandigarh are implementing licensing frameworks for such private de-addiction centres.

The state government of Punjab has also endeavoured to follow a three-tiered system (primary, secondary and tertiary) of provision of de-addiction services. Apart from services of PGIMER, three more model drug de-addiction centres in Patiala, Jalandhar and Faridkot are planned with an outlay of Rs. 10 crores for setting up these centres. Also, Rs. 15 crore has been sanctioned for setting 31 ten-bedded de-addiction units at district and sub-division levels. Trained medical personnel are allocated for delivering the services in these de-addiction centres. To acknowledge the issue of de-addiction in jails, it has been decided to screen the entire inmate population as well as staff for drug use in the course of a general medical examination. It has been planned to create de-addiction facilities in all eight central jails with separate barracks with 50 beds for initial treatment and 100 beds for recovering patients. Training of the physicians who tend to the inmate population has already been started at PGIMER for management of substance use disorders.

Infrastructure for dealing with substance use disorders has been lacking, given the extent of the problem of substance use disorders in the country. The services are being provided by de-addiction centres, government hospitals, private centres and others. That they are grossly inadequate is well recognised by all the stake holders. But there is no reliable data about the deficit between the requirement of de-addiction services and that actually provided. The relative lack of services is not surprising, considering that the overall healthcare systems in the country are inadequate. Though suggestions have been made about requirement of basic infrastructure at de-addiction centres (Arya and Dube 2009), whether these standards are met need to be looked at. Concrete data are not available at present to discern the needs deficit of the de-addiction services in the community.

7 Special Situations and Populations

7.1 Migrants and Drug Use

Migrant populations present as a unique challenge among the substance users. It is because of their mobile nature that these populations are in a flux and hence difficult to provide services to. Migrants can include rural to rural, rural to urban and state to state migrants moving in search of work. Due to the stress of the reasons of shift, acculturation to the new community and often living alone and without the customary social support systems, this population may have higher rates of substance use. This applies not only to males, but also to females (Verma et al. 2010). Substance use disorders have been reported to concur with the spread of sexually transmitted diseases in this population (Gupta et al. 2010). Again, difficulties may be experienced in accessing care by the migrants due to unfamiliarity with healthcare facilities and nuances of accessing in the newer place of residence. Providing appropriate services to this population not only would help in controlling substance use disorders, but might also stop the spread of other communicable illnesses.

7.2 North Eastern Scenario

Drug abuse has become a major problem in the North East. High rates of unemployment coupled with the easy availability of opioids from the Golden Triangle region has led to the surge in the rates of use of heroin and other opioids in states of Manipur, Nagaland and Mizoram (Kermode et al. 2009). Given the proximity to Myanmar, one of the largest producers of heroin in the world, trafficking in drugs is common, which is used to fuel arms procurement for insurgent activities (Lama 2001). Heroin is commonly referred to 'number 4' in the region, and people resort to injectable drug use as a cheaper option for this highly addictive drug. The problem of injecting drug use is substantial, with approximately 2 % of the population injecting drugs, both heroin and pharmaceutical agents (Kermode et al. 2010). Injecting drug use has added the problem of transmission of HIV, leading to high rates of HIV positivity in the region. This area has received concerted attention from the government, and NGOs in the form of active work of providing opioid substitution therapy as well as promoting safe injecting practices (Kumar et al. 2009). But further work needs to be undertaken to improve the outcomes of patients in the region and control the epidemic of drug abuse and HIV.

8 Legal Framework for Services

Legal provisions are available for management of substance use disorders. The Narcotic Drugs and Psychotropic Substances (NDPS) act of 1985 has provisions for treatment of substance users in lieu of their imprisonment. The Section 64A of the Act provides for medical treatment of the person charged under the provisions of the act for possession of small quantities of substances in lieu of immediate conviction. However, the treatment can be carried out only for detoxification or de-addiction from a hospital or an institution maintained or recognised by the Government, and then the court decides whether the conviction should be annulled.

Apart from this, the NDPS also has provisions that empower the government to establish centres for identification, treatment, education, after care, rehabilitation, social reintegration of substance users and for supply, of any narcotic drugs and psychotropic substance (as prescribed by concerned Government) to the users registered with government, and to others where such supply is a medical necessity. This falls under Section 71 of the Act and provides for treatment with substances like buprenorphine, where it is considered a necessity and beneficial in patients' and community's interest.

9 Conclusions

De-addiction services have been provided through a variety of pathways and in different settings ranging from outpatient, inpatient, community outreach and therapeutic communities. The extent and variety of substance using population necessitates different formats of services being available as one size does not fit all. The different services, pathways and models complement and supplement each other. However, the existing de-addiction services are grossly inadequate to meet the needs of the population, and further planning and implementation of effective and acceptable de-addiction services is likely to help to curtail the scourge of substance use disorders.

References

Abou-Saleh, M. T. (2006). Substance use disorders: Recent advances in treatment and models of care. *Journal of Psychosomatische Research, 61*, 305–310.

Arya, S., & Dube, S. (2009). Minimum standards of care at de-addiction centres: Infrastructure. In B. Tripathi & A. Ambekar (Eds.), *Minimum standards of care for the Government de-addiction centres* (pp. 18–24). All India Institute of Medical Sciences, New Delhi: National Drug Dependence Treatment Centre.

Bruckner, T. A., Scheffler, R. M., Shen, G., Yoon, J., Chisholm, D., Morris, J., et al. (2011). The mental health workforce gap in low- and middle-income countries: A needs-based approach. *Bulletin of the World Health Organization, 89*, 184–194.

Charles, M., & Britto, G. (2002). Culture and the drug scene in India. *Globalization, drugs and criminalization: Part 3—Social and cultural dimensions of drug trafficking* (pp. 6–39). Paris: UNESCO MOST and UNDP.

Chavan, B. S., Gupta, N., & Raj, L. (2003). Camp approach-an effective, alternate inpatient treatment setting for substance dependence: A report from India. *German Journal of Psychiatry, 6*, 17–22.

Cherry, A. L., Dillon, M. E., & Rugh, D. (2002). *Substance abuse: A global view*. California: Greenwood Publishing Group.

Chopra, R. N., & Chopra, I. C. (1965). *Drug addiction; with special reference to India*. New Delhi: Council of Scientific and Industrial Research.

Dutra, L., Stathopoulou, G., Basden, S. L., Leyro, T. M., Powers, M. B., & Otto, M. W. (2008). A meta-analytic review of psychosocial interventions for substance use disorders. *American Journal of Psychiatry, 165*, 179–187.

Fareed, A., Vayalapalli, S., Casarella, J., & Drexler, K. (2012). Effect of buprenorphine dose on treatment outcome. *Journal of Addictive Diseases, 31*, 8–18.

Ganguly, K. (2008). Pattern and process of drug and alcohol use in India. *ICMR Bulletin, 38*, 1–8.

Gupta, K., Vaidehi, Y., & Majumder, N. (2010). Spatial mobility, alcohol use, sexual behavior and sexual health among males in India. *AIDS and Behavior, 14*(1), 18–30.

Kermode, M., Deutschmann, P., Arunkumar, M. C., & Manning, G. (2010). Injecting drug use and HIV in northeast India: Negotiating a public health response in a complex environment. *South Asian History and Culture, 1*, 239–249.

Kermode, M., Longleng, V., Singh, B. C., Bowen, K., & Rintoul, A. (2009). Killing time with enjoyment: A qualitative study of initiation into injecting drug use in north-east India. *Substance Use Misuse, 44*, 1070–1089.

Kumar, M. S., Natale, R. D., Langkham, B., Sharma, C., Kabi, R., & Mortimore, G. (2009). Opioid substitution treatment with sublingual buprenorphine in Manipur and Nagaland in Northeast India: What has been established needs to be continued and expanded. *Harm Reduct J, 6*, 4.

Lama, M. P. (2001). India's north-east states: Narcotics, small arms and misgovernance. *Ethnic Studies Report, 19*, 243–258.

Minozzi, S., Amato, L., Vecchi, S., Davoli, M., Kirchmayer, U., & Verster, A., 2011. Oral naltrexone maintenance treatment for opioid dependence. *Cochrane Database Systematic Review*, CD001333.

Murthy, R. (2004). The national mental health programme: Progress and problems. In S. Agarwal, D. Goel, & R. Ichhpujani (Eds.), *Mental health an Indian perspective 1946–2003* (pp. 75–91). New Delhi: Directorate General of Health Services Ministry of Health and Family Welfare.

Murthy, P., Manjunatha, N., Subodh, B. N., Chand, P. K., & Benegal, V. (2010). Substance use and addiction research in India. *Indian Journal of Psychiatry, 52*, 189–199.

Patel, V., & Thara, R. (2003). *Meeting the mental health needs of developing countries NGO innovations in India*. New Delhi/Thousand Oaks: Sage Publications.

Purohit, D. R., & Razdan, V. K. (1988). Evolution and appraisal of community camp-approach to opium detoxification in North India. *Indian Journal of Social Psychiatry, 4*, 15–21.
Ray, R., (2004). The extent, patterns and trends of drug abuse in India—national survey.
Ray, R. (2009). Drug de-addiction Programme in India. In R. Lal & A. Ambekar (Eds.), *Substance Use Disorders: A Manual for Paramedical Staff* (pp. 17–21). All India Institute of Medical Sciences, New Delhi: National Drug Dependence Treatment Centre.
Rehm, J., Gmel, G., Sempos, C. T., & Trevisan, M. (2003). Alcohol-related morbidity and mortality. *Alcohol Research and Health, 27*, 39–51.
Rehm, J., Taylor, B., & Room, R. (2006). Global burden of disease from alcohol, illicit drugs and tobacco. *Drug Alcohol Review, 25*, 503–513.
Rösner, S., Hackl-Herrwerth, A., Leucht, S., Vecchi, S., Srisurapanont, M., Soyka, M. (2010). Opioid antagonists for alcohol dependence. *Cochrane Database Systematic Review*, CD001867.
Thavorncharoensap, M., Teerawattananon, Y., Yothasamut, J., Lertpitakpong, C., & Chaikledkaew, U. (2009). The economic impact of alcohol consumption: A systematic review. *Substance Abuse Treatment Prevention Policy, 4*, 20.
United Nations Office on Drugs and Crime. (2012). World drug report 2012. United Nations, New York.
Verma, R. K., Saggurti, N., Singh, A. K., & Swain, S. N. (2010). Alcohol and sexual risk behavior among migrant female sex workers and male workers in districts with high in-migration from four high HIV prevalence states in India. *AIDS and Behavior, 14*(1), 31–39.

Part VI
Developments in Community Psychiatry

Chapter 21
From Institutions, to Clinics to Community: Development of Community Mental Health in the Last 50 Years and Looking to the Future

R.S. Murthy

1 Introduction

The celebration of the Golden Jubilee of the Department of Psychiatry, Postgraduate Institute of Medical Education and Research (PGIMER), Chandigarh, is a special occasion for the department and in the lives of all of us associated with the institution. The theme of the International CME, 'The journey from madness to mental health: the next 50 years of psychiatry' is an opportunity to look back to the road taken and think ahead for the future. Of the many aspects of psychiatry, community mental health is closest to the theme of the CME. The present chapter covers this vast canvas of the past developments and presents a personal view towards mental health in the next 50 years.

In India, among the developments in various sectors of the society during the last 65 years of independent India, lack of adequate development in the health sector would be the most significant. Reviewing the scene, a recent book, 'An Uncertain Glory' (Dreze and Sen 2013), refers to this as follows: '*the lack of effective public involvement with health matters in India has played no small part in the resilience of India's health predicament*' (p. 148). Further, calling for 'the need for impatience' (p. 276), they note the need for '*the struggle against injustice has to be clearly connected with constructive demands for essential public services and basic entitlements*' (p. 281) and identify this as '*one of the principal challenges facing India today*' (p. 287). The authors call for 'the need for impatience' as follows: '*and yet the*

R.S. Murthy, Former Professor and Head

R.S. Murthy (✉)
Department of Psychiatry, National Institute of Mental Health and Neurosciences, Bangalore, India
e-mail: smurthy030@gmail.com

R.S. Murthy
Association for the Mentally Challenged, Hosur Road, Bangalore, India

S. Malhotra and S. Chakrabarti (eds.), *Developments in Psychiatry in India*,
DOI 10.1007/978-81-322-1674-2_21

democratic policies of India do offer opportunities for the most deprived Indians to reflect on their own strength, and to demand that the critically important inequalities that ruin the lives of so many people in the country be rapidly remedied. This is, of course, partly a matter of political organisation, but there is also an important role for a clear-headed understanding of the extensive reach and peculiar nature of deprivation and inequality in India. This is surely one of the principle challenges facing India today' (p. 287). Further, they emphasise that 'there is a strong case for forceful public demand for much larger allocations to basic public services…' (p. 276).

The importance of the public demand and individual initiatives was considered one of the defining themes of the twenty-first century by Mr. Gopalakrishnan of Infosys, Bangalore, in a BBC programme on 'Changing Fortunes' (July 20, 2013), where he referred to the current century as one of 'individual capacities and power'. These two themes of demand creation and individual empowerment are relevant to the community mental health movement of India.

Much of what is said about health care in particular and social services in general could be said about the mental health care in the country. The current account reviews the progress and identifies the way forward for the coming years and decades. The progress of mental health care in independent India and the community mental health has been extensively documented (Chavan et al. 2012; Agarwaal et al. 2004; Srinivasa Murthy 2004a, b, 2007a, b, 2008, 2011, 2012a, b). The details are not repeated here, and the following is a summary of the developments as the background for looking to the future, which is the theme of this book. The Department of Psychiatry, PGIMER, has been a pioneer in the development of the community mental health in the country, and this rich contribution of the department makes this chapter special on the occasion of the golden jubilee of the department.

2 Historical Developments

Community psychiatry is an important approach to the organisation of mental health care in both economically rich and in low- and middle-income (LAMI) countries. This development of the community psychiatry movement, all over the world, is part of series of phases of development of mental health care over the last 200–300 years, starting from setting up special institutions for the care of the persons with mental disorders (asylums), to the humane treatment of the ill persons, deinstitutionalisation and recognition of the rights of the ill persons with mental disorders (WHO 2001; Thornicroft and Szmukler 2001; Thornicroft et al. 2011; Srinivasa Murthy 2011).

3 Challenging Mental Health Situation in India

Throughout the period of independent India, there have a number of challenges faced by the professionals in organising the care programmes (Box 1), (Dube 1963; Gururaj and Issac 2004; Srinivasa Murthy 2011, 2012a, b). The story of community mental health is the way India has addressed the key mental health barriers in the country, namely lack of access, affordability, acceptability and stigma of mental disorders.

Box 1: Challenges for mental health care in India

1. There is a large 'unmet need' for mental health care in the community;
2. There is poor understanding of the psychological distress as requiring medical intervention in the general population;
3. There is limited acceptance of the modern medical care for mental disorders in the general population;
4. There are severe limitations in the availability of mental health services (professionals and facilities) in the public health services;
5. There is poor utilisation of the available services by the ill population and their families;
6. There are problems in recovery and reintegration of the persons with mental illnesses.
7. Institutionalised mechanisms for organisation of mental health care are not adequate in the country.

4 Development of Mental Health Services in India

In contrast to the economically rich countries, the development of community psychiatry in India occurred against the background of almost no mental health services, and special challenges of lack of awareness in the community, existing systems of traditional care, stigma and poorly functioning institutions (NHRC 1999, 2008). Almost all of the persons with mental disorders are living in the community, most often without any organised services, with the family providing the care in whatever form they are able to do (ranging from isolation to committed care). In a way, community psychiatry has developed in India as 'the service' and not as an 'alternative' to institutionalised care. This distinction of the development of community psychiatry is important to understand the developments in the movement (Srinivasa Murthy 2004a, b, 2008, 2011, 2012a, b).

At the time of India's Independence, there were almost no mental health services in the country. For a population of about 300 million, there were only 10,000 psychiatric beds, in contrast to over 150,000 psychiatric beds for about 30 million in United Kingdom at that time. The initial period of 1947–1966 focussed on doubling of the psychiatric beds (Dube 1963; Sharma 1990), along with development of training centres to train psychiatrists, clinical psychologists, psychiatric social workers and psychiatric nurses. The period of 1960s to the 1970s saw the emergence of general hospital psychiatric units (GHPUs) in a big way both as service providers and training centres (Wig 1978). Community psychiatry initiatives were taken up initially in the 1970s, and in a big way from the 1980s, following the adoption of the National Mental Health Programme (NMHP) in August 1982 (DGHS 1982).

A striking aspect of the developments of mental health services in India is as much the location of the care in the community (where most of the ill persons were already living), as the utilisation of a wide variety of community resources. For example, in the initial phase, family members were the focus, followed by the utilisation of the existing general health care infrastructure through integration of mental health services with general health services. This was followed by increased use of school teachers, volunteers, counsellors, mentally ill persons, survivors of disasters, parents of children with mental disorders and personnel of the education system (Srinivasa Murthy 2006). In this way, the three principles of community psychiatry—meeting population based needs, use of range of resources and accessibility—were partially addressed.

5 Community Mental Health Initiatives in India

5.1 Family Support

At the time of independence, in India, there were only 10,000 psychiatric beds for over 300 million population. This was in contrast to over 190,000 psychiatric beds in the UK for less than one-tenth of the population of India. In this context, most of the ill patients were living with their families or in the community. What challenged the psychiatric community was the need to provide care with almost no specialised resources. Recognising the cultural factor of commitment of the families to their ill family members, psychiatrists looked to the family members of the ill persons as the answer. India is a pioneer in involving the family members in the care of their ill relatives from the early 1950s. It is significant to recall that at that time period in the development of psychiatry in the rest of the world, families were thought to be 'toxic' to the patient and excluded from the mental health interventions. In India, the story is different. This occurred first at the Amritsar Mental Hospital (Vidya 1973) and soon followed by the Mental Health Centre at Vellore (Kohmeyler and Fernandes 1963; Chacko 1967; Verghese 1971) and mental hospital at Bangalore (Narayanan and Reddy 1968; Narayanan et al. 1972; Narayanan 1977; Geetha et al. 1980; Bhatti 1980; Bhatti et al. 1982). In India, family involvement was started in the 1950s (Vidya 1973; Carstairs 1974, 1980; Srinivasa Murthy 2007a, b). Indian initiatives relating to families and mental health care have depended on the family support for the mentally ill persons. Since 1950s, families have been formally included to supplement and support the psychiatric care by professionals. During this period, literally, family members were admitted along with mentally ill to be part of the care of the patients. This has largely been the pattern in most of the LAMI countries. During the 1970s and 1980s, efforts were made to understand the functioning of families with an ill person in the family and their needs (Bhatti 1980; Bhatti et al. 1980, 1982; Bhatti and Verghese 1995).

Two centres, namely PGIMER, Chandigarh, and the National Institute of Mental Health and Neurosciences (NIMHANS), Bangalore, systematically studied the needs of the families, and the role of non-medical professionals in providing support to the families (Suman et al. 1980). In the NIMHANS, Bangalore, (Pai and Kapur 1982, 1983; Pai et al. 1983, 1985), two similar groups of patients with schizophrenia undergoing two treatment modalities, namely hospital admission and home treatment through a nurse, were compared for the outcome in terms of symptoms, social dysfunction, burden on the family, cost of treatment and outcome at the end of 6 months. A nurse trained in patient follow-up and counselling visited the home regularly for the purpose of patient assessment and treatment. The results found that the home treatment through a visiting nurse gives a better clinical outcome and better social functioning of the patient and greatly reduces the burden on the patients' families. Further, the treatment modality is also more economical. A follow-up study observed that the home care group of patients had maintained significantly better clinical status than the controls, and this group had been admitted less often. In a subsequent study, the focus of family care by visiting nurses was patients with a diagnosis of chronic schizophrenia; this found that only two of the home care group were admitted to hospital over 2 years in comparison with eight patients in routine care. Along with this, there was study of factors contributing positively or negatively to the course and outcome of schizophrenia. Research into the special needs of mentally retarded and their families has also been studied (Russell et al. 1999, 2004).

During the last 15 years, a more active role for families is emerging in the form of formation of self-help groups and professionals accepting to work with families in partnership (Srinivasan 2008). However, many of the leads provided by pilot studies and successes of family care programmes have not received the support of professionals and planners to the extent it could become a routine part of psychiatric care in the twenty-first century. It is very interesting that in the last decade there is recognition of the value of family involvement in mental health care in developed countries (Selis 2007; Shimazu et al. 2011).

However, it is important to recognise that there are large unfinished tasks to make families a part of the community mental health movement. Reviewing the scene, Shankar and Rao (2005) opine that 'professional inputs have not kept pace' and conclude that the 'family movement in India is one of 'unfulfilled promises or great expectations for the future' as follows: '***the vision for the family movement in India would see families from passive carers to informed carers, from receiving services to proactive participation, from suffering stigma to fighting stigma. And it is the responsibility of the mental health system to facilitate this journey of care givers from burden to empowerment***' (p. 285).

Many of the leads provided by pilot studies and successes of family care programmes have not received the support of professionals and planners to the extent it could become a routine part of psychiatric care. In the coming years, moving from passive utilisation of the families to partnership and true empowerment of the families has the greatest potential in organising mental health care in India. The advances in communication technology (mobile phones) and the widening availability of information technology (Internet) should be used creatively to share the caring skills with families, to bridge gap in professional resources. This will be building mental health care from the 'bottom of the pyramid' as it has happened in the other developmental and commercial areas in developing countries (Prahlad 2006). This area should receive the highest importance in future efforts.

5.2 General Hospital Psychiatry (GHP)

Addressing the challenges of limited treatment facilities (mental hospitals), their location limiting access to majority of the population, and the stigma associated with care in these facilities, the GHP movement emerged. The development of organised mental health care is essentially a post-independence phenomenon. Though the first 15 years of the independence saw doubling of the mental hospital beds to 20,000, pharmacological advances in the treatment of mentally ill persons and the closing down of the mental hospitals in Western countries gave a big push to the development of general hospital-based psychiatric services. The initial GHPUs in Calcutta and Bombay came in the 1930s and the 1940s (IPS 1964). The big spurt in the GHPUs occurred in the 1960s at academic centres at Chandigarh, Delhi, Madurai, and Lucknow. These centres also became centres for training of psychiatrists and for mental health research (Wig 1978). It is relevant to note that the generation of psychiatrists in the 1960s and 1970s faced the challenge of moving mental health care beyond the isolated mental hospitals and bringing mental health care to the general medical care settings (liaison psychiatry). It was these two forces that led to the development of the GHPU. Another striking aspect of Indian GHPUs is their function as primary centres for mental health care. It has been a slow and silent change but in many ways a major revolution in the whole approach to psychiatric treatment. The GHPUs offered numerous advantages over traditional mental hospitals, like accessibility, decreased stigma to seek care, multidisciplinary care, limited legal restrictions, active involvement of the family members in day-to-day care and shorter duration of stay. In the last decade, psychiatric units in all major hospitals has become a reality. This shifting of the place of care to the general hospital setting has contributed significantly to the process of destigmatisation of psychiatric illnesses and psychiatric care. The research contributions of Prof. N.N. Wig and the Department of Psychiatry, PGIMER, Chandigarh, have been significant (Srinivasa Murthy 2010, 2011).

5.3 Integration of Mental Health with General Health Care

Increasing access to care has called for decentralisation and deprofessionalisation of mental health care. As an effort at taking services beyond the isolated and centralised mental hospitals, to GHPUs, the integration of mental health with general health services is the next major innovation. This measure is one of the most important community mental health initiatives in India.

India was the first developing country to formulate a NMHP in 1982 (DGHS 1982). Twenty-five years later, the WHO again re-emphasised the approach through the recommendation in the World Health Report, 2001 (WHO 2001), to '*provide treatment in primary care*'.

In India, training primary health care workers for mental health and integrating mental health with general health care was started in 1975 at centres in Bangalore and Chandigarh (Srinivasa Murthy et al. 1978; Wig and Srinivasa Murthy 1980; Wig et al. 1981; Chandrashekar et al. 1981; Parthasarathy et al. 1981; Issac et al. 1982, 1986; Sartorius and Harding 1983; Srinivasa Murthy and Wig 1983; Srinivasa Murthy et al. 1988). These experiences formed the basis of the NMHP formulated in 1982. Currently, the government supports over 125 district-level programmes in 22 states, covering a population of over 200 million (GOI 2007).

to see each and every mentally ill, rather than allow the non-specialists to treat them'. The second meeting of 30 professionals reviewed the draft document and finalised the same on 2 August 1982. Following the two tumultuous meetings, there was less than a month for the Central Council of Health and Family Welfare (CCH & FW) meeting (18–20 August 1982). It is historical fact that the CCH&FW did debate and recommend the NMHP as follows: '***Mental health must form an integral part of the total health programme and as such should be included in all national policies and programmes in the field of Health, Education and Social Welfare. Realising the importance of mental health in the course curricula for various levels of health professionals, suitable action should be taken in consultation with the appropriate authorities to strengthen the Mental Health Education components. While appreciating the efforts of the Central Government in pursuing legislative action on Mental Health Bill, the joint Conference expressed its earnestness to see that the bill takes a legal shape at the earliest***.' The formulation of the NMHP, the passion with which Prof. Wig pursued the same is a creditable national-level contribution.

Prof. Wig continued his interest in this area following his move to AIIMS, New Delhi, addressing the problem of mental disorders in an urban slum and its implications for mental health care at primary health care, assessment of functioning of non-psychiatric physicians in the management of psychiatric emergencies and a manual for primary health care physicians. Further, when he moved to work with the WHO as Regional Advisor on Mental Health at the Eastern Mediterranean Regional office, in 1984, he carried this mission to the 22 countries of the Middle East (from Pakistan to Morocco). He has contributed richly with technical and administrative support to the development of community mental health in Pakistan and school mental health programmes in Egypt.

Prof. Wig has written extensively about the need and approaches to organising mental health care in India and developing countries on 'Rational treatment in psychiatry: perspective on psychiatric treatment by level of care', 'Evaluation of the progress in mental health in India since independence' and 'Development of regional and national mental health programmes'. He continues to share his thoughts, as in his article in The Tribune 2009, on the occasion of World Mental health day (Mental health care-need to expand the reach, Wig and Srinivasa Murthy 2009).

Prof. Wig's Vision of Mental Health Psychiatry in India by the year 2020 (Wig 1989):

1. To make the benefits of modern psychiatry available to all sections of the population, rich and poor, urban and rural, men and women.
2. To combine both the biomedical and psychosocial approaches in psychiatric practice.
3. To effectively utilise emerging technologies to solve our national problems.
4. To make psychiatry more relevant for Indian cultural needs.
5. To keep a balance between psychiatry and mental health.

Prof. R. Srinivasa Murthy, who moved from PGI in 1982, to NIMHANS, Bangalore, took on a number of responsibilities for the implementation of the NMHP. He received financial support for 5 years, from ICMR, New Delhi, for a Centre for Advanced Research in Community Mental Health (1985–1990). He was part of the team lead by Prof. Mohan Issac, who developed the Bellary District Mental Health Programme (DMHP) (1985–1991), which has formed the model for the development of the over 120 DMHP in the country. Prof. Murthy worked with a number of developing countries to share the Indian experiences and support the mental health programmes in those countries like Yemen, Iran, Pakistan, Bhutan, Afghanistan, Sudan, Somalia and Iraq. He was the chief editor of the historic WHO Report of 2001 on 'Mental Health-New Understanding and New Hope'. Most recently, he has authored the chapter in the Oxford Textbook of Psychiatry (2011) on development of mental health care in LAMI countries (Srinivasa Murthy 2011).

A very important recent initiative of the Department headed by Prof. Savita Malhotra is the 'telepsychiatry' programme. This programme has the great potential to reach the largest numbers of care providers using the modern technology. In this project, funded by the Dept. of Science and Technology, Government of India, the department, in collaboration with the Tata Consultancy Services, has developed a model telepsychiatry application for diagnosis and treatment of psychiatric disorders. This application has been used in over a thousand patients in PGIMER and three peripheral sites in the neighbouring hill states.

Similarly, the new leadership provided by Prof. Ajit Avasthi and Dr. Debhasish Basu in developing deaddiction services in Punjab is in the best traditions of the department of psychiatry. The Punjab Government has approved setting up of five new deaddiction centres in the state. It was decided that all government hospitals at district level and all the health centres at subdivision and block levels would be strengthened by providing training to all the doctors and other supporting staff members in a phased manner. Suggestions to bring reforms in the health set-up in the jails in Punjab were also accepted.

5.10 Personal Reflections of the Last Six Decades (Srinivasa Murthy 2012a, b)

I have been a part of the community psychiatry movement in the country from the 1970s.

I have been a participant of many of the initiatives and witness to other developments. In reviewing the progress, it would be inappropriate to view the wide variety of developments from the current time perspective. Each of the successes and failures have to be placed in their historical perspective-realities, policies, socio-economic factors, personalities, national and international developments. An overview of the community psychiatry developments of the last six decades, presents a picture of a large number of initiatives. These initiatives have been largely the response to a specific need at a specific time period. For example, in the 1950s, the lack of human resources in mental hospitals was addressed by bringing the families to become part of the care programmes. In the 1960s, the availability of the psychopharmacological agents for the treatment of mental disorders and the growing general hospitals, resulted in the setting up of GHPUs. During the 1970s, the growth of the public sector health services, the influence of the Alma Ata declaration guided the development of the community mental health programmes and the formulation of the NMHP in 1982. During the decades of 1980s and 1990s, the need for non-mental hospital facilities for rehabilitation resulted in setting up of a number of community care facilities in different parts of India, mainly by the voluntary organisations. The recognition of the human rights of the mentally ill persons is reflected not only in the improvement of the mental hospitals, but also with revision of the mental health legislation. Each of these initiatives have been started and guided by visionary professionals and have occurred at a particular time period and to address a specific need perception.

One striking aspect is the innovativeness of the professionals and voluntary agencies to address the multiple needs using the available community resources. This has occurred in a number of areas. This, I consider is the strength of Indian mental health movement. The negative side of these developments is the lack of depth in most of the initiatives. Even when the initial results have been very positive (e.g. nurse involvement in community care) the innovations has not received the type of expansion and in depth understanding that should have occurred. The lack of evaluation is seen uniformly in all the programmes, and I have considered the need for this aspect in each of the sections. The other aspect of significance is the largely person-centred specific nature of the initiatives. There has been limited effort to join hands, carry forward to work beyond the initial initiators. A result of all of these factors is the lack of theory building and influencing the policies at the national level. It is important that the next phase of development will address some of these in a focussed manner.

6 Future of Community Psychiatry in India

In the beginning of the chapter, I referred to the story of community mental health is the way India has addressed the key mental health barriers in the country, namely lack of access, affordability, acceptability and stigma of mental disorders. The progress of the last half century has partially addressed these challenges, and much needs to be solved in the coming 50 years.

There are two important areas for future development of community mental health in the country. Firstly, the many areas of community mental health reviewed in the earlier sections need greater attention and increased clarity and depth, especially about evaluation and study of outcomes.

Secondly, there is need to shift focus from delivering services to '**empowerment of the people for mental health**'.

The following are some of the components of this shift from professionals to people. The recent developments in the areas of information technology, mobile connectivity, the explosion of the mass media and the many people movements to address social issues make this the most appropriate approach to take mental health forward in the country. Towards this goal, there are many initiatives that need to be undertaken by the mental health professionals.

Firstly, **we must move from 'madness' to 'mental health'** (the theme of the deliberations) so that we are referring to 'mental health needs of all, rather than few ill persons'. There is no doubt about the changing world that we are living in (technology, social, political, economic, philosophical changes and the breakdown of social institutions etc.). The changing world has implications for mental health, both in terms of increasing demand for mental health services with a wide range of the mental health needs of the community and possibilities for interventions. In a way, mental health has reached from the mental hospitals to psychiatric clinics to the people in the community, somewhat similar to what happened when the shift occurred from mental hospitals to the clinics in the middle of the last century. Our future professional work will have 'people' as the focus of all of our work.

Secondly, **mental health has to be a movement of 'people'**. The persons intervening to address the multiple mental health needs in the community will be not only be the mental health professionals. Today, in India, everyone is doing mental health interventions, whether it is the celebrities on their chat shows, the help lines or the number of voluntary organisations providing 'counselling services'. Currently, most of these initiatives are based on emotional responses and not on sound mental health knowledge and skills. It will take some time for some order to come to these 'quick fix' responses. It is important for mental health professionals to recognise this growing army of 'persons in mental health field'.

Thirdly, **mental health professionals have to take up leadership** of the movement. Professionals have an opportunity to take mental health people to the people riding on the wave of raised awareness and explosion of help giving avenues. Leadership from the professionals would require a sense of openness to share mental health skills, innovation and partnership between professionals and 'people'. Sharing of knowledge cannot be only scientific information but a mixture of information and entertainment (often referred to as infotainment). This embracing of the 'others' in mental health has to be a proactive and planned activity.

Fourthly, there is need for **innovation** in all of our activities. The chief responsibility of the mental health professionals would be to undertake the following activities: (i) continuous review, synthesis and simplification of mental health information to share with the general population; (ii) study of impact of social changes and mental health; (iii) compilation of the social coverage of mental health issues in different parts of the country and in the different forms of mass media; (iv) systematic examination and recording of the mental health professionals' work with the community; and (v) identification of the areas for collaboration between professionals, non-professionals and people.

Fifthly, the **interventions using community resources** have to be a continuous effort and not a one-time activity. We have to create structures and mechanisms for such long-term involvement, interactions and evaluation of people-level interventions.

Sixthly, **networking with other disciplines** to utilise the strengths of the different sectors and disciplines. For example, life skills education initiatives have demonstrated the important role education sector can play towards advancement of mental health of students (Srikala Bharath and Kishore Kumar 2010).

Seventhly, **advocacy for mental health** with the different institutions of the society like the central and state governments, local governments, religious organisation, special population groups and all manner of stakeholders in the society. Our role would be to sensitise and support these groups to mental health issues of the society.

In conclusion, in the last 50 years, there have been many advances that changed the way mental health care is practiced. The building of mental hospitals, the discovery of the pharmacological interventions, the community mental health movement and recognition of the human rights of the mentally ill persons are some of these milestones. We are on the cusp of a similar milestone with the growing importance of information and communication technology (ICT). It is for us mental health professionals to utilise these opportunities for the good of the community. Economically rich countries have addressed the community psychiatry movement from the institutionalised care to community care building on the strengths of their social institutions. India has begun this process more recently and has made significant progress utilising the strengths of the community. There is need to continue the process by widening the scope of the mental health interventions, increasing the involvement of all available community resources and rooting the interventions in the historical, social and cultural roots of India. This is a continuing challenge for professionals and people in the coming years.

References

Agarwaal, S. P., Goel, D. S., Ichhpujani, R. L., Salhan, R. N., & Shrivatsava, S. (2004). *Mental health—An Indian perspective (1946–2003)*. New Delhi: Directorate General of Health Services, Ministry of Health and Family Welfare.

Bhatti, R. S. (1980). Psychiatric family ward treatment I. An appraisal. II. How to select a relative to stay with the patient. *Family Process, 19*, 193–200.

Bhatti, R. S., Janakiramiah, N., Channabasavanna, S. M., & Shobha Devi, R. S. (1980). Descriptive and manifestation of multiple family group interaction. *Indian Journal of Psychiatry, 22*, 51.

Bhatti, R. S., Janakiramiah, N., & Channabasavanna, S. M. (1982). Group interaction as a method of family therapy. *International Journal of Group Therapy, 32*, 103–114.

Bhatti, R. S., & Verghese, M. (1995). Family therapy in India. *Indian Journal of Social Psychiatry, 11*, 30–34.

Carstairs, G. M. (1974). In community action for mental health care. WHO/SEARO/MENT/22.

Carstairs, G. M. (1980). Development of psychiatric care in India. *Bulletin Royal College of Psychiatry*, 146–148.

Chacko, R. (1967). Family participation in the treatment and rehabilitation of the mentally ill. *Indian Journal of Psychiatry, 9*, 328–333.

Chandrashekar, C. R., Issac, M. K., Kapur, R. L., & Parthasarathy, R. (1981). Management of priority mental disorders in the community. *Indian Journal of Psychiatry, 23*, 174–178.

Chatterjee, S., Patel, V., Chatterjee, A., & Weiss, H. A. (2003). Evaluation of a community based rehabilitation model for chronic schizophrenia in India. *British Journal of Psychiatry, 182*, 57–62.

Chatterjee, S., Pillai, A., Jain, S., Cohen, A., & Patel, V. (2009). Outcomes of people with psychotic disorders in a community-based rehabilitation programme in rural India. *British Journal of Psychiatry, 195*, 433–439.

Chavan, B. S., Gupta, N., Arun, P., Sidana, A., & Jadhav, S. (2012). *Community mental health in India*. New Delhi: Jaypee.

Chisholm, D., Sekar, K., Kishore Kumar, K., Saeed, K., James, S., Mubbashar, M., et al. (2000). Integration of mental health care into primary health care: Demonstration cost-outcome study in India and Pakistan. *British Journal of Psychiatry, 176*, 581–588.

Director General of Health Services (DGHS). (1982). National Mental Health Programme for India. New Delhi: Ministry of Health and Family Welfare.

Dreze, J., & Sen, A. (2013). *An uncertain glory: India and its contradictions*. New York: Allan Lane.
Dube, K.C. (1963). Unlocking of wards—an Agra Experiment. *Indian Journal of Psychiatry, 5*, 2–7.
Gautam, S. (1985). Development and evaluation of training programmes for primary mental health care. *Indian Journal of Psychiatry, 27*, 51–62.
Geetha, P. R., Channabasavanna, S. M., & Bhatti, R. S. (1980). The study of efficacy of family ward treatment in hysteria in comparison with the open ward and the out-patient treatment. *Indian Journal of Psychiatry, 22*, 317–323.
Government of India. (2007). *Annual Report of Ministry of Health and Family Welfare, 2006–2007*, New Delhi.
Gururaj, G., & Issac, M. K. (2004). Psychiatric epidemiology in India: Moving beyond numbers. In S. P. Agarwaal, D. S. Goel, R. N. Salhan, R. L. Ichhpujani, S. Shrivatsava (Eds.), *Mental health—An Indian perspective* (1946–2003), (pp. 37–61). New Delhi: Directorate General of Health Services, Ministry of Health and Family Welfare.
Indian Council of Marketing Research. (2009). *Evaluation of the District Mental Health Programme-Final report*, New Delhi.
Indian Council of Medical Research—Department of Science and Technology (ICMR-DST). (1987). *A collaborative study of Severe Mental Morbidity*. New Delhi: ICMR.
Indian Psychiatric Society (IPS). (1964). *First report of the Standing Committee on Public Education in Mental Health*, (pp. 1–22) IPS.
Issac, M. K., Kapur, R. L., Chandrasekar, C. R., Kapur, M., & Parthasarathy, R. (1982). Mental health delivery in rural primary health care—development and evaluation of a pilot training programme. *Indian Journal of Psychiatry, 24*, 131–138.
Issac, M. K., Chandrasekar, C. R., & Srinivasa Murthy, R. (1986). Decentralised training for PHC medical officers of a district—The Bellary approach. In A. Verghese (Ed.), *Continuing medical education*, (Vol. 6). Calcutta: Indian Psychiatric Society.
Issac, M. K., Chandrasekar, C. R., & Srinivasa Murthy, R. (1984). *Manual of mental health care for medical officers*. Bangalore: National Institute of Mental Health and Neurosciences.
Issac, M. K., Chandrasekar, C. R., & Srinivasa Murthy, R. (1994). *Mental health care by primary care doctors*. Bangalore: National Institute of Mental Health and Neurosciences.
James, S., Chisholm, D., Srinivasa Murthy, R., Kishore Kumar, K., Sekar, K., Saeed, K., et al. (2002). Demand for, access to and use of community mental health care: Lessons from a demonstration project in India and Pakistan. *International Journal of Social Psychiatry, 48*, 163–176.
Jadhav, S., & Jain, S. (2009). Pills that swallow policy: Clinical ethnography of a Community Mental Health Program in northern India. *Transcultural Psychiatry, 46*, 60–85.
Kapur, R. L. (2004). The story of community mental health in India. In S. P. Agarwaal, D. S. Goel, R. L. Ichhpujani, R. N. Salhan, S. Shrivatsava (Eds.), *Mental Health—An Indian perspective* (1946–2003) (pp. 92–100). New Delhi: Directorate General of Health Services, Ministry of Health and Family Welfare.
Kohmeyler, W. A., & Fernandes, X. (1963). Psychiatry in India: Family approach in the treatment of mental disorders. *American Journal of Psychiatry, 119*, 1033–1038.
Naik, A. N., Parthasarathy, R., & Issac, M. K. (1996). Families of rural mentally ill and treatment adherence in district mental health programme. *International Journal of Social Psychiatry, 42*, 168–172.
Narayanan, H. S., & Reddy, G. N. N. (1968). Review of treatment in family ward. *Indian Journal of Psychiatry, 14*, 123.
Narayanan, H. S., Embar, P., & Reddy, G. N. N. (1972). Review of treatment in family wards. *Indian Journal of Psychiatry, 14*, 23–25.
Narayanan, H. S. (1977). Experience of group and family therapy in India. *International Journal of Group Psychotherapy, 1*, 517.
National Human Rights Commission. (1999). *Quality assurance in mental health*. New Delhi: NHRC.
National Human Rights Commission (NHRC). (2008). In D. Nagaraja, P. Murthy (Eds.), *Mental health care and human rights*. New Delhi: NHRC-NIMHANS.
Parthasarathy, R., Chandrasekar, C. R., Issac, M. K., & Prema, T. P. (1981). A profile of the follow-up of the rural mentally ill. *Indian Journal of Psychiatry, 23*, 139–141.

Pai, S., & Kapur, R. L. (1982). Impact on treatment intervention on the relationship between the dimensions of clinical psycho-pathology, social dysfunction and burden on families of schizophrenic patients. *Psychological Medicine, 12*, 651–658.

Pai, S., Kapur, R. L., & Roberts, E. J. (1983). Follow up study of schizophrenic patients initially treated with home care. *British Journal of Psychiatry, 143*, 447–450.

Pai, S., & Kapur, R. L. (1983). Evaluation of home care treatment for schizophrenic patients. *Acta Psychiatrica Scandinavica, 67*, 80–88.

Pai, S., Channabasavanna, S. M., Nagarajiah, Pai, S., & Raghuram, R. (1985). Home care for chronic mental illness in Bangalore: An experiment in the prevention of repeated hospitalisation. *British Journal of Psychiatry, 147*, 175–179.

Patel, V., & Thara, R. (Eds.). (2003). Meeting mental health needs in developing countries: NGO innovations in India. New Delhi: Sage (India).

Prahlad, C. (2006). *The future at the bottom of the pyramid—eradicating povertythrough profits*. Wharton Publishing House.

Reddy, G.N.N., Channabasavanna, S.M., & Srinivasa Murthy, R. (1986). Implementation ofNational Mental Health Programme, *NIMHANS Journal,4*, 77–84.

Russell, P. S., John, J. K., & Lakshmanan, J. (1999). Family intervention for intellectually disabled children. Randomised controlled trial. *British Journal of Psychiatry, 174*, 254–258.

Russell, P. S., John, J. K., Lakshmanan, J., Russell, S., & Lakshmidevi, K. M. (2004). Family intervention and acquisition of adaptive behaviour among intellectually disabled children. *Journal of Learning Disabilities, 8*, 383–395.

Sartorius, N., & Harding, T. (1983). The WHO collaborative study on strategies for extending mental health care, I: The genesis of the study. *American Journal of Psychiatry, 140*, 1470–1479.

Selis, S. (2007). Making treatment for bipolar disorder a family affair. http://psychiatrictimes.com/show Article.jhtml?articleId=201001634.

Sharma, S. D. (1986). *Psychiatry in primary care*. Ranchi: Central Institute of Psychiatry.

Sharma, S. (1990) Mental hospitals in India. Director General of Health Services, New Delhi.

Shimazu, K., Shimodera, S., Mino, Y., Nishida, A., Kamimura, N., Sawada, K., et al. (2011). Family psychoeducation for major depression: Randomised controlled trial. *British Journal of Psychiatry, 198*, 385–390.

Srikala Bharath & Kishore Kumar, K.V. (2010). Empowering adolescents with life skills education in schools-school mental health programme: Does it work. *Indian Journal of Psychiatry*, *52*, 344–349.

Srinivasa Murthy, R., Kaur, R., & Wig, N. N. (1978). Mentally ill in a rural community: Some initial experiences in case identification and management. *Indian Journal of Psychiatry, 20*, 143–147.

Srinivasa Murthy, R., & Wig, N. N. (1983). The WHO Collaborative study on strategies for extending mental health care, IV: A training approach to enhancing the availability of mental health manpower in a developing country. *American Journal of Psychiatry*, *140*, 1486–1490.

Srinivasa Murthy, R., Issac, M. K., Chandrasekar, C. R., & Bhide, A. (1987). Manual of mental health for medical officers-Bhopal disaster. New Delhi: Indian Council of Medical Research.

SrinivasaMurthy, R., Chandrasekar, C. R., Nagarajiah, Issac, M. K., Parthasathy, R., & Raghuram, A. (1988). *Manual of mental health care for multi-purpose workers*. Bangalore: National Institute of Mental Health and Neurosciences.

Srinivasa Murthy, R., & Wig, N. N. (1993). Evaluation of the progress in mental health in India since independence. In M. Purnima, K. Gandevia (Eds.), *Mental health in India*, (pp. 387–405). Mumbai: Tata Institute of Social Sciences.

Srinivasa Murthy, R., Kishore Kumar, K. V., Chisholm, D., Thomas, T., Sekar, K., & Chandrasekar, C. R. (2004). Community outreach for untreated schizophrenia in rural India: A follow-up study of symptoms, disability, family burden and costs. *Psychological Medicine, 34*, 1–11.

Srinivasa Murthy, R. (2004a). The National Mental Health Programme: Progress and problems. In S. P. Agarwaal, D. S. Goel, R. L. Ichhpujani, R. N. Salhan, & S. Shrivatsava (Eds.), *Mental health—An Indian perspective (1946–2003)* (pp. 75–91). New Delhi: Directorate General of Health Services, Ministry of Health and Family Welfare.

Srinivasa Murthy, R. (2004b). Mental health research in India. *Indian Journal of Medical Research, 120*, 63–66.

Srinivasa Murthy, R. (Ed.). (2006). *Mental health by the people*. Bangalore: Peoples Action for Mental Health.

Srinivasa Murthy, R. (2007a). Mental health programme in the 11 five year plan. *Indian Journal of Medical Research, 125*, 707–712.

Srinivasa Murthy, R. (2007b). Family and mental health care in India. *Alumni Journal of Christian Medical College, 41*(2), 19–30.

Srinivasa Murthy, R. (2008). Organisation of mental health services—Universal challenge. In Varma, V. K., Gupta, N., Kala, A. K. (Eds.), *Culture, Personality and mental illness: A perspective of traditional societies*, (pp. 414–446). New Delhi: B.I. Publications.

Srinivasa Murthy, R. (2010). Schizophrenia: Epidemiology and community aspects, In P. N. Kulhara, A. Avasthi, S. Grover (Eds.), *Schizophrenia-the Indian scene* (Chap. 4, pp. 57–112). Chandigarh: PGIMER.

Srinivasa Murthy, R. (2011). Mental health services in low and middle income countries, Chapter 39. In G. Thornicroft, G. Szmukler (Eds.), *Oxford textbook of community psychiatry* (pp. 325–336). Oxford: Oxford University Press.

Srinivasa Murthy, R. (2012a). Relevance of community mental health in India. In B. S. Chavan, N. Gupta, P. Arun, A. Sidana, S. Jadhav (Eds.), *Community mental health in India*. New Delhi: Jaypee.

Srinivasa Murthy, R. (2012b). Public mental health education. In Chavan, B. S., Gupta, N., Arun, P., Sidana, A., Jadhav, S. (Eds.) *Community mental health in India*. New Delhi: Jaypee.

Srinivasan, T. N., Thara, R., & Padmavati, R. (2004) Duration of psychosis and treatment outcome in schizophrenia patients untreated for many years. *Australian New Zealand Journal of Psychiatry, 38*, 339–343.

Srinivasan, N. (2008). *We are not alone-family care for persons with mental illness*. Bangalore: Action for Mental Illness (ACMI).

Shankar, R., & Rao, K. (2005). From burden to empowerment: The journey of family caregivers in India. In N. Sartorius, J. Leff, J. J. Lopez-Ibor, M. Maj, A. Okasha (Eds.), *Families and mental disorders* (pp. 259–290). Chichester: Wiley.

Suman, C., Baldev, S., Srinivasa Murthy, R., & Wig, N. N. (1980). Helping chronic schizophrenics and their families in the community—Initial observations. *Indian Journal of Psychiatry, 22*, 97–102.

Thara, R., Padmavati, R., Aynkran, R. A., & John, S. (2008). Community mental health in India: A rethink. *International Journal of Mental Health Systems, 2*, 11.

Thirthahalli, J., Venkatesh, B. K., Kishorekumar, K. A., Arunachala, U., Venkatasubramaniam, G., Subbukrishna, D. K., & Gangadhar, B. N. (2009). Prospective comparison of course of disability in antipsychotic treated and untreated schizophrenia patients. *Acta Psychiatrica Scandinavica, 119*, 209–217.

Thirthahalli, J., Venkatesh, B. K., Naveen, M. N., Venkatasubramaniam, G., Arunachala, U., Kishorekumar, K. A., et al. (2009b). Do antipsychotics limit disability in schizophrenia? A naturalistic comparative study in community. *Indian Journal of Psychiatry, 52*, 37–41.

Thiruvanakarasu, M., & Thiruvanakarasu, P. (2010). Training and national deficit in psychiatrists—A critical analysis. *Indian Journal of Psychiatry, 52*, S83–S88.

Thornicroft, G., Szmukler, G. (2001). *Textbook of community psychiatry*. New York: Oxford.

Thornicroft, G., Szmukler, G., Mueser, K. T., & Drake, R. E. (2011). *Oxford textbook of community mental health*. Oxford: Oxford University Press.

Verghese, A. (1971). Development of families in mental health care. *Journal of Christian Medical Association of India, 46*, 83–87.

Vidya, S. (1973). Presidential address: Challenge of our times. *Indian Journal of Psychiatry, 15*, 1–7.

Wig, N. N. (1978). General hospital psychiatry units: Right time for evaluation. *Indian Journal of Psychiatry, 20*, 1–3.

Wig, N. N., & Srinivasa Murthy, R. (1980). Manual of mental disorders for peripheral health personnel. Chandigarh: Department of Psychiatry, PGIMER (2nd printing 1993).

Wig, N. N., Srinivasa Murthy, R., & Harding, T. W. (1981). A model for rural psychiatric services—Raipur Rani experience. *Indian Journal of Psychiatry, 23*, 275–290.

Wig, N. N., & Parhee, R. (1984). *Manual of mental disorders for primary health care physicians*. New Delhi: Indian Council of Medical Research.

Wig, N. N. (1989). The future of psychiatry in developing countries—The Need For National Programmes of Mental Health. *NIMHANS Journal, 7*(1), 1–11.

Wig, N. N. (1987). Stigma against mental illness (Editorial). *Indian Journal of Psychiatry, 39*(3), 187–189.

Wig, N. N., & Srinivasa Murthy, R. (2009, Oct 10). Mental health care—need to expand its reach, The Tribune.

World Health Organisation. (2001). World Health Report 2001—Mental health—New understanding, New Hope, Geneva.

Chapter 22
Psychiatry in Primary Health Care: Indian Perspectives

V.K. Sharma

1 Introduction

1.1 The Need for Primary Health Care

The Alma-Ata declaration of 1978 (Primary Health Care 1978) affirmed that health, including mental health and social well-being, is a fundamental human right, and primary health care is the key to attain this worldwide goal. The World Health Organization (WHO) in its World Health Report of 2008 stressed the urgent need to strengthen primary health care worldwide. The existing health delivery systems fail to meet the populations' health care needs. People all over the world deserve a health system that is person centred and comprehensive, provides continuity, and is well integrated. A well-planned primary-care health system can meet all these objectives.

1.2 The Need for Integrating Mental Health in Primary Care and General Health Care

Mental health despite being a leading cause of disability worldwide is not well incorporated at the primary-care level even in the most developed countries. Patients with mental illnesses remain under-treated in both low- and high-income countries (Ormel

V.K. Sharma, Professor

V.K. Sharma (✉)
International Health Development, University of Chester, Chester, UK
e-mail: v.sharma@chester.ac.uk

V.K. Sharma
Early Intervention in Psychosis Services, Cheshire and Wirral Partnership NHS Trust, Chester, UK

S. Malhotra and S. Chakrabarti (eds.), *Developments in Psychiatry in India*,
DOI 10.1007/978-81-322-1674-2_22

et al. 2008; Sharma and Copeland 2009). Most people with mental illness seek help from their primary-care doctors and many of them present with physical symptoms. Health professionals in general often fail to recognise mental illnesses, especially when they coexist with physical conditions. It is worth noting that people with physical illness have a raised psychiatric morbidity. A cross-national study (Scott et al. 2009) of the joint effect of mental and physical conditions on disability found that co-morbidity exerts detrimental synergistic effects. It therefore recommended that clinicians need to deal with both mental and physical conditions giving them equal priority, if they are to manage co-morbidity and reduce disability. Overall, about one-third of patients admitted to medical wards also suffer from diagnosable mental illness ranging from acute organic brain syndrome, dementia, depression, anxiety, and psychosis and somatisation disorder to adjustment disorders and alcohol abuse. However, only a few of them undergo a mental health assessment or receive appropriate treatment. This is consistently reported in different parts of the world and among patients of all age groups (Sim et al. 2001; Hansen et al. 2001; Ames and Tuckwell 1994; Ndetei et al 2009). Untreated mental illness leads to longer times spent in the hospital with increased health care costs (Verbosky et al. 1993).

2 Barriers to Recognition and Treatment of Mental Illness in Primary Care

It is important to understand the reasons for poor recognition and treatment of mental disorders in general so that positive steps can be taken at all levels to address this issue effectively. The main barriers occur at three levels. Firstly, patients may find it hard to acknowledge that their problems are mental health related, especially if they are experiencing the problem for the first time (Olsson and Kennedy 2010). Equally, people find it hard to accept they have a mental illness, even if they acknowledge that they suffer from mental health problems. The findings of the National Co-morbidity Survey-Replication of people with common mental disorders in the USA (Mojtabai et al. 2010) concerning patients' perceived barriers to mental health treatment revealed that (a) a low perceived need for treatment was the main reason for not seeking help especially among those who only had mild to moderate problems; (b) the majority of people with more severe disorders reported they wished to handle their problems on their own. About a quarter felt that the problem was not severe enough to seek help or would be likely to recover spontaneously; (c) Over one-third of respondents who dropped out of treatment altogether reported an "attitudinal/evaluative barrier" such as stigma, negative therapeutic experience, or poor quality of treatment.

Secondly, barriers occur at service provider level, mainly due to the primary-care and general health-care service providers' attitudes towards mental illness, their knowledge, training, and experience of dealing generally with mental disorders. A meta-analysis of 36 studies (Cepoiu et al. 2008) of patients in a general hospital ward showed that barriers due to service providers' included their concerns about the ill effects of potential patient stigma, their own time pressures, a belief that making a proper diagnosis of mental illness was burdensome, inadequate knowledge about diagnostic criteria or treatment options, general lack of a psychosocial orientation, and inadequate insight into the different cultural presentations of mental disorders. It could be concluded that general health professionals' inadequate training in mental illness, recognition and management coupled with a lack of available user-friendly clinical facilities for the diagnosis, and treatment of mental disorders in general hospital settings could be an important service barrier.

The third barrier, the most important one occurs at an organisational level due to the State's mental health related policies and those created by local systems. The priorities directed at mental health care are sometimes half-hearted, ranging from public health policy to the resources provided for care, for the "hard to reach" groups (Dowrick et al. 2009). Local system barriers include productivity pressures, limitations of third-party mental health coverage, restrictions on specialists, psychotropics, and psychotherapeutic care, lack of a systematic method for detecting and managing such patients, and inadequate continuity of care.

3 Primary Health Care in India

3.1 Current State

India has a complex system of health-care delivery ranging from largely unregulated indigenous practitioners to highly equipped private hospitals. People have the complete freedom to choose between these services depending on their beliefs, access to services, and their ability to pay for these services. The health delivery system is far from a comprehensive and well integrated one. In that context, the primary-care health service is largely underdeveloped in most parts of the country, and there is no universal health-care coverage for its population as compared to developed countries such as the UK, where primary care is the backbone of its National Health Service.

The 12th Five Year Plan (2012–2017) of the Planning Commission of India highlights the following weaknesses of health-care system:

Inadequate resources and coverage: Health-care services from the public and private sectors put together are quantitatively inadequate. The numbers of doctors is only half, and the numbers of nurses and auxiliaries merely one-fourth of the expected numbers required to provide adequate services. Rural areas are served even worse (Khandelwal et al. 2004).

Variable quality of care: The quality of service provided by qualified as well as many unqualified doctors and other health professionals varies considerably in both the public and private sector. Standards and regulatory systems are not properly defined, and as result the health-care services are poorly regulated.

Lack of affordability: The vast majority of the population is unable to pay the cost of adequate health care, especially in tertiary care. This is largely due to lack of extensive and adequately funded public health services. This results in people having to access private health services at a great personal expense. Even in public sector hospitals, patients may have to pay for their medicines in many places. The families are put through a very high financial burden, especially when affected by a chronic and severe illness. Only a small proportion of the population is covered by health insurance and that too fails to cover outpatients and expenses on medicines.

Future trends of health-care needs: The problems are likely to worsen in future due to several factors e.g. rising life expectancy with increasing long-term medical conditions, increase in public awareness of treatment possibilities leading to rise in demand for quality medical care, increase in lifestyle related diseases such as diabetes and heart conditions with rising prosperity, and an increase in accidents and injuries.

Very low base of public expenditure on health: The public expenditure on health was on only 27 % of overall expenditure on health in 2008–2009. This is very low by any standards.

These enormous challenges have led the commission to formulate a health planning and delivery strategy under the 12th Five Year Plan that may take two or three planning cycles to implement. The new strategy focuses on universal health coverage. Addressing all the key issues, the strategy emphasises on the efficient and effective use of resources, a holistic approach of care delivery, public–private partnerships, and greater integration in health delivery systems. The health planning and delivery strategy also proposes a major role for primary health care in its national health package, i.e. a high quality primary care provided free at the point of delivery.

Good quality primary-care health services are lacking in both rural as well as urban communities in India. The National Rural Health Mission (NRHM), (National Rural Health Mission 2010) a government funded public health system set up subcentres with health workers serving 5–6 villages, primary health centres with doctors (PHCs) for 30–40 villages, and community health centres (CHCs), based on a polyclinic model to serve about 100 villages. In addition private qualified and non-qualified health workers fill the gap to large extent. In urban areas, the lion's share of diagnostic and treatment services is provided by private clinics and hospitals with limited training in primary care (Rao and Mant 2012).

4 Mental Health and Primary Care in India

Public mental health services are traditionally provided by mental health institutions or psychiatric departments of teaching hospitals. In recent years, an increasing number of psychiatrists are working at the level of district hospitals. At the same time, there are increasing numbers of private psychiatric clinics and hospitals, usually based in urban areas, which provide direct care to people with mental illnesses. Rural communities in India still have poor access to mental health services.

The Department of Psychiatry at the Postgraduate Institute of Medical Education and Research (PGIMER), Chandigarh is one of the leading centres in India that has provided vision and leadership in taking mental health to the community and primary-care level (Wig 2001). One of the recognised models is based on the Raipur Rani Project lead by Dr. Murthy and Dr. Wig, based at the psychiatry department of the PGIMER (Murthy and Wig 1983). In this model, primary-care health workers received training in mental health and were supported by a team of psychiatrists from the department, in detecting and treating patients in rural and urban centres, located in a district near the hospital (Ambala). The programme resulted in a large number of patients being recognised and treated for their mental illness in the community.

Murthy in a review of mental health initiatives in India from 1947 to 2010 (Wig 2000) described the progress made in developing community mental health services, especially in recent years (Murthy 2011). The National Mental Health Programme (NMHP) is the main framework to foster integration of mental health services in primary care, through its District Mental Health Programmes (DMHPs). A number of states have taken initiatives in introducing mental health training at the primary-care level through their DMHPs. Recently a primary-care project in Goa (Pereira et al. 2011) found that training lays counsellors in common mental disorders and linking them to primary-care physicians supported by a visiting psychiatrist assisted patients in accessing services for their mental health problems. This also helped in integrating mental health in general health care at the primary-care level.

Rao and Mant (2012) in their recent review of strengthening primary care in India sharing the experience of the National Health Service in the UK recommended that such services are best delivered by a multidisciplinary team of professionals. Multi-skilling (training individuals to perform tasks within their capacity, but beyond their traditional professional roles) allows the available workforce in the team to be deployed most efficiently. Enhancing skills of frontline health workers in diagnosing and treating people with mental illness at primary-care level is important part of this multi-skilling process.

5 The UK Experience

The author has a special interest in mental health service development at the primary-care level. Working within the National Health Service in the UK, he led the Primary Care Mental Health Project in Liverpool to develop a model of integrated mental health service delivery with primary health care.

The Liverpool Primary Care Mental Health Project (Sharma et al. 2000) has demonstrated that a specialist mental health team can work closely with general practice. The model of working appears beneficial for patients as well as for general practitioners. This project has given us an opportunity to examine the process of integrating services between primary and secondary care. The project demonstrated several advantages of integration of mental health with general health in primary care. These included patients attended in their familiar place and were seen by their known practice staff; complete health records were readily available, particularly the information about investigations and treatments they were receiving; any new prescription or change of medication was done straight away; face to face contact with the primary-care doctors (GPs) gave the opportunity to discuss their patients' management in some detail; this contact also has an educational value for GPs, primary health care members, as well as mental health team members; a new and enhanced role of community mental health nurse linked to the general practice assisted in integration of the services and provided continuity of care; the team provided a seamless service by accepting patients of common mental disorders for assessments, yet concentrating on the care of severely mentally ill people; integration of mental health services with primary care helped in reducing the stigma attached to the mental illness.

(Description of models, their principles, efficacy, and their limitations could be added.)

6 Mental Health Delivery Models

Specialist service model: In that mental health services are provided by specialist mental health professionals and teams using a top–down approach. Specialised mental health institutes are centres of excellence for service provision as well as training. They then extend their services to district and village level through mental health workers through mental health clinics. They may raise awareness of mental illness in primary-care teams as well as in public, but retain service provision as their responsibility. This approach appears attractive, as it can easily be managed and monitored. In addition, people with mental illness get treatment from experts in mental health. But the benefits come with serious limitations. This requires huge numbers of trained mental health personnel to serve the whole population that is not possible to recourse in any country. Besides, this keeps mental health to be separate from the mainstream health. In addition, primary-care and general health care professionals get deskilled in identifying and managing mental health problems. Retaining mental health separate also adds to reinforcing stigma attached to mental illness.

Integrated service model: In this model, mental health is a part of overall health provision for the community (Balarajan et al. 2011). The primary-care services become the backbone of identifying and managing mental illness with the support of mental health specialists. The role of specialists becomes supportive to all health professionals especially to primary-care health teams. The primary-care workers are trained in detecting and managing mental illness along with other conditions. This is a preferred service delivery model to meet the population need but not without huge challenges. The barriers include willingness for primary-care workers to learn and apply skills in detecting and managing mental illness as well as commitment from mental health specialists to train, support, and work with primary-care workforce. This model requires a huge shift in the mindset of health professionals as well as policy makers.

7 Can Mental Health Services Be Integrated with Primary Health Care in India?

Recent successful projects of training health-care workers in detecting and managing mental disorders in primary care in different states of India (Pereira et al. 2011; Jayaram et al. 2011; Chisholm et al. 2000; Armstrong et al. 2011) reveals the real scope of such integration. The real challenge is in reaching vast majority of remote rural communities. The size of the mental health problem keeps increasing and new problems keep appearing, e.g. Behere and Behere (2008) have recently reported a raised suicide rate among farmers in India. At the same time, rapid economic and technological development raises opportunities to strengthen the workforce by increasing the number of mental health staff who can take part in training and supporting primary-care health workers.

Malhotra et al. (2013) from PGIMER have suggested an innovative approach of telepsychiatry using modern technology to fill the enormous diagnostic and treatment gap that exists for sufferers of mental disorders in India. The technology could make training and expert advice for primary-care health workers readily available and accessible.

The author (Sharma) has developed a computer-assisted assessment, diagnostic, treatment and training tool—the Global Mental Health Assessment Tool/Primary Care (GMHAT/PC) (Sharma et al. 2004). The GMHAT/PC has been developed to assist general practitioners and other health professionals to carry out a quick, convenient, and comprehensive standardised mental health assessment. It has proved to be a reliable and valid tool based on the number of research studies in primary-care and general health settings (Sharma et al. 2004, 2008, 2010, 2013; Krishna et al. 2009). The GMHAT/PC has now being translated into other European, Asian, and African languages. Further studies (done in India, UAE, and Belgium) have proved that this can be used in different cultures. The average time taken for the interview is around 15 min. Any health professional with training can administer the GMHAT/PC. It gives useful output including diagnosis, ratings of symptoms, and treatment guidelines. Following validation of its Hindi version, studies are underway in Maharashtra and Rajasthan of its use in primary-care and in general health settings. The GMHAT/PC may be a useful addition to other training and diagnostic methods available to frontline workers to diagnose and treat mental disorders in primary care.

8 Future Challenges and Proposed Solutions

There are number of practical challenges in providing integrated mental health services at the primary-care level including the following: (a) an inadequate workforce, specially of dedicated mental health trainers (leaders) and support staff with a mindset for improving community mental health and well-being, (b) the lack of acceptance of such services by the community, especially in the rural areas where people still rely on faith healers, and (c) the willingness for primary-care health workers to learn about mental illness and treat such patients without considering this as an extra burden placed on them. One has to look at all other community resources in achieving this objective; that may include voluntary workers and NGOs. A "fit for purpose" training on mental health for nursing and medical students highlighting the importance that managing mental health problems are everybody's business will certainly help in long run in bringing mental health in mainstream health. Such a programme for medical undergraduates is in progress in Delhi (Sood and Sharan 2011). There is a need for incorporating training in family medicine and mental health in these programmes for doctors. The government should take the responsibility of funding mental health services for all; arrangements should be made with the private sector to allow it to work in concert with public sector to fill the service gap. Generic medications for mental illness should be made available free or at a minimal cost at the primary-care level.

References

Ames, D., & Tuckwell, V. (1994). Psychiatric disorders among elderly patients in a general hospital. *The Medical Journal of Australia, 160*(11), 671–675.

Armstrong, G., Kermode, M., Raja, S., Suja, S., Chandra, P., & Jorm, A. F. (2011). A mental health training program for community health workers in India: Impact on knowledge and attitudes. *International Journal of Mental Health System, 5*(1), 17.

Balarajan, Y., Selvaraj, S., & Subramanian, S. V. (2011). Health care and equity in India. *The Lancet, 377*(9764), 505–515.

Behere, P. B., & Behere, A. P. (2008). Farmers' suicide in Vidarbha region of Maharashtra state: A myth or reality? *Indian Journal of Psychiatry, 50*(2), 124–127.

Cepoiu, M., McCusker, J., Cole, M. G., Sewitch, M., Belzile, E., & Ciampi, A. (2008). Recognition of depression by non-psychiatric physicians—A systematic literature review and meta-analysis. *Journal of General Internal Medicine, 23*(1), 25–36.

Chisholm, D., Sekar, K., Kumar, K. K., Saeed, K., James, S., Mubbashar, M., et al. (2000). Integration of mental health care into primary care. Demonstration cost-outcome study in India and Pakistan. *British Journal of Psychiatry, 176*, 581–588.

Dowrick, C., Gask, L., Edwards, S., Aseem, S., Bower, P., Burroughs, H., et al. (2009). AMP Group. Researching the mental health needs of hard-to-reach groups: Managing multiple sources of evidence. *Health Services Research, 10*(9), 226.

Government of India Planning Commission—Twelfth five year plan. (2012–2017). Social Sectors. http://planningcommission.gov.in/plans/planrel/12thplan/pdf/vol_3.pdf.

Hansen, M. S., Fink, P., Frydenberg, M., Oxhøj, M., Søndergaard, L., & Munk-Jørgensen, P. (2001). Mental disorders among internal medical inpatients: Prevalence, detection, and treatment status. *Journal of Psychosomatic Research, 50*(4), 199–204.

Jayaram, G., Goud, R., & Srinivasan, K. (2011). Overcoming cultural barriers to deliver comprehensive rural community mental health care in Southern India. *Asian Journal of Psychiatr, 4*(4), 261–265.

Khandelwal, S. K., Jhingan, H. P., Ramesh, S., Gupta, R. K., & Srivastava, V. K. (2004). India mental health country profile. *International Review of Psychiatry, 16*(1–2), 126–141.

Krishna, M., Lepping, P., Sharma, V. K., Copeland, J. R., Lockwood, L., & Williams, M. (2009). Epidemiological and clinical use of GMHAT-PC (global mental health assessment tool—primary care) in cardiac patients. *Clinical Practice and Epidemiology in Mental Health, 5*, 7.

Malhotra, S., Chakrabarti, S., & Shah, R. (2013). Telepsychiatry: Promise, potential, and challenges. *Indian Journal of Psychiatry, 55*(1), 3–11.

Mojtabai, R., Olfson, M., Sampson, N. A., Jin, R., Druss, B., Wang, P. S., et al. (2010). Barriers to mental health treatment: Results from the national comorbidity survey replication. *Psychological Medicine, 7*, 1–11.

Murthy, R. S. (2011). Mental health initiatives in India (1947–2010). *National Medical Journal of India, 24*(2), 98–107.

Murthy, R. S., & Wig, N. N. (1983). The WHO collaborative study on strategies for extending mental health care, IV: A training approach to enhancing the availability of mental health manpower in a developing country. *American Journal of Psychiatry, 140*, 1486–1490.

National Rural Health Mission. (2010). Annual review. http://mohfw.nic.in/NRHM.htm.

Ndetei, D. M., Khasakhala, L. I., Kuria, M. W., Mutiso, V. N., Ongecha-Owuor, F. A., & Kokonya, D. A. (2009). The prevalence of mental disorders in adults in different level general medical facilities in Kenya: A cross-sectional study. *Annals of General Psychiatry, 148*, 1–8.

Olsson, D. P., & Kennedy, M. G. (2010). Mental health literacy among young people in a small US town: Recognition of disorders and hypothetical helping responses. *Early Intervention in Psychiatry, 4*(4), 291–298.

Ormel, J., Petukhova, M., Chatterji, S., Aguilar-Gaxiola, S., Alonso, J., Angermeyer, M. C., et al. (2008). Disability and treatment of specific mental and physical disorders across the World. *British Journal of Psychiatry, 192*(5), 368–375.

Pereira, B., Andrew, G., Pednekar, S., Kirkwood, B. R., & Patel, V. (2011). The integration of the treatment for common mental disorders in primary care: Experiences of health care providers in the MANAS trial in Goa, India. *International Journal of Mental Health System, 5*(1), 26.

Primary Health Care. (1978). Report of the International Conference on Primary Health Care, Alma-Ata, USSR. Geneva, World Health Organization. September 6–12, 1978.

Rao, M., & Mant, D. (2012). Strengthening primary healthcare in India: White paper on opportunities for partnership. *BMJ: British Medical Journal, 15*(344), e3151. doi:10.1136/bmj.e3151.

Scott, K. M., Von Korff, M., Alonso, J., Angermeyer, M. C., Bromet, E., Fayyad, J., et al. (2009). Mental-physical co-morbidity and its relationship with disability: Results from the world mental health surveys. *Psychological Medicine, 39*(1), 33–43.

Sharma, B. B., Singh, S., Sharma, V. K., Choudhary, M., Singh, V., Lane, S., et al. (2013). Psychiatric morbidity in chronic respiratory disorders in an Indian service using GMHAT/PC. *General Hospital Psychiatry, 35*(1), 39–44.

Sharma, V. K., & Copeland, J. R. (2009). Detecting mental disorders in primary care. *Mental Health in Family Medicine, 6*(1), 11–13.

Sharma, V. K., Lepping, P., Cummins, A. G., Copeland, J. R., Parhee, R., & Mottram, P. (2004). The global mental health assessment tool—primary care version (GMHAT/PC). Development, reliability and validity. *World Psychiatry, 3*(2), 115–119.

Sharma, V. K., Lepping, P., Krishna, M., Durrani, S., Copeland, J. R., Mottram, P., et al. (2008). Mental health diagnosis by nurses using the Global mental health assessment tool: A validity and feasibility study. *British Journal of General Practice, 58*(551), 411–416.

Sharma, V. K., Jagawat, S., Midha, A., Jain, A., Tambi, A., Mangwani, L. K., et al. (2010). The global mental health assessment tool-validation in Hindi: A validity and feasibility study. *Indian Journal of Psychiatry, 52*(4), 316–319.

Sharma, V. K., Wilkinson, G., Dowrick, C., Church, E., & White, S. (2000). Developing mental health services in a primary care setting: Liverpool primary care mental health project. *International Journal of Social Psychiatry, 47*(4), 16–19.

Sim, K., Rajasoorya, C., Sin Fai Lam, K. N., Chew, L. S., & Chan, Y. H. (2001). High prevalence of psychiatric morbidity in a medical intensive care unit. *Singapore Medical Journal, 42*, 522–525.

Sood, M., & Sharan, P. (2011). A pragmatic approach to integrating mental health in undergraduate training: The AIIMS experience and work in progress. *National Medical Journal of India, 24*(2), 108–110.

Verbosky, L. A., Franco, K. N., & Zrull, J. P. (1993). The relationship between depression and length of stay in the general hospital patient. *Journal of Clinical Psychiatry, 54*(5), 177–181.

Wig, N. N. (2000). WHO and mental health—A view from developing countries. *Bulletin of the World Health Organization, 78*(4), 502–503.

Wig, N. N. (2001). Bringing mental health into the mainstream. *Journal of the Association of Physicians of India, 49*, 405–407.

WHO World Health Report. (2008). Primary health care—now more than ever.

Part VII
Developments in Liaison Psychiatry

Chapter 23
Psycho-oncology: Indian Experiences and Research

S.K. Chaturvedi

1 Introduction: Psycho-oncology—A Specialty of Oncology and Psychiatry

Psycho-oncology is the study of psychiatric and psychosocial aspects of cancer, which may be related to the development, course, or outcome of cancer. Psychiatric oncology as a sub-speciality focuses on a number of issues, which include the role of life events, stress, and other psychological factors in the causation, maintenance, and prognosis of cancer; psychological and emotional reactions to the diagnosis of cancer, its recurrence, metastasis; psychiatric disorders in relation to cancer and its treatment; psychological methods of treatment, and counselling, communicating with cancer patients and their relatives; terminal care and palliative care; study and management of grief and bereavement related to cancer; and staff stress and burnout among professionals treating cancer patients. This chapter discusses some of these aspects.

2 Psychiatric Morbidity in Cancer Patients

The commonest psychiatric disorder observed in cancer patients is depression. Depression was considered as the only emotional response to cancer for a long time. A patient with cancer is expected to have a certain level of psychological distress. Assessing distress has now become routine as the sixth vital sign (Chaturvedi 2012a).

S.K. Chaturvedi, Professor

S.K. Chaturvedi (✉)
Department of Psychiatry, National Institute of Mental Health and Neurosciences, Bangalore 560029, India
e-mail: skchatur@gmail.com

S. Malhotra and S. Chakrabarti (eds.), *Developments in Psychiatry in India*,
DOI 10.1007/978-81-322-1674-2_23

A majority of the studies report a significant level of psychiatric morbidity among patients with cancer. Generally, these studies have found adjustment disorder as the commonest psychiatric syndrome among patients with cancer, with major depression, delirium, and anxiety disorders as the next common diagnoses. Conditions such as personality disorders, psychoses, and substance abuse are comparatively infrequent. In clinical practice, and in epidemiological studies of patients with cancer, depression and anxiety disorders have been noted in 20–60 % of the (Chaturvedi and Uchitomi 2012). In the Indian setting, 38 % of patients with cancer were found to have identifiable DSM-III-R anxiety or depressive disorder (Chaturvedi et al. 1994a, b, c). Recent meta-analytical-pooled prevalence for DSM-defined major depression was about 16.5 % in palliative care, haematological, and oncological settings (Mitchell et al. 2011). The common psychiatric disorders related to cancer are described below.

Adjustment disorders: These are the commonest psychiatric syndrome seen among patients with cancer. A majority of these patients are found to have adjustment disorder mainly with depressed mood, anxious mood, and mixed emotional disturbances. The prevalence of adjustment disorder alone was 15.4 % in palliative care settings and 19.4 % in oncological and haematological settings (Mitchell et al. 2011).

Major depression: Depressive symptoms can be caused by the disease process directly, by the various chemotherapeutic agents used for the treatment of cancer, or as a functional response to the disabilities. Feelings of worthlessness and guilt were found to be powerful discriminants between normal sadness seen in cancer and major depression. Recurrent thoughts of suicide are common in patients with cancer, but morbid intensity of the desire to commit suicide, if present, helps to differentiate major depression from a normal reaction.

A number of risk factors for developing depression in patients with cancer have been identified. These include uncontrolled pain and low performance status. Abnormalities in electrolyte levels (sodium, potassium, and calcium), nutritional deficiencies (vitamin B12 and folate levels), and abnormalities in levels of hormones such as parathyroid and thyroid hormones, ACTH, and cortisol have also been found to increase the risk of developing depression. Other physical states or conditions that raise the risk of depression are cachexia, paraneoplastic syndrome, primary and metastatic brain tumours, vascular vulnerability, and. Parkinsonism. Medications such as corticosteroids, interferon, interleukin-2, vincristine, vinblastine, procarbazine, paclitaxel are common risk factors. Additionally, a history of depression and suicide, and substance abuse contribute to the onset of depression. Finally, social factors such as young age, living alone, recent life events, recent loss of spouse, poor social support, and financial breakdown also have a role to play in the onset of depression among patients with cancer (Chaturvedi and Uchitomi 2012).

Anxiety disorders: Anxiety symptoms are observed as part of depression in patients with cancer. Anxiety can also be a part of the normal stress response, adjustment disorder, or delirium. Patients with cancer become anxious when there is uncertainty and communication with the health-professional has not been appropriate or satisfactory. Other situations, which can make a patient with cancer anxious, are costs of their treatment, the future of their family members, lack of adequate response to cancer treatment, and other unfinished businesses they may have. Effective communication skills and breaking the bad news properly can reduce or minimise much of this anxiety.

Delirium: Delirium can be produced either by cancer directly and its treatment, or because of associated mental disorders and their treatment. The commonly used medications, which produce delirium, are narcotic analgesics such as morphine and methadone, sedatives, hypnotics mainly benzodiazepines, drugs with anti-cholinergic effects, and drugs with psychoactive side effects such as digitalis and anti-hypertensives. Metabolic encephalopathies, organ failure, electrolyte, imbalance, nutritional deficiencies, infection, and hypoxia are some of the related medical disorders causing delirium (Chaturvedi and Uchitomi 2012). Besides delirium, other organic mental syndromes such as dementia are also seen among patients with cancer.

Post-traumatic stress disorders: A number of patients have post-traumatic stress disorder (PTSD) like experiences in relation to discovery of an abnormal growth, which can turn out to be cancer, when the bad news of having developed cancer is broken to them, when they have to be hospitalised, and when they have unpleasant experiences during their treatment. Patients get distressing memories, flashbacks of these unpleasant experiences, panic attacks, and symptoms of hyper-arousal when they have PTSD.

Somatoform disorders and abnormal illness behaviour: Somatoform symptoms and somatisation are noted in patients who have recovered from their cancer, or those who have residual symptoms of the disease. These are in the form of fatigue, tiredness, and pain. These take the form of abnormal illness behaviour and are usually misinterpreted by the patients as signs of the disease coming back, a relapse, or spread of the disease. Presence of a somatoform disorder in cancer can create management problems resulting either in delaying the treatment or over treating psychosomatic symptoms (Chaturvedi and Maguire 1998; Chaturvedi et al. 1993, 2006).

Psychosexual dysfunctions: Sexuality and intimacy are altered following mastectomy. Wellisch et al. (1978) found that approximately 36 % husbands reported that mastectomy had a 'bad' or 'somewhat bad' influence on their sexual relationships. Maguire et al. (1980) found that one year after their wives' mastectomy, 29 % of the husbands reported moderate to severe sexual difficulties.

Anticipatory nausea and vomiting (*as a conditioned response to chemotherapy*): Such conditioned side effects to chemotherapeutic treatment are thought to develop through classical conditioning. These conditioned responses can occur before, during, or after chemotherapy. Anticipatory nausea and vomiting were found to be associated with a higher anxiety level in one study (Ingle et al. 1984). Post-chemotherapy nausea and vomiting are also reliable predictors of such anticipatory side effects.

Miscellaneous disorders: Other psychiatric syndromes worth mentioning are substance abuse-related problems such as alcohol, narcotic, and other drug withdrawal syndromes.

3 Psychiatric Disorders Related to Disease and Treatments

(a) **Effect of the cancer**: Psychiatric symptoms sometimes occur due to the direct effect of the disease process. Psychiatric symptoms are seen in almost all patients with supratentorial tumours and are the presenting symptoms in 25 % of patients. A common presentation of carcinoma of pancreas is depression. Physiologically active tumours of endocrine glands such as the thyroid, pituitary, and the parathyroid can also manifest as psychiatric syndromes. In the advanced stage, cancer can produce psychiatric symptoms by metastasis and other modes as paraneoplastic syndromes (Chaturvedi 2012a, b).

Impact of the diagnosis: Diagnosis of cancer evokes a far greater emotional reaction than diagnosis of any other disease, regardless of mortality rate or treatment modality. The normal reaction can vary from person to person. The intensity and duration of emotional distress and the degree to which it interferes with the patient's life seem to determine whether the emotional response is normal or abnormal. The role of relatives and collusion about disclosure of diagnosis, complicates the picture, and needs cautious handling.

(b) **Morbidity associated with treatment modalities**: Differentiation of psychiatric morbidity related to the cancer as such or from its treatment is rarely clear. Psychiatric morbidity associated with cancer therapies ranges from 18 to 40 %.

Due to surgery: Cancer surgery often generates fear of the procedure and grief over the lost body parts. Mastectomy, which has been studied extensively, causes a negative body image and persistent negative feelings among patients about their bodies. Colostomy, laryngectomy, and hysterectomy are the other surgical treatments studied. Patients who have undergone colostomy have significantly more depression, sexual dysfunctions, and other social problems than patients undergoing bowel resection without colostomy. Depression, anxiety, and disturbances in familial and social relationships have been noted as main problems among patients who have had laryngectomy done (Chaturvedi et al. 1994a, b, c, 1996a, b). In a comparison of pre-operative and post-,operative laryngeal and oral cancers in India, concerns about disease and its treatment significantly reduced following laryngectomy, but the concerns about speech and communication were reported by 76 % of laryngectomees following surgery. These needed the attention of a speech therapist (Chaturvedi et al. 1996a, b, 1999).

Due to radiotherapy: Radiation treatment (RT) is associated with highly unpleasant side effects. These side effects include nausea, vomiting, and increasing fatigue. A prospective study of patients receiving radiotherapy had shown significant psychiatric problems in first three months (Chaturvedi et al. 1996a, b; Chandra et al. 1998a). The unpleasant fatigue usually seen among patients undergoing radiotherapy has a high correlation with psychiatric morbidity. Radiotherapy has also been reported to cause nausea, a peculiar enervating kind of fatigue, poor psychosocial adjustment, and unrealistic expectations about the outcome and non-engagement with the physician. In a prospective study on the levels of anxiety and depression in patients receiving RT in a cancer hospital in India (Chandra et al. 1998a), anxiety and depressive disorders were detected frequently both prior to treatment and later during follow-up. The frequency of anxiety increased significantly after initiating RT, but later reduced during follow-up assessments after a few months.

Due to chemotherapy: In some of the neoplastic disorders such as Wilm's tumour or Hodgkin's disease, chemotherapy produces dramatic improvement. However, most often prolongation of life is achieved at the cost of distressing adverse effects and a negative impact on quality of life (QOL). In fact, the concept of QOL has gained momentum and significance with the developments of newer life saving, but toxic chemotherapeutic agents.

Psychiatric morbidity in advanced cancer: Advanced cancer is associated with increased psychiatric morbidity due to physical symptoms such as pain, nausea, vomiting, and weakness causing emotional distress; fear of death and disfigurement; and disease process or its spread and metastasis.

4 Management of Psychiatric and Psychosocial Problems in Cancer

Psychopharmacological management: There are several reports on the efficacy of antidepressants in depressed patients with major physical disorder and on the usefulness of antidepressants in patients with cancer who suffer from depression. Although the use of antidepressants in patients with cancer has grown, there is still some reluctance to use these medications in these patients (Chaturvedi et al. 1994a, b, c). Selective serotonin reuptake inhibitors (SSRIs), such as citalopram and sertraline, can be the preferred medications while initiating antidepressant treatment, because of their better safety profiles and lower incidence of adverse effects. Mirtazapine, duloxetine, and venlafaxine are also considered especially for patients with cancer pain. Although SSRIs and selective non-adrenergic reuptake inhibitors (SNRIs) have been shown to be effective in treating hot flushes in women with a history of breast cancer, paroxetine (an irreversible inhibitor of CYP2D6) use during tamoxifen treatment is recently reported to be associated with an increased risk of death from breast cancer. Tricyclic antidepressants are usually avoided because of their anti-cholinergic and anti-alpha-adrenergic properties, except for patients with neuropathic cancer pain. Vulnerable and elderly patients should be started at low doses with careful dose escalation and monitored every 1–2 weeks for adverse effects and response (Chaturvedi and Uchitomi 2012).

Psychosocial methods of treatment: The types of psychological interventions used in cancer patients are many and diverse, such as behaviour therapy, cognitive therapy, and supportive psychotherapy. The aims of the psychological interventions are as follows: to reduce anxiety, depression, and other emotional distresses, to improve the psychological adjustment to cancer by imparting a positive attitude, to promote a sense of personal control over cancer and its treatment, to improve the patient's communications with the spouse or other family members, and to encourage the open patients to openly express their emotions expression of emotions. Supportive psychotherapy can be done in individual as well as group settings.

Individual supportive therapy: Here, a one-to-one format helps develop a relationship of trust, so that patient can talk freely. Efforts should be made to reduce denial, but maintain hope. Meaningful activities should be encouraged for as long as possible. Simply listening, understanding, and sometimes just sitting quietly with the patient also prove to be helpful and are described as important components of individual supportive therapy.

Group supportive therapy: Support groups are frequently employed in psychosocial intervention to provide emotional support. Groups of patients with cancer, those who have recovered from cancer and those who have undergone surgery, chemotherapy, or radiotherapy can be very effective in alleviating distress among participants. Spouses or family members also benefit from attending such groups (Chaturvedi 1990a).

Counselling: While counselling a patient with cancer, the therapist should be on the lookout for 'cues' to emotional distress, which are likely to be given out by the patient. The aim is to optimise the therapeutic environment, to enable the patient to disclose his or her distress, and to facilitate emotional expression by patients. Counselling sessions may progress through several levels before becoming effective. At the first level, the patient will give a lot of information about the physical condition, physical symptoms, family or other issues, but not anything about emotions. On reaching the second level, the patient besides giving information about physical aspects may talk about emotional distress, but would not express or show the feelings. The third level would have not only information about physical and psychological aspects, but it would also have the expression of emotional distress. The therapist should attempt to achieve this third level to be effective in his role.

5 Indian Contributions to Psycho-oncology

The research on psycho-oncology in our country has focused on the areas of cancer pain (Chaturvedi 1986a, b, 1989), detection of psychiatric morbidity, QOL measurements, and issues related to communications. Somatisation in cancer has been another area of work.

Coping methods: Though the different coping methods described in Western literature are also noted in Indian patients with some modifications and variations, the common coping methods noted in our studies in Indian settings have been denial, resort into religion, putting it on to fate / or *karma*, and sheer helplessness. Using these mechanisms, however, resolution was noted in less than 40 % of the frequent concerns (Chaturvedi et al. 1996a, b). In the Indian setting, 38–53 % of patients with cancer were found to have identifiable DSM-III-R psychiatric disorder. In a large study including 903 cancer patients attending a hospice, a general hospital and the neurosurgery department of NIMHANS, psychiatric disorders were identified in 48 %, of which 44 % had adjustment disorders, whereas the prevalence of psychiatric disorders in a cancer hospital was 53 % (depressive disorders 22 %, sleep disorders 15 %, adjustment disorders 9 %, mixed anxiety and depression 6 %, and anxiety disorders in 1 %) (Chaturvedi et al. 1994a, b, c; Chaturvedi 2012a, b). The substitution of physical symptoms to diagnose depression in medical disorders needs to be considered (Chaturvedi 1990b).

The coping and concerns checklist developed in the Cancer Research Campaign's Cancer Research Centre and adapted for use in India which helps in detecting common physical and psychosocial problems among patients with cancer. In the NIMHANS study, 90 % of the patients' cancer had at least one concern, of which 44 % had 1–3 concerns and 46 % had 4 or more concerns (Chaturvedi et al. 1994a, b, c, 1996a, b).

Detection: For rapid assessment of psychiatric morbidity in cancer patients, the Hospital Anxiety and Depression Scale (HADS) has been adapted to screen Indian patients with cancer. The cut-off score of 7 on the anxiety subscale gives a sensitivity of 87 % and specificity of 79 %; for the depression subscale the cut-off score of 8 gives a sensitivity of 75 % and specificity of 76 %. If one uses the total scale scores, the cut-off of sixteen gives a sensitivity of 85 % and a specificity of 88 % (Chaturvedi et al. 1994a, b, c, 1996a, b). The HADS scale, though simple and convenient, has problems for use among Asian populations and with its factor structures (Chaturvedi 1990a, 1991a). In a prospective study on levels of anxiety and depression in patients receiving RT in a cancer hospital in India (Chaturvedi et al. 1996a, b), anxiety and depressive disorders were detected frequently, both prior to treatment and later during follow-up. The frequency of anxiety disorders increased significantly after initiating RT, but later reduced during follow-up assessments after a few months. Similarly, subjective well-being changed as the RT progressed (Chandra et al. 1998a).

Somatisation in cancer: Expecting functional or nonorganic symptoms in an established medical disease is not easily accepted by health professionals. In a study conducted during my Commonwealth Fellowship at Christie Hospital and Cancer Research Campaign, Manchester, common somatic complaints in a study were sensory symptoms (30 %), tiredness or exhaustion (30 %), multiple symptoms (27 %), weakness (22 %), reduced energy (19 %), pain (19 %), and fatigue or lethargy (17 %). In this group, depressive disorders were diagnosed in 53 %, anxiety disorders in 12 %, and atypical somatoform disorders in 27 % of the patients with cancer; somatic concern and preoccupation were noted in 40 %. During follow-up, somatisers with depression showed clinical improvement, whereas those with atypical somatoform disorder showed no improvement or deteriorated (Chaturvedi et al. 1993, 1998, 2006).

Communication related: Communicating with cancer patients is very challenging, especially in our culture. In one of our studies (Chandra et al. 1998), it was surprising to note that, even in patients attending a cancer hospital for treatment, the awareness about diagnosis was noted in 54 %, whereas 46 % were unaware that they had cancer, though they were regularly coming for treatment and were aware about the name of the cancer hospital.

Breaking the bad news is a skill, which most doctors and nurses are not trained in, and this is an integral part of cancer care. Psychiatrists are called upon to train cancer specialists in skills of breaking the bad news (Chaturvedi and Chandra 2010; Chaturvedi et al. 2008).

Family members urge the doctor not to discuss diagnosis with the patients, due to fear of upsetting the patient, while the patient who is aware of the diagnosis does not want this to be shared with the family members due to a similar fear (Chaturvedi et al. 2009). Dealing with collusion and breaking collusion sensitively is important to maintain trust and communication between patient and family members without the conspiracy of silence. Handling difficult questions like, “What will happen in future, will one become alright, How long will one live, Why me?” and talking about death and dying (Chandra et al. 1999; Chaturvedi and Chandra 2010; Chaturvedi et al. 2008) also requires a great degree of skill.

It has been reported that antidepressants are grossly underused in cancer patients for fear of addiction or dependence, and the fear of adverse side effects and drug interactions (Chaturvedi et al. 1994a, b, c). Another reason for this underuse is the frequently held, but mistaken belief that depression among patients with cancer is a natural reaction and will disappear with time, without the need for antidepressants (Chaturvedi and Chandra 1996).

Quality of life and cancer: QOL has emerged as the most important outcome factor in cancer care and palliative care (Chaturvedi 1994, 1998). In a study on what is important for QOL among Indian patients with cancer, it was noted that satisfaction with functioning, rather than the level of functioning, was more important. Further, peace of mind, spiritual satisfaction, and social satisfactions were considered to be very important by nearly two-thirds of the subjects. Individual's functioning and level of physical and psychological health were given much less significance. Level of satisfaction was valued much higher than the level of functioning (Chaturvedi 1991b).

Due to non-availability of a satisfactory measure of QOL for patients with cancer in India, the relationship between number of concerns and QOL was explored, and it was noted that the number of concerns was a clear indication of poorer QOL. The finding that the number of key concerns indicates the QOL was replicated. Patients with cancer in a general hospital had 2.6 concerns, whereas those in a hospice had an average of 4.7 concerns. QOL was poorest among the hospice patients as expected. On the positive side, QOL improved following interventions (Chaturvedi 2012a, b). QOL studies show relatively better QOL for patients with brain tumours (Chaturvedi et al. 2000a; Pathak et al. 2000), despite appreciable psychiatric morbidity (Chaturvedi et al. 2000; Sharma et al. 2000), and difficulties faced by their caregivers (Jacob and Chaturvedi 2000).

Ethical aspects: Psychosocial care of patients with cancer is full of ethical dilemmas for professionals, including communication issues such as disclosing the diagnosis to patients or their relatives (Chaturvedi 2008). This invariably leads to collusion, a conspiracy of silence and an atmosphere of mistrust in the family (Chaturvedi et al. 2009). Another issue in a financially impoverished family is to decide whether to spend hard earned money on the family or invest on expensive cancer care. Decision-making and making choices can be very stressful for all. The role of traditional healers and complementary and alternative medicine providers, qualified and unqualified, is another issue in our country, where such traditional methods are relatively inexpensive and accepted by the public and popular press (Chaturvedi and Chandra 1998). Ethical dilemmas are also common in dealing with requests for euthanasia, caring for the dying person, answering questions about death and dying, and about how to provide spiritual care (Chandra et al. 1999; Chaturvedi 2007; Chaturvedi et al. 2008; Kandaswamy et al. 2011).

A number of important studies on psychological aspects of cancer have been conducted at the Department of Psychiatry of the Postgraduate Institute of Medical Education and Research (PGIMER), Chandigarh. These have been very informative. These studies have focused on cervical cancer (Kulhara et al. 1988; Sharma et al. 2003), haematological malignancies (Kulhara et al. 1990, 1998), breast cancer (Mattoo et al. 1985a, b), and children suffering from leukaemias (Rao et al. 1992; Sharan 1995, 1999a, b).

6 Current and Future Prospects of Development of the Area in India

Thus, in India, psycho-oncology has made some advances in the understanding of psychiatric disturbances and care of patients with cancer. The role of psychopharmacological and psychological intervention in increasing survival of patients with cancer, or influencing the outcome among such patients, is far from convincing from the point of view of the oncologists. Research on psychiatric oncology is gradually overcoming the methodological deficiencies, and hopefully, the coming years would yield results acceptable to the scientific community. Psychiatric oncology relevant to Indian conditions has been described in some of the recent publications (Chaturvedi 2012a, b; Chaturvedi and Venkateswaran 2008).

For the future, predictors of treatment response among cancer patients to psychiatric intervention will be of clinical significance. Research in psycho-oncology is an exciting area despite numerous challenges and the principles are as applicable for consultation liaison psychiatry. India does not have an active society or a group of psychiatrists or mental health professionals who could form an association. Most cancer centres still do not have a full-time psychiatrist or a psychologist. Some do have social workers. Nevertheless, research would continue in the area of psycho-oncology. It would, however, be a challenge to educate the medical, surgical, and radiation oncologists about this field.

References

Chandra, P. S., Akhileswaran, R., Chaturvedi, S. K., & Shinde, U. (1999). *Caring at home: frequently asked questions by persons with advanced cancers and their caregivers*. Bangalore: BHT Center for Palliative Care Education.

Chandra, P. S., Chaturvedi, S. K., Channabasavanna, S. M., Reddy, B. K. M., & Anantha, N. (1998a). Awareness of diagnosis and psychiatric morbidity among cancer patients—A study from South India. *Journal of Psychosomatic Research, 45*, 257–262.

Chandra, P. S., Chaturvedi, S. K., Channabasavanna, S. M., Reddy, B. K. M., Anantha, N., & Sharma, S. (1998b). Psychological well being in patients receiving radiotherapy—A prospective study. *Quality of Life Research, 7*, 495–500.

Chaturvedi, S. K. (1986a). Psychiatric aspects of chronic pain in cancer patients. *Indian Journal of Pain, 1*, 42–45.

Chaturvedi, S. K. (1986b). Coping with cancer pain. *Acta Psychiatrica Scandinavica, 74*, 112.

Chaturvedi, S. K. (1989). Pain relief in active patients with cancer. *British Medical Journal, 298*, 461.

Chaturvedi SK (1990) Psychosocial intervention and survival of breast cancer patients. Lancet, ii, 1209.

Chaturvedi, S. K. (1990b). Asian patients and the HAD scales. *British Journal of Psychiatry, 156*, 133.

Chaturvedi, S. K. (1990c). Substituting non-somatic symptoms for somatic symptoms (for diagnosing depression in cancer). *American Journal of Psychiatry, 147*, 958.

Chaturvedi, S. K. (1991a). What quality of Life means for Indians—in relation to cancer. *Social Science and Medicine, 33*, 91–99.

Chaturvedi, S. K. (1991b). Clinical irrelevance of HADS factor structure (for use in cancer patients). *British Journal of Psychiatry, 159*, 298.

Chaturvedi, S. K. (1994). Exploration of concerns and the role of psychosocial intervention in palliative care. *Annals of Medicine, Singapore, 23*, 756–760.

Chaturvedi, S. K. (1998). Quality of life in advanced cancer: Psychosocial aspects. *Indian Journal of Palliative Care, 4*(2), 17–23.

Chaturvedi, S. K. (2007). Spirituality issues at end of life. *Indian Journal of Palliative Care, 13*, 48–52.

Chaturvedi, S. K. (2008). Ethical dilemmas in palliative care in a traditional developing society, with special reference to Indian setting. *Journal of Medical Ethics, 34*, 611–615.

Chaturvedi, S. K. (2012). Psychiatric oncology-cancer in mind. *Indian Journal of Psychiatry, 54*, 111–118.

Chaturvedi S. K. (2012a) Distress and depression in cancer. *Journal of Health and Human Behaviour*, 58–64.

Chaturvedi, S. K., & Chandra, P. (1996). Rationale of psychotropic medications in palliative care. *Progress in Palliative Care, 4*, 39–44.

Chaturvedi, S. K., & Chandra, P. (1998). Palliative care in India. *Supportive Care in Cancer, 6*, 81–84.

Chaturvedi, S. K., & Chandra, P. S. (2010). Breaking bad news—issues critical for psychiatrists. medical education corner. *Asian Journal of Psychiatry, 3*, 87–89.

Chaturvedi, S. K., Chandra, P., & Channabasavanna, S. M. (1994a). Detection of anxiety and depression in cancer patients. *NIMHANS Journal, 12*, 141–144.

Chaturvedi, S. K., Chandra, P., Channabasavanna, S. M., Reddy, B. K. M., Anantha, N., & Sharma, S. (1996a). Levels of anxiety and depression in patients receiving radiotherapy. *Psycho Oncology, 5*, 343–346.

Chaturvedi, S. K., Chandra, P., Shenoy, A., & Premalatha, B. S. (1999). Assessment of quality of life of oral cancer patients. In A. K. Varma (Ed.), *Oral oncology* (pp. 509–512). New Delhi: MacMillan India Ltd.

Chaturvedi, S. K., Chandra, P. S., & Simha, S. (2008). *Communication skills in palliative care*. New Delhi: Voluntary Health Association of India.

Chaturvedi, S. K., Gandhi, A., Lopes, C., Chandramouli, B. A., & Sastry, K. V. R. (2000a). Psychiatric psychosocial problems in neurosurgical patients with specific reference to brain tumors. *NIMHANS Journal, 18*(3,4), 165–176.

Chaturvedi, S. K., Hopwood, P., & Maguire, G. P. (1993). Somatisation in cancer patients. *European Journal of Cancer, 29*(7), 1006–1008.

Chaturvedi, S. K., Hopwood, P., & Maguire, G. P. (1994b). Antidepressant medications in cancer patients. *Psycho Oncology, 3*, 57–60.

Chaturvedi, S. K., Loiselle, C. G., & Chandra, P. S. (2009). Communication with relatives and collusion in palliative care—A cross cultural perspective. *Indian Journal of Palliative Care, 15*, 2–9.

Chaturvedi, S. K., & Maguire, P. (1998). Persistent somatization in cancer: A follow up study. *Journal of Psychosomatic Research, 45*, 249–256.

Chaturvedi, S. K., Maguire, P., & Somashekhar, B. S. (2006). Somatization in cancer. *International Review of Psychiatry, 18*(1), 49–54.

Chaturvedi, S. K., Prasad, K. M. R., Senthilnathan, S. M., Shenoy, A., & Premkumari, B. S. (1994c). Quality of life of oral cancer patients. *Oral cancer: therapy IIIB* (pp. 528–531). New Delhi: MacMillan India Ltd.

Chaturvedi, S. K., Sastry, K. V. R., Chandra, P. S., & Chandramouli, B. A. (2000b). Quality of life of patients with brain tumours: Observations of the pilot study. *NIMHANS Journal, 18*(3,4), 191–196.

Chaturvedi, S. K., Shenoy, A., Prasad, K. M. R., Senthilnathan, S. M., & Premakumari, B. S. (1996b). Concerns, coping and quality of life in head and neck cancer patients. *Supportive Care in Cancer, 4*, 32–36.

Chaturvedi, S. K., & Uchitomi, Y. (2012). Psychosocial and psychiatric disorders. In L. Grassi & M. Riba (Eds.), *Clinical psycho oncology*. New York: Wiley Publications.

Chaturvedi, S. K., & Venkateswaran, C. (2008). New research in psycho oncology. *Current Opinion in Psychiatry, 21*(3), 306–310.

Ingle, R. J., Burish, T. G., & Wallston, K. A. (1984). Conditionability of cancer chemotherapy patient. *Oncology Nursing Forum, 11*, 97–102.

Jacob, A., & Chaturvedi, S. K. (2000). Caregivers of neurotumor patients. *NIMHANS Journal, 18*(3,4), 239–245.

Kandasamy, A., Chaturvedi, S. K., & Desai, G. (2011). Spirituality, distress, depression, anxiety and quality of life in patients with advanced cancer. *Indian Journal of Cancer, 48*, 55–59.

Kulhara, P., Ayyagiri, S., & Nehra, R. (1988). Psychological aspects of cancer cervix. *Indian Journal of Psychological Medicine, 11*, 79–83.

Kulhara, P., Marwaha, R., Das, K., & Aga, V. M. (1998). Burden of care in parents of children suffering from hematological malignancies. *Indian Journal of Psychiatry, 40*, 13–20.

Kulhara, P., Verma, S. C., Bambery, P., & Nehra, R. (1990). Psychological aspects of hematological malignancies. *Indian Journal of Psychiatry, 32*, 279–284.

Maguire, G. P., Lee, E. G., & Bevington, D. J. (1980). Psychiatric problems in the first year after mastectomy. *British Medical Journal, 1*, 963–965.

Mattoo, S. K., Varma, V. K., & Bose, S. M. (1985a). Psychosocial adjustment to breast cancer: Pre-operative assessment. *PGI Bulletin, 17*, 121–125.

Mattoo, S. K., Varma, V. K., & Bose, S. M. (1985b). Psychosocial adjustment to breast cancer: Post operative assessment. *PGI Bulletin, 19*, 19–24.

Mitchell, A. J., Chan, M., Bhatti, H., Halton, M., Grassi, L., Johansen, C., et al. (2011). Prevalence of depression, anxiety, and adjustment disorder in oncological, haematological, and palliative-care settings: a meta-analysis of 94 interview-based studies. *Lancet Oncology, 12*, 160–174.

Pathak, M., Sharma, M. P., Chaturvedi, S. K., & Sastry, K. V. R. (2000). Quality of life in brain tumours. *NIMHANS Journal, 18*(3,4), 197–204.

Rao, G. P., Malhotra, S., & Marwaha, R. K. (1992). Psychosocial study of leukemic children and their parents. *Indian Journal of Pediatrics, 29*(8), 985–990.

Sharan, P., Mehta, M., & Choudhry, V. P. (1995). Coping and adaptation in parents of children suffering from acute lymphoblastic leukemia. *Indian Journal of Pediatrics, 62*(6), 737–741.

Sharan, P., Mehta, M., & Choudhry, V. P. (1999a). Psychiatric morbidity in children suffering from acute lymphoblastic leukemia. *Pediatric Hematological Oncology, 16*(1), 49–54.

Sharan, P., Mehta, M., & Choudhry, V. P. (1999b). Psychiatric disorders among parents of children suffering from acute lymphoblastic leukemia. *Pediatric Hematological Oncology, 16*(1), 43–47.

Sharma, Y., Mattoo, S. K., Kulhara, P., Sharma, S. C., & Sharan, P. (2003). Stress and coping in women with cervical and breast cancer in India. *German Journal of Psychiatry, 2*, 40–48.

Sharma, M. P., Pathak, M., Chaturvedi, S. K., & Sastry, K. V. R. (2000). Symptom distress in patients with brain tumors. *NIMHANS Journal, 18*(3,4), 177–186.

Wellisch, D. K., Jamison, K. R., & Pashau, R. O. (1978). Psychological aspects of mastectomy: II. The man's perspective. *American Journal of Psychiatry, 135*, 543–546.

Chapter 24
Delirium Research: Contribution from India

S. Grover and N. Kate

1 Introduction

Delirium is a complex neuropsychiatric syndrome characterized by disturbances of consciousness, attention, cognition, perception, emotions, sleep, and psychomotor activity. It develops acutely or subacutely and fluctuates through its course. It usually lasts from few days to as long as few months, but typically resolves in 10–12 days (American Psychiatric Association 1999). Delirium has also been shown to be independently associated with significant increases in the length of hospital stay, inpatient mortality, long-term mortality, cognitive decline, requirement for institutional care, functional decline, health-care costs, and distress to the patient and family (Trzepacz and Meagher 2005; Siddiqi et al. 2006; Inouye et al. 1998; McCusker et al. 2002; Tennen et al. 2009; Grover and Shah 2011; Grover et al. 2012c). Taking all these facts into consideration, it is very important to identify and manage delirium as early as possible to improve the morbidity and mortality and reduce the associated distress in patients and caregivers.

Although studies from the West have addressed delirium for quite some time, most of the studies from India have come over the last decade.

In contrast to the studies from the West, which have focussed on delirium mainly in the elderly, those admitted to Intensive Care Unit (ICU), or those suffering from terminal illnesses, studies from India have evaluated patients of delirium who are mostly young and seen in the consultation liaison psychiatry services. However, some of the studies have also evaluated patients admitted into various intensive care settings and

---

S. Grover, Assistant Professor; N. Kate, Formerly Senior Resident

---

S. Grover (✉) · N. Kate
Department of Psychiatry, Postgraduate Institute of Medical Education and Research, Chandigarh, India
e-mail: drsandeepg2002@yahoo.com

S. Malhotra and S. Chakrabarti (eds.), *Developments in Psychiatry in India*,
DOI 10.1007/978-81-322-1674-2_24

have evaluated delirium in children and adolescents. In this chapter, the global literature on delirium, as well as research data emerging from India, is reviewed.

2 Epidemiology of Delirium

Many studies from West have evaluated the incidence and prevalence of delirium in different settings. Folstein et al. (1991) using the DSM-III criteria reported a prevalence rate of 0.4 % in community sample aged more than 55 years. With regard to incidence and prevalence of delirium in hospitalized patients, in a review of mostly prospective studies, Fann (2000) reported that incidence of delirium ranged from 3 to 42 %, and the prevalence ranged from 5 to 44 % in hospitalized patients. However, the incidence and prevalence rate figures are much higher in patients admitted to ICU (Ely et al. 2001a, b, c, 2004a, b; Bergeron et al. 2001; Kishi et al. 1995). Some of the recent studies, which have evaluated the prevalence of delirium throughout the period of hospital stay, especially in severely ill patients, have reported the prevalence of delirium to be as high as 82 % (Ely et al. 2004a, b). Overall, it is said that 50–80 % of ventilated patients develop delirium and 20–50 % of subjects with less severe physical problems develop delirium during the ICU stay. Further, delirium persists in 10 % of subjects at discharge (Ely et al. 2001a, b, c, 2004a, b; Bergeron et al. 2001; Kishi et al. 1995). Onset of ICU delirium occurs commonly on 2 ± 1.7 days after being admitted to ICU and commonly lasts 4.2 ± 1.7 days (Ely et al. 2001a, b, c; McNicoll et al. 2003).

With regard to epidemiology of delirium in India, Chaudhury et al. (1991) reported an incidence of 4.3 % in a 1-year prospective study of post-cataract surgery patients. Two studies from different centers have evaluated prevalence rate of delirium in patients aged more than 65 years admitted to medical wards and have reported 27–27.42 % prevalence rate of delirium (Khurana et al. 2002, 2011). In their study, Khurana et al. (2002) reported that 19 % (70 % of total found to have delirium) of patients had delirium at first assessment done within 24 h of admission and 8 % developed delirium more than 24 h after admission. In the other study, evaluating the elderly patients, 85.5 % of patients were found to have delirium at admission, while the remaining 14.5 % developed it after hospitalization (Khurana et al. 2011). Sood et al. (2006) reported delirium in 3 % of 528 inpatients aged more than 65 years. A study from PGIMER, Chandigarh, which reviewed psychiatric referrals received over a 6-year period from different wards of a multi-specialty hospital, reported 1,050 out of the 3,092 cases as having delirium; each year delirium constituted the single largest diagnostic category accounting for 30.77–38.95 % for all ages and 48.72 % for those aged more than 60 years (Grover et al. 2009b). Another study reported 21 % (17/81) cases of hip fracture developing delirium in postoperative period (Chrispal et al. 2010).

Studies have also evaluated the incidence and prevalence of delirium in various ICUs. A study from PGIMER, Chandigarh, which evaluated patients admitted to the respiratory ICU, reported a prevalence rate of 53.57 % and the incidence rate to be 24.41 %. However, the prevalence rate of delirium was higher (64 %) in mechanically ventilated patients (Sharma et al. 2012). When the prevalence of delirium was assessed according to the age of the patients, the prevalence rate in those less than 65 years of age was 44.82 %, while 95.83 % of those more than 65 years of age had delirium (Sharma et al. 2012). Another study from the same center evaluated the epidemiology of delirium in patients admitted to coronary care unit (CCU) and reported a prevalence rate of 26.21 % and an incidence rate of 9.27 % for delirium (Lahariya et al. 2014).

Thus, it can be concluded that the epidemiology of delirium in India is similar to that reported from the West.

3 Etiology and Risk Factors Associated with Delirium

In general, there is some overlap in the risk factors and etiological factors associated with delirium. According to the literature, these have been described together or separately.

Researchers have divided the risk factors for delirium into predisposing and precipitating factors. Predisposing factors are conceptualized as those that are present in the individual at the time of admission and reflect the underlying vulnerability to delirium. Precipitating factors are those noxious insults or hospital-related factors that contribute to the development of delirium. Studies have shown that the predisposing risk factors tend to have a relatively greater contribution to the development of delirium than for the precipitating factors. The various predisposing factors discussed in the literature include the visual impairment, poorer functional ability, older age, male gender, severity of illness, comorbid illnesses, alcohol abuse, and use of medications (prescribed or non-prescribed). The various precipitating factors include malnutrition, any iatrogenic event during hospitalization, physical restraints or bladder catheter, more than three newly prescribed medications, high number of procedures during early hospitalization (X-rays, blood tests, etc.), intensive care treatment, prolonged waiting time before surgery, type and duration of operation, type of anesthetic, intra-operative blood loss, postoperative pain and problems in pain management, infection and use of drugs with a high anticholinergic activity, opiates, benzodiazepines, and corticosteroids (Mattoo et al. 2010). Among the various risk factors, certain risk factors such as increased age, preexisting cognitive impairment, severe coexisting illnesses, and exposure to medication are considered as robust risk factors (Mattoo et al. 2010). Few studies from India have also looked at the risk factors associated with development of delirium. A study with 100 general medical ward geriatric inpatients identified preexisting cognitive deficits, neurological illnesses, urinary tract infections, visual impairment, hearing impairment, current pneumonia, leukocytosis, raised blood ammonia, hyponatremia, and hypo-/hyperkalemia as important risk factors for development of delirium (Khurana et al. 2002). Another study identified various predisposing factors for development of delirium during the postoperative phase in patients with hip fracture as the presence of underlying dementia, longer duration of surgery (>2.5 h), and use of preoperative packed cell volume; and various precipitating causes such as postoperative infections, metabolic abnormalities, and vascular events (Chrispal et al. 2010).

Studies from the West have specifically looked at the factors associated with development of delirium in patients undergoing cardiac surgery. A recent review looked at the data for risk factors leading to development of delirium in patients undergoing cardiac surgery and identified 27 risk factors—12 predisposing and 15 precipitating factors for delirium after cardiac surgery (Koster et al. 2011). The predisposing risk factors that were related to development of delirium were atrial fibrillation, cognitive impairment, ongoing episode of depression, history of stroke, older age, peripheral vascular disease, presence of diabetes mellitus, elevated Euroscore, and preoperative cardiogenic shock. Of these, atrial fibrillation and depression are factors that can be modified in some way. The precipitating risk factors that were identified included red blood cell transfusion, an abnormal albumin level, low cardiac output and the use of an intra-aortic balloon pump (IABP) or inotropic medication, acute infection, electrolyte imbalance, hemocrit less that 30 %, intra-operative hemofiltration, longer duration of cardiac bypass surgery, operating time >3 h, low cardiac output after surgery, subjective memory complaints, postoperative cardiogenic shock, prolonged ionotropic support (>12 h), and urgent operation. Recent studies evaluating the patients admitted to CCU or cardiothoracic unit have also alluded to the role of hemodynamic instability and impaired cardiac output, electrolyte abnormalities, frequent occult infections, high serum cortisol level, number of comorbidities, history of delirium, alcohol use, and type of surgery (Mu et al. 2010; Koster et al. 2013).

One study from India evaluated the risk factors associated with delirium in patients admitted to CCU (Lahariya et al. 2014). In the multivariate analysis, the risk of development of delirium was found to be highest with hypokalemia (highest odds ratio) and this was followed by sequential organ failure assessment (SOFA) score. Other risk factors for which odds ratio was more than 10 included presence of cognitive deficits, receiving more than 3 medications, sepsis, and hyponatremia. The variables with odds ratio between 6 and 10 included presence of cardiogenic shock, having undergone coronary artery bypass grafting, left ventricular ejection fraction <30, and currently receiving opioids. Other variables with odds ratio of more than one included age more than 65 years, presence of diabetes mellitus, presence of uncontrolled diabetes mellitus, history of seizures, presence of congestive cardiac failure, having undergone angioplasty, presence of atrial fibrillation, ongoing depression, currently receiving/taking benzodiazepines, warfarin, ranitidine, steroids, nonsteroidal anti-inflammatory drugs, higher total number of medications, presence of raised creatinine, anemia, hypoglycemia, high acute physiology and chronic health evaluation-II (APACHE-II) score, and high Charlton score (Lahariya et al. 2014).

Other studies from India, especially PGIMER, Chandigarh, have evaluated the etiological factors associated with delirium, using self-designed checklists or the Delirium Etiology Checklist. Irrespective of the assessment instrument and treatment setting (i.e., consultation–liaison services or ICU), studies suggest that development of delirium is most commonly associated with metabolic and endocrine disturbances and the mean number of etiologies associated with delirium vary from 3 to 5.39. The other commonly associated etiologies include sepsis, organ insufficiency, substance withdrawal, and postoperative stage (Sharma et al. 2012; Aarya et al. 2013; Jain et al. 2011; Mattoo et al. 2012; Grover et al. 2013a). A study from another center reported sepsis to be the most common etiology followed by metabolic abnormalities (Khurana et al. 2011).

4 Symptom Profile of Delirium

The symptoms of delirium include a constellation of physical, biological, and psychological disturbances. Many studies have looked at the symptom profile of delirium. However, one of the major limitations of studying phenomenology was lack of instruments covering the broad range of symptoms of delirium till recently. In recent times, Delirium Rating Scale-Revised-98 version has emerged as one of the standard instrument for assessment of symptom profile of delirium. Further, another limitation of study of phenomenology of delirium has been the fact that in many studies, the diagnosis of delirium is based on screening instruments which can be useful in making a diagnosis of delirium in the hands of non-psychiatrists, but many of these are not sufficient to study the phenomenology of delirium. To further characterize the symptoms of delirium, many studies have used factor analysis to study the symptom clusters of delirium, whereas other studies have tried to assess the relationship of cognitive and non-cognitive symptoms of delirium.

Broadly, the symptoms of delirium are divided into cognitive and non-cognitive symptoms. The cognitive deficits in delirium involve domains of attention, memory, orientation, comprehension, vigilance, visuospatial abilities, and executive functioning (Gupta et al. 2008). Inattention is a consistent feature and is an important diagnostic criterion. Attention is impaired in all its aspects, and studies have shown that subjects with delirium have difficulty in mobilizing, shifting, and sustaining attention. Both short- and long-term memory are also impaired with particular disruption of recent memory due to diminished capacity to incorporate new experience. Disorientation to time, place, and person is also common and is often used to screen for disturbed cognition in clinical settings, but it is prone to inaccuracy due to its fluctuating nature. Visuospatial disturbances impair patient functionality in ward environments (Marquis et al. 2007).

The non-cognitive symptoms of delirium include speech and language disturbances (Trzepacz and Meagher 2005). Sleep–wake cycle disturbances range from napping and nocturnal disruptions to severe disintegration of the normal circadian cycle. Motoric disturbances often encountered range from hyperactive to hypoactive presentations. Other symptoms include psychotic features and affective lability (Gupta et al. 2008).

In a review of 21 studies from the West, Gupta et al. (2008) reported the frequency of different symptoms of delirium. Most of the studies from India which have studied the frequency of different symptoms have come from PGIMER, Chandigarh, and are based on DRS-R-98 and have assessed patients of delirium seen in psychiatry consultation–liaison services and ICUs (respiratory ICU and CCU).

Additionally, these studies have also tried to compare the DRS-R-98 profile across different age groups, like children and adolescents, and adults and elderly. As is evident from Table 1, the findings from India are comparable to that reported from the West, with minor differences. In general studies, from the respiratory ICU have reported much lower prevalence of psychotic symptoms such as delusions and hallucinations (Sharma et al. 2012); however, the prevalence of these symptoms has been comparable across different studies involving patients seen in CLP services.

Phenomenology in special populations: Very few studies from the West have evaluated delirium in children and adolescents (Hatherill and Flisher 2010). Two studies from India have evaluated the clinical profile of delirium in children and adolescents. One of these was a retrospective study which included patients seen by the CL psychiatry team and reported that sleep–wake cycle disturbance, impairment in orientation, attention, short-term memory, and agitation are the common symptoms of delirium in children and adolescents (Grover et al. 2009b). In another study, authors rated 30 children and adolescents (age 8–18 years) diagnosed with delirium on DRS-R-98 and showed that delirium commonly manifests in children and adolescents in the form disturbance in attention, orientation, sleep–wake cycle disturbances, fluctuation of symptoms, disturbance of short-term memory, and motor agitation. Delusions and motor retardation were the least commonly observed symptoms (Grover et al. 2012b). In another retrospective study, the authors studied the clinical profile of delirium in elderly and reported that delirium in elderly commonly manifests in the form of sleep–wake cycle disturbance, disturbance in orientation, attention and short-term memory impairments, fluctuation of symptoms, temporal onset of symptoms, and a physical disorder (Grover et al. 2012a).

Comparison of symptoms across different age groups: Occasional study from the West has compared the symptom profile of delirium across different age groups. A study that compared children and adolescents with adults showed that compared to adults, the children and adolescent had higher average scores for acute onset, hallucinations, delusions, psychomotor symptom, and lability of mood, but lower scores for cognitive deficits, fluctuation, and sleep–wake disturbance. Further, when compared to the elderly, the children and adolescent had higher average scores for acute onset, hallucinations, delusions, psychomotor symptoms, and lability of mood, but lower scores for cognitive deficits, fluctuation, and sleep–wake disturbance (Leentjens et al. 2008). A study from Chandigarh compared children and adolescents with adults and elderly and showed that compared to adults, children and adolescents had lower frequency of long-term memory and visuospatial disturbances, whereas, compared to the elderly, children and adolescents had higher frequency of lability of affect. In terms of severity of symptoms, children and adolescents had lower severity of sleep–wake disturbances, motor agitation, orientation, attention, short-term memory, long-term memory, and visuospatial abilities compared to the adults. When compared to the elderly group, children and adolescents had higher severity of lability of affect and lower severity of short-term memory and visuospatial abilities (Grover et al. 2012b). Another study compared symptom profile of adults and elderly in a larger sample size and reported that the prevalence and

Table 1 Frequency of DRS-R-98 items in various studies

	Gupta et al. (2008) (%)	Grover et al. (2011a) $N = 151$ (CLP) (%)	Grover et al. (2012b) $N = 109$ elderly (CLP) (%)	Jain et al. (2011) $N = 85$ (CLP) (%)	Mattoo et al. (2012) $N = 100$ (CLP) (%)	Aarya et al. (2013) $N = 64$ (CLP) (%)	Grover et al. (2012c) $N = 30$ (CAP-CLP) (%)	Grover et al. (2013a) Adult $N = 245$ (%)	Grover et al. (2013a) Elderly $N = 76$ (%)	Grover et al. (2013d) AWD $N = 112$ (%)	Lahariya (2012) $N = 81$ (CCU) (%)	Sharma et al. (unpublished) $N = 75$	Indian studies range (%)
Sleep–wake cycle disturbances	92–97	100	97.2	100	99	100	96.7	98.8	96.1	100	100	94.7	94.7–100
Perceptual disturbance	50–63	76.2	78.9	76.7	35	84.4	80	79.2	80.3	75	70	5.3	5.3–80.3
Delusions	21–31	27.8	35.8	37.2	14	67.2	33.3	46.5	40.8	48.2	22	0	14–67.2
Lability of affect	43–86	77.5	62.4	59.3	94	92.2	90	87.8	78.9	87	100	73.3	59.3–100
Language	57–67	76.8	79.8	73.3	90	93.8	73.3	88.2	85.8	85.7	59	90.6	59–90.6
Thought process abnormality	54–79	69.5	74.3	89.5	92	73.4	73.3	87.3	76.3	87	90	100	69.5–100
Motor agitation	24–94	94	89.0	89.5	94	85.9	93.3	90.2	90.8	94.6	73	46.6	73–94.6
Motor retardation		39.1	32.1	31.4	9	56.2	33.3	51.0	50.0	25	40	53.3	25–56.2
Disorientation	76–96	100	95.4	100	100	100	100	99.2	97.4	99.1	94	81.3	81.3–100
Attention deficits	97–100	100	97.2	97.7	100	100	100	99.6	100	100	100	100	97.2–100

(continued)

Table 1 (continued)

	Gupta et al. (2008) (%)	Grover et al. (2011a) $N = 151$ (CLP) (%)	Grover et al. (2012b) $N = 109$ elderly (CLP) (%)	Jain et al. (2011) $N = 85$ (CLP) (%)	Mattoo et al. (2012) $N = 100$ (CLP) (%)	Aarya et al. (2013) $N = 64$ (CLP) (%)	Grover et al. (2012c) $N = 30$ (CAP-CLP) (%)	Grover et al. (2013a) Adult $N = 245$ (%)	Grover et al. (2013a) Elderly $N = 76$ (%)	Grover et al. (2013d) AWD $N = 112$ (%)	Lahariya (2012) $N = 81$ (CCU) (%)	Sharma et al. (unpublished) $N = 75$	Indian studies range (%)
Short-term memory	88–96	97.4	91.8	97.7	91	96.9	93.3	94.7	98.7	92.9	100	73.3	73.3–100
Long-term memory		93.4	65.1	40.7	97	48.4	53.3	53.1	51.3	65.2	86	57.3	40.7–97
Visuospatial ability		96.7	63.3	98.8	93	75	60	64.9	57.9	68.8	66	58.6	58.6–98.8

CLP Source of patients was consultation–liaison psychiatry services
RICU Source of patients was respiratory intensive care unit
CAP-CLP Children and adolescents referred to consultation liaison team
CCU Coronary care unit
AWD Alcohol withdrawal delirium

severity of various symptoms of delirium as assessed on DRS-R-98 were similar across the two age groups except for the fact that adult group had higher prevalence and severity scores for thought process abnormality and lability of affect (Grover et al. 2013a). From the above, it can be concluded that there are more similarities than differences in terms of prevalence and severity of different symptoms of delirium across different age groups. This suggests that delirium manifest similarly across all age groups.

Factor analytic studies: Factor analysis as a tool has been extensively used to delineate the phenomenology of delirium. It is thought that factor analysis can help in understanding the correlations among different symptoms (Trzepacz and Dew 1995). Studies from the West have been limited to the elderly (Camus et al. 2000; Trzepacz et al. 1998; Saravay et al. 2004; de Jonghe et al. 2005), critically ill (van der Mast 1994), or those with malignancies (Trzepacz and Dew 1995; Franco et al. 2009). Many of these studies have small sample size as a limitation (Trzepacz et al. 1998; Saravay et al. 2004; de Jonghe et al. 2005; Fann et al. 2005).

The factor analytic studies from India (Table 2) have used larger sample sizes and have mostly involved DRS-R-98; however, occasional study has carried out factor analysis of the Memorial Delirium Assessment Scale (MDAS) (Shyamsundar et al. 2009) and another study used 3 scales, i.e., DRS-R-98, MDAS, and Confusion State Evaluation (CSE) (Jain et al. 2011). A study evaluated the factor structure of Intensive Care Delirium Screening Checklist (ICDSC) (George et al. 2011). Studies from India have more consistently showed 3-factor structure (except 2 studies), with minor differences across the composition of symptoms across different factors. In most of these studies, the cognitive symptoms cluster together, the motoric and psychotic symptoms cluster together, and the third factor consists of language, thought process abnormality, and diagnostic items. In general, the motoric and psychotic symptoms factor appears to be more consistent across different studies. However, it is important to remember that most of these studies have included patients with heterogenous etiologies for delirium.

Relationship between cognitive and non-cognitive symptoms: Very few studies from West have evaluated the relationship between cognitive and non-cognitive symptoms and motoric subtypes of delirium. Meagher et al. (2007) reported that among the cognitive symptoms of delirium, inattention was the most frequent and disorientation the least frequent. About one-fourth of subjects had no evidence of disorientation on the DRS-R-98, and only half had evidence of a greater than mild disturbance of orientation on the Cognitive Test for Delirium (CTD). The authors concluded that use of disorientation as a key indicator of delirium may lead to missed cases, and the use of inattention would be a more reliable way of screening cases for suspected delirium. They also reported that poor performance on attention and vigilance items on CTD was significantly related to the degree of disturbance on all other cognitive items on both the CTD and DRS-R-98, though much less so for non-cognitive items. The level of functioning on the CTD comprehension item (comprising a combination of language and executive function) was associated with more

Table 2 Factor analytic studies of delirium from India

	Sample size	Treatment setting	Scales used	Percentage of variance explained (%)	Factor structure
Shyamsundar et al. (2009)	120	ICU	MDAS	62.7	**Factor I (‘*cognitive disturbance*’)**—impaired digit span, short-term memory impairment, disorientation, and inattention
					Factor II (‘*behavioral abnormality*’)—altered psychomotor activity, perceptual disturbances, delusions, disorganized thinking, sleep–wake cycle disturbances, and reduced awareness
George et al. (2011)	53	ICU	ICDSC	56.2	**Factor I** (altered sensorium/psychopathology)—altered level of consciousness, inattention, disorientation, hallucination/delusion/psychosis, psychomotor agitation, and inappropriate speech or mood
					Factor II (sleep–wake cycle problems)—sleep–wake cycle disturbances, and fluctuation of symptoms
Jain et al. (2011)	86	CLP	DRS-R-98 separately and DRS-R-98, MDAS, CSE combined	47.8	**Factor I (‘*cognitive*’)**—abnormalities of language, thought process, orientation, attention, short-term memory, long-term memory, visuospatial ability, reduced level of consciousness (awareness), and perseveration or prolonged latency
					Factor II (‘*behavioral*’)—sleep–wake cycle disturbances, delusions, perceptual disturbances including hallucinations, motor agitation, inverse of motor retardation, lability of affect, distractibility, irritability, and temporal onset of symptoms
Grover et al. (2011a)	151	CLP, drug naive	DRS-R-98	47.32	**Factor I (cognitive)—**attention, orientation, short-term memory, long-term memory, and visuospatial ability
					Factor II (sleep and motoric disturbances)—sleep–wake cycle disturbances, delusions, perceptual disturbances, lability of affect, motor agitation, and inverse of motor retardation
					Factor III (thought, language, and fluctuations)—language, thought process abnormality, temporal onset of symptoms, and fluctuations

(continued)

Table 2 (continued)

	Sample size	Treatment setting	Scales used	Percentage of variance explained (%)	Factor structure
Grover et al. (2012b)	112	CLP, elderly	DRS-R-98	43.5	**Factor I (cognitive)**—thought disturbance, short-term memory, long-term memory, and visuospatial disturbance
					Factor II (cognitive and diagnostic factor)—disturbance of attention and concentration and the three items of diagnostic significance (temporal onset, fluctuation, and presence of physical disorder)
					Factor III (psychotic and motoric symptoms)—perceptual disturbances, delusions, and the motoric disturbances
Mattoo et al. (2012)	100	CLP, mixed adult and elderly	DRS-R-98	48.5	***2-factor model***
					Factor I (cognition and thinking)—delusions, language disturbances, thought process abnormality, attention, orientation, short-term memory, long-term memory, visuospatial ability, and temporal onset of symptoms
					Factor I (circadian)—motoric disturbances, fluctuations
				59	***3-factor model***
					Factor I (cognition)—attention, orientation, short-term memory, long-term memory, visuospatial ability, and fluctuation
					Factor II (circadian and psychosis)—sleep disturbances, delusions, hallucinations, and motoric disturbances
					Factor III (higher order thinking)—language disturbances, thought process abnormality, and temporal onset of symptoms
Grover et al. (2013a)	321	CLP, mixed adult and elderly	DRS-R-98	45.8	**Factor I (psychotic and motoric disturbances)**—sleep–wake cycle disturbances, delusions, perceptual disturbances, lability of affect, motor agitation, inverse of motor retardation, and fluctuation
					Factor II (cognitive)—language, thought process abnormality, short-term memory, long-term memory, and visuospatial ability
					Factor III (diagnostic factor)—attention, orientation, temporal onset of symptoms, and physical disorder

(continued)

Table 2 (continued)

	Sample size	Treatment setting	Scales used	Percentage of variance explained (%)	Factor structure
Grover et al. (2013a)	245	CLP, adult	DRS-R-98	46.75	**Factor I (psychotic and motoric disturbances)**—sleep–wake cycle disturbances, delusions, perceptual disturbances, lability of affect, motor agitation, inverse of motor retardation, and fluctuation
					Factor II (cognitive)—language, thought process abnormality, short-term memory, long-term memory, and visuospatial ability
					Factor III (diagnostic factor)—attention, orientation, temporal onset of symptoms, and physical disorder
Grover et al. (2013a)	76	CLP, elderly	DRS-R-98	48.53	**Factor I (cognitive-1)**—delusions, language disturbance, thought process abnormality, long-term memory, and visuospatial ability
					Factor II (psychotic and motoric disturbances)—sleep–wake cycle disturbances, perceptual disturbances, motor agitation, inverse of motor retardation, fluctuation, and physical disorder
					Factor III (cognitive-2)—inverse of lability of affect, attention, orientation, short-term memory, and temporal onset of symptoms
Sharma et al. (Unpublished)	75	RICU	DRS-R-98	54.6–63.4	**Factor I (cognitive factor)**—attention, orientation, short-term memory, long-term memory, and visuospatial ability
					Factor II (motoric disturbances)—motor agitation, inverse of motor retardation, and lability of affect
					Factor III (behavioral disturbances)—language disturbance, thought process abnormality, temporal onset of symptoms, and fluctuation

DRS Delirium Rating Scale, *MDAS* Memorial Delirium Assessment Scale, *MMSE* Mini-Mental State Examination, *DRS-R-98* Delirium Rating Scale-Revised-1998, *CSE* Confusional State Evaluation, *ICU* intensive care unit, *ICDSC* Intensive Care Delirium Screening Checklist non-cognitive DRS-R-98 items than the other CTD items. Among the non-cognitive symptoms, neither delusions nor hallucinations were associated with cognitive impairments. The authors did not find any relationship between psychotic symptoms and motoric items, highlighting the fact that patients with quieter presentations also experience disturbing psychotic symptoms. Another prospective study of stem cell transplantation patients found that non-cognitive features dominated in the early stages of delirium, while cognitive impairment peaked after 1 week and dominated thereafter (Fann et al. 2005). Grassi et al. (2001) evaluated subjects with delirium on MMSE, DRS, and MDAS scale and reported high correlations between individual MDAS items and the MMSE total score than individual DRS items and the MMSE score. Non-cognitive items (e.g., perceptual disturbances, sleep–wake cycle disturbances) of both scales and certain specific DRS items (i.e., lability of mood, physical disorder) showed lower correlations with the MMSE.

A study from PGIMER, Chandigarh, evaluated the relationship of cognitive and non-cognitive symptoms of delirium as assessed on DRS-R-98 and CTD in 64 patients seen by the consultation liaison psychiatry services (Aarya et al. 2013). This study showed that poor attention on DRS-R-98 is associated with significantly higher motor retardation and higher DRS-R-98 severity scores. On CTD, higher attention deficits were associated with higher dysfunction on all other domains of CTD. Further, the study showed significant correlations between individual cognitive domains as assessed on CTD and total DRS-R-98 score (except for vigilance), DRS-R-98 severity score and DRS-R-98 severity score without the attention item score. Significant correlations also emerged between the total CTD scores and DRS-R-98 total scores, DRS-R-98 severity scores, DRS-R-98 severity score minus attention scores, total score of cognitive items of DRS-R-98, and total score of non-cognitive items DRS-R-98. Further, all these correlations persisted even when total CTD scores minus attention deficits score was used for correlations. On the basis of the findings of this study, it can be concluded that with the increase in severity of delirium, there is increase in cognitive deficits. This relationship is not dependent on attention deficits alone. Additionally, the relationship between severity of delirium exists with each domain of cognitive function (Aarya et al. 2013).

5 Subtypes of Delirium

Several attempts have been made to subclassify delirium based on phenomenological or etiological differences. Candidates for subtyping delirium include hyperactive versus hypoactive, cortical versus subcortical, anterior versus posterior cortical, right versus left hemisphere, psychotic versus non-psychotic, acute versus chronic, etc. (Meagher 2009). The most commonly used classification of subtypes of delirium is the one proposed by Lipowski (1983). Lipowski (1989) suggested 'hyperactive' and 'hypoactive' as labels for delirium subtypes, before adding a third 'mixed' category in recognition that many patients experience elements of both within short time frames (Lipowski 1989). Later, some of the authors have added another subtype to the above three subtypes. Liptzin and Levkoff (1992) described hyperactive, hypoactive, mixed, and neither subtype of delirium. O'Keefe and Lavan (1997) described hyperactive, hypoactive, mixed, and no subtype of delirium.

In view of the above described subtypes, studies from the West have used the descriptions of agitation and retardation from the MDAS, the Delirium Rating Scale, the Delirium Rating Scale-Revised-98, or visual analog scales, clinical observation, and agitation/sedation scale ratings to define motor subtypes.

Prevalence of various subtypes: Studies that have tried to characterize the subtype of delirium suggest that hyperactive delirium is the most common subtype in patients seen in CL psychiatry services (Mittal et al. 2006). In contrast, studies done in various other treatment settings suggest that mixed or hypoactive subtypes are more common compared to hyperactive subtype (Stagno et al. 2004). Studies that have evaluated subtypes of delirium using Delirium Motor Subtype Scale (DMSS) in palliative care setting suggest that hypoactive delirium is the most common subtype of delirium (Meagher et al. 2012, 2011). It has been suggested that some of the differences in incidence and clinical profile of motor subtypes can be attributed to assessment methods and population studied. Meagher et al. (2008) highlighted the inconsistency of current approaches by reporting concordance of motor subtype attribution with four different approaches applied to a single population as being a mere 34 %. Following this, Meagher et al. (2008) collated 30 clinical features used in different subtyping methods to define motor subtypes and developed a Delirium Motoric Checklist (DMC). Next, they identified 11 items that by virtue of frequency, correlation with independent measures of motor behavior, and relative specificity for delirium and constructed the DMSS (Meagher et al. 2008), which can be rated by both medical and non-medical staff and has been shown to have good concurrent and predictive validity (Leonard et al. 2003; Godfrey et al. 2010).

In contrast to the studies from the West, most of the studies from India have used DMSS to study the prevalence of various motoric subtypes of delirium. In a small sample study, Aarya et al. (2013) classified 64 patients of delirium using DMSS and reported nearly equal prevalence of hyperactive (39.1 %) and hypoactive delirium 35.93 %. One-eighth (12.5 %) of patients had mixed subtype of delirium, and 11 % of patients could not be classified into any of the three motoric subtypes. Sharma et al. (2012) subtyped patients of delirium admitted to RICU using RASS scores as suggested by Peterson et al. (2006) and reported hypoactive delirium (45.33 %) to be the most common subtype, followed by hyperactive (37.33 %) subtype, and only a small proportion (17.33 %) of patients were found to have mixed subtype. In the study which evaluated patients admitted to CCU for delirium, based on the DMSS, hyperactive (56.8 %) was the most common subtype of delirium, followed by hypoactive subtype (26 %). Only about 10 % of patients were categorized into mixed subtype, and 5 % could be categorized into any of the 3 subtypes and were defined as 'no subtype.' On further analysis, it was seen that incidence cases more commonly had hyperactive delirium (70 %), with no case of mixed subtype, whereas half (51 %) of the prevalence cases were categorized into hyperactive subtype, 26 % had hypoactive delirium, 15 % had mixed subtype, and 7 % had no subtype (Lahariya 2012). Another study evaluated motor subtypes in a large sample ($N = 321$) seen in CL psychiatry services showed that hyperactive subtype (50.15 %) was the most common motoric subtype of delirium, followed by mixed subtype (24.61 %), hypoactive subtype (19.93 %), and 'no subtype' (5.3 %) being the least common (Grover et al. 2014b).

Relationship between motor subtypes with other features of delirium: Studies from West suggest that psychosis is more common in the hyperactive subtype (Sandberg et al. 1999), while others report no difference in occurrence of psychosis between hyperactive and hypoactive subtypes (Breitbart et al. 2002) and no difference in antipsychotic responsiveness between the 2 groups (Platt et al. 1994). Greater sleep–wake cycle disturbance (Gupta et al. 2005) and mood lability (Gupta et al. 2005; de Rooij et al. 2006) have been reported in hyperactive subtype, while higher prevalence of language disturbance has been reported in hypoactive patients (Gupta et al. 2005). Evidence also suggests that there is no difference in mood alteration (Sandberg et al. 1999) between the hyperactive and hypoactive subtypes. Studies have also shown that motoric subtypes share core elements of delirium with similar degrees of cognitive impairment (Koponen et al. 1989; Meagher et al. 2000; Ross et al. 1991). However, the earlier studies from the West which evaluated cognitive impairment had done so using Delirium Rating Scale, which had only one item for assessment of all the cognitive domains (O'Keeffe and Lavan 1997). Meagher et al. (2000) using DMSS reported that subjects with hypoactive delirium scored lower than the hyperactive group for delusions, mood lability, sleep–wake cycle disturbances, and variability of symptoms, but lower than the mixed group only for mood lability. However, the three groups did not differ on cognitive functions.

Few studies from India have also tried to characterize the relationship of motor subtypes with other features of delirium. A study that evaluated delirium subtypes in small sample reported that lability of affect and motor agitation are more common in hyperactive subtype, whereas language disturbances, thought process abnormality, and motor retardation are more common in the hypoactive subtype. On CTD, different motor subtypes do not differ on various cognitive domains except that patients with hyperactive subtype had higher mean scores for memory (Aarya et al. 2013). A recent large sample study compared the symptoms of delirium as assessed on DRS-R-98 across different motor subtypes and showed that hyperactive and hypoactive groups differed significantly in terms of prevalence of perceptual disturbances, delusions, thought process abnormality, motor agitation, and motor retardation. All the symptoms were more common in hyperactive subtype but for thought process abnormality and motor retardation. When the hyperactive and mixed motoric subtype groups were compared, it was seen that patients with mixed subtype had significantly higher prevalence of thought process abnormality and motor retardation. When the mixed and hypoactive subtypes were seen, significant differences were seen for perceptual disturbances, delusions, and motor agitation, all more commonly seen in patients with mixed subtype. No significant differences emerged across the different motor subtypes in terms of cognitive symptoms as assessed on DRS-R-98, i.e., disorientation, attention, short-term memory, and long-term memory (Grover et al. 2014b). The lack of difference across different motor subtypes supports the finding from the West and supports the notion that delirium is primarily a cognitive disorder.

Another study that evaluated the patients admitted to CCU found that compared to those with hypoactive delirium, patients with hyperactive delirium have significantly higher prevalence of motor agitation and lower prevalence of motor retardation and deficits in visuospatial ability. Those with hyperactive delirium were also more likely to have total DRS-R-98 score of 18 or more. In terms of severity, those with hyperactive delirium had significantly higher severity score on the item of motor agitation and significantly lower scores on the items of motor retardation, deficits in visuospatial ability, and total DRS-R-98 cognitive score (Lahariya 2012).

Motoric subtypes and risk factors for delirium: A study from India, which involved patients admitted to CCU, evaluated the relationship of motoric subtypes with risk factors for delirium and showed that those with hypoactive delirium had higher prevalence of diabetes mellitus, uncontrolled diabetes mellitus and were less frequently receiving opioids, frusemide and steroids. Further, those with hypoactive delirium more frequently had cardiogenic shock, hypocalcemia, hypoglycemia, and acid base imbalance and less frequently had history of alcohol and tobacco use (Lahariya 2012).

Motoric subtypes and outcome of delirium: Studies from West have variedly reported that prognosis of delirium is similar across different subtypes, whereas other studies have reported poorer prognosis for hypoactive, hyperactive, and mixed subtypes (Meagher 2009). The study from India which evaluated patients admitted to RICU showed that hypoactive subtype was more common in patients who did not survive (Sharma et al. 2012). Similarly, another study that evaluated predictors of mortality of patients seen in CL psychiatry services reported that hypoactive subtype was one of the predictor of mortality in patients of delirium (Grover et al. 2012c). The study that involved patients admitted in CCU also showed that hypoactive subtype of delirium was more frequently associated with mortality at the time of discharge or at 1-year follow-up (Lahariya 2012).

6 Etiological Models

In contrast to the West, in India, family is the major support for patients with severe illnesses, both mental and physical. When a medically ill patient develops mental symptoms of delirium (especially misrecognition, delusions, and hallucinations) which are associated with stigma, it leads to a panic in the caregivers and they tend to seek alternate modalities of treatment and cure, which at times may be harmful for the patient. Hence, in the Indian context, it is important to recognize the causal models held by them, as this can influence their help seeking. A study from our center evaluated the cause of delirium as perceived by the caregivers. Half of the caregivers had poor understanding about the cause of delirium in their patients. About one-third of the caregivers attributed the symptoms of delirium to non-organic causes such as supernatural causation, mental stress due to physical illness, tension due to social causes, attention seeking, religious disobedience, and homesickness, rather than an organic cause, and another 8.3 % of the caregivers could not give any reason for the altered mental state of the patient (Grover and Shah 2012). This causal belief pattern of caregivers of patients with delirium was similar to the causal models for schizophrenia existing in our community (Charles et al. 2007; Srinivasan and Thara 2001). On the basis of the findings, the authors suggested that the consultation–liaison psychiatrist and the treating physicians should always explain the caregivers about the organic etiology of symptoms of delirium and its short lasting nature. This can reduce the distress of caregivers and help them cope better with the crisis and act in an informed manner (Grover and Shah 2012).

7 Distress in Patients and Caregivers

Although studies have evaluated the impact of delirium with respect to physical morbidity and mortality, very few studies have evaluated the psychological impact of delirium on the patients and their caregivers who stay with the patients during the acute delirious phase.

Studies from the West which have addressed the issue of psychological consequences in patients suggest that a significant proportion (53.5–94 %) of patients recall their experiences during the episode of delirium (Breitbart et al. 2002; Cohen et al. 2009) and describe these experiences as distressing and disturbing (Laitinen 1996; Minnick et al. 2001; Asbury 1985; Holland et al. 1997; Stein-Parbury and McKinley 2000; Jones et al. 2000). The dominant emotions are of fear, anxiety, and feeling threatened (Schofield 1997). The commonly remembered experiences include perceptual disturbances such as illusions and hallucinations, and short verbal commands from nurses during these periods of altered perception (O'Malley et al. 2008), others described their delirium as incomprehensible experience for them.

Only one small study from India has evaluated this aspect (Grover and Shah 2011). This study suggested that only 28.3 % of patients are able to remember the experience of being confused. Those who remembered their experience, in general, described it as a state of fearfulness, anxiety, confusion, and feeling strange. Other experiences, which were recollected, were those of visual hallucinations and illusions. About one-fourth of those who could remember their experience had moderate level of distress, another 40 % had severe distress, and one-third had very severe level of distress. Among those who could not remember their delirium experience, most of them had moderate (44.7 %) to severe (26.3 %) distress (Grover and Shah 2011). Keeping these facts in mind, it is very important for the treating team to take appropriate measures to reduce the distress.

Very few studies from the West have evaluated the impact of delirium on the caregivers and nurses, and those that have suggest high level of distress (Breitbart et al. 2002; Cohen et al. 2009; Bruera et al. 2009). These studies suggest that the level of distress is significantly higher for spouses or caregivers than the patients themselves (Breitbart et al. 2002; Bruera et al. 2009). A study, which evaluated hospitalized patients with cancer and delirium, reported severe distress in 76 % of spouses or caregivers and in 73 % of nurses (Breitbart et al. 2002). Predictors of family distress were hyperactive delirium and poor functional status, while severe delirium and perceptual disturbances were the strongest predictors of nurses' distress (Breitbart et al. 2002). However, these studies have been limited by the fact that they do not provide any information about the symptoms of delirium, which are associated with higher levels of distress. To overcome this limitation, one study from PGIMER, Chandigarh, evaluated the distress experienced by the caregivers of delirium due to symptoms of delirium (Grover and Shah 2013). For this, the authors designed a scale called the caregiver experience and distress due to delirium scale (CEDDDS), which was a semi-structured interview designed specifically for this study by the authors. It has 32 items, based on the commonly seen symptoms of delirium and items of the DRS-R98 and the Delirium Motor Checklist. Symptoms of delirium which were associated with severe or very severe distress in more than two-thirds of the caregivers included the following: decreased sleep, increased motor activity, attempts to remove intravenous lines or tubes, and attempts to get out of bed when they were actually required to lie down. In terms of mean distress scores, highest level of distress was associated with sleep disturbances, hyperactivity, trying to pull out the tubes or lines inserted as part of the treatment, trying to get out of the bed, low frustration tolerance and irritability, confusion, distraction, excessive reactivity to the surroundings, and lack of awareness about the surroundings. Further, it was seen that the distress associated with most of the behaviors of the patients correlated positively with baseline DRS-R98 severity score. The authors concluded that the finding of negative correlation between DRS-R98 scores and items suggestive of hypoactive delirium can have important clinical implications with respect to the fact that hypoactive delirium may be considered as a respite by the burdened caregivers and hence may lead to poor care and neglect of the patient. Taking this into consideration, the authors suggested that medically ill patients should be routinely screened for delirium, and when found to have delirium, appropriate management strategies should be instituted as early as possible to reduce the symptoms/severity of symptoms and resultant distress in the caregivers (Grover and Shah 2013).

8 Pharmacological Treatment of Delirium

Besides treating the underlying illness, which contributes to delirium, pharmacological treatment of delirium largely consists of antipsychotics and benzodiazepines. Although antipsychotics, especially haloperidol, continue to be the most commonly used medications for management of delirium, till recently, data arising from randomized controlled trials were sparsely available. Further, in recent times, due to tolerability issues with haloperidol, many authors have tried to use atypical antipsychotics in the management of delirium.

An open-label trial from India evaluated the effectiveness of risperidone in 7 patients with delirium (hyperactive subtype in 6 cases). Most of these patients were young with a mean age of 32 years (range: 24–67 years) and had delirium of 5.29-day duration prior to institution of risperidone. The mean daily starting does was 1.14 mg (range: 0.5–2.0 mg), and the average dose used in the study was 1.07 mg (range: 0.5–1.5 mg). It was seen that over the period of 48 h, all patients, except one with hypoactive delirium, significantly improved or recovered; none developed extrapyramidal symptoms or any other serious side effects (Gupta et al. 2005).

In a randomized controlled single-blind study from India, the authors compared haloperidol with olanzapine and risperidone. This study included 64 patients with 20 in the haloperidol group, 21 in the risperidone group, and 23 subjects in the olanzapine group. The patients were evaluated at the baseline, at 3 days and at 6 days. The primary efficacy measure used in the study was the DRS-R-98, and the MMSE was used as a secondary measure of efficacy. It was seen that all the three antipsychotics were efficacious. No significant difference was seen in the reduction in DRS-R98 severity scores and significant improvement in the MMSE scores over the period of 6 days between the three groups. Very few patients (4 in haloperidol group, 6 in risperidone group, and 2 patients in olanzapine group) experienced some side effects. On the basis of their findings, the authors concluded that olanzapine and risperidone are as effective as haloperidol in the management of delirium and can be used in the management of delirium (Grover et al. 2011b).

Besides these studies, data from India suggest that haloperidol is the most commonly used antipsychotic in patients of delirium (Grover et al. 2009b), and this is followed by use of risperidone (Grover et al. 2009a), even in the children and adolescents (Grover et al. 2009b).

9 Mortality and Outcome

Studies from the West have indicated a high mortality rate among patients with delirium. Most of these studies have evaluated the inpatient and follow-up mortality rates in patients with delirium who are elderly or admitted to the ICUs (Inouye et al. 1998; McCusker et al. 2002; Tennen et al. 2009; Ely et al. 2004; Leslie et al. 2005; Adamis et al. 2006; Curyto et al. 2001). Very few studies have evaluated the mortality rates of medical–surgical inpatients with delirium referred for psychiatric consultation. Studies have shown that 9–34.5 % of patients with delirium die during their inpatient stay (Inouye et al. 1998; McCusker et al. 2002). Tennen et al. (2009) studied the 1-year mortality rate of medical–surgical inpatients referred for psychiatric consultation and reported that 15.2 % died within 1 year of referral for psychiatric consultation. Among the various predictors of mortality, delirium was the only psychiatric diagnosis which was associated with higher 1-year mortality (52.2 % vs. 29.9 %, $p = 0.01$; hazard ratio = 1.7).

In the initial retrospective study from India, which involved data of psychiatric referrals over the period of 6 years, the authors reported a mortality rate of 6.6 % (Grover et al. 2009b). This study also shows that about three-fourths of patients with delirium (74.7 %) improve or recover from their delirium episode during the inpatient stay (Grover et al. 2009b). However, in one of the first longitudinal studies from India, which evaluated the outcome of patients with delirium referred to the consultation-liaison psychiatry team, it was seen that 12.1 % expired during their hospital stay, which was higher than the mortality seen in other patients referred to consultation-liaison psychiatric services during the same period, and diagnosed with other psychiatric disorders (4.43 %), or who had no psychiatric diagnosis (no death) and were referred to consultation-liaison psychiatry services. The mortality rate in patients of delirium was also significantly higher than that seen in all admissions to the hospital during the study period (6.79 %; 2,119 deaths in 31,190 admissions; chi-square value 4.73; $p = 0.02$). At 3-month follow-up, another 12 out of 54 patients and at 6-month follow-up another 3 out of 42 contactable patients died. Overall mortality associated with delirium at 6 months was 27.83 %, which was in the range reported in studies from the West. None of the demographic or clinical factors were found to predict mortality (Grover et al. 2012c).

Another recent study evaluated the inpatient mortality rate and the predictors of mortality of patients referred to psychiatric liaison team and diagnosed to have delirium. The study included 321 patients of delirium diagnosed to have delirium. The inpatient mortality rate was 12.4 %, and it was seen that mortality was associated with younger age group (i.e., age <65 years), alcohol dependence and use of restrains prior to development of delirium. However, in logistic regression analysis, only age less than 65 years emerged as the significant predictors of mortality (Grover et al. 2013b).

A study evaluated the mortality associated with delirium in patients admitted to respiratory ICU (Sharma et al. 2012). None of the patient without delirium during the RICU stay died. In contrast, 30.7 % of patients with delirium died during the RICU stay (Sharma et al. 2012). It was seen that those who died were younger than those who survived. Further, it was seen that mortality was higher in those who more frequently had malignancy and multi-organ failure. Among the delirium variables, mortality was associated with higher DRS-R-98 severity scores, higher DRS-R-98 total score, and hypoactive delirium (Sharma et al. 2012).

Another recent study evaluated patients admitted to CCU for delirium and outcome. It was seen that about one-fourth (27 %) of patients with delirium died during their CCU/hospital stay, this was in contrast to 2 patients (0.8 %) in the non-delirium group, and the difference between the two groups was statistically significant. At 1-year follow-up of these patients, additionally 23 % patients who had delirium during their CCU stay died, in contrast to 9.2 % in the non-delirium group. In total, half (50.6 %) of patients who developed delirium died at the end of 1 year, in contrast to 10 % mortality in those who did not develop delirium, and this difference was statistically significant. Most of the existing literature has not evaluated the role of phenomenology/symptoms of delirium in predicting mortality. This study evaluated the same and showed that the predictors of mortality during the hospital/CCU stay in patients of delirium were presence of perceptual disturbances, disturbance in language, motor retardation, long-term memory, visuospatial ability all being more common in those who died in the hospital and motor agitation being more common in those who were alive. In terms of severity of symptoms, it was seen that those who died in the hospital in general had higher severity for cognitive symptoms as seen on DRS-R-98 and MDAS, thought abnormality and language disturbances on DRS-R-98, reduced level of consciousness on MDAS, and overall severity of delirium. All these findings were also true when the frequency and severity of symptoms were compared between those who were alive at 1 year and those who died. On the basis of this, the authors concluded that clinical picture of delirium can also predict mortality. In terms of other predictors of mortality, it was seen that presence uncontrolled diabetes mellitus, cardiogenic shock, and sepsis had highest odds ratio for predicting in-hospital/CCU mortality. Other predictors of mortality in the hospital/CCU were presence of diabetes mellitus, higher APACHE-II score, higher SOFA score, and higher Charlton comorbidity score (Lahariya et al. 2014).

10 Validation and Development of Scales for Delirium

Most of the instruments used for assessment of various aspects of delirium have been developed in the West (Grover and Kate 2012).

Very few studies from India have evaluated the psychometric properties of different scales used in delirium research. One study reported the reliability and validity of diagnosing delirium with the MDAS in 121 consecutive patients admitted to medical and cardiac ICUs, who were neither mute nor intubated. Interrater agreement and test–retest reliability of MDAS were 0.92 (95 % confidence interval, 0.81–0.96) and 0.93 (95 % confidence interval, 0.83–0.97), respectively. The internal consistency of the scale was good, with Cronbach's alpha of 0.89 and Guttman split-half coefficient of 0.71. Factor analysis revealed a 2-factor structure, namely cognitive disturbances and behavioral abnormalities. The sensitivity (100 %), specificity (95.45 %), positive predictive value (75 %), and negative predictive value (100 %) of the scale were also found to be very high (Shyamsundar et al. 2009).

In a study from south India, authors validated the ICDSC in non-intubated ICU patients in a resource-poor medical intensive care setting in south India. The authors proposed a cutoff of 3 or more for delirium, which had a sensitivity of 90 % and specificity of 61.54 %. Interrater reliability of the scale was found to be 0.947, and the internal consistency was found to be good with Cronbach α of 0.754 and Guttman split-half coefficient of 0.71. Factor analysis revealed a

2-factor structure, namely altered sensorium/psychopathology and sleep–wake cycle problems (George et al. 2011). Another recent study evaluated the validity of DMSS in assessment of motor subtypes of delirium in patients seen in consultation–liaison psychiatry services. Using factor analysis, the authors replicated the findings of original DMSS and additionally described certain items, which were combined with the original scale with overlap of 3 hyperactive items and 6 hypoactive items. Additional items were also found to load on the hyperactive and hypoactive factors. On the basis of the replication and comparison with the original DMSS scale, the authors described the amended DMSS scale, which has 13 items (5 hyperactive and 8 hypoactive). The amended DMSS has 1 item substituted in the hyperactive subtype of the original DMSS and 1 additional item for describing the hypoactive subtype compared to the original DMSS. After addition of few items to the original scales, the authors concluded that the amended DMSS may have broader generalizability than the original DMSS (Grover et al. 2013).

Another study that assessed the distress associated with symptoms of delirium, the authors developed an instrument called *CEDDDS*. It is a semi-structured interview with 32 questions, which were designed based on the phenomenology of delirium commonly seen in consultation–liaison psychiatry setting, items of DRS-R98 and Delirium Motor Checklist. Each question has provision for the following ratings: Did the patient have these symptoms (e.g., did he become confused as to where he was?)—this is rated as yes/no based on the presence or absence of the symptoms throughout the period of delirium, and if the symptom is present, the caregivers are further required to rate the duration of the symptom taking the whole duration of delirium into consideration on a five-point Likert scale with 'not at all' rated as 0 and 'almost always' rated as 4. Then, the caregivers are asked to rate their distress due to these symptoms on a five-point Likert scale with 'not at all' rated as 0 and 'very severe' rated as 4. The distress score is analyzed as frequency count, and mean distress score can also be calculated (Grover and Shah 2013c).

11 Delay in Psychiatry Referral for Delirium

Evidence from the West suggests that physicians and surgeons fail to identify the patients with delirium in the early phase, and this leads to delay in psychiatric referral. However, only occasional studies have evaluated the predictors of delay in psychiatry referral for delirium. A study from PGIMER, Chandigarh, showed that presence of delirium at the time of hospitalization, presence of sleep–wake disturbance, and surgical specialty of referral were significant predictors of delayed diagnosis (Gupta et al. 2010). Another study from the same center, which included much larger sample, showed that older age, presence of and higher severity of sleep disturbance, presence of and higher severity of motor retardation, presence of visuospatial disturbances, presence of fluctuation of symptoms, being admitted to medical ward/medical ICUs, and absence of comorbid axis-1 psychiatry diagnoses were associated with longer duration of psychiatric referral after the onset of delirium. Of these, only 4 variables (presence of sleep disturbance, presence of motor retardation, being admitted to medical ward/medical ICUs, and absence of comorbid axis-1 psychiatry diagnoses) were associated with longer duration of psychiatric referral in the regression analysis. On the basis of their findings, the authors concluded that efforts should be made to inform the primary team members about the signs and symptoms and risk factors of delirium to reduce the referral delay and improve the outcome of delirium (Grover et al. 2014a).

12 Conclusions

Over the years, many studies from India have evaluated the various aspects of delirium. Findings suggest that delirium is the most common diagnosis in patients seen in psychiatry consultation–liaison psychiatry services. The phenomenology of delirium in India is similar to that reported from the west, and in general, there is no difference in the frequency of various symptoms and severity of symptoms of delirium across different age groups. However, the phenomenology of delirium in ICU patients is different from those seen in the consultation–liaison psychiatry services. Findings also suggest that the symptoms of delirium cluster into 2–3 groups in various factor analytic studies. Delirium is a multifactorial disorder associated with multiple etiologies, with metabolic causes being the most common. Findings also suggest that delirium is associated with excessive mortality, both inpatient mortality and mortality after 6 month to 1 year after development of delirium. Data also indicate that as a syndrome, delirium is very distressing for the caregivers and also for those patients who remember their experiences of delirium. As reported by studies from other parts of the world, evidence from India also suggests that atypical antipsychotics such as risperidone and olanzapine are as efficacious as haloperidol in management of delirium.

References

Aarya, A., Mattoo, S. K., & Grover, S. (2013). Relationship between cognitive and non-cognitive symptoms of delirium. *Asian Journal of Psychiatry, 6*, 106–112.

Adamis, D., Treloar, A., Martin, F. C., & Macdonald, A. J. D. (2006). Recovery and outcome of delirium in elderly medical inpatients. *Archives of Gerontology and Geriatrics, 43*, 289–298.

American Psychiatric Association. (1999). Practice guideline for the treatment of patients with delirium. American Psychiatric Association. *American Journal of Psychiatry, 156*(5 Suppl), 1–20.

Asbury, A. J. (1985). Patients' memories and reactions to intensive care. *Care Critically Ill, 1*, 62–65.

Bergeron, N., Dubois, M. J., & Dumont, M. (2001). Intensive care delirium screening checklist: Evaluation of a new screening tool. *Intensive Care Medicine, 27*, 859–864.

Breitbart, W., Gibson, C., & Tremblay, A. (2002a). The delirium experience: Delirium recall and delirium-related distress in hospitalized patients with cancer, their spouses/caregivers, and their nurses. *Psychosomatics, 43*, 183–194.

Breitbart, W., Tremblay, A., & Gibson, C. (2002b). An open trial of olanzapine for the treatment of delirium in hospitalized cancer patients. *Psychosomatics, 43*, 175–182.

Bruera, E., Bush, S. H., Willey, J., Paraskevopoulos, T., Li, Z., Palmer, J. L., et al. (2009). Impact of delirium and recall on the level of distress in patients with advanced cancer and their family caregivers. *Cancer, 115*, 2004–2012.

Camus, V., Burtin, B., Simeone, I., Schwed, P., Gonthier, R., & Dubos, G. (2000). Factor analysis supports the evidence of existing hyperactive and hypoactive subtypes of delirium. *International Journal of Geriatric Psychiatry, 15*, 313–316.

Charles, H., Manoranjitham, S. D., & Jacob, K. S. (2007). Stigma and explanatory models among people with schizophrenia and their relatives in Vellore, South India. *International Journal of Social Psychiatry, 53*, 325–332.

Chaudhury, S., Mahar, R. S., & Augustine, M. (1991). Post-cataractomy delirium a prospective study. *Medical Journal Armed Forces India, 47*, 286–290.

Chrispal, A., Mathews, K. P., & Surekha, V. (2010). The clinical profile and association of delirium in geriatric patients with hip fractures in a tertiary care hospital in India. *Journal of the Association of Physicians of India, 58*, 15–19.

Cohen, M. Z., Pace, E. A., Kaur, G., & Bruera, E. (2009). Delirium in advanced cancer leading to distress in patients and family caregiver. *Journal of Palliative Care, 25*, 164–171.

Curyto, K. J., Johnson, J., TenHave, T., et al. (2001). Survival of hospitalized elderly patients with delirium: A prospective study. *The American Journal of Geriatric Psychiatry, 9*, 141–147.

de Jonghe, J. F. M., Kalisvaart, K. J., Timmers, J. F. M., Kat, M. G., & Jackson, J. C. (2005). Delirium-O-Meter: A nurses' rating scale for monitoring delirium severity in geriatric patients. *International Journal of Geriatric Psychiatry, 20*, 1158–1166.

De Rooij, S. E., van Munster, B. C., Korevaar, J. C., Casteelen, G., Schuurmans, M. J., van der Mast, R. C., et al. (2006). Delirium subtype identification and the validation of the delirium rating scale-revised-98 (Dutch version) in hospitalized elderly patients. *International Journal of Geriatric Psychiatry, 21*, 876–882.

Ely, E. W., Gautam, S., Margolin, R., Francis, J., May, L., & Speroff, T. (2001a). The impact of delirium in the intensive care unit on hospital length of stay. *Intensive Care Medicine, 27*, 1892–1900.

Ely, E. W., Inouye, S. K., & Bernard, G. R. (2001b). Delirium in mechanically ventilated patients: validity and reliability of confusion assessment methods for the intensive care unit (CAM-ICU). *JAMA, 286*, 2703–2710.

Ely, E. W., Margolin, R., & Francis, J. (2001c). Evaluation of delirium in critically ill patients: validation of the confusion assessment method for the intensive care unit (CAM-ICU). *Critical Care Medicine, 29*, 1370–1379.

Ely, E. W., Shintani, A., & Truman, B. (2004a). Delirium as a predictor of mortality in mechanically ventilated patients in the intensive care unit. *JAMA, 291*, 1753–1762.

Ely, E. W., Stephens, R. K., & Jacson, J. C. (2004b). Current opinions regarding the importance, diagnosis, and management of delirium in the intensive care unit: A survey of 912 healthcare professionals. *Critical Care Medicine, 32*, 106–112.

Fann, J. R. (2000). The epidemiology of delirium: A review of studies and methodological issues. *Seminars in Clinical Neuropsychiatry, 5*, 64–74.

Fann, J. R., Alfano, C. M., Burington, B. E., Roth-Roemer, S., Katon, W. J., & Syrjala, K. L. (2005). Clinical presentation of delirium in patients undergoing hematopoietic stem cell transplantation. *Cancer, 103*, 810–820.

Folstein, M. F., Bassett, S. S., & Romanoski, A. J. (1991). The epidemiology of delirium in the community: The eastern baltimore mental health survey. *International Psychogeriatrics, 3*, 169–176.

Franco, J. G., Trzepacz, P. T., Mejia, M. A., & Ochoa, S. B. (2009). Factor analysis of the Colombian translation of the delirium rating scale (DRS), revised-98. *Psychosomatics, 50*, 255–262.

George, C., Nair, J. S., Ebenezer, J. A., Gangadharan, A., Christudas, A., Gnanaseelan, L. K., et al. (2011). Validation of the intensive care delirium screening checklist in non-intubated intensive care unit patients in a resource-poor medical intensive care setting in South India. *Journal of Critical Care, 26*, 138–143.

Godfrey, A., Leonard, M., Donnelly, S., Conroy, M., Olaighin, G., & Meagher, D. (2010). Validating a new clinical subtyping scheme for delirium with electronic motion analysis. *Psychiatry Research, 178*, 186–190.

Grassi, L., Caraceni, A., Beltrami, E., Borreani, C., Zamorani, M., Maltoni, M., et al. (2001). Assessing delirium in cancer patients. The Italian versions of the Delirium Rating Scale and the Memorial Delirium Assessment Scale. *Journal of Pain and Symptom Management, 21*, 59–68.

Grover, S., Agarwal, M., Sharma, A., Mattoo, S. K., Avasthi, A., Chakrabarti, S., et al. (2013a). Symptoms and etiology of Delirium: A comparison of elderly and adult patients. *East Asian Archives of Psychiatry, 23*, 56–64.

Grover, S., Chakrabarti, S., Shah, R., & Kumar, V. (2011a). A factor analytic study of the delirium rating scale-revised-98 in untreated patients with delirium. *Journal of Psychosomatic Research, 70*, 473–478.

Grover, S., Ghormode, D., Ghosh, A., Avasthi, A., Chakrabarti, S., Mattoo, S. K., et al. (2013b). Risk factors for delirium and inpatient mortality rate in patients with delirium. *Journal of Postgraduate Medicine, 59*(4), 263–270.

Grover, S., & Kate, N. (2012). Assessment scales for delirium: A review. *World Journal of Psychiatry, 2*, 58–70.

Grover, S., Kate, N., Aggarwal, M., Mattoo, S. K., Avasthi, A., Malhotra, S., et al. (2012a). Delirium in elderly: A study from a psychiatric liaison service in North India. *International Psychogeriatrics, 24*, 117–127.

Grover, S., Kate, N., Malhotra, S., Chakrabarti, S., Mattoo, S. K., & Avasthi, A. (2012b). Symptom profile of delirium in children and adolescent—Does it differs from adults and elderly? *General Hospital Psychiatry, 34*, 626–632.

Grover, S., Kate, N., Mattoo, S. K., Chakrabarti, S., Malhotra, S., Avasthi, A., et al. (2014a). Predictors of delay in referral to consultation-liaison psychiatry services. *Indian Journal of Psychiatry. 56*, 171–175.

Grover, S., Kumar, V., & Chakrabarti, S. (2011b). Comparative efficacy study of haloperidol, olanzapine and risperidone in delirium. *Journal of Psychosomatic Research, 71*, 277–281.

Grover, S., Malhotra, S., Bharadwaj, R., Subodh, B. N., & Kumar, S. (2009a). Delirium in children and adolescents: A study from India. *International Journal of Psychiatry in Medicine, 39*, 179–187.

Grover, S., Mattoo, S. K., Aarya, K. R., Pratim Das, P., Chakrabarty, K., Trzepacz, P., et al. (2013c). Replication analysis for composition of the delirium motor subtype scale (DMSS) in a referral cohort from Northern India. *Psychiatry Research, 206*, 68–74.

Grover, S., & Shah, R. (2011). Distress due to delirium experience. *General Hospital Psychiatry, 33*, 637–639.

Grover, S., & Shah, R. (2012). Perceptions among primary caregivers about the etiology of delirium: A study from a tertiary care centre in India. *African J Psychiatry, 15*, 193–195.

Grover, S., & Shah, R. (2013c). Delirium related distress in caregivers: A study from a tertiary care centre in India. *Primary Care Perspectives, 49*, 21–29.

Grover, S., Shah, R., & Aarya, K. R. (2012c). The mortality rate among patients with delirium 6 months after diagnosis by a consultation-liaison psychiatric team. *Turkish Journal of Psychiatry, 23*, 189–192.

Grover, S., Sharma, A., Agarwal, M., Mattoo, S. K., Chakrabarti, S., Malhotra, S., et al. (2014b). Comparison of symptoms of delirium across various motoric subtypes. *Psychiatry and Clinical Neurosciences, 68*(4), 283–291.

Grover, S., Sharma, A., Kate, N., Mattoo, S. K., Basu, D., Chakrabarti, S., et al. (2013d). Symptom profile and outcome of delirium associated with alcohol withdrawal syndrome: A study from India. *The American Journal on Addictions, 22*(5), 503–509.

Grover, S., Subodh, B. N., Avasthi, A., Chakrabarti, S., Kumar, S., Sharan, P., et al. (2009b). Prevalence and clinical profile of Delirium: A study from a tertiary care hospital in north India. *General Hospital Psychiatry, 31*, 25–29.

Gupta, N., de Jonghe, J., Schieveld, J., Leonard, M., & Meagher, D. (2008). Delirium phenomenology: What can we learn from the symptoms of delirium? *Journal of Psychosomatic Research, 65*, 215–222.

Gupta, A. K., Saravay, S. M., Trzepacz, P. T., & Chiray, P. (2005a). Delirium motoric subtypes. *Psychosomatics, 46*, 158.

Gupta, N., Sharma, P., & Mattoo, S. K. (2005b). Effectiveness of risperidone in delirium. *Canadian Journal of Psychiatry, 50*, 75.

Gupta, N., Sharma, P., & Meagher, D. (2010). Predictors of delayed identification of delirium in a general hospital liaison psychiatry service: A study from North India. *Asian Journal of Psychiatry, 3*, 31–32.

Hatherill, S., & Flisher, A. J. (2010). Delirium in children and adolescents: A systematic review of the literature. *Journal of Psychosomatic Research, 68*, 337–344.

Holland, C., Casson, C. L., & Prater, L. R. (1997). Patients' recollections of critical care. *Dimensions of Critical Care Nursing, 16*, 132–141.

Inouye, S. K., Rushing, J. T., Foreman, M. D., Palmer, R. M., & Pompei, P. (1998). Does delirium contribute to poor hospital outcomes? A three-site epidemiologic study. *Journal of General Internal Medicine, 13*, 234–242.

Jain, G., Chakrabarti, S., & Kulhara, P. (2011). Symptoms of delirium: An exploratory factor analytic study among referred patients. *General Hospital Psychiatry, 33*, 377–385.

Jones, C., Griffiths, R. D., & Humphris, G. (2000). Disturbed memory and amnesia related to intensive care. *Memory, 8*, 79–94.

Khurana, V., Gambhir, I. S., & Kishore, D. (2011). Evaluation of delirium in elderly: A hospital based study. *Geriatr and Gerontol International, 11*, 467–473.

Khurana, P., Sharma, P. S. V. N., & Avasthi, A. (2002a). Prevalence of delirium in geriatric hospitalized general medical population. *Indian Journal of Psychiatry, 44*, 41–46.

Khurana, P. S., Sharma, P. S., & Avasthi, A. (2002b). Risk factors in delirious geriatric general medical inpatients. *Indian Journal of Psychiatry, 44*, 266–272.

Kishi, Y., Iwasaki, Y., & Takezawa, K. (1995). Delirium in critical care unit patients admitted through an emergency room. *General Hospital Psychiatry, 17*, 371–379.

Koponen, H., Stenbåck, U., Mattila, E., Soininen, H., Reinikainen, K., & Riekkinen, P. J. (1989). Delirium among elderly persons admitted to a psychiatric hospital: Clinical course during the acute stage and one-year follow-up. *Acta Psychiatrica Scandinavica, 79*, 579–585.

Koster, S., Hensen, A. G., Schuurmans, M. J., & Van der Palen, J. (2011). Risk factor of delirium after cardiac surgery: A systematic review. *European Journal of Cardiovascular Nursing, 10*, 197–204.

Koster, S., Hensens, A. G., Schuurmans, M. J., & van der Palen, J. (2013). Prediction of delirium after cardiac surgery and the use of a risk checklist. *European Journal of Cardiovascular Nursing, 12*, 284–292.

Lahariya, S. (2012). A study of incidence, prevalence and risk factors for delirium in patients admitted to coronary care unit. MD Thesis, PGIMER.

Lahariya, S., Grover, S., Bagga, S., Sharma, A. (2014). Delirium in patients admitted to a cardiac intensive care unit with cardiac emergencies in a developing country: incidence, prevalence, risk factor and outcome. *General Hospital Psychiatry, 36*, 156–164.

Laitinen, H. (1996). Patients' experience of confusion in the intensive care unit following cardiac surgery. *Intensive Critical Care Nursing, 12*, 79–83.

Leentjens, A., Schieveld, J., Leonard, M., Lousberg, R., Verhey, F., & Meagher, D. (2008). A comparison of paediatric, adult and geriatric delirium. *Journal of Psychosomatic Research, 64*, 219–223.

Leonard, M., Godfrey, A., Silberhorn, M., Conroy, M., Donnelly, S., Meagher, D., et al. (2003). Motion analysis in delirium: A novel method of clarifying motoric subtypes. *Neurocase, 13*, 272–277.

Leslie, D. L., Zhang, Y., Holford, T. R., et al. (2005). Premature death associated with delirium at 1-year follow-up. *Archives of Internal Medicine, 165*, 1657–1662.

Lipowski, Z. J. (1983). Transient cognitive disorders (delirium, acute confusional states) in the elderly. *American Journal of Psychiatry, 140*, 1426–1436.

Lipowski, Zbigniew J. (1989). Current concepts—geriatrics: Delirium in the elderly patient. *The New England Journal of Medicine, 320*, 578–582.

Liptzin, B., & Levkoff, S. E. (1992). An empirical study of delirium subtypes. *British Journal of Psychiatry, 161*, 843–845.

Marquis, F., Ouimet, S., Riker, R., Cossette, M., & Skrobik, Y. (2007). Individual delirium symptoms: Do they matter? *Critical Care Medicine, 35*, 2533–2537.

Mattoo, S. K., Grover, S., Chakravarty, K., Trzepacz, P., Meagher, D. J., & Gupta, N. (2012). Symptom profile and etiology of delirium in a referral population in northern india: factor analysis of the DRS-R98. *Journal of Neuropsychiatry and Clinical Neurosciences, 24*, 95–101.

Mattoo, S. K., Grover, S., & Gupta, N. (2010). Delirium in general practice. *Indian Journal of Medical Research, 131*, 387–398.

McCusker, J., Kakuma, R., & Abrahamowicz, M. (2002). Predictors of functional decline in hospitalized elderly patients: A systematic review. *Journals of Gerontology. Series A, Biological Sciences and Medical Sciences, 57*, M569–M577.

McNicoll, L., Pisani, M. A., Zhang, Y., Ely, E. W., Siegel, M. D., & Inouye, S. K. (2003). Delirium in the intensive care unit: Occurrence and clinical course in older patients. *Journal of the American Geriatrics Society, 51*, 591–598.

Meagher, D. (2009). Motor subtypes of delirium: Past, present and future. *International Review of Psychiatry, 21*, 59–73.

Meagher, D. J., Leonard, M., Donnelly, S., Conroy, M., Adamis, D., & Trzepacz, P. T. (2011). A longitudinal study of motor subtypes in delirium: Relationship with other phenomenology, etiology, medication exposure and prognosis. *Journal of Psychosomatic Research, 71*, 395–403.

Meagher, D. J., Leonard, M., Donnelly, S., Conroy, M., Adamis, D., & Trzepacz, P. T. (2012). A longitudinal study of motor subtypes in delirium: Frequency and stability during episodes. *Journal of Psychosomatic Research, 72*, 236–241.

Meagher, D., Moran, M., Raju, B., Gibbons, D., Donnelly, S., Saunders, J., et al. (2007). Phenomenology of delirium: Assessment of 100 adult cases using standardized measures. *British Journal of Psychiatry, 190*, 135–141.

Meagher, D. J., Moran, M., Raju, B., Gibbons, D., Donnelly, S., Saunders, J., et al. (2008a). Motor symptoms in 100 patients with delirium versus control subjects: Comparison of subtyping methods. *Psychosomatics, 49*, 300–308.

Meagher, D., Moran, M., Raju, B., Leonard, M., Donnelly, S., Saunders, J., et al. (2008b). A new data-based motor subtype schema for delirium. *Journal of Neuropsychiatry and Clinical Neurosciences, 20*, 185–193.

Meagher, D. J., O'Hanlon, D., O'Mahony, E., Casey, P. R., & Trzepacz, P. T. (2000). Relationship between symptoms and motoric subtype of delirium. *Journal of Neuropsychiatry and Clinical Neurosciences, 12*, 51–56.

Minnick, A., Leipzig, R. M., & Johnson, M. E. (2001). Elderly patients' reports of physical restraint experiences in intensive care units. *American Journal of Critical Care, 10*, 168–171.

Mittal, D., Majithia, D., Kennedy, R., & Rhudy, J. (2006). Differences in characteristics and outcome of delirium as based on referral patterns. *Psychosomatics, 47*, 367–375.

Mu, D. L., Wang, D. X., Li, L. H., Shan, G. J., Li, J., Yu, Q. J., et al. (2010). High serum cortisol level is associated with increased risk of delirium after coronary artery bypass graft surgery: A prospective cohort study. *Critical Care, 14*, R238.

O'Keeffe, S., & Lavan, J. (1997). The prognostic significance of delirium in older hospital patients. *Journal of the American Geriatrics Society, 45*, 174–178.

O'Malley, G., Leonard, M., Meagher, D., & O'Keeffe, S. T. (2008). The delirium experience: A review. *Journal of Psychosomatic Research, 65*, 223–228.

Peterson, J. F., Pun, B. T., Dittus, R. S., et al. (2006). Delirium and its motoric subtypes: a study of 614 critically ill patients. *Journal of the American Geriatrics Society, 54*, 479–484.

Platt, M. M., Breitbart, W., Smith, M., Marotta, R., Weisman, H., & Jacobson, P. B. (1994). Efficacy of neuroleptics for hypoactive delirium. *Journal of Neuropsychiatry and Clinical Neurosciences, 6*, 66–67.

Ross, C. A., Peyser, C. E., Shapiro, I. R. A., & Folstein, M. F. (1991). Delirium: Phenomenologic and etiologic subtypes. *International Psychogeriatrics, 3*, 135–147.

Sandberg, O., Gustafson, Y., Brannstrom, B., & Bucht, G. (1999). Clinical profile of delirium in older patients. *Journal of the American Geriatrics Society, 47*, 1300–1306.

Saravay, S. M., Kaplowitz, M., Kurek, J., Zeman, D., Pollack, S., Novik, S., et al. (2004). How do delirium and dementia increase length of stay of elderly general medical inpatients? *Psychosomatics, 45*, 235–242.

Schofield, I. (1997). A small exploratory study of the reaction of older people to an episode of delirium. *Journal of Advance Nursing, 25*, 942–952.

Sharma, A., Malhotra, S., Grover, S., & Jindal, S. K. (2012). Incidence, prevalence, risk factor and outcome of delirium in intensive care unit: A study from India. *General Hospital Psychiatry, 34*, 639–646.

Sharma, A., Malhotra, S., Grover, S., Jindal, S. K. (Unpublished). Symptom profile as assessed on DRS-R-98 of delirium in respiratory intensive care unit: A study from India.

Shyamsundar, G., Raghuthaman, G., Rajkumar, A. P., & Jacob, K. S. (2009). Validation of memorial delirium assessment scale. *Journal of Critical Care, 24*, 530–534.

Siddiqi, N., House, A. O., & Holmes, J. D. (2006). Occurrence and outcome of delirium in medical inpatients: A systematic literature review. *Age and Ageing, 35*, 350–364.

Sood, A., Singh, P., & Gargi, P. D. (2006). Psychiatric morbidity in non-psychiatric geriatric inpatients. *Indian Journal of Psychiatry, 48*, 56–61.

Srinivasan, T. N., & Thara, R. (2001). Beliefs about causation of schizophrenia: do Indian families believe in supernatural causes? *Social Psychiatry and Psychiatric Epidemiology, 36*, 134–140.

Stagno, D., Gibson, C., & Breitbart, W. (2004). The delirium subtypes: A review of prevalence, phenomenology, pathophysiology, and treatment response. *Palliat Support Care, 2*, 171–179.

Stein-Parbury, J., & McKinley, S. (2000). Patients' experiences of being in an intensive care unit: A select literature review. *American Journal of Critical Care, 9*, 20–27.

Tennen, G. B., Rundell, J. R., & Stevens, S. R. (2009). Mortality in medical-surgical inpatients referred for psychiatric consultation. *General Hospital Psychiatry, 31*, 341–346.

Trzepacz, P. T., & Dew, M. A. (1995). Further analyses of the delirium rating scale. *General Hospital Psychiatry, 17*, 75–79.

Trzepacz, P. T., & Meagher, D. J. (2005). Delirium. In J. L. Levenson (Ed.), *Textbook of psychosomatic medicine* (pp. 91–130). Washington, DC: American Psychiatric Association.

Trzepacz, P. T., Mulsant, B. H., Dew, M. A., Pasternak, R., Sweet, R. A., & Zubenko, G. S. (1998). Is delirium different when it occurs in dementia? A study using the delirium rating scale. *Journal of Neuropsychiatry and Clinical Neurosciences, 10*, 199–204.

van der Mast, R. C. (1994). Delirium after cardiac surgery: A prospective study. PhD dissertation, Rotterdam.

Part VIII
Developments in Other Psychiatric Specialities

Chapter 25
Geriatric Psychiatry in India: Developments and Future Directions

Sudhir K. Khandelwal and Raman Deep Pattanayak

For age is opportunity no less
Than youth itself, though in another dress,
And as the evening twilight fades away
The sky is filled with stars, invisible by day

(HW Longfellow-Morituri Solutamus. L. 281)

1 Introduction

Population ageing is a global phenomenon as a result of declining trends in fertility and mortality rates over the past century. In 2000, for the first time ever in history, people aged 60 years or above exceeded the number of children below 5 years of age. This demographic transition is unprecedented, pervasive and likely to be enduring in future with profound implications, especially for developing countries (United Nations 2002, 2013; Census of India 2011).

The health care needs of an ageing population are likely to be different, with a higher prevalence of chronic non-communicable diseases and neuropsychiatric disorders compared to adult population. Further, several age-related risk factors may increase the likelihood of psychiatric morbidity. The care and support of elderly in India has been a prerogative of families rather than the state. However, in recent times, with a gradual breakdown of joint families, changing value systems and urbanization, there is an emerging need to pay greater attention to elderly care and elderly mental health issues (Ageing in India 2003; Krishnaswamy et al. 2008).

S.K. Khandelwal, Professor vand Head; R.D. Pattanayak, Assistant Professor

S.K. Khandelwal (✉) · R.D. Pattanayak
Department of Psychiatry, All India Institute of Medical Sciences,
New Delhi, India
e-mail: sudhir_aiims@yahoo.co.uk

S. Malhotra and S. Chakrabarti (eds.), *Developments in Psychiatry in India*,
DOI 10.1007/978-81-322-1674-2_25

This chapter discusses the sociocultural context of ageing, reviews the geriatric psychiatric research from India and provides future directions for elderly mental health services, research and policy. A vast amount of Western literature is available but has not been covered as the present chapter aims to focus on the Indian contributions in geriatric psychiatry.

2 Elderly in India

2.1 Demographics

In India, the legal and policy framework considers those aged 60 years or above as *senior citizens,* and most geriatric studies from India have also used a similar cut-off.

Elderly (aged $\geq$ 60 years) comprise 8.3 % of the Indian population as per the provisional data from latest census (Census of India 2011). The elderly population in some states like Kerala, Himachal Pradesh and Tamil Nadu had crossed 10 % about a decade back (Census of India 2001). In absolute numbers, India has world's second largest elderly population (100 million). Further, the 60 years plus age group is the fastest growing segment of Indian population, with a projected increase of 3.5 times in their percentage between 2000 and 2050 (United Nations 2013). There are more females in the elderly age group (1,022 per 1,000 males), with a considerable increase among the oldest old due to a relatively higher life expectancy for females (Census of India 2011).

These numbers indicate that India has a huge burden to look after its elderly population, which may have mental health needs. Unfortunately, India is still not well geared to the burden of elderly mental morbidities, and this burden is likely to increase in future too with more and more people surviving well in old age.

2.2 Socio-economic Profile and Health Status

The National Sample Survey (60th round) was devoted to assess the socio-economic and health status of elderly in the country (National Sample Survey 2004). It will be useful to have a quick look at the elderly situation in order to better understand their mental health aspects.

Only 50 % of elderly men and 20 % of elderly women have any formal education. About 65 % of elderly have to depend on others for day to day maintenance. Elderly women often face a triple jeopardy, that of being old, female and financially insecure (National Sample Survey 2004).

Nearly one-third reported suffering from an ailment, and 5.6–9.1 % were hospitalized over past year. Approximately 6 % of elderly live with a physical disability. It is noteworthy, however, that the subjective perception of health was reported to be fair or good by a vast majority of elderly. More than half of those with a sickness also perceived their health to be fair or good, indicating a possible acceptance of ailments as part of normal ageing (National Sample Survey 2004).

The socio-economic status creates a major challenge among the elderly group coupled with the health status also being compromised. This has to be seen in the light of the fact that the health expenditure in India is borne by the individuals to the tune of 80 %, and the state spends only 20 % of total expenses. This kind of expenditure erodes into the meagre savings of the elderly people and pushes them further into the cycle of poverty and debt.

3 Ageing in India: Sociocultural Perspectives

3.1 Religious–Philosophical Perspectives

Prevalent religions of India e.g. Hinduism and Buddhism offer a cyclical view of human existence (*sāmsāra*), with a belief in an endless cycle of birth, ageing, death and rebirth. Old age is met with a gradual preparation and acceptance in India and several other Asian societies, in contrast to Western societies with denial or postponement of ageing for as long as one can.

In India, an element of detachment from worldly pursuits (*māyā)* and engagement in a meditative and contemplative life is prescribed for later years. Upanishads state that the anxiety associated with ageing helps to drive the sensitive thinker to break out of the condition of being human and transcend it. Ancient texts encourage the pursuit of appropriate tasks for each stage of life, which facilitate a smooth and easy transition to old age. Hindu Vedic philosophy conceptualizes the life as four stages (*āśramas)*, each with its own goals and purpose (Lipner 2010). The latter two stages, that is *vanaprastha* (forest dweller) and *sannyasa* (ascetic), are particularly relevant for elderly years.

During *vānaprastha* (50–75 years), a person gradually moves away from materialistic ties and starts living in a simple and detached way. The main components of this stage include a personal spiritual quest, involvement in religious activities and sharing the wisdom with others. This is considered as a phase of partial renunciation, in preparation for next phase of complete renunciation.

During *sannyasa* (75 years onwards), one renounces the world and detaches from all emotional and social relations. All activities are directed purely towards attainment of *mokśa* (liberation) through self-realization.

In his writings, Prof. Wig reflected on the relevance of *vānaprastha āśrama* in the modern times and suggested that its core features are as relevant and meaningful today as they were during the ancient times. An adaptation is required, where instead of retreating to the forest, one can still try to withdraw from rush of life, contribute to societal welfare and pursue a spiritual path during the life after retirement (Wig 2010).

3.2 Cultural Practices, Joint Family System and Changing Scenario

Indian culture, like several other Asian cultures, has a strong sense of filial piety and duty. The elderly are considered as head of the families and continue to make several important decisions (Krishnaswamy et al. 2008). They usually have strong familial and social networks which provide them support and care. A wide range of social traditions, cultural practices and religious beliefs reinforce the respect and authority for older people. Looking after one's parents in their old age is akin to paying a debt (*pitra karz*) one owes to parents for the rearing and paves the way for salvation. Culturally, the outlook of Indian elderly is also different. Most elderly in India prefer less to be independent and perceive their children as their old age security, even in face of conflicts and differences.

In contemporary India, there has been a gradual decline of extended family systems due to various factors e.g. urbanization, migration, female workforce participation and changes in cultural values and beliefs. There is a gradual shift towards individualism and materialistic culture leading to isolation and alienation of elderly. The unconditional respect, power and authority that older people used to enjoy in rural extended traditional families are gradually being undermined by a multitude of these changes (Krishnaswamy et al. 2008; Jamuna 2000). The global trend towards having fewer children assures that there will be less elder care and support by the families in the future.

4 Psychological Aspects in Elderly

Elderly people have to deal with a variety of stressors and issues which are unique to old age. Individuals in late adulthood may face a crisis of 'integrity versus despair' as proposed by Newton and Erikson (2007). Retirement from active work life may be one of first psychosocial stressors of old age. It may entail a search for an alternate identity especially if work had occupied a central position in life earlier. Elderly may have to cope with reduced income, change of status and power, lot of free unstructured time and, at times, unfinished familial tasks such as marriage of daughter. Decline in health status, income insecurity, problems of isolation, loneliness and the 'generation gap' are other prominent areas of frustration among Indian elderly (Raju 2011). Many elderly turn to religion for overcoming the feelings of anxiety or isolation during old age. Even though Indian culture is oriented towards respect and care for the elderly group, but some elders do suffer verbal, psychological or physical abuse from family members which adds to psychological ill health (Soneja 2013).

5 Geriatric Psychiatric Research in India

5.1 Epidemiological Studies

The geriatric psychiatric research in India began with the pioneering studies of Ramachandran and Venkoba Rao on prevalence and pattern of morbidity in older persons. Several epidemiological studies have been conducted in community (Table 1) (Ramachandran et al. 1979; Seby et al. 2011) as well as in hospital settings (Prasad et al. 1996; Prakash et al. 2007). The prevalence of psychiatric morbidity among elderly ($\geq$60 years) residing in community has ranged between 8.5 and 42.2 %. Recent surveys from Lucknow, supported by Indian Council of Medical Research (ICMR), found that 17.3 % of rural elderly and 23.5 % of urban elderly suffer from a psychiatric illness (Tiwari et al. 2010; Seby et al. 2011).

Mood disorders especially depression is the commonest disorder among the elderly.

Table 1 Community-based epidemiological surveys for geriatric psychiatric morbidity

References/place of study	Instruments	Setting	Sample	Prevalence	Profile
Ramachandran et al. (1979) (Tamil Nadu)	Clinical interview	Sub-urban area Field survey	$n = 406$ aged ≥ 50 years	35 %	General illness, isolation and low family cohesion (nuclear families/widowhood) seen
Ramachandran et al. (1982) (Tamil Nadu)	Clinical interview	Sub-urban area Field survey	$n = 183$ aged ≥ 60 years	33.3 %	Functional disorders: 27.6 % (including depression in 20.8 %); organic psychosis: 6.4 %; functional psychosis: 1.7 %
Venkoba Rao et al. (1982)	Clinical interview	Sub-urban area	$n = 686$ Aged ≥ 60 years	8.9 %	Depression seen in 5.9 % 50 % had a physical illness; sensory handicap in 85 %
Venkoba Rao, ICMR task force project, 1984–1988 (Tamil Nadu) (ICMR 2005) ICMR - Indian Council of Medical Research	Use of a screening schedule by trained multi-purpose workers and project staff	Rural PHC attendees and Field visits	$n = 1910$ aged ≥ 60 years	8.5 %	Depression (6.9 %) was commonest diagnosis Co-occurring physical illness in almost all
Nandi et al. (1997) (West Bengal)	Case detection schedule (in regional language)	Rural house to house survey	$n = 183$ aged ≥ 60 years	61.2 %	Prevalence more in women(77.6 %) than men (44.2 %) Depression commonest diagnosis (55.2 %)
Tiwari et al. (1998) (Uttar Pradesh)	Screening by mental health item sheet & ICD-9 diagnosis by a psychiatrist	Rural house to house survey of randomly selected 5 villages	$n = 488$ Aged ≥ 60 years	42.2 % (vs. 4 % in non-geriatric sample from same survey)	Neurotic depression, bipolar depression, anxiety disorder were commonest diagnosis

(continued)

Table 1 (continued)

References/place of study	Instruments	Setting	Sample	Prevalence	Profile
Tiwari et al. (2009) (Uttar Pradesh)	Screening (HMSE, SPAS/MDQ) & diagnosis by CAMDEX-R, SCAN	Urban, house to house survey	Aged $\geq$ 60 years	17.3 %	Depression commonest diagnosis Cognitive disorders: 5.6 %
Tiwari et al. (2010) (Uttar Pradesh)	Screening (HMSE, SPAS/MDQ) & diagnosis by CAMDEX-R, SCAN	Rural, house to house survey	$n = 2324$ (aged $\geq$ 60 years) and $n = 390$ (55–59 years)	23.5 % in elderly (vs. 18.2 % in pre-elderly)	Among elderly, affective disorders (7.6 %), MCI (4.6 %), organic mental disorders (2.7 %), substance use disorders (4.1 %), neurotic/stress-related (2 %)
Seby et al. (2011) (Maharashtra)	GHQ-12; geriatric depression scale, CAGE; MMSE	Urban house to house survey	$n = 202$ aged $\geq$ 65 years	26.7 %	Depression(16.3 %), cognitive impairment(15 %), anxiety (6.4 %), bipolar (2.5 %), alcohol use disorder (4 %), schizophrenia (1.5 %) Physical illness in over two-third

5.2 Studies on Mental and Behavioural Disorders in Indian Elderly

5.2.1 Depression

Some community surveys have specifically looked for depression among elderly population (Rajkumar et al. 2009; Barua and Kar 2010; Deshpande et al. 2011; Reddy et al. 2012). These are summarized in Table 2. Between 21.7 and 47 % of elderly screened positive for depression, while a more definitive diagnosis of depression was found in 12.7–19 % of elderly.

Depression is also common among elderly users visiting the general health settings and those residing in old age homes (Dey et al. 2001; Tiwari et al. 2012 Ganguli et al. 1999). For use in illiterate elderly, Ganguli et al. (1999) developed and validated a Hindi version of the geriatric depression scale (GDS-H).

The prevalence rates of depression in elderly are considerably higher than the general population rates in India (very low to 15 %) (Reddy and Chandrashekhar 1998; Poongothai et al. 2009). Further, the prevalence is also higher than the elderly residing in other countries of Asia, America and Europe. A meta-analysis of 74 community-based surveys of elderly population across the world (including 6 Indian surveys) found that the proportion of depressed elderly in India was higher compared to rest of the world (Barua et al. 2010). Further, there appears to be an upward trend in prevalence of elderly depression in India.

Female gender and an advanced age are two non-modifiable risk factors for elderly depression. Several other factors have been found to increase the likelihood of depression, which include illiteracy, financial difficulties, living alone, low social/emotional support, widowhood, economic or physical dependency and presence of chronic physical illnesses or disability of any kind (Barua et al. 2010).

Studies also found that life events, including a perceived family crisis, are an important precipitating event for depression (Agrawal and Jhingan 2002). Venkoba Rao et al. observed that the stressors were related to 'bereavement', 'occupation' and 'family and social relationships' in the 2 years preceding onset. Living in joint families does not, by itself, guarantee a good social integration, as old ones in family can be 'lonely islands' (Venkoba Rao 1981). Having a good social support and having more confidants emerged as protective factors for elderly depression.

Not much work is available on biological aspects of elderly depression. A recent study reported that persons with ApoE4 allele have 4.7 times more risk of developing depression in old age (Sureshkumar et al. 2012).

Some phenomenological differences have been observed in elderly depression, which include an increased agitation, restlessness rather than retardation, rarity of ideas of sin and guilt and a higher somatic presentation. The commonest symptoms of depression in elderly using the 40-item WHO assessment schedule were sadness (93.3 %), somatic symptoms (71 %), suicidal ideas (66.6 %), and among others (Venkoba Rao 1981, 1983). The other manifestations of adult depression, viz. depressed mood, lack of energy and fatigue, decline in work and interest and anorexia have poor discriminatory power for the diagnosis of elderly depression

Table 2 Community surveys for depression in elderly population

Reference and place of study	Instruments	Setting	Sample	Prevalence of depression	Additional findings
Rajkumar et al. (2009) (Tamil Nadu)	Screening by NPI followed by ICD-10 diagnosis	Rural	$N = 1{,}000$ aged $\geq$ 65 years	12.7 %	Low income, hunger, physical illnesses increased the risk of depression
Barua et al. (2010a) (Karnataka)	Screening by WHO—wellbeing index	Rural	$N = 627$ aged $\geq$ 60 years	21.7 %	The study also validated the WHO-wellbeing index against the ICD-10 depression inventory
Deshpande et al. (2011) (Maharashtra)	Screening by 15-item geriatric depression scale (GDS)	Rural, community-based	$N = 180$ aged $\geq$ 60 years	41.1 % likely depression 19 % definite depression	Stressful events, systemic illness/disability and low emotional support seen in depressed elderly
Reddy et al. (2012) (Tamil Nadu)	Geriatric depression scale-short version; MMSE	Rural, ten randomly selected villages	$N = 800$ aged $\geq$ 60 years	47 % depression	More in females, lower social class, oldest old, alone and dependent subjects Cognitive (43 %) and sleep(36 %) impairments common

References Rajkumar et al. (2009), Barua and Kar (2010), Deshpande et al. (2011), Reddy et al. (2012)

(Khandelwal 1995, 2001). The depressed elderly are more likely to have undiagnosed physical disorders and multiple illnesses compared to controls (Sagar et al. 1992). The use of a substance or abuse of a prescription medication should be asked specifically from elderly patients. The medications used for physical conditions need an enquiry for their potential to cause or aggravate depression (Sagar et al. 1990).

The course and outcome of depression remain under-researched in Indian elderly. In a one-year follow-up of 50 elderly patients with depression, 28 % had recovered, 30 % partially recovered, 23 % had intermittent relapses, 6 % had been continuously ill, 11 % had died, and 6 % had dementia (Jhingan et al. 2001). Factors predicting a good outcome were shorter duration of episode and those living in joint families.

5.2.2 Mania

Mania appears to be uncommon in elderly surveys. In a recent descriptive study of 30 elderly with mania, 50 % had delusions and/or hallucinations (Prakash et al. 2009). The psychotic and cognitive symptoms were higher in elderly mania compared to depression. A significant proportion had neurological disorders (10 %), substance abuse (53.3 %) and medical comorbidity (66.6 %). Venkoba Rao (1983), in his series of elderly patients with affective disorders, found that depression occurred thrice more common after 60 years than mania (3:1) (Venkoba Rao 1983). Few case reports are available which have described an unusually late age of onset or an association with hyperthyroidism (Aggarwal et al. 2010; Nath and Sagar 2001). A thorough examination and investigations are required in late-onset cases of mania to rule out secondary causes. Safety profile appeared to be main consideration in choosing a medication.

Overall, mania in elderly is an uncommon clinical presentation and needs more research attention.

5.2.3 Anxiety Disorders

Anxiety disorders were common in community surveys of elderly, point prevalence ranging between 6.4 and 10.4 % (refer Table 1). The clinic-based studies have reported neurotic disorders in 5–19.8 % of elderly, a significant proportion of which are likely to be anxiety disorders (Prasad et al. 1996; Singh et al. 2004; Prakash et al. 2007). Not much original research from India is available on other aspects of anxiety disorders in the elderly.

5.2.4 Elderly Suicide

The data derived from various sources e.g. Government of India statistics, suicide prevention centres, suicide autopsies, geropsychiatric clinics and surveys indicate an upward trend in suicide among the elderly. The average annual suicide rate among elderly ($\geq$55 years) is 189 per 100,000 in a study from South India, which is considerably higher than the national average. The male:female ratio was 1.5:1. Further, the age-specific suicide rates increased with advanced age (Abraham et al. 2005).

Among the autopsy cases of elder suicide over a 10-year period ($n = 43$) at a tertiary care centre, the age range was 60–87 years, commonest being 60–69 years age group. Males were over-represented (60 %) in this sample. Hanging, followed by poisoning, appear to be common methods of suicide by elderly (Abraham et al. 2005; Behera et al. 2007). Depressive illness is the leading cause for suicide, and nearly two-thirds of depressed elderly had suicide ideation (Venkoba Rao and Madhavan 1983). Lack of family and social integration is more important risk factor rather than 'living alone'. Certain ethical, religious and familial factors [described as *suicide counters* by Venkoba Rao (1985)] may hold back the person from attempting suicide. Suicides in older people are often associated with high intent, long planning and involve highly lethal methods. Further, elderly are medically fragile and may live alone, thereby increase the probability of a fatal outcome (Suicidal Behaviour in Special Population 2007).

5.2.5 Psychotic Disorders

Very few Indian studies have described psychotic disorders among the elderly population. Venkoba Rao reported a series of patients with *late paraphrenia* (onset after 60 years), which formed about 4 % of geropsychiatric clinic patients. Most had accompanying visual or hearing impairment (Venkoba Rao and Madhavan 1981). The late-onset cases (defined as onset ≥45 years) formed nearly 2 % of all schizophrenia patients presenting to a tertiary care centre in North India over a two-year period. Further, female preponderance was seen in the late-onset cases, with female to male ratio being 1.67:1 among those with onset after 40 years and 10: 1 among those with an onset after 45 years of age (Jayaswal et al. 1987; Jayaswal et al. 1988; Adityanjee et al. 1989; Khandelwal 1999). Another study described the profile of late-onset schizophrenia (mean age: 53.5 years), majority being treatment-naive. Delusion of persecution was universal, followed by delusions of reference in 85 % and, less commonly, hallucinations (Bhuyan et al. 2009; Kulhara et al. 1999; Shaji et al. 2009). Follow-up study of *late paraphrenia* series revealed a sustained remission for 4–5 years in 75 % of patients with treatment (Khandelwal 1999). There is a need for more hospital-based studies for late-onset psychosis.

5.2.6 Substance Use Disorders

Studies on elderly substance use are relatively infrequent. Among rural elderly, the overall prevalence of smoking is 51–71.8 % among males and 5–41 % among females (Goswami et al. 2005; Jotheeswaran et al. 2010; Shaji 2002). In a large-scale population study, the current use of alcohol varied between 10 and 28 % among 50 years plus age groups, majority being current heavy users (Mohan et al. 2002; Gupta et al. 2003). In a clinic-based review, alcohol (60 %) and opioid (35 %) were commonly misused substances (Grover et al. 2005). Individuals over 60 years should be routinely screened for substance use, especially in the presence of depressive symptoms.

In the oldest-old group, substance use is likely to decline. Isolated reports have described continued use of substances e.g. poppy tea dependence in octogenarian age group (Subodh et al. 2010).

5.2.7 Delirium in Elderly

Only a few Indian studies have separately focused on delirium occurring in the geriatric patients (Grover et al. 2009; Pinto 2010). Available studies on delirium in elderly had sample sizes ranging between 100 and 400, from hospital settings. Nearly two-thirds had hospital-emergent delirium (Grover et al. 2012). Hypoactive delirium was relatively common than other forms. Most patients had sleep–wake cycle disturbance, disturbance in orientation, attention and short-term memory impairments, fluctuation of symptoms, temporal onset of symptoms and a physical disorder. Most common aetiologies were sepsis followed by metabolic. The mortality rate was nearly 15–16.5 % (Grover et al. 2012; Chrispal et al. 2010).

There are no specific Indian studies on treatment aspects or long-term course and outcome of elderly post-discharge.

5.2.8 Dementia

Nearly two-thirds of the world's elderly with dementia reside in developing countries (Alzheimer's & Related Disorders Society of India 2010). Several community surveys from India, with samples ranging from 740 to 24,000, have found the prevalence to range between 0.8 and 4.9 % among those aged 65 years and above (Shaji et al. 1996; Rajkumar et al. 1997; Chandra et al. 1998; Vas et al. 2001; Shaji et al. 2005; Mathuranath et al. 2009; Saldanha et al. 2010). Concerns have been raised that milder cases may be missed out, pointing to a need to operationalize the criteria to diagnose dementia in community (Prince et al. 2003). Using the 10/66 dementia research group algorithm, a higher prevalence rate for dementia was found (urban Chennai: 7.5 % and rural Vellore: 10.6 %) (Llibre Rodriguez et al. 2008). Vellore screening instrument was developed after employing the 'activities of daily living', which are not influenced by education and culture and can reduce the false-positive rates in community studies (Stanley et al. 2009).

Few studies are available on the incidence of dementia in Indian settings. It varies between 1.74 and 11.67 per 1,000 person years, which is lower than the Western figures (Chandra et al. 2001; Mathuranath et al. 2009; Raina et al. 2009).

Alzheimer's disease appears to be more common than vascular dementia in some studies, though results are conflicting in Indian studies. The risk factors found in Indian studies include an advanced age, female gender, low socio-economic status, low education, family history, urban living, lack of exercise, depression, presence of diabetes, hypertension and hyperlipidemia. Living in joint families, being married and increased intake of polyunsaturated fats were protective factors (Shaji et al. 1996; Rajkumar et al. 1997; Mathuranath et al. 2009; Saldanha et al. 2010).

The behavioural and psychological symptoms of dementia (BPSD) were described by Khandelwal et al. (1992) in one of the earliest studies from India. The delusion that 'people are stealing thing' was most common (27 %) followed by believing that 'one's house is not one's own' (10 %). Depressive and anxiety, features, agitation, wandering and paranoid ideation were observed to be common features in patients with dementias (Khandelwal et al. 1992; 10/66 dementia research group 2004). BPSD appear to be more common in Alzheimer's disease compared to vascular dementia and have been associated with an increase in caregiver burden (Shaji et al. 2009).

Presence of dementia in elderly is associated with twice the risk of mortality after adjusting for age and gender. The mortality risk is linearly correlated to the severity of cognitive impairment (Jotheeswaran et al. 2010).

Given the huge deficits of mental health resources in country, there is a need to develop locally based, low-cost models of dementia identification, care and support. The local community health workers in rural Kerala could identify the possible dementia cases in community after being trained for 2.5 h only (Shaji 2002). Another study from Goa described a randomized trial of a low-cost home-based intervention, which was feasible, acceptable and led to significant improvements in caregiver mental health and burden (Dias et al. 2008).

5.3 Informal Care Resources: Dementia Caregivers

Family members caring for a disabled elderly may themselves suffer adverse mental health consequences. In a preliminary study on dementia caregivers, Khandelwal and colleague (1996) described reduction of leisure time, social restriction, embarrassment and financial difficulties. The caregiver burden and deterioration in their physical/mental health have been reported in subsequent studies (Shaji et al. 2003; Pattanayak et al. 2010). Females in a household were more often the primary caregivers for elderly with dementia. The multiplicity of roles and responsibilities for a female in a traditionally oriented household may lead to a higher perception of stress among female caregivers, even among those caring for otherwise healthy elderly (Soneja 2013).

The family-based care of elderly is rooted in Indian tradition, but in view of considerable strain on families, there is a need to take steps towards supporting, empowering and strengthening the caregivers.

6 Elderly Welfare in India: Policy and Legal Aspects

The geriatric issues were not high in priority till late 1990s. The year 1999 was declared as the International Year of Older persons by UN general Assembly, and to coincide with the same year, the Ministry of Social Justice and Welfare, Government of India, developed and adopted the National Policy for Older Persons in India (National Policy on Older Persons 1999). The ensuing year (2000) was declared as the National Year of Older Persons by the Government of India.

Various schemes and programmes have been launched under National Policy for Older Persons (National Policy on Older Persons 1999; Panda and Nayak 2012) (see Box 1). The more challenging aspect is the implementation and the extent of coverage of elderly under these schemes.

A recently introduced legislative provision, the Maintenance and Welfare of Parents and Senior Citizens Act (2007) makes it obligatory for children and relatives to provide need-based maintenance for senior citizens, with penal provisions for elder neglect (Maintenance and Welfare of Parents and Senior Citizens Act 2007).

Box 1: Governmental programmes, schemes and initiatives for elderly welfare in India

Ministry of Health

- Linking geriatric health care to National Rural Health Mission (NRHM)
- Separate registration queues for elderly in public hospitals
- Establishment of geriatric medicine clinics in several hospitals
- National Programme for Health Care of Elderly in 11th five-year plan (2007–2012)
  - (a) strengthening of geriatrics centres
  - (b) dedicated facilities at PHC/CHC and at the district hospital, including 10 beds
  - (c) community-based health care, home visits by trained workers under NRHM
  - (d) mainstreaming of AYUSH for geriatric care

Ministry of Social Justice and Welfare

- Setting up of old age pension fund for unorganized sector workers
- Free food grain distribution (10 kg/month) for destitute elderly under Annapurna scheme
- Old age pension for elderly below poverty line (proposed increase from Rs 200/- to Rs 500/- per month, with an equal amount of contribution from state) under National Pension Scheme
- Training and orientation of health professionals (e.g. geriatric care courses by National Institute of Social Defence)
- Assistance for production and distribution of material on geriatric care
- Promotion of healthy ageing and preventive aspects
- Under the Integrated Programme for Older Persons (2008), the capacity building of Panchayati raj institutions/NGOs/self-help groups/voluntary organizations is done through a one-time financial aid meant for any of following:
  - Old age homes; Respite care/continuous care; Dementia care centres; Multi-service centres
  - Mobile medicare units, Physiotherapy clinics, Disability aids
  - Mental health care and specialized care for older persons
  - Helplines and counselling centres; Community awareness and sensitization of younger generation
  - Training of caregivers to older persons
  - Regional resource and training centres
  - Formation of *vridha sangha* (senior citizen associations)

Ministry of Railways (and roadways of some states)

- Concessional railway and air fares
- Reserved/fare concession in some states for bus travel

Ministry of Finance

- Taxation and savings benefits
- Allowing entry into general health insurance schemes till 65 years of age.

7 Future Directions for Geriatric Mental Health in India

The characteristics of Indian elderly population can be summarized as:

- most residing in rural areas, females over-represented
- many participate in workforce well beyond 60 years of age
- a large percentage live in poverty and have no pension/insurance benefits
- majority reside in joint/extended families with children and grandchildren
- subjective health reported to be fair to good in vast majority in spite of physical ailments or disabilities
- mental and behavioural disorders are common (10–40 %), especially depression, anxiety disorders and dementia.
- physical comorbidities are frequent
- inadequate coverage and implementation of welfare policies

The state of geriatric mental health care has to be seen in the context of general mental health care which is still evolving and struggling with a huge deficit of resources and inadequate infrastructure (Soneja 2013; Lipner 2010). The District Mental Health Programme is struggling with issues related to implementation. The future road involves a multi-sectoral collaboration and broad-based approach to elderly care. There is something for all the stakeholders to contribute towards the welfare of elderly mental health. Several different measures are needed at various levels from policy to research to community care (Tiwari and Pandey 2012; Shaji 2004).

As far as geriatric mental health measures are concerned, some of the critical elements are emphasized here:

- *Provision and strengthening of mental health care services which are 'closer to home'*
  Treatment seeking is generally low among elderly. As two-thirds of elderly reside in rural areas, while specialized geriatric care is available only at select few places. Therefore, it is paramount that the availability of mental health services should be closer to the doorsteps at the primary care level. Most elderly suffer from common mental disorders, and the trained primary care staff can provide basic care and counselling. The next 12th five-year plan proposes an expansion of services to all districts and strengthening the primary care. Following would be useful for strengthening of services in community:
  - Awareness and health camps (aimed at both physical and mental health)
  - Local support networks of the caregiver
  - Collaboration with NGOs working in the communities
  - Collaboration with local bodies (panchayati/social sector agencies)
  - Provision/distribution of free essential medicines for mental disorders in elderly
  - Home visits, as needed
- *Integration with National Rural and Urban Health Missions (NRHM/NUHM)*
  There can be some amount of integration with other flagship programmes e.g. NRHM which are already functional. The primary health workers can be sensitized to identify elderly problems. It has been previously observed that, with as little training, these workers can detect dementia in elderly residing in

communities [124] . The early diagnosis can help in early treatment seeking and delay of disability. Similarly, other professionals e.g. physicians can detect and intervene for the mental morbidities after a basic orientation and training.

- *Manpower and resource development*
  It is the most crucial step in ensuring long-term geriatric care. There is a need to incorporate the geriatric care in the curriculum of all professional courses (e.g. MBBS, B.Sc Nursing). Further, there is a need to have separate multi-disciplinary geriatric-specific services in medical colleges and teaching hospitals, which can facilitate the training of students across various disciplines. For professionals already working in the field, there is a need to organize regular short-term training courses (2 weeks) to sensitize and empower them to geriatric care. Dementia care is a specialized area which can be taken up as a diploma course. These teaching/training activities shall need a national coordinating centre as well as resource centres at the regional levels.
- *Research aspects and development of low-cost models of elderly care*
  Most of available research is on epidemiological aspects, and very few studies have evaluated the course and outcomes. The patient and caregiver needs continue to remain under-explored. Further, there is a dearth of studies aimed at evaluating the mental health interventions for elderly patients and their families. Research evidence is needed not only for improving the mental health services, but also to influence policy decisions. There is a need to focus on developing the culturally acceptable, easily deliverable, low-cost models of care of geriatric patients, preferably with involvement of local community.
- *Need for a policy framework for geriatric mental health care*
  There is a need to have a policy framework under which various programmes for mental health of elderly can be initiated and facilitated. The National Policy on Older Persons is geared mainly towards welfare aspects, but not mental health aspects per se. It remains to be seen that how much emphasis has been given to the geriatric aspects in the mental health policy draft.
- *Community participation*
  There are a lot of untapped resources in the community which can be utilized for generating support for the elderly mental health activities. Any community-based programme is successful only if it can be sustained at very low cost and becomes self-sustaining after a while with active contribution of members of community. Dignity Foundation, a not-for-profit non-governmental organization in Mumbai, is such an example. It is a non-profit organisation, committed to changing the way people look at ageing in India. It enables senior citizens to lead active lives through easy access to trusted information, opportunities for productive ageing and social support services. Similarly, HelpAge India is another not-for-profit organization which has been actively working towards elder care, protection of their rights, promotion of awareness and advocacy for issues related to aged population.
- *Support and strengthen the family-based caregiving for elderly*
  Indian family system is supportive and extends care to elderly, both during health and illness. However, there is a need to strengthen these informal care resources which are providing almost all of geriatric chronic care in the country. The local NGOs can be involved for empowering the caregivers to carry out

caregiving activities by providing information/technological help devices and caregiver networks can be strengthened to extend emotional support to each other. Certain governmental initiatives are needed for supporting the caregivers who take on the role of caring for chronically disabled elderly.

- *Promotion of elderly as a useful resource rather than burden*
  In the long term, the younger generations in India will be providing care to elderly of future. There is a need to promote the value of aged as a repertoire of experience and wisdom. Often, there is a tendency to view elderly as a burden on society, which is not true. Many elderly males continue to be a part of workforce, working part time or full time. Elderly contribute to supervision of household, child-rearing functions, social welfare activities and participate in local community matters. It is pertinent that elderly are protected and promoted as valuable resources in the coming generations as well.

8 Conclusion

Families form the backbone of elderly care in India, but with familial and societal changes, the elderly care may pose a problem in the times to come. Further, caregivers do experience considerable burden and receive very little external support. There is a need for a broad-based, multi-sector approach to geriatric mental health care. The elderly welfare measures initiated by government are far from adequate. The critical elements for future geriatric mental health care would involve strengthening of primary care services, integration and collaboration, training and manpower development, community involvement and most importantly, strengthening the traditional family-based system of care of elderly.

The ages roll
Forward; and forward with them, draw my soul
Into time's infinite sea.
And to be glad, or sad, I care no more;
But to have done, and to have been, before I cease to do and be.

Owen Meredith (Lord Lytton), The Wanderer, Book IV, A Confession and Apology, Stanza 9.

References

Census of India. (2011). *Office of Registrar General and Census Commissioner of India*. New Delhi: Ministry of Home Affairs, Government of India.

10/66 dementia research group. (2004). Behavioral and psychological symptoms of dementia in developing countries. *International Psychogeriatrics, 16*, 441–459.

Abraham, V. J., Abraham, S., & Jacob, K. S. (2005). Suicide in the elderly in Kaniyambadi block, Tamil Nadu, South India. *International Journal of Geriatrics Psychiatry, 20*, 953–955.

Adityanjee, J. S. K., Lal, K. P., & Khandelwal, S. K. (1989). Late-onset schizophrenia: An Asian study. *Schizophrenia Bulletin, 15*, 171–173.

Ageing in India. (2003). In A. B Dey (Ed.), *Situation analysis and planning for the future*. Ministry of Health and Family Welfare, New Delhi.

Aggarwal, A., Kumar, R., Sharma, R. C., & Sharma, D. D. (2010). First episode mania at 75 years of age. *Indian Journal of Psychological Medicine, 32*, 144–145.

Agrawal, N., & Jhingan, H. P. (2002). Life events and depression in elderly. *Indian Journal of Psychiatry, 44*, 34–40.

Alzheimer's & Related Disorders Society of India. (2010). In K. S. Shaji, A. T. Jotheeswaran, N. Girish, S. Bharath, A. Dias, M. Pattabiraman, et al. (Eds.), *The dementia India report: Prevalence, impact, costs and services for Dementia*. New Delhi: ARDSI.

Barua, A., Ghosh, M. K., Kar, N., & Basilio, M. A. (2010a). Distribution of depressive disorders in the elderly. *Journal of Neurosciences in Rural Practice, 1*, 67–73.

Barua, A., Ghosh, M. K., Kar, N., & Basilio, M. A. (2010b). Socio-demographic factors of geriatric depression. *Indian Journal of Psychological Medicine, 32*, 87–92.

Barua, A., & Kar, N. (2010). Screening for depression in elderly Indian population. *Indian Journal of Psychiatry, 52*, 150–153.

Behera, C., Rautji, R., & Sharma, R. K. (2007). Suicide in elderly: A study in South Delhi (1996–2005). *Indian Journal of Forensic Medicine and Toxicology, 1*, 13–18.

Bhuyan, M., Khandelwal, S. K., & Gupta, S. (2009). A Study of late onset schizophrenia: Clinical characteristics with review of literature. *Delhi Psychiatry Journal, 12*, 84–93.

Census of India. (2001). *Office of registrar general and census commissioner of India*. New Delhi: Ministry of Home Affairs, Government of India.

Chandra, V., Ganguli, M., Pandav, R., Johnston, J., Belle, S., & DeKosky, S. T. (1998). Prevalence of Alzheimer's disease and other dementias in rural India: The Indo-US study. *Neurology, 51*, 1000–1008.

Chandra, V., Pandav, R., Dodge, H. H., Johnston, J. M., Belle, S. H., DeKosky, S. T., et al. (2001). Incidence of Alzheimer's disease in a rural community in India: The Indo-US study. *Neurology, 25*(57), 985–989.

Chrispal, A., Mathews, K. P., & Surekha, V. (2010). The clinical profile and association of delirium in geriatric patients with hip fractures in a tertiary care hospital in India. *Journal of the Association of Physicians of India, 58*, 15–19.

Deshpande, S. S., Gadkari, M., & Raje, S. S. (2011). Screening for depression and its risk factors in geriatric population: A rural community based study. *Asian Journal of Psychiatry, 4*, 284–287.

Dey, A. B., Soneja, S., Nagarkar, K. M., & Jhingan, H. P. (2001). Evaluation of the health and functional status of older Indians as a prelude to the development of a health programme. *National Medical Journal of India, 14*, 135–138.

Dias, A., Dewey, M. E., D'Souza, J., Dhume, R., Motghare, D. D., Shaji, K. S., et al. (2008). The effectiveness of a home care program for supporting caregivers of persons with dementia in developing countries: A randomized controlled trial from Goa, India. *PLoS ONE, 3*(6), e2333.

Ganguli, M., Dube, S., Johnston, J. M., Pandav, R., Chandra, V., & Dodge, H. H. (1999). Depressive symptoms, cognitive impairment and functional impairment in a rural elderly population in India: A Hindi version of the geriatric depression scale (GDS-H). *International Journal of Geriatric Psychiatry, 14*, 807–820.

Goswami, A., Reddaiah, V. P., Kapoor, S. K., Singh, B., Dwivedi, S. N., & Kumar, G. (2005). Tobacco and alcohol use in rural elderly Indian population. *Indian Journal of Psychiatry, 47*, 192–197.

Grover, S., Irpati, A. S., Saluja, B. S., Basu, D., Mattoo, S. K. (2008). Drug dependence in the geriatric age group: A clinic-based study. *German Journal of Psychiatry, 11*, 10–15.

Grover, S., Kate, N., Agarwal, M., Mattoo, S. K., Avasthi, A., Malhotra, S., et al. (2012). Delirium in elderly people: A study of a psychiatric liaison service in north India. *International Psychogeriatrics, 24*(1), 117–127.

Grover, S., Subodh, B. N., Avasthi, A., Chakrabarti, S., Kumar, S., Sharan, P., et al. (2009). Prevalence and clinical profile of delirium: A study from a tertiary care hospital in north India. *General Hospital Psychiatry, 31*, 25–29.

Gupta, P. C., Saxena, S., Pednekar, M. S., & Maulik, P. K. (2003). Alcohol consumption among middle-aged and elderly men: A community study from western India. *Alcohol and Alcoholism, 38*, 327–331.

Jamuna, D. (2000). Ageing in India: Some key issues. *Ageing International, 25*, 16–31.

Jayaswal, S. K., Praveenlal, K., Khandelwal, S. K., & Mohan, D. (1987). Sex difference in the age at symptom onset in schizophrenia. *Indian Journal of Psychological Medicine, 10*, 68–74.

Jayaswal S. K., Adityanjee, J. S. K., & Khandelwal, S. K. (1988). Age of onset of schizophrenia. *The British Journal of Psychiatry, 152*, 428.

Jhingan, H. P., Sagar, R., & Pandey, R. M. (2001). Prognosis of late onset depression in the elderly: A study from India. *International Psychogeriatrics, 13*, 51–61.

Jotheeswaran, A. T., Williams, J. D., Prince, M. J. (2010). Predictors of mortality among elderly people living in a south Indian urban community; a 10/66 Dementia Research Group prospective population-based cohort study, *BioMed Central public health, 10*, 366, doi:10.1186/1471-2458-10-366.

Khandelwal, S. K. (1995). Management of psychogeriatric disorders. In P. Kulhara (Ed.), *Proceedings of the Annual Continuing Medical Education of Indian Psychiatric Society* (pp. 41–50).

Khandelwal, S. K. (1999). Late onset schizophrenia in a developing country. In R. Howard, P. V. Rabins, D. J. Castle (Eds.), *Late onset schizophrenia*. Petersfield UK & Philadelphia USA: Wrightson Biomedical Publishing Ltd.

Khandelwal, S. K. (2001). Depressive disorders in old age. *Journal of the Indian Medical Association, 99*(39), 42–44.

Khandelwal, S. K., Ahuja, G. K., & Gupta, S. (1992). Behavioural symptoms in dementia: Nature and treatment. *Indian Journal of Psychiatry, 34*, 36–40.

Khandelwal, S. K., & Gupta, S. (1996). Caring for dementia suffers: Impact on caregivers (psychological and social consequences). *Journal of Mental Health Human Behavior, 1*, 41–48.

Krishnaswamy, B., Than Sein, U., Munodawafa, D., Varghese, C., Venkataraman, K., & Anand, A. (2008). Aging in India. *Ageing International, 32*, 258–268.

Kulhara, P., Avasthi, A., Sharan, P., Gupta, N., & Rao, S. A. (1999). Late onset schizophrenia versus early onset schizophrenia: A comparison of clinical features. *Indian Journal of Psychiatry, 41*, 333–335.

Lipner, J. (2010). *Hindus: Their religious beliefs and practices*. Abingdon, Oxon. Routledge: Library of Religious Beliefs and Practices.

Llibre Rodriguez, J. J., Ferri, C. P., Acosta, D., Guerra, M., Huang, Y., Jacob, K. S., et al. (2008). Prevalence of dementia in Latin America, India, and China: A population-based cross-sectional survey. *The Lancet, 372*,464–474.

Maintenance and Welfare of Parents and Senior Citizens Act. (2007). *Ministry of social justice and empowerment*, Government of India. Available at: http://socialjustice.nic.in/oldageact.php. Accessed on Jan 30, 2013.

Mathuranath, P. S., Cherian, P. J., Mathew, R., Kumar, S., George, A., Alexander, A., et al. (2009). Dementia in Kerala, South India: Prevalence and influence of age, education and gender. *International Journal of Geriatric Psychiatry, 25*, 290–297.

Mathuranath, P. S., George, A., Ranjith, N., Justus, S., Kumar, M. S., Menon, R., et al. (2012). Incidence of Alzheimer's disease in India: A 10 years follow-up study. *Neurology India, 60*, 625–630.

Mohan, D., Chopra, A., & Sethi, H. (2002). The co-occurrence of tobacco and alcohol in general population of metropolis Delhi. *Indian Journal of Medical Research, 116*, 150–154.

Nandi, P. S., Banerjee, G., Mukherjee, S. P., Nandi, S., & Nandi, D. N. (1997). A study of psychiatric morbidity of the elderly population of a rural community in West Bengal. *Indian Journal of Psychiatry, 39*, 122–129.

Nath, J., & Sagar, R. (2001). Late-onset bipolar disorder due to hyperthyroidism. *Acta Psychiatrica Scandinavica, 104*, 72–75.

National Policy on Older Persons. (1999). Ministry of social justice and empowerment, Government of India. Available at: socialjustice.nic.in/hindi/pdf/npopcomplete.pdf. Accessed on Jan 30, 2013.

National Sample Survey. (2004). *Morbidity, health care and the condition of the aged. 60th round (Jan–June 2004): National Sample Survey Office*. Ministry of Statistics and Programme Implementation, Government of India.

Newton, D., Erikson, E. (2007). In: B. J. Sadock, V. A. Sadock, P. Ruiz (Eds.), *Kaplan and Sadock's comprehensive textbook of psychiatry* (9th ed.). (pp. 838–847). Philadelphia: Wolter Kluwer/Lippincott Williams & Wilkins.

Panda, B., Nayak, L. M. (2012). National and international approaches to reduce vulnerability among elderly in India. *Indian Streams Research Journal*. Available at: http://www.isrj.net/publishArticles/883.pdf. Accessed on Jan 30, 2013.

Pattanayak, R. D., Jena, R., Tripathi, M., & Khandelwal, S. K. (2010). Assessment of burden in caregivers of Alzheimer's disease from India. *Asian Journal of Pyschiatry, 3*, 112–116.

Pinto, C. (2010). Indian research on acute organic brain syndrome. *Delirium, 52*, 139–147.

Poongothai, S., Pradeepa, R., Ganesan, A., & Mohan, V. (2009). Prevalence of depression in a large urban South Indian population—The Chennai urban rural epidemiology study (CURES-70). *PLoS ONE, 4*, E7185.

Prakash, O., Gupta, L. N., Singh, V. B., Singhal, A. K., & Verma, K. K. (2007). Profile of psychiatric disorders and life events in medically ill elderly: Experiences from geriatric clinic in Northern India. *International Journal of Geriatric Psychiatry, 22*, 1101–1105.

Prakash, O., Kumar, C. N., Shivakumar, P. T., Bharath, S., & Varghese, M. (2009). Clinical presentation of mania compared with depression: Data from a geriatric clinic in India. *International Psychogeriatrics, 21*, 764–767.

Prasad, K. M. R., Sreenivas, K. N., Ashok, M. V., & Bagchi, D. (1996). Psychogeriatric patients—A sociodemographic and clinical profile. *Indian Journal of Psychiatry, 38*, 178–181.

Prince, M., Acosta, D., Chiu, H., Scazufca, M., & Varghese, M. (2003). Dementia diagnosis in developing countries: A cross-cultural validation study. *The Lancet, 361*, 909–917.

Raina, S., Pandita, K. K., & Razdan, S. (2009). Incidence of dementia in a Kashmiri migrant population. *Annals of Indian Academy of Neurology, 12*, 154–156.

Rajkumar, S., Kumar, S., & Thara, R. (1997). Prevalence of dementia in a rural setting: A report from India. *International Journal of Geriatric Psychiatry, 12*, 702–707.

Rajkumar, A. P., Thangadurai, P., Senthilkumar, P., Gayathri, K., Prince, M., & Jacob, K. S. (2009). Nature, prevalence and factors associated with depression among the elderly in a rural south Indian community. *International Psychogeriatrics, 21*, 372–378.

Raju, S. S. (2011). Studies on ageing in India: A Review, BKPAI Working Paper No. 2, United Nations Population Fund (UNFPA), New Delhi.

Ramachandran, V., Sarda Menon, M., & Arunagiri, S. (1982). Sociocultural factors in late onset depression. *Indian Journal of Psychiatry, 24*, 268–273.

Ramachandran, V., Sarda Menon, M., & Ram Murthi, B. (1979). Psychiatric disorders in subjects aged over fifty. *Indian Journal of Psychiatry, 21*, 193–198.

Reddy, M. V., & Chandrashekhar, C. R. (1998). Prevalence of mental and behavioural disorders in India: A metaanalysis. *Indian Journal of Psychiatry, 40*, 149–157.

Reddy, N. B., Pallavi, M., Reddy, N. N., Reddy, C. S., Singh, R. K., & Pirabu, R. A. (2012). Psychological morbidity status among the rural geriatric population of Tamil Nadu, India: A cross-sectional study. *Indian Journal of Psychological Medicine, 34*, 227–231.

Sagar, R. S., Mohan, D., Kumar, V., & Khandelwal, S. K. (1990). Elderly depressives: Use of medicines with a potential to cause depression. *Indian Journal of Psychiatry, 32*, 64–68.

Sagar, R. S., Mohan, D., Kumar, V., Khandelwal, S. K., & Nair, P. G. (1992). Physical illnesses among elderly psychiatric out-patients with depression. *Indian Journal of Psychiatry, 34*, 41–45.

Saldanha, D., Mani, M. R., Srivastava, K., Goyal, S., & Bhattacharya, D. (2010). An epidemiological study of dementia under the aegis of mental health program, Maharashtra, Pune. *Indian Journal of Psychiatry, 52*, 131–139.

Seby, K., Chaudhury, S., & Chakraborty, R. (2011). Prevalence of psychiatric and physical morbidity in an urban geriatric population. *Indian Journal of Psychiatry, 53*, 121–127.

Shaji, K. S., Arun Kishore, N. R., & Lal, P. (2002). Revealing a hidden problem: An evaluation of a community dementia case-finding program from the Indian 10/66 dementia research network. *International Journal of Geriatric Psychiatry, 17*, 222–225.

Shaji, K. S., Arun Kishore, N. R., Praveen Lal, K., Pinto, P., & Trivedi, P. K. (2004). Better mental health care for older people in India. *Indian Journal of Psychiatry, 46*, 367–372.

Shaji, S., Bose, S., & Kuriakose, S. (2009a). Behavioral and psychological symptoms of dementia: A study of symptomatology. *Indian Journal of Psychiatry, 51*, 38–41.

Shaji, S., Bose, S., & Verghese, A. (2005). Prevalence of dementia in an urban population in Kerala, India. *The British Journal of Psychiatry, 186*, 136–140.

Shaji, K. S., George, R. K., Prince, M. J., & Jacob, K. S. (2009b). Behavioral symptoms and caregiver burden in dementia. *Indian Journal of Psychiatry, 51*, 45–49.

Shaji, S., Promodu, K., Abraham, T., Roy, K. J., & Verghese, A. (1996). An epidemiological study of dementia in a rural community in Kerala, India. *The British Journal of Psychiatry, 168*, 745–749.

Shaji, K. S., Smitha, K., Lal, K. P., & Prince, M. J. (2003). Caregivers of people with Alzheimer's disease: A qualitative study from the Indian 10/66 Dementia Research Network. *International Journal of Geriatric Psychiatry, 18*, 1–6.

Singh, G. P., Chavan, B. S., Arun, P., & Lobraj, S. A. (2004). Geriatric out-patients with psychiatric illnesses in a teaching hospital setting—A retrospective study. *Indian Journal of Psychiatry, 46*, 140–143.

Soneja, S. (2013). Elder abuse in India. Country report for World Health Organization. Helpage India. Available at: http://www.who.int/ageing/projects/elder_abuse/alc_ea_ind.pdf. Accessed on Jan 30, 2013.

Stanley, R., Kuruvilla, A., Kumar, S., Gayathri, K., Mathews, P., Abraham, V., et al. (2009). The Vellore screening instruments and strategies for the diagnosis of dementia in the community. *International Psychogeriatrics, 21*, 539–547.

Subodh, B. N., Murthy, P., Chand, P. K., Arun, K., Bala, S. N., Benegal, V., et al. (2010). A case of poppy tea dependence in an octogenarian lady. *Drug and Alcohol Review, 29*, 216–218.

Suicidal Behaviour in Special Population. (2007). Elderly, women and adolescent in special reference to India. *Delhi Psychiatry Journal, 10*, 106–118.

Sureshkumar, R., Bharath, S., Jain, S., Prakash, O., Purushottam, M., Thennarasu, K., et al. (2012). ApoE4 and late onset depression in Indian population. *Journal of Affective Disorders, 136*, 244–248.

Tiwari, S. C., Kar, A. M., Singh, R., Kohli, V. K., & Agarwal, G. G. (2009). *An epidemiological study of prevalence of neuro-psychiatric disorders with special reference to cognitive disorders, amongst (urban) elderly—Lucknow study*. New Delhi: ICMR Report.

Tiwari, S. C., Kar, A. M., Singh, R., Kohli, V. K., & Agarwal, G. G. (2010). *An epidemiological study of prevalence of neuro-psychiatric disorders with special reference to cognitive disorders, amongst (rural) elderly-Lucknow study*. New Delhi: ICMR Report.

Tiwari, S. C., & Pandey, N. M. (2012). Status and requirements of the geriatric mental health services in India. *Indian Journal of Psychiatry, 54*, 8–14.

Tiwari, S. C., Pandey, N. M., & Singh, I. (2012). Mental health problems among inhabitants of old age homes: A preliminary study. *Indian Journal of Pyshicatry, 54*, 144–148.

Tiwari, S. C., & Srivastava, S. (1998). Geropsychiatric morbidity in rural Uttar Pradesh. *Indian Journal of Psychiatry, 40*, 266–273.

United Nations. (2002). *World Population Ageing: 1950–2050*. United Nations, Washington, DC: Department of Economic and Social Affairs.

United Nations. (2013). *World population prospects*: *The 2010 revision* (population division, department of economic and social affairs, United Nations, Washington DC). Available at: http://esa.un.org/wpp/. Accessed on Jan 30, 2013.

Vas, C. J., Pinto, C., Panikker, D., Noronha, S., Deshpande, N., Kulkarni, L., et al. (2001). Prevalence of dementia in an urban Indian population. *International Psychogeriatrics, 13*, 439–450.

Venkoba Rao, A. (1981). Mental health and aging. *Indian Journal of Psychiatry*, *23*,11–20.

Venkoba Rao, A. (1983). Depression and suicide behavior in the aged. *Indian Journal of Psychiatry*, *25*, 251–259.

Venkoba Rao, A. (1985). Suicide in the elderly. *Indian Journal of Social Psychiatry*, *1*, 3–10.

ICMR (2005). ICMR task force project, A Study on Health care of the rural aged. 1984–1988. *Mental Health Research in India* (pp. 13–15). Technical monograph on ICMR mental health services. Division of non-communicable diseases, Indian Council of Medical Research.

Venkoba Rao, A. & Madhavan,T. (1981). Late Paraphrenia (A report from geropsychiatric clinic, Madurai, India). *Indian Journal of Psychiatry, 23,* 291–297.

Venkoba Rao, A. & Madhavan, T. (1982). Geropsychiatric morbidity survey in a semi-urban area near Madurai. *Indian Journal of Psychiatry. 24*, 258–262.

Venkoba Rao, A. & Madhavan, T. (1983). Depression and suicide behaviour in the aged. *Indian Journal of Psychiatry*, *25,* 251–259.

Wig, N. N. (2010). In K. J. S Chatrath (Ed.) *The joy of mental health*: *Some popular writings of Dr NN Wig*. Mental Health Forum Servants of the People Society, Chandigarh.

Chapter 26
A Perspective on Marital and Psychosexual Disorders in India

A. Avasthi, S. Sarkar and S. Grover

1 Introduction

Marital and psychosexual problems are among the more common disorders, but are infrequently brought to clinical attention. Issues of privacy and a general embarrassment in discussing marital and psychosexual problems often lead to overlooking these problems and disorders in clinical settings. The patient may not volunteer information, particularly if adequate efforts are not made to put the patient at ease. At the same time, marital and psychosexual disorders are a cause of intense distress to the patient as well as his or her partner. These disorders are a cause of concern for patients for several reasons and affect their day-to-day functioning. Hence, there is a need for dealing with these disorders in an appropriate manner.

Sexual problems are common in both males and females (Simons and Carey 2001). These disorders are present in populations who seek medical help, as well in those who do not seek medical help. Initial studies from India suggested a rate of sexual dysfunction of around 10 % in psychiatric outpatient services (Bagadia et al. 1972; Nakra 1971). The rates may be even higher in patients being treated with psychotropic medications (Krishna et al. 2011). Patients with psychosexual disorders are often referred from other specialties like urology. A large proportion of these patients can be helped effectively.

Similarly, marital problems are common in cohabitating couples. When two people live together, there are bound to be instances when opinions differ, and differences expressed verbally and non-verbally. A successful marriage requires a considerable

A. Avasthi, Professor; S. Sarkar, Senior Resident; S. Grover, Assistant Professor

A. Avasthi (✉) · S. Sarkar · S. Grover
Department of Psychiatry, Postgraduate Institute of Medical Education and Research, Chandigarh, India
e-mail: drajitavasthi@yahoo.co.in

S. Malhotra and S. Chakrabarti (eds.), *Developments in Psychiatry in India*,
DOI 10.1007/978-81-322-1674-2_26

degree of adjustment, and either of the partners may be unwilling or unable to adjust. The difficulties in adjustment can manifest in many ways—as an outburst on the other partner, or a silent displeasurable suffering, or a combination of the two. Though intermittent tiffs are common among most couples, matters spiral downwards when relations deteriorate, at times to physically alarming proportions. Marital functioning has been seen to be impaired in psychiatric patients (those suffering from depression or dysthymia), as compared to healthy controls (Subodh et al. 2008).

This chapter primarily discusses the research arising from India on various aspects of psychosexual disorders and marital problems. The epidemiology of psychosexual disorders is discussed, and sexual attitudes and knowledge in the Indian scenario are delved into. Thereafter, the *Dhat syndrome*, a culture-bound sexual neurosis of India, is explored. Other issues, which are covered, include the effect of psychosexual disorders on the spouses and on marital functioning, women's sexual issues and role of psychotropics in causing sexual dysfunction. Finally, psychological and pharmacological treatments for the psychosexual and marital disorders are touched upon.

2 Epidemiology of Psychosexual Disorders

Having an estimate of the problem of sexual dysfunction would help in understanding the gravity of the situation and would also help in planning concerted efforts made to deal with the issue. However, drawing accurate inferences about the prevalence of sexual disorders is a challenging task. Patients with sexual disorders may not be forthcoming due to a general secrecy about the matter. Also, the quality of sexual experience is a subjective concept and comparing sexual functioning between individuals poses difficulties in ascertainment. Moreover, some conditions, which are encountered in clinical settings in India (e.g. apprehension about sexual potency), do not find mention in the current diagnostic systems (Kulhara and Avasthi 1995). Nonetheless, many clinic-based studies (Bagadia et al. 1972; Nakra 1971; Nakra et al. 1978, 1977) have been conducted in India looking at the rates of sexual disorders, primarily erectile dysfunction and premature ejaculation.

In one of the earlier studies, Bagadia et al. (1972) evaluated cases coming with complaints of sexual dysfunction to a teaching hospital in the general outpatient setting. They found that in the married group of patients, impotence, premature ejaculation and passage of semen in the urine were the most frequent presenting complaints. In the unmarried group, nocturnal emission and passage of semen in urine were the commonest presenting complaints.

Nakra and colleagues (Nakra 1971; Nakra et al. 1978, 1977) studied sexual disorders in male subjects and found that these were present in 9.2 % of all patients seen in the psychiatric outpatient. The commonest disorder was impotence, followed by premature ejaculation. Nearly 20 % of the patients were diagnosed as having the *Dhat syndrome*. Sexual behaviours of patients prior to the development of sexual problems were also explored (Nakra et al. 1978). It was found that nearly 75 % of the patients had practiced masturbation before developing the sexual problems, and a sizeable number of them had associated guilt. Nocturnal emissions were reported by 95 % of the subjects with 60 % of them having associated guilt feelings. Loss of semen was thought to be injurious to health by 64 % of the participants.

A study from the Postgraduate Institute of Medical Education and Research (PGIMER) explored the prevalence of various sexual disorders in 66 patients attending a marital and psychosexual clinic (MPC) (Avasthi et al. 1994). Erectile dysfunction was the main diagnosis in 30 % of the cases, premature ejaculation in 12 % of cases and a combination of erectile dysfunction and premature ejaculation in 45 % of the cases. Nearly 38 % of the patients dropped out even before treatment was instituted. Initial dropout was associated with chronic and continuous sexual dysfunction. Of those patients who could be treated, about 44 % had improvement. It was observed that better outcome was associated with the greater number of visits to the clinic. Better short-term outcome (within 1 year) indicated good long-term outcome (at 7 years). Another study examined the prevalence of various sexual disorders in a set of 464 new patients examined in the MPC of PGIMER over a period of 7 years (Avasthi et al. 1998a). It was observed that erectile dysfunction was the most common disorder encountered, closely followed by a combination of erectile dysfunction and premature ejaculation. Marital discord was present in 8 % of the patients. A fifth of the patients dropped out of treatment after evaluation, before therapy could be instituted. Of the patients who followed up, about 30 % had partial and complete improvement, while no improvement was noticed in about 40 % of the patients.

In another study from Ranchi, Kar and Varma (1978) looked at the sexual and marital functioning in patients with psychiatric disorders and compared them to controls who were the healthy relatives of these patients. They found that patients with psychiatric disorders had greater rates of premature ejaculation and erectile dysfunction at the time of consummation of marriage. The state of marriage was described to be unpleasant by a considerably greater number of patients than controls. In another clinical sample attending a psychosexual clinic, premature ejaculation was reported to be the commonest disorder encountered, followed by erectile dysfunction study (Kendurkar et al. 2008). Certain other studies focusing on specialised groups like opioid- and alcohol-dependent patients have found significant rates of sexual dysfunction in these group of patients (Arackal and Benegal 2007; Mattoo et al. 2010; Ramdurg et al. 2012). It is thus evident from the literature that sexual dysfunction is a common reason for seeking psychiatric consultation in India and that premature ejaculation and erectile dysfunction are the commonest disorders encountered.

3 Sexual Knowledge and Attitudes

In any culture, the way sexuality is discussed or remains a taboo determines the knowledge people have about sexual matters. Inadequate sexual knowledge can give rise to misconceptions and doubts, leading to untamed curiosity or frustration. It may also cause embarrassment or confusion about sexual matters. Since a degree of apprehension surrounds any discussion of sexuality, more so in the Indian culture, the knowledge about sexual matters in both the genders may be questionable. Also, the attitude towards sexual matters, which includes beliefs, liking–disliking as well as action tendencies, may differ between people with the same degree of knowledge. Clinical experience suggests that in many cases of psychosexual disorders, sexual ignorance, misconceptions and attitudes play a significant role in the causation and perpetuation of the disorder. Hence, understanding a person's knowledge and attitude towards sexuality is useful for treatment planning.

One of the earlier studies (Singh et al. 1987) aimed to find the differences in sexual attitudes and knowledge in medical and non-medical postgraduate students. The investigators assessed sexual knowledge and attitude using a modified version of Sexual Knowledge and Attitude Test (SKAT) among male hostel-residing students at Panjab University and PGIMER, Chandigarh. The results showed that as compared to medical students, non-medical students had poorer knowledge and a relatively conservative attitude towards sexual matters. This suggested that knowledge and attitude differences existed between medical and non-medical students, presumably due to exposure to accurate anatomical and physiological information among medical students.

Various scales have been in vogue for measuring sexual knowledge and attitude. The Sex Knowledge and Attitude Questionnaire II (SKAQ II) was among the first such validated instrument developed in India. It was developed after Hindi translation of SKAT was done to create SKAQ I. The numbers of items were reduced further to yield a 55-item scale in Hindi. This well-validated scale measures sexual knowledge and attitudes (Avasthi et al. 1992). Out of the 55 items, 35 pertain to sexual knowledge (rated in a 'yes' or 'no' format) and 20 to sexual attitudes (rated on a Likert scale). The scale is easy to administer and score. Higher scores reflect a greater knowledge and a liberal attitude. Test–retest reliability of the test has been evaluated in a sample of 60 subjects (20 with psychosexual disorder, 20 normal males and 20 normal females) and was found to be fair. The validity of the scale was checked in 80 subjects (20 experts, 20 patients with psychosexual disorders, 20 normal males and 20 normal females). It was seen that males were more liberal in their attitudes towards sex than females, and experts had the most liberal attitudes among all the groups (Avasthi et al. 1992).

A scale has also been developed to assess the knowledge and attitude towards condoms (Avasthi et al. 1998b). This scale has a special relevance with the increasing number of patients with sexually transmitted diseases (STDs) and acquired immunodeficiency syndrome (AIDS). The scale was developed by pooling items relating to the awareness and attitudes towards condoms. The final form of the scale had 62 items: 26 items pertaining to knowledge and answered in a 'yes' or 'no' format, and 36 items relating to attitudes rated on 5-point Likert format. The scale was field-tested in a set of 60 healthy controls, 30 patients with STDs and 15 resident doctors. The scale was found to have good validity and reliability (Avasthi et al. 1998b).

A study was conducted at the PGIMER (Avasthi et al. 2005) to evaluate the impact of sexual knowledge and attitude on treatment outcome. The sample comprised of patients with premature ejaculation, erectile dysfunction or the combination of two. Knowledge and attitude was measured using the SKAQ. It was seen that patients in all the three groups had poor knowledge and a conservative attitude towards sexual matters. There were no significant relationship between the overall knowledge and attitude scores and the outcome. In an effort to improve the sexual knowledge of subjects attending the clinic, a guide book on sex education was developed by Avasthi and Banerjee (2002).

4 Dhat Syndrome: A Culture-Bound Neurosis in India

The term *Dhat syndrome* was coined by Prof Wig (1960), referring to a common culture-bound preoccupation with loss of semen in the Indian subcontinent. It is considered a form of culture-bound sexual neurosis (Bhatia and Malik 1991), which commonly affects young adult and adolescent males.

The evolution of the concept of *Dhat syndrome* can be traced to the teachings of Ayurveda. Ayurveda states that there are seven essential components of the body (the seven *Dhatus*). Semen is considered as the most concentrated and precious of these components. It is said that 40 meals make one drop of blood, 40 drops of blood make one drop of marrow and 40 drops of marrow make one drop of semen. *Sushrut samhita* writes that loss of semen in any form leads to draining of physical and mental energy. *Charak samhita* describes a disorder of *shukrameha* (draining of the semen), an entity similar to the present-day *Dhat syndrome*. Thus, ancient scriptures give paramount importance to conservation of semen.

The *Dhat syndrome* is usually presented as the loss of semen in young men, while passing urine or straining for stools. The associated symptoms commonly include vague and multiple somatic and psychological complaints like fatigue, listlessness, loss of appetite, lack of physical strength, poor concentration and forgetfulness (Avasthi and Jhirwal 2005). These symptoms are usually accompanied by anxious or dysphoric mood. These patients may also have other disorders of sexual dysfunction, like premature ejaculation or erectile dysfunction. The patient ascribes his symptoms, including sexual dysfunction, to the passage of *Dhat* (semen or some whitish substance presumed to be semen) in the urine, or excessive indulgence in sexual activity, masturbation or nocturnal emissions. Apart from a whitish discharge with urine, there are no other urinary symptoms. The patient may insist on passage of semen in the urine, though there is no objective evidence of the presence of semen. Neurotic depression (dysthymia) and generalised anxiety disorder are the commonest disorders encountered in patients with the *Dhat syndrome* (Avasthi and Jhirwal 2005).

The *Dhat syndrome* is encountered not only in India, but also in other countries in the subcontinent like Nepal, Bangladesh and Pakistan (De Silva and Dissanayake 1989; Mumford 1996). Masturbation, excessive indulgence in sexual activities, venereal diseases, urinary tract infections, overeating, constipation, worm infestation, disturbed sleep or genetic factors are believed to be the main aetiological factors (Bhatia and Malik 1991). A majority of the patients get information about the *Dhat syndrome* from friends, colleagues or relatives, whereas some from posters, advertisements in mass media, magazines or quacks. The *Dhat syndrome* has also been described in females (Rajpal et al. 2013; Singh et al. 2001).

Standardised instruments have been developed for the assessment of the *Dhat syndrome* (Grover et al.; Sharan et al. 2003). The Dhat Syndrome Questionnaire (DSQ) is a comprehensive instrument looking at various aspects of the *Dhat syndrome*, including situations of passage of semen, reasons for passage, consequences of passage, accompanying symptoms and common comorbidities (Grover et al. n.d.). The other instrument comprises of 13-item semi-structured questionnaire and is meant to be used as an interview schedule (Sharan et al. 2003).

The treatment of *Dhat syndrome* poses some challenges. Explanation and reassurances do not prove to be of much use as they do not match with the culturally ingrained beliefs. Hence, some workers have recommended emphatic listening, a non-confrontational approach, reassurance and correction of mistaken beliefs, along with the use of placebo, anti-anxiety and anti-depressant medications, wherever required (Wig 1998). A standardised treatment package for single males presenting with the *Dhat syndrome* has been developed (Avasthi and Gupta 2002), which mainly includes sex education and relaxation exercises. Sex education mainly focuses on anatomy and physiology of sexual organs, with reference to masturbation, semen, nocturnal emissions and the functioning of genito-urinary system. Relaxation therapy includes the Jacobson's Progressive Muscular Relaxation Technique along with biofeedback. If there is the presence of associated anxiety or depressive symptoms that may impede the process of therapy, anxiolytics and/or antidepressants can be added for the minimum possible time and in minimum possible doses. This kind of treatment has been found to be quite useful for patients with the *Dhat syndrome*. A cognitive behavioural model of treatment has also been developed and tested for patients with the *Dhat syndrome* and comprises of assessment, psycho education and cognitive behavioural interventions (Abdul Salam et al. 2012).

Occasional case reports have also reported a female counterpart of the *Dhat syndrome,* which is characterised by subjective complaints of excessive passage of discharge per vaginum, associated with complaints of weakness and lethargy. These symptoms are attributed to passage of discharge per vaginum (Singh et al. 2001; Rajpal et al. 2013).

5 Psychosexual Disorders and Effect on Spouses

Sexual intimacy can be considered an integral part of married life and can be a mutually satisfying experience. Hence, sexual disorders are likely to have an impact on the well-being of the marital unit and the spouse may also be affected. Moreover, various forms of marital and sexual therapies require the active cooperation of spouses. Here, we enumerate some studies that have assessed the impact of psychosexual disorders on spouses.

Kumar et al. (1999a, b) assessed the level of distress among wives of patients with psychosexual dysfunction and its relationship to marital adjustment. Their sample comprised of wives of 30 male patients with psychosexual dysfunction. The PGI Health Questionnaire N1 was used to ascertain the physical and psychological distress, the Dyadic Adjustment Scale was used to assess marital functioning, and the Dysfunctional Analysis Questionnaire was used to assess the dysfunction. A majority of the male patients suffered from combination of premature ejaculation and failure of genital response. Wives were found to be significantly more distressed than husbands and exhibited higher degree of psychosocial dysfunction. However, wives still had normal marital adjustment. There was a significant and positive association between distress and psychosocial dysfunction. Marital adjustment showed a significant negative association with both the distress experienced and psychosocial dysfunction. These findings have important implications for the management of these disorders, as wives with more distress were likely to have poorer marital functioning and greater dysfunction.

A study by Avasthi et al. (2010) aimed to examine the psychosexual functioning of spouses of men with non-organic erectile dysfunction in terms of their sexual satisfaction, psychological problems, marital adjustment, quality of life and level of dysfunction. This study was a methodological advancement over the previous study (Kumar et al. 1999a, b). Fifty spouses of men with erectile dysfunction were compared with fifty spouses of men without any psychosexual dysfunction. A wide variety of variables, which could affect sexual functioning were taken into consideration in this study. The Marital Questionnaire was used for assessing marital adjustment, the Quality of Life Enjoyment and Satisfaction Questionnaire was used to assess the degree of enjoyment and satisfaction, the Symptom Questionnaire was used to measure degree of distress and hostility, the Dyadic Adjustment Scale was used to assess marital adjustment, the Dysfunction Analysis Questionnaire was used to measure present level of functioning, and the Sexuality Scale was utilised to assess sexuality. It was seen that spouses of men with erectile dysfunction had significantly lower levels of marital and sexual satisfaction, and higher levels of psychiatric symptoms than controls. Furthermore, spouses of men with non-organic erectile dysfunction also reported poor quality of life in most domains and had a greater level of dysfunction. The study emphasised that spouses of men with erectile dysfunction faced many difficulties, which also need to be recognised and attended to in clinical practice.

From the above studies, it can be postulated that if the psychosexual disorders are treated effectively, it is likely that the psychiatric symptoms, the marital adjustment and the quality of life of the spouse may all improve. In case it is not possible to ameliorate the psychosexual disorders completely, it may still be worthwhile to attempt to reduce the distress and dysfunction in the spouses and offering medical assistance when needed.

6 Female Sexual Health

Female sexual health has been a relatively understudied area in India. Agarwal (1977) reported a case series of 17 females who had frigidity as one of their main complaints. All these patients had sought treatment for neurotic or somatic complaints, except 1 patient who had sought treatment for frigidity. Ignorance regarding sexual activity, fear of pregnancy, marital disharmony, lack of proper residential accommodation, tiredness and poor precoital attention were cited as the factors responsible for frigidity.

Avasthi et al. (1998a) in their descriptive study of the attendees of a special clinic dealing with marital and sexual dysfunctions found that the number of female patients was only 13 out of a total sample of 464 patients (i.e. about 3.5 % of the total attendees). Vaginismus, dyspareunia and lack of sexual desire were the main problems reported.

Singh et al. (2009) assessed the sexual dysfunction in women attending a tertiary care medical clinic in south India. The researchers administered a Tamil version of the Female Sexual Function Index to 149 married women. A high degree of sexual dysfunction was found, and scores above the cut-off were present in two-thirds of the sample. Difficulties with desire were present in 77.2 % subjects; arousal in 91.3 %; lubrication in 96.6 %; orgasm in 86.6 %; satisfaction in 81.2 %; and pain during sexual intercourse in 64.4 %. Greater sexual dysfunction was present with increasing age. Sexual dysfunction was attributed by these women to physical illness in themselves or the partner, relationship problems and cultural taboos. Varghese et al. (2012) evaluated 150 young married clinic-attending women in South India. They found that a third of the sample met DSM-IV criteria for female sexual dysfunction. The common disorders were hypoactive desire (16.67 %), decreased arousal (14.67) and orgasmic disorders (18 %). Women with a diagnosis of sexual disorder had poorer quality of life and impaired social relationships.

Avasthi et al. (2008) conducted a study to assess the sexual functioning in young married women attending the paediatrics outpatient clinic of the PGIMER with non-critically ill children. They found that out of the 100 subjects assessed with the Brief Index of Sexual Functioning for Women and the SKAQ II, most subjects considered sex as an important aspect of life. A majority of the participants were able to communicate their sexual desires to their spouses. More than half of the sample admitted having inhibition or anxiety while performing sexual activity. Most subjects revealed that both partners were satisfied with their sexual relationship. Peno-vaginal intercourse was considered as the most frequent mode of sexual behaviour followed by kissing, foreplay, mutual masturbation and oral sex. A total of 17 % participants encountered one or more difficulties during sexual activities, and the study showed that the females had adequate knowledge and liberal attitudes.

Though there is some literature on female sexual functioning, more comprehensive data in this area are required as women constitute about half of the world population.

7 Impact of Psychotropics and Medical Disorders on Sexual Functioning

Psychotropic medications and medical conditions are known to cause sexual dysfunction. There have been a few studies assessing the impact of psychotropic medications in the Indian population. These have focused upon antipsychotics as well as antidepressants, the two common classes of drugs known to cause sexual dysfunction.

Grover et al. (2012) studied female patients attending the psychiatric outpatient and receiving a single antidepressant. It was seen that 21 % of the women taking antidepressants reported decreased sexual functioning after the initiation of antidepressants. Sexual dysfunction assessed using a structured instrument (the Female Sexual Function Index) revealed that 95 % of the sample had decreased desire, 60 % had decreased arousal, 37.5 % had decreased lubrication, 63.8 % had decreased orgasm, 55 % had decreased satisfaction and 25 % had pain during sexual activity. Problem with lubrication were most frequent with tricyclic antidepressants and problems of orgasm with mirtazapine. Another cross-sectional study of impact of antidepressants on sexual functioning in married women [measured with the Arizona Sexual Experience Scale (ASEX)] showed that sexual dysfunction was present in four-fifths of the sample of 76 patients (Kate et al. 2013).

Nebhinani et al. (2012) assessed the rate and typology of sexual dysfunction in male subjects with psychotic disorders at the PGIMER receiving trifluoperazine, risperidone or olanzapine. This is one of the few studies worldwide, which have assessed sexual dysfunction with more than one scale, i.e. the ASEX, the Psychotropic Related Sexual Dysfunction Questionnaire (PRSexDQ), and the sexual function section of the modified Udvalg for Kliniske Undersøgelser Side Effect Rating Scale (UKU) in the same study population. The rate of sexual dysfunction varied from scale to scale among the subjects (25 % on the ASEX, 37 % on the PRSexDQ and 40 % on the UKU). The rate of sexual dysfunction was highest for risperidone, followed by trifluoperazine and olanzapine. In a study from south India involving 102 subjects using Sexual Functioning Questionnaire (SFQ), Nagaraj et al. (2009) also found that risperidone was associated with greatest extent of sexual dysfunction.

Krishna et al. (2011) attempted to estimate the prevalence and impact of sexual dysfunction in patients with depression in remission and receiving antidepressants. Sexual functioning was assessed in 100 patients using the ASEX. Twenty-three percentage of subjects were found to have sexual dysfunction. 9 subjects had dysfunction in the domain of desire, 5 had arousal difficulty, 6 subjects had problem with erection, and 8 had a problem with orgasm. Sexual dysfunction was associated with poor dyadic adjustment and quality of life. Sexual dysfunction did not translate into impairment in global assessment of functioning scores or poor compliance.

Another study evaluated the quality of life (QoL) of men (using World Health Organization Quality of Life-Bref version-WHOQOL-BREF) with type 2 diabetes mellitus (T2DM) suffering from erectile dysfunction and compared the same for men with diabetes mellitus without erectile dysfunction. Patients with erectile dysfunction had poorer QoL in all domains (except the physical domain); however, the differences between the two groups were significant only for the environmental domain (Avasthi et al. 2011).

Male sexual dysfunction has also been studied in patients attending the Department of Urology at the PGIMER. Lokanadham (1993) studied sexual functioning in patients undergoing prostatectomy and compared them to controls undergoing abdominal surgery. It was found that sexual functioning decreased and impotence occurred more frequently in those undergoing prostatactomy as compared to that of controls. Jagadeesha (1995) compared sexual functioning in males undergoing procedures for urethral strictures. It was observed that optical internal urethrotomy was associated with considerable improvement in a significant proportion of cases.

Thus, over the years, evidence is being consolidated regarding the extent of sexual dysfunction in patients with psychiatric disorders receiving psychotropic medications and patients with medical problems.

8 Treatment Aspects

Treatment of psychosexual and marital disorders requires careful assessment. It is important to undertake detailed assessment of the patient and ascertain the presence of additional psychiatric disorders, which may contribute to the disorder or impair recovery. For psychosexual disorders, it is important to assess for medical causes like diabetes and arteriosclerosis which can explain or contribute to the causation of the disorder. Treatment approaches vary with the type of sexual disorder being encountered and include both pharmacological and psychotherapeutic means. Indian guidelines are available which have been developed on behalf of the Indian Psychiatric Society (Avasthi et al. 2006).

9 Pharmacological

A wide array of pharmacological options is available for treatment of erectile dysfunction. Among the oral agents, sildenafil citrate, a Phosphodiesterase E (PDE5) inhibitor (Avasthi and Biswas 2004), seems to be the most commonly used first-line drug for erectile dysfunction. The medication can be utilised on as-needed basis, about half an hour before the intercourse, and it has a short duration of action. The medication acts on non-adrenergic and non-cholinergic neurons of the corpus cavernosa and releases nitric oxide. It has been shown to be fairly safe and efficacious in many randomised-controlled trials. However, it can cause hypotension in patients with coronary heart diseases receiving nitrates. Other longer-acting PDE5 inhibitors like vardenafil and taladafil are also being used. Lodenafil, mirodenafil, udenafil, sulfoaildenafil and nitrosoprodenafil are the other PDE5 inhibitors that are available.

Other oral drugs that have been used for treatment of erectile dysfunction include yohimbine, trazodone, apomorphine and phentolamine mesylate. Certain intracavernosal injections have been tried for treatment of erectile dysfunction and include phentolamine mesylate, papaverine, vasoactive intestinal peptide and alprostadil (Fallon 1995). Combinations of these agents have been suggested as they might improve outcomes and require lesser amounts of the individual drugs. The intracavernosal injections have the potential side effects of priapism, pain, corporal fibrosis and scar tissue formation. Intraurethral therapy using alprostadil has also been tried in the treatment of erectile dysfunction.

For treatment of premature ejaculation, lidocaine has been utilised among the topical agents and SSRIs and tricyclic antidepressants among the oral medications. Among the SSRIs, fluoxetine and paroxetine have been found to be effective in treatment of premature ejaculation. Meta-analytic data support the efficacy of paroxetine in increasing the intravaginal latency time. Dapoxetine, a newer SSRI with a relatively short duration of action, has been widely utilised in recent times for treatment of premature ejaculation (Buvat et al. 2009). The medication can be used half an hour prior to intercourse on as-needed basis and can be combined with oral erectogenic drug like sildenafil. The drug can avoid the side effects of long-term use of SSRIs. There is some suggestion that PDE5 inhibitors can also be useful in increasing ejaculatory latency.

Judicious use of pharmacological agents can help in effective treatment of psychosexual disorders, especially when combined with psychotherapeutic interventions. However, it must be emphasised that there is a relative lack of studies from India to evaluate patient preference, efficacy and tolerability of these pharmacological agents in India.

10 Psychotherapeutic Measures

Various forms of martial therapy and counselling are available for treating the problems and interpersonal issues encountered in the marital unit (Avasthi and Khurana 2005). The approach can be psychodynamic, cognitive–behavioural, interpersonal, eclectic and others. The techniques used in therapy vary from situation to situation. Psychodynamic therapy would include interpretation of behaviours in the light of past experiences and relationships of each of the partners. Cognitive behavioural measures would typically include emphasis on clear communication between the couple, spending quality time with each other, and trying to resolve contentious issues in an amicable manner. The type of intervention delivered in practice depends upon the theoretical background. Given the wide variety of marital units in different cultural backgrounds in India, ranging from the traditional to the modern, the type of intervention would need to be tailored.

Therapy for psychosexual disorders also often involves the couple. The Masters and Johnson's technique is the most studied technique worldwide for psychosexual disorders, wherein the couple is dealt with by a pair of male and female therapists. Psycho education and selected exercises like caressing, foreplay and sensate focusing are utilised. For premature ejaculation, exercises like the 'start and stop' technique are used. The results of this therapy seem to be quite promising. In the Indian setting, the Masters and Johnson's technique is likely to be utilised in high-income group patients, with liberal attitudes, and with stable partners (Avasthi et al. 2003). Due to peculiar challenges faced in the Indian scenario and high rates of dropout, variations of the Masters and Johnson's technique have been tried. It has been suggested that the dual-sex therapist team as well as the requirement for daily sessions can be dispensed with (Avasthi et al. 2003). However, no systematic studies are available from India exploring efficacy of marital therapy.

Apart from the above, standardised manuals have been developed for the treatment of psychosexual disorders in single males (Avasthi and Gupta 2002). As single men quite often present to the outpatient and are reluctant to bring in sexual partners, or approach for sexual 'weakness', manuals focusing on treatment on single males have significant empirical use. These manuals provide session-wise guidance for intervention with these patients.

Yoga has been tried in India for treatment of psychosexual disorders in both males and females with promising results (Dhikav et al. 2010a, b, 2007). Male and female sexual functioning had improved after a course of yoga in a camp in non-controlled trials (Dhikav et al. 2010a, b). In a comparative trial, it was seen that yoga was as effective, if not better than fluoxetine for premature ejaculation (Dhikav et al. 2007).

11 Further Research and Training

Comparatively less attention has been focused upon marital and psychosexual disorders in the Indian setting. The need and importance of these disorders is reflected in the suggestion to establish a section in Indian Psychiatric Society dealing with sexual medicine (Sathyanarayana Rao and Avasthi 2008). Further research in these disorders is needed.

At present, many studies at the PGIMER are evaluating sexual dysfunction in alcohol- and opioid-dependent patients, and those patients being maintained on pharmacoprophylactic medications like naltrexone, disulfiram and acamprosate. These studies would further our knowledge about sexual dysfunction in these special groups of patients. Studies are also evaluating sexual dysfunction association with mood stabilisers, and impact of sexual dysfunction on drug compliance is also being assessed. Phenomenology of the *Dhat syndrome* and its relationship with alexithymia is being looked into.

Qualitative studies about taboo, practices and biases regarding sexuality can help in enlightening about the cultural aspects of sexuality in India. Large-scale community studies on sexual disorders as well as normal sexuality can help in better understanding of psychosexual functioning in the country. The course of the sexual problems can be better studied from clinic-based cohorts followed up at regular intervals. Treatment studies looking at impact of each component of therapeutic approach (suggestion, education and pharmacotherapy) can be undertaken. Treatment studies of the *Dhat syndrome* can be undertaken with blinded ratings on predefined efficacy measures. Marital issues can be explored in research settings, especially focusing on the distinction that differentiates pathological and normal. The marital typology can be dissected to know what interventions delivered would help a particular marital unit.

Effective help for treatment of psychosexual and marital problems requires some degree of training. Training of personnel, including psychiatrists, general practitioners, nurses as well as paramedical staff, should include awareness about sexual issues and problems. Training should also include ensuring privacy and confidentiality and showing sensitivity in dealing with sexuality and marital discord. Hopefully, with adequate impetus, the distress and dysfunction arising due to psychosexual and marital disorders can be ameliorated and those persons in need can be helped effectively.

References

Abdul Salam, K., Sharma, M., & Prakash, O. (2012). Development of cognitive-behavioral therapy intervention for patients with Dhat syndrome. *Indian Journal of Psychiatry, 54*, 367.

Agarwal, A. (1977). Frigidity—A clinical study. *Indian Journal of Psychiatry, 19*, 31–37.

Arackal, B. S., & Benegal, V. (2007). Prevalence of sexual dysfunction in male subjects with alcohol dependence. *Indian Journal of Psychiatry, 49*, 109–112.

Avasthi, A., Arora, A., Kulhara, P., & Banerjee, S. T. (1998a). A study of psychosexually disordered patients attending a special clinic. *Archives of Indian Psychiatry, 4*, 92–96.

Avasthi, A., & Banerjee, S. T. (2002). *Guide-Book on Sex Education*. PGIMER, Chandigarh: Department of Psychiatry.

Avasthi, A., Basu, D., Kulhara, P., & Banerjee, S. T. (1994). Psychosexual dysfunction in Indian male patients: revisited after seven years. *Archives of Sexual Behavior, 23*, 685–695.

Avasthi, A., & Biswas, P. (2004). Pharmacotherapy of sexual dysfunctions: current status. *Indian Journal of Psychiatry, 46*, 213–220.

Avasthi, A., Grover, S., Bhansali, A., Dash, R. J., Gupta, N., Sharan, P., et al. (2011). Erectile dysfunction in diabetes mellitus contributes to poor quality of life. *International Review of Psychiatry, 23*, 93–99.

Avasthi, A., Grover, S., Kaur, R., Prakash, O., & Kulhara, P. (2010). Impact of nonorganic erectile dysfunction on spouses: A study from India. *The Journal of Sexual Medicine, 7*, 3666–3674.

Avasthi, A., & Gupta, N. (2002). *Standardized management of single males with sexual disorders*. PGIMER, Chandigarh: Department of Psychiatry.

Avasthi, A., Gupta, N., Sharma, P., & Gupta, R. (2005). A study to examine relationship of sexual knowledge and attitude with diagnosis and treatment adherence in male sexual dysfunction. *Journal of Health and Human Behavior, 21*, 12–24.

Avasthi, A., & Jhirwal, O. (2005). The concept and epidemiology of dhat syndrome. *Journal of Pakistan Psychiatric Society, 2*, 6–8.

Avasthi, A., Kaur, R., Prakash, O., Banerjee, A., Kumar, L., & Kulhara, P. (2008). Sexual behavior of married young women: A preliminary study from north India. *Indian Journal of Community Medicine, 33*, 163–167.

Avasthi, A., & Khurana, H. (2005). Family and marital therapies. In J. N. Vyas & S. S. Nathawat (Eds.), *Essentials of Postgraduate Psychiatry* (pp. 842–853). Delhi: Paras Medical Publisher.

Avasthi, A., Nehra, R., Kumar, B., & Persad, D. (1998b). Quantification of knowledge and attitude towards use of condom. *Indian Journal of Clinical Psychology, 25*, 159–164.

Avasthi, A., Rao, T. S. S., Grover, S., Biswas, P., & Kumar, S. (2006) Clinical practice guidelines for management of sexual dysfunctions. *Indian Psychiatric Society*, 114–231.

Avasthi, A., Sharan, P., & Nehra, R. (2003). Practicing behavioral sex therapy in India: Selection, modifications, outcome, and dropout. *Sexuality and Disablity, 21*, 107–112.

Avasthi, A., Varma, V. K., Nehra, R., & Das, K. (1992). Construction and standardization of a sex knowledge and attitude questionnaire (SKAQ), in simple Hindi, for north Indian population. *Indian Journal of Psychiatry, 34*, 24–27.

Bagadia, V., Dave, K., Pradhan, P., & Shah, L. (1972). A study of 258 male patients with sexual problems. *Indian Journal of Psychiatry, 14*, 143–151.

Bhatia, M. S., & Malik, S. C. (1991). Dhat syndrome—A useful diagnostic entity in Indian culture. *British Journal of Psychiatry, 159*, 691–695.

Buvat, J., Tesfaye, F., Rothman, M., Rivas, D. A., & Giuliano, F. (2009). Dapoxetine for the treatment of premature ejaculation: results from a randomized, double-blind, placebo-controlled phase 3 trial in 22 countries. *European Urology, 55*, 957–968.

De Silva, P., & Dissanayake, S. A. W. (1989). The loss of semen syndrome in Sri Lanka: A clinical study. *Sexual and Marital Therapy, 4*, 195–204.

Dhikav, V., Karmarkar, G., Gupta, M., & Anand, K. S. (2007). Yoga in premature ejaculation: a comparative trial with fluoxetine. *Journal of Sexual Medicine, 4*, 1726–1732.

Dhikav, V., Karmarkar, G., Gupta, R., Verma, M., Gupta, R., Gupta, S., et al. (2010a). Yoga in female sexual functions. *Journal of Sexual Medicine, 7*, 964–970.

Dhikav, V., Karmarkar, G., Verma, M., Gupta, R., Gupta, S., Mittal, D., et al. (2010b). Yoga in male sexual functioning: a noncompararive pilot study. *Journal of Sexual Medicine, 7*, 3460–3466.

Fallon, B. (1995). Intracavernous injection therapy for male erectile dysfunction. *The Urologic Clinics of North America, 22*, 833.

Grover, S., Shah, R., Dutt, A., & Avasthi, A. (2012). Prevalence and pattern of sexual dysfunction in married females receiving antidepressants: An exploratory study. *Journal of Pharmacology and Pharmacotherapeutics, 3*, 259–265.

Jagadeesha, B. V. C. (1995). A study of sexual functions in patients of urethral stricture before and after treatment. Thesis submitted to PGIMER, Chandigarh.

Kar, G., & Varma, L. (1978). Sexual problems of married male mental patients. *Indian Journal of Psychiatry, 20*, 365–370.

Kate, N., Grover, S., & Avasthi, A. (2013). Prevalence and type of sexual dysfunction in female patients receiving psychotropic medications. *Indian Journal of Psychiatry*. p.14.17, 55, S117.

Kendurkar, A., Kaur, B., Agarwal, A. K., Singh, H., & Agarwal, V. (2008). Profile of adult patients attending a marriage and sex clinic in India. *The International Journal of Social Psychiatry, 54*, 486–493.

Krishna, K., Avasthi, A., & Grover, S. (2011). Prevalence and psychological impact of antidepressant-associated sexual dysfunction: a study from North India. *Journal of Clinical Psychopharmacology, 31*, 457–462.

Kulhara, P., & Avasthi, A. (1995). Sexual dysfunction on the Indian subcontinent. *International Review of Psychiatry, 7*, 231–239.

Kumar, P., Avasthi, A., & Basu, D. (1999a). Distress in wives of patients with psychosexual dysfunction: an exploratory study. *Indian Journal of Psychiatry, 41*, 24–29.

Kumar, P., Avasthi, A., & Basu, D. (1999b). Distress in wives of psychosexually dysfunctional patients: a correlational study. *Journal of Mental Health and Human Behaviour, 4*, 11–20.

Lokanadham, S. (1993). Impact of prostatectomy on sexual functioning. Thesis submitted to PGIMER, Chandigarh.

Mattoo, S. K., Kumar, V., Aarya, K. R., & Basu, D. (2010). Sexual functioning in substance dependent men attending a deaddiciton centre. *Indian Journal of Psychiatry, 52*, S40.

Mumford, D. B. (1996). The "Dhat syndrome": A culturally determined symptom of depression? *Acta Psychiatrica Scandinavica, 94*, 163–167.

Nagaraj, A. K. M., Pai, N. B., & Rao, S. (2009). A comparative study of sexual dysfunction involving risperidone, quetiapine, and olanzapine. *Indian Journal of Psychiatry, 51*, 265–271.

Nakra, B. (1971). A psychosocial study of male potency disorders. Thesis submitted to PGIMER, Chandigarh.

Nakra, B., Wig, N., & Varma, V. K. (1977). A study of male potency disorders. *Indian Journal of Psychiatry, 19*, 13–18.

Nakra, B., Wig, N., & Varma, V. K. (1978). Sexual behaviour in the adult north Indian male (a study of 150 patients of male potency disorders). *Indian Journal of Psychiatry, 20*, 178–182.

Nebhinani, N., Grover, S., & Avasthi, A. (2012). Sexual dysfunction in male subjects receiving trifluoperazine, risperidone, or olanzapine: Rates vary with assessment questionnaire. *The Primary Care Companion to CNS Disorders, 14*.

Rajpal, N., Kate, N., & Grover, S. (2013). Female dhat syndrome precipitating obsessive compulsive disorder: A case report. *Indian Journal of Psychiatry, 55*, S125.

Ramdurg, S., Ambekar, A., & Lal, R. (2012). Sexual dysfunction among male patients receiving buprenorphine and naltrexone maintenance therapy for opioid dependence. *Journal of Sexual Medicine, 9*, 3198–3204.

Sathyanarayana Rao, T. S., & Avasthi, A. (2008). Roadmap for sexual medicine: Agenda for Indian Psychiatric Society. *Indian Journal of Psychiatry, 50*, 153–154.

Sharan, P., Avasthi, A., Gupta, N., Mohanty, M., Gill, S., & Jain, A. (2003). Development of Dhat syndrome interview schedule. *Indian Journal of Psychiatry, 45*, 88.

Simons, J. S., & Carey, M. P. (2001). Prevalence of sexual dysfunctions: Results from a decade of research. *Archives of Sexual Behavior, 30*, 177–219.

Singh, G., Avasthi, A., & Pravin, D. (2001). Dhat syndrome in a female—A case report. *Indian Journal of Psychiatry, 43*, 345–348.

Singh, R., Malhotra, S., Avasthi, A., & Persad, D. (1987). Sexual knowledge and attitude of medical and non-medical students. *Indian Journal of Social Psychiatry, 3*, 126–136.

Singh, J. C., Tharyan, P., Kekre, N. S., Singh, G., & Gopalakrishnan, G. (2009). Prevalence and risk factors for female sexual dysfunction in women attending a medical clinic in south India. *Journal of Postgraduate Medicine, 55*, 113–120.

Subodh, B. N., Avasthi, A., & Chakrabarti, S. (2008). Psychosocial impact of dysthymia: a study among married patients. *Journal of Affective Disorders, 109*, 199–204.

Varghese, K. M., Bansal, R., Kekre, A. N., & Jacob, K. S. (2012). Sexual dysfunction among young married women in southern India. *International Urogynecology Journal, 23*, 1771–1774.

Wig, N. N. (1960). Problem of mental health in India. *Journal of Clinical Social Psychiatry, 17*, 48–53.
Wig, N. N. (1998). Dhat syndrome. In R. Brahmbhatt (Ed.), *Therapy of common sexual problems—A hand book*. Mumbai: Family Planning Association of India.
Grover S, Avasthi A, Aneja J, Shankar G, Mohan M, Nehra R, et al. (2014). Comprehensive questionnaire for assessment of Dhat syndrome: Development and use in patient population. *Journal of Sexual Medicine, 11*, 2485–2495.

Part IX
Developments in Treatment

Chapter 27
Electroconvulsive Therapy: Research from India

K. Deka and S. Balachander

1 Introduction

This chapter contains a review of the practice electroconvulsive therapy (ECT) and research from around the world, but focuses mainly on the Indian developments from around the 1980s to the present.

ECT has been an effective, safe, evidence-based, but most controversial treatment method in psychiatry for past few decades. The technique of ECT has undergone several modifications over the years to minimize the adverse effects of the procedure. The practice of ECT has also been extensively investigated, as have the mechanisms underlying its effect.

ECT has been quite frequently used for the treatment of psychiatric disorders in developing countries. There is a considerable body of Indian research on the different aspects of ECT. Approximately 250 research papers have been published in different journals, and more than half have been in the Indian Journal of Psychiatry (Gangadhar et al. 2010). Of note is the fact that Dr. DLN Murthy Rao published first ever article in 1958, describing the "Ectonus" method ECT stimulation with positive results. This method however became obsolete after newer developments in ECT administration. In India, there has been an ongoing debate regarding the recent ban on the use of unmodified ECT by the Health Ministry. Nevertheless, many psychiatrists believe in effectiveness of ECT and have opined that it must be continued as a method of treatment. A brief discussion on this vsubject has also been included as part of this chapter.

K. Deka, Professor; S. Balachander, Junior Resident

K. Deka (✉)
Department of Psychiatry, Assam Medical College, Dibrugarh, India
e-mail: drkamala_99@yahoo.co.in

S. Balachander
Department of Psychiatry, Postgraduate Institute of Medical Education and Research (PGIMER), Chandigarh, India

S. Malhotra and S. Chakrabarti (eds.), *Developments in Psychiatry in India*,
DOI 10.1007/978-81-322-1674-2_27

2 History

The journey of ECT began in 1938, when Ugo Cerletti and Lucio Bini started the practice of electrically inducing convulsions in people who had schizophrenia and noted startling improvements among these patients. This method quickly replaced the earlier insulin coma therapy and camphor-induced convulsive therapies. Though it was initially tried only in patients with schizophrenia, its effectiveness in depression was established soon after. Throughout the 1940s, the use of ECT quickly became widespread, and it was used as a first-line therapy for schizophrenia and major depression.

Several modifications to the procedure quickly ensued during the 1950s, to enhance its safety and acceptability, such as the use of monitoring, anaesthesia and oxygenation. Its use however declined in the 1970s and the 1980s, when there came about several new developments in psychopharmacology. With the widespread use of pharmacological agents as first-line treatments for major psychiatric disorders, ECT is now more commonly used for patients with resistance to pharmacotherapy, except in the case of life-threatening illness due to inanition, severe suicidal symptoms or catatonia.

Work continues to explore the underlying mechanisms and biological characteristics of effective ECT treatments, with interest in having the treatment focus on appropriate neural networks with a more efficient stimulus as a method of reducing cognitive side effects.

Despite the advent of several newer forms of somatic treatments, the efficacy of ECT has been unparalleled, and it continues to remain the most predominant method of brain stimulation till date.

3 Practice Parameters

Over the last few decades, several controlled trials have been done, which have measured the effect of various aspects of ECT administration on response rates and adverse cognitive effects, most frequently the types of electrode placement and stimulus dosing strategies.

Several guidelines have been published, which have evidence-based recommendations about all aspects of the ECT technique. The most comprehensive and widely accepted amongst these are the American Psychiatric Association's guidelines (Weiner 2001) and the Royal College of Psychiatrists' guidelines (Scott 2005).

Leiknes et al. (2012) reviewed use and practice of ECT worldwide. A systematic literature search from 1990 to 2010 was carried out by the authors. The authors of this review have concluded that there is a considerable variation in administration of ECT worldwide. Unmodified ECT is substantially used today, not only in Asia (Over 90 %), Africa and Latin America, but is also practiced in Europe (Russia, Turkey and Spain). The authors found that the most common electrode placement is bilateral, but some places in Europe and Australia/New Zealand prefer unilateral ECT as first choice. Brief-pulse wave current devices are used worldwide. In Western countries (Europe, USA, Australia and New Zealand), unilateral ECT is preferably administered to elderly females with depression. In some places (Africa, Asia, Latin America and Russia), unmodified ECT is still administered to young and male patients with schizophrenia.

4 Modified and Unmodified ECT

Earlier, unmodified ECT was practiced everywhere, but in this decade, modified ECT using general anaesthetic agents and muscle relaxants is the internationally accepted standard (Weiner 2001; Scott 2005) Despite this, many patients continue to receive unmodified ECT. Reasons has put forth for not practicing modified ECT include lack of anaesthetists, contraindication for anaesthesia and the cost involved in administering modified ECT. Some have suggested that there are circumstances, in which unmodified ECT is to be preferred than no ECT (Andrade 2010). A decade earlier, a postal questionnaire survey of members of the Indian Psychiatric Society found that only 42 % of respondents who practiced ECT always administered modified ECT, while 24 % always practiced unmodified ECT (Andrade 1992, 1993). Another survey of teaching hospitals in 2001–2002, found that of 66 hospitals surveyed, 44(67 %) reported use of muscle relaxant (Andrade 2010). So trend towards using modified ECT has been noted.

5 Electrode Placement

There have been many studies worldwide on facilitation of ECT response with electrode placement, but conclusive results are lacking. Bilateral ECT is more effective than unilateral, though cognitive side effects are found to be higher in bilateral ECT. Unilateral ECT requires a much higher stimulus in order to maintain efficacy, and this may nullify the advantage of having lesser cognitive adverse effects. Bi-temporal electrode placements are the most common method of administration. Although there has long been a theoretical interest in greater localization of the effects produced by electroconvulsive stimulation in brain tissue, neurophysiological and clinical findings related to the interaction of electrode placement and stimulus intensity have rekindled interest in concentrating current density in prefrontal areas by manipulating electrode placement. Viswanath et al. (2011) compared bi-frontal with bi-temporal electrode placements and found lesser cognitive side effects with bi-frontal electrode placement.

6 Type of Stimulus

The original sine wave form of delivering current was replaced with constant-current brief-pulse machines in 1976, due to significant cognitive side effects with sine wave current. However, Andrade 1988 found that significantly more patients responded to Sine wave than to Brief pulse ECT. The last decade has seen the advent of an ultra-brief-pulse stimulus, which when used in right unilateral ECT has been shown in controlled trials to be as effective as both unilateral and bilateral brief-pulse ECTs, with almost no effect on cognitive functioning. Ultra-brief right unilateral ECT at six times the seizure threshold is equally effective as both brief-pulse bilateral ECT and brief-pulse right unilateral ECT. Ultra-brief bilateral ECT at 2.5 times the seizure threshold was, however, an ineffective treatment. Patients with Schizophrenia and Depression when treated with ECT -Bilateral 1.5 times the threasold level require similar ECT sessions as in threasold level but patients with Mania showed clinical improvement at lesser ECT sessions when suprathreasold dose was used (Thirthalli et al. 2009).

7 Stimulus Dosing

According to American Psychiatric Association Task Force, on ECT 1990, the seizure threshold can help guide the selection of the electrical stimulus dose at ECT. This threshold is smallest dose that can produce seizure.

A study by Janakirammaih et al. (1992) shows decrease in seizure duration reflecting increased seizure threshold, when compared between thrice weekly and twice weekly ECT treatments.

Gangadhar et al. (2003) examined the low and high pulse frequencies of stimulus on seizure threshold and physiological response to ECT. The seizure threshold and no of sub-convulsive stimulation were lower with 50 pulses per second (PPS), compared to 200 PPS. Lower stimulus frequencies were more efficient in inducing a seizure without compromising the physiological response to ECT. Gogoi et al. (2009, Unpublished) studied 21 patients on "stimulus dose, seizure duration, post-ictal disorientation and cognitive status following modified ECT" and found that as the number of ECT increased, the stimulus dose required also increased, more so in those who had received ECT earlier, while seizure duration decreases and post-ictal duration to reorient decreased; those with greater seizure duration took longer time to reorient. This study did not find any cognitive impairment with ECT; rather improvement was noted in domains of attention and concentration, immediate and delayed recall, visual retention and recognition and recent and remote memory among patients with schizophrenia.

8 Utilization Rates

There has been a large variation in the ECT utilization rates and clinical practice. The worldwide review on these parameters by Leikenes et al. (2012) found that

1. The treated person rate (number of ECTs per 10,000 population) ranges from 0.11 to 5.1
2. Inpatient prevalence rate (i.e. inpatients who received ECT) was highest in Africa (21–28 %), in Asia it ranged from less than 9–26 % and in USA it was lowest at 0.4–1.3 %.

Average number of ECTs administered in Asia remains between 6 and 8, while in other countries it is higher. With regard to frequency of ECT administration, twice weekly seems to have better balance between therapeutic outcome and adverse effect in depressive disorder using bilateral ECT. Increasing frequency though associated with increase improvement in depression but would cause cognitive adverse effect reviewed by Gangadhar and Thirthalli (2010)

9 Efficacy of ECT

Evidence for ECT's efficacy derives from several different sources. In the 1940s, open clinical series and case studies cited response rates of 80–90 % with the use of ECT as a first-line treatment. Decreased chronicity of illness, decreased morbidity and the suggestion of decreased mortality were frequently cited as benefits of ECT. From the 1950s through the 1980s, ECT was subjected to randomized clinical trials with sham ECT and psychotropic medications as comparators. In the sham versus real ECT trials, anaesthesia alone was used for comparison groups, because of a concern that there were benefits from its repeated use. ECT was shown to be consistently superior, and the further use of sham conditions has been abandoned in studies of major depression.

10 Indications

In the West, the most common indication for ECT is affective disorders, particularly major depression (Leikenes et al. 2012), a survey of major teaching hospitals in India (Chanpattanna et al. 2007) found the most common indication for ECT in India is schizophrenia (36.5 %), major depression (33.5 %) and mania (17.9 %).

11 Schizophrenia

A review by Sackeim (1989), of double-blind studies at England from 1970 till 1980, found that real ECT is more effective than sham ECT in schizophrenia. Abraham and Kulhara, in 1987, studied 22 patients of schizophrenia, randomly allocated to real ECT and sham ECT. Patients with real ECT showed more improvement than simulated ECT as measured by BPRS. But at the end of 6 months, superiority of real ECT was not confirmed. A double-blind study conducted on response of ECT in treatment-resistant schizophrenia from India found favourable results (Goswami et al. 2003). The authors concluded that the recovery may be maintained with maintenance ECT. Non-affective catatonia which did not respond with lorazepam 6–8 mg per day for 5 days showed good response to ECT administered in a double-blind trial; hence, ECT was proposed to have superior efficacy compared to lorazepam in non-affective catatonia (Girish and Gill 2003). Painuly and Chakrabarti (2006) conducted a review and metaanalysis all the Indian research, which had examined the combination of ECT and antipsychotics in schizophrenia. They found that the ECT–antipsychotic combination was more efficacious than drugs used alone in the first few weeks of treatment. The effect, however, was short-lasting, and there was no significant difference between the two groups (ECT and antipsychotics vs. antipsychotics alone) after more than 5 weeks of treatment. Tharyan and Adams in 2005 published a systematic review of all double-blinded RCTs done worldwide on ECT in schizophrenia. The findings suggested that ECT, combined with treatment with antipsychotic drugs, may be considered an option for people with schizophrenia, particularly when rapid global improvement and reduction of symptoms is desired. There was no evidence however that this early advantage for ECT is maintained over the medium to long term, except in some cases where there was resistance to medications.

Phutane et al. (2011) studied indications of schizophrenia prescribed ECT in a 1 year period and did a frequency analysis. The authors found that among 202 patients with schizophrenia, the most common indication was "to argument pharmacotherapy" ($n = 116$), and the most common target symptoms were catatonic symptoms ($n = 72$). Overall, ECT appears to be effective in schizophrenia and may improve response to medication. Catatonic as well as paranoid symptoms and other positive symptoms respond the best. Bilateral high-dose treatments are preferable, titrating their number to response. Augmenting medication (even clozapine) with ECT and using ECT for prevention of relapse appears justified by existing research, but there is a need for more specifically designed studies to provide conclusive data in this regard.

12 Depression

From the 1950s onward, there has also been interest in the relative efficacy of antidepressants and ECT. In these reports, ECT has been found to be 20–40 % more effective than medications, and there has not been a study that found medication to be superior to ECT.

Many of the antidepressants investigated in the past have been superseded by newer compounds, such as the specific serotonin reuptake inhibitors and pharmacologically unique agents such as bupropion and mirtazapine. Unfortunately, there is little data to inform comparisons of ECT and modern pharmaceuticals.

Janakiramaiah et al. (1992) studied seizure duration over ECT sessions in melancholic depression and found that the thrice weekly ECT failed to have adequate response and later cumulatively increased the seizure duration. Moreover, the add-on the third ECT treatment cost more; also treatment outcome did not differ between twice weekly and thrice weekly groups.

13 Mania

With the advent of pharmacological agents, particularly lithium and anticonvulsants and atypical antipsychotics, which have become the mainstay of management of manic episodes, the use of ECT is generally reserved for patients with very severe symptoms of mania or patients resistant to medications.

Evidence of ECT use in mania has reported 75–80 % response rates, most of the evidence being in the form of uncontrolled case series. Mixed states, rapid-cycling disorder and delirious manic states are known to particularly show good response to ECT.

Sikdar et al. (1994) compared real ECT with sham ECT in patients of mania, among patients simultaneously treated with chlorpromazine in a double-blind controlled study. They demonstrated that a combination of ECT and a moderate dose of an antipsychotic was extremely effective in rapidly aborting an acute episode of mania.

A double-blinded randomized controlled trial compared the efficacy and safety of bi-frontal with bi-temporal electrode positioning in patients of acute mania (Hiremani et al. 2008). It found that patients in the bi-frontal placement group had significantly more rapid improvement rates, compared to the bi-temporal placement group. In addition, there were no significant differences in cognitive functioning between the two groups after the fifth ECT.

ECT in Bipolar disorder has been reviewed by Bharadwaj et al. 2012 and found that nearly 90 % of patients of bipolar disorder especially mania with psychotic symptoms and severe depression with psychotic symptoms showed >50 % improvement in standard rating scales and 3/4th of them achieved remission.

14 Others Diagnoses

Neurological conditions such as the neuroleptic-induced extrapyramidal symptoms improved when ECT was used to treat underlying psychiatric conditions (Gangadhar et al. 1983; Goswami et al. 1989). Bilateral ECT was used in psychosis associated with Parkinson's disease with good improvement of psychosis and had no cognitive side effects (Muralidharan et al. 2011). ECT in mental retardation in patients with different psychiatric disorders was studied, and a favourable outcome was found among those resistant to pharmacotherapy (Chopra and Sinha 2002). A pre-pubertal (11 years) patient of catatonia was prescribed ECT with effective results that reported in a case study by Thakur and Dutta in 2001.

15 Maintenance ECT

Continuation and maintenance ECT has been found to be safe and effective treatment for relapse and recurrence prone patients who have responded to a course of ECT. Few prospective as well as retrospective studies are available from India (Table 1).

Table 1 Prospective and retrospective studies available from India

Author	Design	Sample	Result
Srinivasan et al. (1995)	Prospective study CM—ECT + DT at low doses (6–24 months) FU/E = 8–24 months after CM-ECT	$N = 4$ 2 MDD and 2 BD	Improved and better response to drugs after CM-ECT
Gupta et al. (2008)	Case–control study CM-ECT versus no CM-ECT administered. FU/E during CM-ECT and 4 years afterwards. Mean interval between session—2.5 weeks	$N = 38$, elderly chronic depressives and recurrent depressives	Significant decrease in the number of admissions and in days of hospitalizations

CM-ECT means weekly for 1st month, every 2 weeks for 2 months and 3rd month, and than monthly
DT = Drug Therapy; FU = Follow up

16 Mechanism of Action

Effects of ECT on platelet serotonin uptake in patients with major depression have been studied by Dalal and Lal in 1998. In this case–control study, platelet serotonin uptake was significantly raised after ECT, which was significantly lower in depression. This was indicative of the role of the serotonergic system in explaining effects of ECT. Jayakumar and Girish in 2001 tried to detect cerebral oedema, 1 day prior to the first ECT and at 2 hours after second ECT. Magnetic resonance imaging T2 relaxation time, which is an indicator of brain water content, was measured in the hippocampus and the thalamus of patients with depression receiving unilateral ECT; no differences were found. The authors concluded that ECT did not produce any brain oedema, and so ECT treatment may be considered safe. An animal model was used to study the effect of single ECT on dopamine autoreceptor down-regulation in the rat brain. The results suggested that ECT did not produce any acute and time dependent dopamine autoreceptor effects (Gangadhar et al. 1990).

17 Side Effects of ECT

Fractures of long bones are evident in many studies in unmodified type of ECT use. This was one main reason for advocating modified ECTs. Side effects associated with direct ECTs are not seen in modified type, although the adverse effects do occur in other areas which are evident in many studies. However, Gangadhar et al. (1983) found that ECT-treated patients reported fewer subjective side effects than imipramine-treated patients.

ECG abnormalities such as sinus tachycardia, ventricular premature beats, minor ST-T wave changes, increased amplitude, prolonged QTC intervals and elevated blood pressure lasting for more than 30 min are seen after ECT.

Cognitive side effects have been the main concern related to ECT. Jain et al. (2008) studied 373 patients who received ECT over 8 years. Of them, 56 (16 %) were more than 60 years of age; 66 % had a comorbid medical illness, and this was associated with higher risk of cognitive side effects. Again cognitive impairment has been found to be associated with ictal increase of blood pressure. 20 patients of depression with melancholic features were administered ECT and assessed before the first and after the second ECT. It was found that ictal systolic blood pressure was negatively correlated with the non-verbal memory score, but not with verbal score. This is hypothesized to be due to generalization of seizure or the stimulus administered.

Andrade et al. in 2000 studied 50 patients who had received bi-fronto temporal unmodified ECT. The results showed that 52 % of the patients complained of backache, of which 14 % had severe backache, and this was found to be more common in older patients. Gender, height or body weight did not predict the presence or severity of backache. One patient had vertebral fracture, which was not of serious kind. This study concluded that incidence of musculoskeletal morbidity is much less than it was thought earlier (20–40 % incidence in earlier studies).

18 Predictors of Response

Several studies have evaluated predictors of response in depression. Melancholic features, psychotic symptoms and catatonic symptoms are some of the clinical predictors of good response to ECT. Gupta et al. 2000 could identify duration of past episode, suicidal thought and somatic symptom that could distinguish good and poor responders of ECT in severe depressives. The effects of duration of the seizure and EEG characteristics have also been evaluated in Indian studies. A smaller post-seizure EEG fractal dimension after the first ECT predicted subsequent response to ECT in the course of depression (Gangadhar et al. 1999).

Cardiovascular changes that occur in ECTs pointed to potency of seizure and indicated the therapeutic efficacy of ECT in another study (Gangadhar et al. 2010). The authors concluded that ictal rate pressure product (RPP = heart rate × systolic blood pressure) can be an additional clinical measure, as ictal RPP increased when there was an adequate cerebral seizure (Gill et al. 2002). Saravanan et al. (2002) reported RPP response to ECT recorded under no Atropine condition predicted therapeutic response in depressive disorder.

Though medication-resistant patients respond to ECT, it predicts poor response to ECT in mania when compared with those in whom ECT was used as first-line treatment (Mukherjee et al. 1994). Symptoms of anger, irritability and suspiciousness are associated with poor response to ECT.

19 Use in Special Populations

19.1 Children and Adolescents

The American Academy of Child and Adolescent Psychiatry (AACAP) issued a guideline titled "Practice parameter for use of ECT with adolescents" (Ghaziuddin et al. 2004). ECT use is recommended for adolescents with serious psychiatric disorders, such as persistent major depression, schizoaffective disorder, schizophrenia or history of manic episodes, with or without psychotic features, catatonia and neuroleptic malignant syndrome. Patient's symptoms must be severe, persistent and significantly disabling, what can include life-threatening symptoms, such as refusal to drink or eat, uncontrollable mania, florid psychosis, severe suicidal risk and lack of treatment response (at least two adequate trials of appropriate drugs, in association with other therapeutic modalities). ECT may be considered earlier in cases when psychopharmacological treatment is not tolerated by the patient, when adolescent is significantly incapacitated, not being able to take medication or when waiting for response of psychopharmacological treatment may put the patient's life at risk.

Despite clear evidence that ECT is as safe and effective in children and adolescents as in adults, its use is much debated and has been restricted. Adolescents subjected to ECT accounted for only 1.4 % of the total in India (Chanpattanna et al. 2005), as compared to around 6 % in Asia overall (Chanpattanna et al. 2010).

A retrospective study in India (Grover et al. 2013) showed this rate to be higher (5.7 %) in one centre, and the most common indication was for schizophrenia and other psychotic disorders, commonly with catatonic symptoms. ECT was effective in 76 % of the cases, and the most common side effects were headache or nausea and prolonged seizures (8 %). There was no significant cognitive impairment following ECTs identified in any of the patients. The same has been reported in Western literature; children and adolescents have less cognitive impairment than adults following a course of ECT.

19.2 Elderly

Depressive disorders are very common in the elderly, are more likely to be severe, with higher risk of suicide, and frequently require hospital admission. Due to the high prevalence of physical comorbidity, problems associated with the concomitant use of several medications and suicidality, ECT remains an important modality for treatment of depression in elderly. Although studies have shown that, treatment with ECT is safe and effective, its use in the elderly population is still mired in controversy. In a study by Jain et al. in 2007, elderly patients made up 15 % of those who received ECT. An overwhelming majority had depression, and most were severely ill and medication resistant. Comorbid physical problems were common and seemed to contribute to cognitive side effects. However, side effects were usually mild and not incapacitating. About 80 % showed some response to treatment. Those who had received more than three ECTs and had inadequate antidepressant treatment prior to ECT were more likely to respond. Thus, ECT appears to be a safe and effective treatment in elderly patients. However, particular caution needs to be exercised in the subgroup with comorbid physical problems, which may be more vulnerable to cognitive adverse effects.

20 Attitudes, Knowledge and Perceptions Among Users

Studies on understanding the factors influencing patient choice of ECT provide a source of insight into the interplay between measures of response and perceived value of this treatment to patients, lending perspective to patient-centred quality improvement efforts.

In a study by Rajagopal et al. in 2012, patients who received ECT were found to be largely unaware of the procedure. Though most did not find the experience of ECT upsetting, sizeable proportions expressed dissatisfaction with aspects such as informed consent, fear of treatment and memory impairment. Although patients were mostly positive about ECT, ambivalent attitudes were also common, but clearly negative views were rare. Relatives were significantly likely to be more aware, more satisfied with the experience and have more favourable attitudes towards ECT, than patients (Grover et al. 2011; Rajagopal et al. 2012, 2013). Patients are many a times not well informed about ECT (Chakrabarti et al. 2010a).

21 Legal Aspects of ECT in India

The draft of the Mental Health Care Bill, 2011 (Thippeswamy et al. 2012), prohibits the administration of unmodified ECT. In several parts of the country, unmodified ECT still continues to be practiced owing to lack of anaesthesiologists, specialized equipment and cost factors. When viewed against the risk of musculoskeletal complications such as fractures, the immediate administration of ECT would be life saving in conditions such as catatonia. Rather than not giving ECT at all, giving a sub-optimal form of treatment may be justifiable in these circumstances. However, it is still debated if such a ban would be reasonable.

The draft also disallows the administration of ECTs in any form to minors. It has however been seen that ECT is the most effective form of treatment in certain situations—such as catatonia and severe suicidality. Several psychiatrists, in view of the fact that it may be a life-saving treatment in these conditions, have opposed such a blanket ban on ECTs in children and adolescents.

22 Future Perspectives

Research definitely shows much evidence for efficacy of ECT rather than its adverse effects. ECT treatment in recent decade is more sophisticated. The ECT machine has EEG and EKG monitoring, stimulus dose can be titrated and seizure may be measured even though debate on prescribing ECT is endless. However, in our opinion, the patient's perspective has a great role in prescribing ECT, as I have seen patients with depression and relatives of patients of depression and schizophrenia in our setup asking for ECT treatment. Perhaps the perception of efficacy with ECT is no longer hidden to the public or misconception of brain damage or stigma with ECT is no more prevalent, but this needs further research in psychiatry setup and in the community as well. The term electroshock (earlier used) must be totally replaced by the term ECT while taking informed consent, even though at times patients and relatives do enquire about whether ECT is a shock therapy. Though unmodified ECT is better than no ECT, modified ECT must be practiced all over India as long as this option is available. For those who cannot afford ECT, treatments may be offered at a subsidized cost. Further research especially in the area of cognition and ECT is needed; double-blind trials on different aspects of efficacy and studies examining the mechanism of ECT will guide us towards a more conclusive opinion about use and practice of ECT.

References

Abraham, K. R., & Kulhara, P. (1987). The efficacy of electroconvulsive therapy in the treatment of schizophrenia. *A comparative study. BJP, 151*, 152–155.

American Psychiatric Association, Committee on Electroconvulsive Therapy, Weiner R. D. (2001). The Practice of Electroconvulsive therapy: Recommendations for Treatment, Training and Privileging: A task force report of the American Psychiatric Association, 2nd Edition, Washington DC: American Psychiatric Association.

Andrade, C. (1992). The practice of electroconvulsive therapy in India: Considerable room for improvement. Editorial. *Indian Journal of Psychology Medicine, 15*, 14.

Andrade, C. (1993). Seizure duration and related issues in ECT for endogenous depression. *Indian Journal of Psychiatry, 35*, 43–47.

Andrade, C. (2010). Variations on a theme of unmodified ECT: Science or heresy? *The Journal of ECT, 26*, 30–31.

Andrade, C., Rele, K., Sutharshan, R., & Shah, N. (2000). Musculoskeletal morbidity with unmodified ect may be less than earlier believed. *Indian Journal of Psychiatry, 42*, 156–162.

Andrade, C., Gangadhar, B. N., Subbakrishna, D. K., Channabasavanna, S. M., & Pradhan, N. (1988). A Double-Blind Comparison of Sinusoidal Wave and Brief-Pulse Electroconvulsive Therapy in Endogenous Depression. *Convulsive Therapy*, *4*(4). http://journals.lww.com/ectjournal/toc/1988/04040

Bharadwaj, V., Grover, S., Chakrabarti, S., Avasthi, A., & Kate, N. (2012). Clinical profile and outcome of bipolar disorder patients receiving electroconvulsive therapy: a study from north India. *Indian Journal of Psychiatry, 54*, 41–47.

Chakrabarti, S., Grover, S., & Rajagopal, R. (2010a). Electroconvulsive therapy: A review of knowledge, experience and attitudes of patients concerning the treatment. *World Journal of Biological Psychiatry, 11*, 525–537.

Chakrabarti, S., Grover, S., & Rajagopal, R. (2010b). Perceptions and awareness of electroconvulsive therapy among patients and their families: a review of the research from developing countries. *The Journal of ECT, 26*, 317–322.

Chanpattana, W., Kramer, B. A., Kunigiri, G., Gangadhar, B. N., Kitphati, R., & Andrade, C. (2010). A survey of the practice of electroconvulsive therapy in Asia. *Journal of ECT, 26*, 5–10.

Chanpattana, W., Kunigiri, G., Kramer, B. A., & Gangadhar, B. N. (2005). Survey of the practice of electroconvulsive therapy in teaching hospitals in India. *Journal of ECT, 21*, 100–104.

Chopra, V. K., & Sinha, V. K. (2002). ECT in mentally retarded subjects with psychiatric illness. *Indian Journal of Psychiatry, 44*, 57–64.

Dalal, P. K., Lal, N., Trivedi, J. K., Seth, P. K., Agarwal, A. K., & Khalid, A. (1998). Active platelet 5-HT uptake in major depression. *Indian Journal of Psychiatry, 40*, 60–66.

Gangadhar, B. N., Choudhary, R. J., & Channabasavanna, S. M. (1983). ECT and drug induced Parkinsonism. *Indian Journal of Psychiatry, 25*, 212–213.

Gangadhar, B. N., Phutane, V. H., & Thirthalli, J. (2010). Research on electroconvulsive therapy in India: An overview. *Indian Journal of Psychiatry, 52*, S362–S365.

Gangadhar, B. N., Ramadevi, G., Andrade, C., & Pradhan, N. (1990). Single electroconvulsive shock and dopamine autoreceptors. *Indian Journal of Psychiatry, 32*, 302–304.

Gangadhar, B. N., Subbakrishna, D. K., Janakiramaiah, N., Motreja, S., NarayanaDutt, D., & Paramehwara, G. (1999). Post-seizure EEG fractal dimension of first ECT predicts antidepressant response at two weeks. *Journal of Affective Disorders, 52*, 235–238.

Gangadhar, B. N., & Thirthalli, J. (2010). Frequency of electroconvulsive therapy sessions in a course. *Journal of ECT, 26*, 181–185.

Gangadhar et. al. (2003). Seizure asymmetry with greater amplitude on the stimulated side in unilateral ECT. *Paper presented at the 51st Annual National Conference of Indian Psychiatric Society*, India:Hyderabad.

Ghaziuddin, N., Kutcher, S., & Knapp, P. (2004). Practice parameter for use of electroconvulsive therapy with adolescents. *Journal of American Academy of Child and Adolescent Psychiatry, 43*, 1521–1539.

Gill, N. S., Girish, K., & Gangadhar, B. N. (2002). Ictal RPP—A supplement to cuff method in detecting ect-induced cerebral seizure. *Indian Journal of Psychiatry, 44*, 29–33.

Girish, K., & Gill, N. S. (2003). Electroconvulsive therapy in lorazepam non-responsive catatonia. *Indian Journal of Psychiatry, 45*, 21–25.

Girish, K., Jayakumar, P. N., Murali, N., Gangadhar, B. N., Janakiramaiah, N., & Subbakrishna, D. K. (2001). ECT and T2 relaxometry: A static walter proton magnetic resonance imaging study. *Indian Journal of Psychiatry, 43*, 22–24.

Goswami, U., Kumar, U., & Singh, B. (2003). Efficacy of electroconvulsive therapy in treatment resistant schizophreinia: A double-blind study. *Indian Journal of Psychiatry, 45*, 26–29.

Goswami, U., Sunil, D., Kuruvilla, K., Eva Papp, Andras, P. (1989). Electroconvulsive therapy in neuroleptic-induced parkinsonism. *Biological Psychiatry, 26*(3), 234–238. http://www.biologicalpsychiatryjournal.com/issue/S0006-3223(00)X0372-1

Grover, S., Chakrabarti, S., Khehra, N., et al. (2011). Does the experience of electroconvulsive therapy improve awareness and perceptions of treatment among relatives of patients? *Journal of ECT, 27*, 67–72.

Grover, S., Malhotra, S., Varma, S., Chakrabarti, S., Avasthi, A., & Mattoo, S. K. (2013). Electroconvulsive therapy in adolescents: A retrospective study from north india. *Journal of ECT, 29*(2), 122–126. http://journals.lww.com/ectjournal/toc/2013/06000

Gupta, S., Tobiansky, R., Bassett, P., & Warner, J. (2008). Efficacy of Maintenance Electroconvulsive Therapy in recurrent depression: A naturalistic study. *Journal of ECT, 24* (3), 191–194.

Gupta, N., Avasthi, A., & Kulhara, P. (2000). Clinical variables as predictors of response to electroconvulsive therapy in endogenous depression. *Indian Journal of Psychiatry, 42*, 60–65.

Hiremani, R. M., Thirthalli, J., Tharayil, B. S., & Gangadhar, B. N. (2008). Double-blind randomized controlled study comparing short-term efficacy of bifrontal and bitemporal electroconvulsive therapy in acute mania. *Bipolar Disorders, 10*, 701–707.

Jain, G., Kumar, V., Chakrabarti, S., & Grover, S. (2008). The use of electroconvulsive therapy in the elderly: a study from the psychiatric unit of a north Indian teaching hospital. *Journal of ECT, 24*, 122–127.

Jain, G., Kumar, V., Chakrabarti, S., & Grover, S. (2007). Use of electroconvulsive treatment in elderly: A clinical audit. *Indian Journal of Psychiatry, 49*, 31.

Janakiramaiah, N., JyotiRao, K. M., Praveen, J., Sujatha, L., Gangadhar, B. N., & Subbakrishna, D. K. (1992). Seizure duration over ECT sessions: Influence of spacing ECTs. *Indian Journal of Psychiatry, 34*, 124–127.

Leiknes, K. A., Schweder, L. J. V., Høie, B., & 283. (2012). Contemporary use and practice of electroconvulsive therapy worldwide. *Brain Behavior, 2*(3), 283–344.

Mukherjee, S., Sackeim, H. A., & Schnur, F. B. (1994). Electroconvulsive therapy of acute manic episodes: A review of 50 years' experience. *American Journal of Psychiatry, 151*, 169–176.

Muralidharan, K., Thimmaiah, R., Chakraborty, V., & Jain, S. (2011). Bifrontal ECT for drug-induced psychosis in Parkinson's disease. *Indian Journal of Psychiatry, 53*, 156–158.

Painuly, N., & Chakrabarti, S. (2006). Combined use of electroconvulsive therapy and antipsychotics in schizophrenia: the Indian evidence. A review and a meta-analysis. *Journal of ECT, 22*, 59–66.

Phutane, V. H., Thirthalli, J., Kesavan, M., Kumar, N. C., Gangadhar, B. N., & 149. (2011). Why do we prescribe ECT to schizophrenia patients? *Indian Journal of Psychiatry, 53*, 149–151.

Rajagopal, R., Chakrabarti, S., & Grover, S. (2013). Satisfaction with electroconvulsive therapy among patients and their relatives. *Journal of ECT, 29*(4), 279–286. (Epub ahead of print).

Rajagopal, R., Chakrabarti, S., Grover, S., & Khehra, N. (2012). Knowledge, experience & attitudes concerning electroconvulsive therapy among patients & their relatives. *Indian Journal of Medical Research, 135*, 201–210.

Sackeim, H.A. (1989 Review). In *The Practice of Electroconvulsive Therapy: Recommendations for Treatment, Training and Privileging*(2nd Edn.). American Psychiatric Association

Saravanan, E. S., Gangadhar, B. N., Janakiramaiah, N., Pandey, R. S., Murthy, H. S., & Subbakrishna, D. K. (2002). Does higher cardiovascular response to ECT predict early antidepressant effect? *Journal of Affective Disorders, 69*, 101–108.

Scott, A. I. F. (2005). The ECT Handbook (2nd Edn). London: Royal College of Psychiatrists.

Sikdar, S., Kulhara, P., Avasthi, A., & Singh, H. (1994). Combined chlorpromazine and electroconvulsive therapy in mania. *British Journal of Psychiatry, 164*, 806–810.

Srinivasan, T. N., Suresh, T. R., & Jayaram, V. (1995). Issues in the use of maintenance electroconvulsive therapy. *Indian Journal of Psychiatry, 37*, 139–142.

Thakur, A., Dutta, S., Jagadheesan, K., & Sinha, V. K. (2001). Electroconvulsive therapy in prepubertal catatonia: A case study. *Indian Journal of Psychiatry, 43*, 354–356.

Tharyan, P., & Adams, C. E. (2005). Electroconvulsive therapy for schizophrenia. *Cochrane Database Systematic Reviews. 18*: CD000076.

Thippeswamy, H., Goswami, K., & Chaturvedi, S. (2012). Ethical aspects of public health legislation: The mental health care bill, 2011. *Indian Journal of Medical Ethics, 9*, 46–49.

Thirthalli, J., Kumar, C. N., Bangalore, R. P., & Gangadhar, B. N. (2009). Speed of response to threshold and suprathreshold bilateral ECT in depression, mania and schizophrenia. *Journal of Affective Disorders, 117*, 104–107.

Viswanath, B., Narayanaswamy, J. C., Thirthalli, J., & Gangadhar, B. N. (2011). Effectiveness of bifrontal ECT in practice: A comparison with bitemporal ECT. *Indian Journal of Psychological Medicine, 33*, 66–70.

Chapter 28
Newer Somatic Treatments: Indian Experience

S.K. Praharaj, R.V. Behere and P.S.V.N. Sharma

1 Introduction

Psychopharmacological and non-pharmacological interventions have inherent limitations in the treatment of neuropsychiatric disorders. The somatic treatment approaches such as modified electroconvulsive therapy (ECT) are associated with risks of anaesthesia and cognitive adverse effects. Therefore, there is a recent surge of interest in newer somatic treatment approaches in psychiatric disorders, which are device-based, circuit-based and which have more focal actions in the key target regions of the brain. Several such approaches are being studied including transcranial magnetic stimulation (TMS) or recurrent transcranial magnetic stimulation (rTMS), transcranial direct current stimulation (tDCS), vagus nerve stimulation (VNS) and deep brain stimulation (DBS). In this chapter, Indian studies using these treatment modalities for various neuropsychiatric disorders have been reviewed.

2 Transcranial Magnetic Stimulation (TMS)

TMS is a non-invasive tool, which is used for studying cortical functions, and it has therapeutic applications in various neuropsychiatric disorders. It works on the principle of electromagnetic induction, involving a bank of capacitors, which discharges very large current (peak current ~5,000 A), which rapidly flows through

S.K. Praharaj, Assistant Professor; R.V. Behere, Assistant Professor; P.S.V.N. Sharma, Professor and Head

S.K. Praharaj · R.V. Behere · P.S.V.N. Sharma (✉)
Department of Psychiatry, Kasturba Medical College, Manipal, Karnataka, India
e-mail: psvn.sharma@manipal.edu

S. Malhotra and S. Chakrabarti (eds.), *Developments in Psychiatry in India*,
DOI 10.1007/978-81-322-1674-2_28

a simple circuit and then through a copper wire coil. This subsequently results in the induction of a brief and pulsed magnetic field (rise time ~0.1 ms, field strength ~2 T), which is perpendicular to the electric current. When the copper coil is held to the head of the subject, this induced magnetic field generates an electrical current, which is parallel to the plane of the coil and of adequate intensity to cause localised depolarisation of superficial, cortical and subcortical neurons, generating a propagating action potential, which is then used to study the various neuronal functions (George et al. 2002). The application of TMS can produce immediate (within seconds) effects, such as quick jerky movements and perception of flashes of light. Different frequencies of TMS have been found to result in divergent intermediate-term (seconds to several minutes) biologic effects. Studies have revealed that repeated stimulation of a single neuron at low frequency produces long lasting inhibition of cell-to-cell communications, which is called as *long-term depression* (LTD; Bear 1999); conversely, repeated high-frequency stimulation can improve cell-to-cell communication by *long-term potentiation* (LTP; Malenka and Nicoll 1999). In low-frequency rTMS (or slow rTMS), stimulation of less than 1 Hz is applied for a longer duration (10–15 min), resulting in LTD of cortical neurons, whereas high-frequency rTMS (or fast rTMS) involves greater 1 Hz frequency stimulation for a shorter duration, manifested as neuronal LTP (Wassermann et al. 1996). Long-term (days to weeks) effects have also been observed with TMS administration, reflected as sustained changes in neurotransmitter release, signalling pathways and gene expression (Post and Keck 2001).

2.1 rTMS in Depression

The therapeutic effects of rTMS have been robust in the field of depression as shown by meta-analysis of the studies, though only small to medium effect sizes have been reported (Berlim et al. 2013a, b). Two major strategies have been used, which have similar antidepressant effect: high-frequency rTMS to the left prefrontal cortex (PFC) and low-frequency rTMS to the right PFC, the latter is better tolerated with lower risk of seizure (Rachid and Bertschy 2006).

Ray et al. (2011) conducted a randomised controlled study on the efficacy of adjunctive high-frequency rTMS of the left PFC in 45 patients with moderate-to-severe depression. These patients received 10 daily sessions of active or sham rTMS (10 Hz, 90 % of resting motor threshold—MT, 20 trains, 6 s duration, 1,200 pulses/day). Depression and psychosis were rated using the Structured Interview Guide for the hamilton depression rating scale (SIGH-D) and brief psychiatric rating scale (BPRS), respectively, before and after rTMS. There was significant effect of treatment over time for both SIGH-D and BPRS scores, with high effect sizes. Similar results were observed with the psychotic subgroup. Another randomised, double-blind, controlled trial by Lingeswaran (2011) on a smaller sample ($n = 23$) using six sessions of rTMS (10 Hz, 100 % of MT, 10 trains, 5 s duration, 1 min inter-train interval) over the left PFC failed to find a difference between active and sham stimulations. The small sample size and fewer rTMS sessions could have resulted in lack of efficacy of active rTMS in their study (Praharaj 2011).

In an open-label study (Jhanwar et al. 2011a, b), 21 patients with treatment-resistant major depressive disorder (defined as failing to respond to an adequate trial of at least 2 antidepressants) received add-on high-frequency rTMS (10 Hz, 110 % of MT) over the left PFC for 4 weeks. An intention-to-treat analysis showed significant reduction in mean HAM-D17 scores from 30.80 (SD 5.00) to 19 (SD 6.37). In a case study, Chatterjee et al. (2012) used high-frequency rTMS over the left PFC in a patient with treatment-resistant depression who went into complete remission following treatment. Although the authors described it as maintenance rTMS, they had used a prolonged course of rTMS (20 sessions) only during the depressive episodes. The number of pulses delivered was high (2,000–3,000 pulses per session), which could have led to the greater than expected improvement. In another single case study, Bagati et al. (2012) used high-frequency rTMS over the left PFC of a patient with treatment-resistant depression, who subsequently developed a seizure during the fourth rTMS session. He received further rTMS sessions under the cover of antiepileptic drug valproate and improved without any recurrence of seizures.

In a novel design, Nongpiur et al. (2011) compared the efficacy of adjuvant, frequency-modulated, active-priming rTMS with sham-priming stimulation in the theta range in patients with moderate-to-severe depression receiving low-frequency rTMS. 40 patients with moderate-to-severe depression were alternately assigned to receive add-on, active-priming rTMS (4–8 Hz; 400 pulses, at 90 % of MT) or sham-priming stimulation followed by low-frequency rTMS (1 Hz; 900 pulses at 110 % of MT) over the right PFC. They were rated with the SIGH-D, the BPRS, and the Clinical Global Impression-Severity of Illness (CGI-S) scale at baseline, after the 5th and 10th rTMS, and 2 weeks post-rTMS treatment. For the SIGH-D scores, there was a significant improvement in the active group over time. Stepwise linear-regression analysis showed that age at onset significantly predicted the SIGH-D scores after the 5th rTMS session in the active-priming group. Pre-stimulation with frequency-modulated priming stimulation in the theta range had greater antidepressant effect than low-frequency stimulation alone.

Venkatesh Babu et al. (2012) studied the efficacy of add-on high-frequency rTMS over the right parietal cortex in patients with moderate-to-severe, unipolar depression. 30 patients were randomly assigned to receive active or sham rTMS (10 Hz; 1,200 pulses at 90 % MT). They were rated with the Structured Interview Guide for the Hamilton Depression Scale (SIGH-D), the Beck's depression Inventory (BDI), the Hamilton Anxiety Scale (HAM–A) and the CGI-S at baseline, after the 5th and the 10th rTMS and 2 weeks post-rTMS treatment. There was a significant effect of treatment over time as shown by changes in the SIGH-D, the BDI and the CGI-S scores in the active group, compared to sham group.

Udupa et al. (2007) examined the effect of rTMS versus treatment with escitalopram on cardiac autonomic parameters, including heart rate variability in 67 patients with major depressive disorder. Heart rate variability measures suggested a significant improvement in sympathovagal balance in the group receiving rTMS, as compared to the escitalopram group. In an extension of this study, which included three patients groups ($n = 94$) receiving either rTMS or tricyclic antidepressants (TCAs) or selective serotonin reuptake inhibitors (SSRIs), Udupa et al. (2011) found that measures of cardiac autonomic function improved in rTMS group, worsened in TCA group, and there was no change in the SSRI group. These preliminary studies suggest a cardioprotective role for rTMS in patients with depression. This finding is important in the context of evidence suggesting enhanced risk of cardiovascular events in patients with depression.

In a single case study, Mehta et al. (2013) found enhanced mirror neuron activity (change in motor evoked potential from resting to observation phase) during catatonia in a patient with bipolar depression, which disappeared after resolution of catatonia.

2.2 rTMS in Schizophrenia

In schizophrenia, hypoactivity of prefrontal cortex plays a role in the pathophysiology of negative symptoms, for which high-frequency rTMS of the prefrontal cortex has been used, whereas for positive symptoms such as hallucinations, which are associated with hyperactivity of temporoparietal areas, low-frequency rTMS has been studied (Mishra et al. 2011).

Goyal et al. (2007) studied the efficacy of adjuvant 10 Hz suprathreshold left prefrontal rTMS in negative symptoms of schizophrenia in a double-blind, controlled design in 10 patients with psychopathology, depression and global improvement ratings before and after the rTMS sessions. Compared to sham treatment control group, active rTMS significantly improved negative symptoms, irrespective of change in depressive symptoms.

Bagati et al. (2009) studied the efficacy of low-frequency left temporoparietal rTMS for auditory hallucinations in schizophrenia. Forty patients were randomised to experimental or control groups. The experimental group received add-on low-frequency rTMS (1 Hz, 90 % MT) over left temporoparietal cortex for 10 days, and the control group received only antipsychotics. The changes in the psychopathology scores for the auditory hallucinations were recorded using the auditory hallucination recording scale. A significant improvement was found in auditory hallucinations in the experimental group as compared to the control group.

Garg et al. (2013a, b) studied high-frequency cerebellar vermal rTMS in a patient with treatment-resistant schizophrenia. This patient received 10 sessions of rTMS in the theta frequency range (5 Hz for the first 7 trains, 6 Hz for the next 7 trains and 7 Hz for the rest 6 trains), at 100 % MT, 20 trains of 30 pulses each to a total of 600 pulses. There was a worsening of auditory verbal hallucinations, whereas an improvement was seen in anergia and thought disorder.

Thirthalli et al. (2008) in a single case study have described use of maintenance rTMS in a patient with treatment-refractory auditory hallucinations. rTMS (1 Hz, 100 % motor threshold) was administered over the left temporoparietal cortex initially once daily, 5 times a week for 2 weeks. Maintenance rTMS was then continued at a frequency of once weekly for 6 weeks, once fortnightly for 6 fortnights and once monthly for 3 months. The patient achieved near total remission in auditory hallucinations, with significant improvement in functioning levels at week 4, which was maintained at the end of 8 months.

In an observational study, Mehta et al. (2012) examined mirror neuron activity using single-pulse TMS in schizophrenia patients ($n = 27$). There was significant correlation between mirror neuron activity (as measured by the per cent change in motor evoked potential from resting to observation stage) and emotion recognition index (a measure of social cognition).

2.3 rTMS in Mania

There are only a few studies on the therapeutic efficacy of rTMS in the manic phase of bipolar disorder. High-frequency rTMS of the right PFC has been found to be effective in mania, suggesting that the therapeutic effect may show a laterality effect opposite to that in depression.

Praharaj et al. (2009) studied the efficacy of adjunctive right prefrontal high-frequency suprathreshold rTMS treatment in patients with bipolar affective disorder, mania, compared to sham stimulation. Forty one right-handed patients with mania were randomised to receive daily sessions of active or sham rTMS (20 Hz, 110 % of MT, 20 trains, 10 s inter-train interval) over the right dorsolateral prefrontal cortex for 10 days. Mania was rated using the Young Mania Rating Scale (YMRS) and the Clinical Global Impression (CGI) at baseline and after the 5th and the 10th rTMS. There was a significant effect of treatment over time for both the YMRS and the CGI-S scores suggestive of add-on therapeutic efficacy.

Pathak and Sinha (2008) examined the efficacy of adjunctive right prefrontal high-frequency (rapid) and left prefrontal low-frequency rTMS treatment in children and adolescents with manic episodes. 28 patients were administered rapid rTMS (20 Hz right prefrontal rTMS, 20 trains per session, each train for 2 s and inter-train interval of 10 s) and 25 low-frequency rTMS (1 Hz left prefrontal rTMS, 20 trains per session, each train for 40 s) for 2 weeks each. In both groups, patients were randomly assigned to active and sham group. They were rated using the YMRS and the CGI at baseline, after the 5th and the 10th rTMS. There was no significant improvement in psychopathology rating scores (YMRS and CGI-S) in the patients receiving active rapid rTMS or low-frequency rTMS as compared to sham controls. The results of this study do not support an active therapeutic effect of add-on rapid right prefrontal or low-frequency left prefrontal rTMS in children and adolescents with mania.

2.4 rTMS in Substance Abuse

Studies have also revealed the potential anticraving effects of rTMS in substance dependence. Muralidharan et al. (2008) explored the differences in the functioning of cortical inhibitory systems in high-risk ($n = 15$) and low-risk ($n = 15$) patients with alcohol dependence using single-pulse TMS. High-risk subjects had significantly shorter contralateral and ipsilateral (iSP) silent periods and a relatively higher prevalence of 'absent' iSP. They had significantly higher mean externalising symptom scores than low-risk subjects, and there was a significant negative correlation between iSP duration and externalising symptom scores. These findings suggest that high-risk subjects have relative impairments in cortico-cortical and transcallosal inhibitory mechanisms resulting in central nervous system hyperexcitability, which may be aetiologically linked to the excess of externalising behaviours. In another study (Muralidharan et al. 2013), resting motor threshold (the minimum stimulus intensity required to elicit a motor evoked potential of greater than or equal to 50 μV in at least 50 % of trials) and motor threshold 1 (defined as the lowest stimulus intensity required to elicit a motor evoked potential greater than 1 mV in at least 50 % of trials) was not significantly different in high-risk ($n = 16$) and low-risk ($n = 12$) patients with alcohol dependence, using single-pulse TMS.

In a similar study, Mishra et al. (2010) examined the anticraving efficacy of high-frequency rTMS in patients with alcohol dependence. 45 patients with alcohol dependence syndrome were allocated to active and sham rTMS in a 2:1 ratio. Stimulation was given over the right PFC (10 Hz, 4.9 s per train, inter-train interval of 30 s, 20 trains per session, total 10 sessions). The Alcohol Craving Questionnaire (ACQ-NOW) was administered to measure the severity of alcohol craving at baseline, after the last rTMS session and 1 month after the last rTMS session. There was a significant reduction in the post-rTMS ACQ-NOW total score and factor scores in the group allocated active rTMS, compared to the sham stimulation, with high effect sizes.

2.5 rTMS in Obsessive Compulsive Disorder (OCD)

Studies evaluating the therapeutic efficacy of rTMS in OCD are limited, and the results have been rather inconsistent. Sarkhel et al. (2010) studied the efficacy of adjunctive right prefrontal high-frequency rTMS treatment in OCD patients. 42 patients were randomly assigned to receive 10 sessions of active rTMS (10 Hz, 110 % of motor threshold, 4 s per train, 20 trains per session) or sham stimulation. They were rated on the Yale Brown Obsessive Compulsive Scale (YBOCS), the Hamilton Rating Scale for Depression (HAM-D), the Hamilton Rating Scale for Anxiety (HAM-A) and the CGI-S at baseline, day 14 and day 28. There was no effect of treatment over time for the YBOCS, but a significant effect of treatment over time was found for both the HAM-D and the HAM-A scores, with medium effect sizes. It was concluded that adjunctive high-frequency right prefrontal rTMS does not have any significant effect in the treatment of OCD. However, it was modestly effective in the treatment of comorbid depressive symptoms in patients with OCD. In a case study, Bishnoi and Jhanwar (2011) administered an extended course of rTMS (60 sessions, initially 5 sessions per week for 6 weeks, then once weekly for 6 months) over the right PFC in a patient with treatment-resistant OCD and found significant reduction in the YBOCS score, which was maintained at 3 months following discontinuation of treatment.

Kumar and Chadda (2011) studied add-on rTMS over the supplementary motor cortex in treatment-refractory OCD patients. 12 right-handed persons with medication-resistant OCD were administered rTMS as an add-on treatment. Stimulation was given at 1 Hz for 10 s followed by 15 s pause and 100 trains of stimulus over the supplementary motor area (SMA) per session for 5 days in a week. Assessments were done on Y-BOCS at baseline and after rTMS. Mean scores on Y-BOCS reduced significantly from 26.17 to 17.17 at the end of treatment.

3 Transcranial Direct Current Stimulation (tDCS)

tDCS involves the continuous passage of a very small current between electrodes at least one of which is placed upon a specific site on the head. The amplitude of the current is usually in the region of 1–3 mA, and the stimulation time is usually about 20 min. tDCS has been found to be efficacious in the treatment for major depression (Berlim et al. 2013). There have been no studies of tDCS in depression from India.

3.1 tDCS in Schizophrenia

Rakesh et al. (2013) in a case study used tDCS as monotherapy for auditory hallucinations in schizophrenia. Stimulation was carried out with the anode over left dorsolateral prefrontal cortex (midway between F3 and FP1) and the cathode over left temporo-parietal junction (midway between T3 and P3) at 2 mA for 20 min. The sessions were conducted twice a day (separated by at least 3 h) on 5 consecutive days. There was cessation of auditory hallucinations after first two tDCS sessions, which was maintained after the last session along with improvement in insight.

Andrade (2013) studied tDCS in a 24-year-old female schizophrenia patient who had severe, clozapine-refractory, continuous auditory hallucinations. The tDCS cathode was placed midway between T3 and P3, and the anode over F3, in the 10–20 electroencephalogram electrode positioning system. Once daily, 20-min tDCS sessions at 1 mA intensity produced noticeable improvement within a week: cognitive and psychosocial functioning improved followed by attenuation in the experience of hallucinations. There was greater than 90 % self-reported improvement within 2 months. Benefits accelerated when the current was raised to 3 mA, treatment duration was increased to 30 min sessions, and session frequency was increased to twice daily. The patient improved from a psychosocially vegetative state to near-normal functioning. Once- to twice-daily domiciliary tDCS was continued across nearly 3 years and is still ongoing. Benefits attenuated or were even lost when alternate day session spacing was attempted or when electrode positioning was changed; benefits were regained when the original stimulation protocol was reintroduced. There was confirmation of benefit in 2 separate on-off-on situations, which occurred inadvertently and under blinded conditions. There were no adverse events attributable to tDCS.

4 Vagus Nerve Stimulation (VNS)

VNS is performed by stimulation of the left cervical vagus nerve using a subcutaneous generator that sends an electrical signal to the nerve. The generator is implanted into the left chest wall, and the bipolar electrodes are wrapped around the left vagus in the neck through a special incision and tunnelled under the skin towards the chest. The stimulation parameters, which can be adjusted by the physician, include current intensity, pulse width, frequency and duration of the on and off periods. VNS has been found to be effective in treatment of depression (Martin and Martín-Sánchez 2012), but there are no reported studies from India.

5 Deep Brain Stimulation (DBS)

DBS is based on the assumption that chronic high-frequency stimulation of the brain areas might be similar to surgical ablation of these areas. The DBS electrodes are implanted in the brain using stereotactic techniques. Stimulation can be programmed to continuous or intermittent firing or to on and off cycles during fixed time intervals. DBS is reversible, and the stimulation parameters can be changed according to patient's symptoms or disease progression. DBS has been suggested as a treatment for psychiatric disorders, such as depression (Anderson et al. 2012) and obsessive-compulsive disorder (Mian et al. 2010).

6 Other Newer Somatic Treatments

Several others methods of focal neuromodulation such as transcranial low-voltage pulsed electromagnetic fields stimulation (Martiny et al. 2010), magnetic seizure therapy (MST; Lisanby et al. 2003) and direct cortical stimulation (Nahas et al. 2010) have been investigated for various psychiatric conditions.

7 Conclusions

TMS and tDCS are promising modes of somatic treatments. These treatment modalities have the advantage of being non-invasive in nature and can provide site specific stimulation of target brain areas. Preliminary evidence from studies performed in India suggests a beneficial role for these treatment modalities in depression, schizophrenia, mania, substance use disorders and OCD. However, larger randomised controlled trials are needed to establish safety and efficacy of the newer somatic treatments, before they can be advocated for routine clinical use in the Indian context. Future research should also focus on DBS and VNS as treatment modalities for psychiatric disorders.

References

Anderson, R. J., Frye, M. A., Abulseoud, O. A., Lee, K. H., McGillivray, J. A., Berk, M., et al. (2012). Deep brain stimulation for treatment-resistant depression: Efficacy, safety and mechanisms of action. *Neuroscience and Biobehavioral Reviews, 36*(8), 1920–1933.

Andrade, C. (2013). Once- to twice-daily, 3-year domiciliary maintenance transcranial direct current stimulation for severe, disabling, clozapine-refractory continuous auditory hallucinations in Schizophrenia. *Journal of Electroconvulsive Therapy*. *29*(3), 239–242.

Bagati, D., Mittal, S., Praharaj, S. K., Sarcar, M., Kakra, M., & Kumar, P. (2012). Repetitive transcranial magnetic stimulation safely administered after seizure. *Journal of Electroconvulsive Therapy, 28*(1), 60–61.

Bagati, D., Nizamie, S. H., & Prakash, R. (2009). Effect of augmentatory repetitive transcranial magnetic stimulation on auditory hallucinations in schizophrenia: Randomized controlled study. *The Australian and New Zealand Journal of Psychiatry, 43*, 386–392.

Bear, M. F. (1999). Homosynaptic long-term depression: A mechanism for memory? *Proceedings of National Academy Sciences of USA, 96*, 9457–9458.

Berlim, M. T., Van den Eynde, F., & Daskalakis, Z. J. (2013a). Clinical utility of transcranial direct current stimulation (tDCS) for treating major depression: A systematic review and meta-analysis of randomized, double-blind and sham-controlled trials. *Journal of Psychiatric Research, 47*(1), 1–7.

Berlim, M. T., Van den Eynde, F., & Daskalakis, Z. J. (2013b). High-frequency repetitive transcranial magnetic stimulation accelerates and enhances the clinical response to antidepressants in major depression: A meta-analysis of randomized, double-blind, and sham-controlled trials. *The Journal of Clinical Psychiatry, 74*(2), e122–e129.

Berlim, M. T., Van den Eynde, F., & Jeff Daskalakis, Z. (2013c). Clinically meaningful efficacy and acceptability of low-frequency repetitive transcranial magnetic stimulation (rTMS) for treating primary major depression: A meta-analysis of randomized, double-blind and sham-controlled trials. *Neuropsychopharmacology, 38*(4), 543–551.

Bishnoi, R. J., & Jhanwar, V. G. (2011). Extended course of repetitive trans-cranial magnetic stimulation therapy and a complicated case of obsessive-compulsive disorder. *Indian Journal of Psychological Medicine, 33*(1), 98–99.

Chatterjee, B., Kumar, N., & Jha, S. (2012). Role of repetitive transcranial magnetic stimulation in maintenance treatment of resistant depression. *Indian Journal of Psychological Medicine, 34*(3), 286–289.

Garg, S., Goyal, N., Tikka, S. K., & Sinha, V. K. (2013a). Exacerbation of auditory verbal hallucinations with adjunctive high-frequency cerebellar vermal repetitive transcranial magnetic stimulation in schizophrenia: A case report. *Journal of Electroconvulsive Therapy, 29*(1), 65–66.

Garg, S., Tikka, S. K., Goyal, N., Sinha, V. K., & Nizamie, S. H. (2013b). Amelioration of anergia and thought disorder with adjunctive high frequency cerebellar vermal repetitive transcranial magnetic stimulation in schizophrenia: A case report. *Schizophrenia Research, 143*(1), 225–227.

George, M. S., Nahas, Z., Kozel, F. A., Li, X., Denslow, S., Yamanaka, K., et al. (2002). Mechanisms and state of the art of transcranial magnetic stimulation. *Journal of Electroconvulsive Therapy, 18*, 170–181.

Goyal, N., Nizamie, S. H., & Desarkar, P. (2007). Efficacy of adjuvant high frequency repetitive transcranial magnetic stimulation on negative and positive symptoms of schizophrenia: Preliminary results of a double-blind sham-controlled study. *Journal of Neuropsychiatry Clinical Neuroscience, 19*, 464–467.

Jhanwar, V. G., Bishnoi, R. J., & Jhanwar, M. R. (2011a). Utility of repetitive transcranial stimulation as an augmenting treatment method in treatment-resistant depression. *Indian Journal of Psychological Medicine, 33*(1), 92–96.

Jhanwar, V. G., Bishnoi, R. J., Singh, L., & Jhanwar, M. R. (2011b). Utility of repetitive transcranial magnetic stimulation as an augmenting treatment method in treatment-resistant depression. *Indian Journal of Psychiatry, 53*(2), 145–148.

Kumar, N., & Chadda, R. K. (2011). Augmentation effect of repetitive transcranial magnetic stimulation over the supplementary motor cortex in treatment refractory patients with obsessive compulsive disorder. *Indian Journal of Psychiatry, 53*(4), 340–342.

Lingeswaran, A. (2011). Repetitive transcranial magnetic stimulation in the treatment of depression: A randomized, double-blind, placebo-controlled trial. *Indian Journal of Psychological Medicine, 33*(1), 35–44.

Lisanby, S. H., Luber, B., Schlaepfer, T. E., & Sackeim, H. A. (2003). Safety and feasibility of magnetic seizure therapy (MST) in major depression: Randomized within-subject comparison with electroconvulsive therapy. *Neuropsychopharmacology, 28*, 1852–1865.

Malenka, R. C., & Nicoll, R. A. (1999). Long-term potentiation—A decade of progress? *Science, 285*, 1870–1874.

Martin, J. L., & Martín-Sánchez, E. (2012). Systematic review and meta-analysis of vagus nerve stimulation in the treatment of depression: Variable results based on study designs. *European Psychiatry: The Journal of the Association of European Psychiatrists, 27*(3), 147–155.

Martiny, K., Lunde, M., & Bech, P. (2010). Transcranial low voltage pulsed electromagnetic fields in patients with treatment-resistant depression. *Biological Psychiatry, 68*, 163–169.

Mehta, U. M., Basavaraju, R., Thirthalli, J., & Gangadhar, B. N. (2012). Mirror neuron dysfunction-a neuro-marker for social cognition deficits in drug naïve schizophrenia. *Schizophrenia Research, 141*(2–3), 281–283.

Mehta, U. M., Basavaraju, R., & Thirthalli, J. (2013). Mirror neuron disinhibition may be linked with catatonic echo-phenomena: A single case TMS study. *Brain Stimulation, 6*, 705–707.

Mian, M. K., Campos, M., Sheth, S. A., & Eskandar, E. N. (2010). Deep brain stimulation for obsessive-compulsive disorder: Past, present, and future. *Neurosurgical Focus, 29*(2), E10.

Mishra, B. R., Nizamie, S. H., Das, B., & Praharaj, S. K. (2010). Efficacy of repetitive transcranial magnetic stimulation in alcohol dependence: A sham-controlled study. *Addiction, 105*, 49–55.

Mishra, B. R., Sarkar, S., Praharaj, S. K., Mehta, V. S., Diwedi, S., & Nizamie, S. H. (2011). Repetitive transcranial magnetic stimulation in psychiatry. *Annals of Indian Academy of Neurology, 14*(4), 245–251.

Muralidharan, K., Venkatasubramanian, G., Pal, P. K., & Benegal, V. (2008). Abnormalities in cortical and transcallosal inhibitory mechanisms in subjects at high risk for alcohol dependence: A TMS study. *Addiction Biology, 13*(3–4), 373–379.

Muralidharan, K., Venkatasubramanian, G., Pal, P. K., & Benegal, V. (2013). Relationship between motor threshold and externalizing symptoms in subjects at high risk for alcohol dependence: A TMS Study. *American Journal of Addiction, 22*(1), 84–85.

Nahas, Z., Anderson, B. S., Borckardt, J., Arana, A. B., George, M. S., Reeves, S. T., et al. (2010). Bilateral epidural prefrontal cortical stimulation for treatment-resistant depression. *Biological Psychiatry, 67*, 101–109.

Nongpiur, A., Sinha, V. K., Praharaj, S. K., & Goyal, N. (2012). Theta-patterned, frequency-modulated priming stimulation enhances low-frequency, right prefrontal cortex repetitive transcranial magnetic stimulation (rTMS) in depression: A randomized, sham-controlled study. *Journal of Neuropsychiatry Clinical Neuroscience 2011*, *23*(3), 348–357. Erratum in: *Journal of Neuropsychiatry Clinical Neuroscience 2012*, *24*(1), 118.

Pathak, V., & Sinha, V. K. (2008). Efficacy of repetitive transcranial magnetic stimulation (high and low frequency) as add on therapy in child and adolescent mania: A randomized sham controlled study. Thesis submitted to Ranchi University for partial fulfilment of MD.

Post, A., & Keck, M. E. (2001). Transcranial magnetic stimulation as a therapeutic tool in psychiatry: What do we know about neurobiologic mechanisms? *Journal of Psychiatry Research, 35*, 193–215.

Praharaj, S. K., Ram, D., & Arora, M. (2009). Efficacy of high frequency (rapid) suprathreshold repetitive transcranial magnetic stimulation of right prefrontal cortex in bipolar mania: A randomized sham controlled study. *Journal of Affective Disorders, 117*, 146–150.

Praharaj, S. K. (2011). Repetitive transcranial magnetic stimulation in depression: Studies from India. *Indian Journal of Psychological Medicine, 33*(2), 216–217.

Rachid, F., & Bertschy, G. (2006). Safety and efficacy of repetitive transcranial magnetic stimulation in the treatment of depression: A critical appraisal of the last 10 years. *Clinical Neurophysiology, 36*, 157–183.

Rakesh, G., Shivakumar, V., Subramaniam, A., Nawani, H., Amaresha, A. C., Narayanaswamy, J. C., et al. (2013). Monotherapy with tDCS for Schizophrenia: A case report. *Brain Stimulation*, *6*, 708–709.

Ray, S., Nizamie, S. H., Akhtar, S., Praharaj, S. K., Mishra, B. R., & Zia-ul-Haq, M. (2011). Efficacy of adjunctive high frequency repetitive transcranial magnetic stimulation of left prefrontal cortex in depression: A randomized sham controlled study. *Journal of Affective Disorders, 128*, 153–159.

Sarkhel, S., Sinha, V. K., & Praharaj, S. K. (2010). Adjunctive high frequency right prefrontal repetitive transcranial magnetic stimulation (rTMS) was not effective in obsessive-compulsive disorder but improved secondary depression. *Journal of Anxiety Disorders, 24*, 535–539.

Thirthalli, J., Bharadwaj, B., Kulkarni, S., Gangadhar, B. N., Kharawala, S., & Andrade, C. (2008). Successful use of maintenance rTMS for 8 months in a patient with antipsychotic-refractory auditory hallucinations. *Schizophrenia Research, 100*(1–3), 351–352.

Udupa, K., Sathyaprabha, T. N., Thirthalli, J., Kishore, K. R., Raju, T. R., & Gangadhar, B. N. (2007). Modulation of cardiac autonomic functions in patients with major depression treated with repetitive transcranial magnetic stimulation. *Journal of Affective Disorder, 104*(1–3), 231–236.

Udupa, K., Thirthalli, J., Sathyaprabha, T. N., Kishore, K. R., Raju, T. R., & Gangadhar, B. N. (2011). Differential actions of antidepressant treatments on cardiac autonomic alterations in depression: A prospective comparison. *Asian Journal of Psychiatry, 4*(2), 100–106.

Venkatesh Babu, G. M., Sinha, V. K., & Gandotra, S. (2012). A randomised double-blind sham-controlled study on efficacy of adjunctive high frequency right parietal cortex repetitive transcranial stimulation in unipolar depression. Thesis submitted to Ranchi University for partial fulfilment of MD.

Wassermann, E. M., Grafman, J., Berry, C., Hollnagel, C., Wild, K., Clark, K., et al. (1996). Use and safety of a new repetitive transcranial magnetic stimulator. *Electroencephalography and Clinical Neurophysiology, 101*, 412–417.

Chapter 29
Psychosocial Interventions: Indian Perspective

S.K. Padhy, A. Kohli and S. Sarkar

1 Introduction

Psychosocial interventions occupy a unique place in the comprehensive care of patients with diagnosable mental health concerns. However, the term 'psychosocial intervention' has been referred to in the published literature in a variety of contexts and with various meanings. The term has been utilised in the field of psychiatry, psychology, sociology, nursing, behavioural medicine and many other allied disciplines. In its simplistic and broad meaning, the term refers to 'a systematic attempt to modify a psychosocial process' (Glass 2000). According to such a definition, any measure undertaken to change a social or psychological attribute may be considered as a psychosocial intervention. Such a broad definition would encompass any intervention at the individual, family, workplace, community and population level that attempts to change the psychological or social situation.

Having such a broad definition is of scant practical use, as this would include interventions such as structured psychotherapy, pharmacotherapy, legislative measures to curb substance use, health insurance regimens and community awareness programmes under the fold of psychosocial interventions. This chapter utilises a narrower definition of psychosocial intervention in the context of mental health services. Those interventions have been considered as psychosocial interventions, which have utilised psychological and social measures delivered in a relatively non-technical setting that act at the individual and family level to improve psychosocial

S.K. Padhy, Assistant Professor; A. Kohli, Professor of Clinical Psychology; S. Sarkar, Senior Resident

S.K. Padhy (✉) · A. Kohli · S. Sarkar
Department of Psychiatry, Postgraduate Institute of Medical Education and Research, Chandigarh, India
e-mail: drsusanta_padhy2001@yahoo.co.in; susanta.pgi30@yahoo.in

S. Malhotra and S. Chakrabarti (eds.), *Developments in Psychiatry in India*,
DOI 10.1007/978-81-322-1674-2_29

functioning of the patient. The present definition is a pragmatic one to limit its scope and differentiate it from interventions like pharmacological management, structured psychotherapy and population-based implementation of policies. Thus, the definition suggests inclusion of measures such as psycho-education, family education, compliance enhancement and others under the purview of psychosocial interventions. Such a differentiation may look artificial on face value, but is necessary to focus upon the important group of interventions which are not of clinically administered 'therapies', but nonetheless may positively impact the psychosocial functioning.

Some related and overlapping terms should be considered while discussing this field. Counselling is defined by Gustad (1953) as a learning-oriented process carried in a one-to-one social environment, in which a counsellor who is professionally competent in psychological skills and knowledge seeks to assist a client by appropriate methods to make the client happier or a more productive member of the society. Social work is defined as a profession that promotes social change, problem-solving in human relationships and the empowerment and liberation of people to enhance well-being (Hare 2004). Psychotherapy has been defined as the treatment by psychological means of problems of an emotional nature in which a trained person deliberately establishes a professional relationship with the patient with the object of removing, modifying or retarding existing symptoms, of mediating disturbed patterns of behaviour and of promoting positive personality growth and development (Wolberg 2005). Appraising these related terms is important for a clearer conceptualisation of the term 'psychosocial intervention'.

2 Salient Attributes of Psychosocial Situation in India

Many factors make the psychosocial milieu in India distinct and unique when compared to the West. This translates to salient distinctions in the manner in which psychosocial interventions can be delivered and are actually done. Firstly, the family set-up and the modes of family function in India are different from those of the some of the Western countries. The family in India has been described as a stable cohesive unit, with patriarchal outlook with multi-generational families being common (Avasthi 2010; Kohlmeyer and Fernandes 1963). Interdependence among the family members is the norm. Personal distance and formality in inter-personal relations are uncommon in the family context. The family due to its closeness has been shown to provide substantial support and care to the mentally ill (Sethi 1989). Due to greater tolerance and better acceptance of the mentally ill patients by the families in India, cohort of patients with schizophrenia showed better outcome (Leff et al. 1990).

The second issue that distinguishes psychosocial scenario in India is with respect to the extent and mechanisms of provision of social security and heath care services. Most people in India do not have health insurance and pay out of pocket for treatment of health conditions or depend upon government hospitals and clinics. The governmental health sector is relatively overburdened, as is often not able to deliver quality services to all the patients. Moreover, there are no disability benefits to patients with chronic mental conditions. Such patients have to depend upon their own resources or those of their family members to make a living and obtain treatment and mental health care services. To fill up the void, non-governmental organizations

(NGOs) have taken commendable initiatives, but the provision of care and services has been patchy, driven by restricted agendas and lack common planning.

Thirdly, the perspective of patients and their family members about the causation and treatment of psychiatric illnesses is at a variance with the west. Magico-religious beliefs are common, and family members often attribute the genesis of the illness to supernatural forces (Kulhara et al. 2000; Srinivasan and Thara 2001). Thus, many patients approach the mental health services after being channelled through the faith healers and are quite often delayed in seeking appropriate care. Taking a second opinion from a faith healer is common for some patients who have shown partial response to treatment, with the hope that complete recovery could be achieved by countering the effects of black magic or by placating the Gods. Such a practice is common not only to the uneducated, but also among the educated.

Fourthly, the willingness to undergo certain forms of treatment, especially psychotherapy, is somewhat different. It has been remarked that the psychological sophistication of patients from India may not be as high, resulting in poor interest, adherence or impact of psychotherapeutic measures (Manickam 2010; Neki 1975; Varma 1982). This could be due to generally lower levels of education in India. However, such a situation does not mean that psychotherapy cannot be practiced at all, but careful selection of patients is required.

Thus, there are certain specific facets, which need to be considered while appraising psychosocial interventions conducted in India, so that interpretation of the findings is made in the right perspective.

3 Research on Psychosocial Interventions from India

A wide variety of psychosocial interventions have been attempted successfully in individuals and families with psychiatric disorders. These have grouped according to the type of intervention and are as follows.

3.1 Involvement of Families in the Care of Hospitalised Patients

Family members can contribute a lot to the management of patients with psychiatric disorders. In fact, in India, they are the primary caregivers at home and are involved in the day-to-day issues of the patients. However, previously, when patients with psychiatric disorders were hospitalised in the psychiatric institutions, the hospital staff looked after the patients and family members had little to do with patient care. The outlook began to change with time, especially with the efforts of Vidyasagar in Amritsar and Narayanan and others in Bangalore, who encouraged active involvement of family members in the treatment process, so that early reintegration with the society could be achieved (Narayanan et al. 1972).

Verghese (1988) systematically studied the role and advantages of family members in the treatment of patients with psychiatric disorders. At his centre in Vellore, two relatives of patients were required to stay during the period of admission in the ward. The assistance of the relatives was taken in the day-to-day care of the patients. Group meetings of the relatives were conducted with the social workers, nurses and occupational therapists discussing about various aspects of mental ailments. In an assessment of 100 relatives who were evaluated at time of admission and at 4 weeks, it was seen that over the course of ward stay, the perception about the illness improved and considerable information was gained by the relatives about the aetiology of the disease, treatment and rehabilitation process.

Other programmes have also suggested that the inclusion of the family members in the treatment process led to better outcomes (Shanker and Menon 1991). Hence, deinstitutionalisation has been suggested to manage the patients at the community level with the active help of the family members (Krishnamurthy et al. 2000).

3.2 Psychoeducation

Psychoeducation refers to a set of measures aimed to increase patients' and the family members' knowledge of the illness and its treatment and to develop some degree of insight in the process (Xia et al. 2011). It can be presented in the form of individual sessions with the patient or the family member or caregiver, a session involving the entire family together, or conducted in groups. It can be delivered in a set of the structured sessions, with each session having a particular agenda, or in the form of unstructured sessions, wherein the queries are answered sequentially.

A few studies have studied psychoeducation of the patients and the family in India. Kulhara et al. (2009) conducted a randomised controlled study comparing nine once-a-month structured psychoeducation sessions with routine care in a cohort of 76 patients. The intervention was delivered by two trained mental health professionals using specific training manuals developed for the study. Structured psychoeducation intervention was found to be significantly better than routine outpatient care on several measures including psychopathology, disability, caregiver support and caregiver satisfaction. The psychoeducation intervention package was simple and was considered quite feasible. The intervention was quite cost effective and required around $25 per patient-family unit.

Other researchers have also carried forth substantive work for exploring the usefulness of individual and family educational programmes in patients with schizophrenia and other psychiatric illness (Ponnuchamy et al. 2005; Shihabuddeen and Gopinath 2005; Thara et al. 2005). Open group formats in which many caregivers aggregate and discuss about the illness under the supervision of a therapist, counsellor or social worker seem to be an easily carried out modality for delivering psychoeducation. Apart from the educational component, these incorporate elements of support among the members of the group. These forums, typically conducted once a month, provide an opportunity to clarify doubts, demystify myths, developed coping, learn from others' experiences and ventilate about their own difficulties and emotional distress.

Many programmes have included psychoeducation as one of the components of the total intervention package (Chatterjee et al. 2003; Patel et al. 2010). Identifying the exclusive role of psychoeducation may be difficult in such studies. Nonetheless, these studies do emphasise the need for psychoeducation for complete and effective programme delivery.

3.3 Community Outreach

Community outreach interventions involve modifications of the standard service delivery by bringing therapeutic processes closer to the patient. It involves provision of service at the doorstep of the patient and reduces dropouts and non-adherence. Such a community outreach usually involves psychosocial inputs.

The Raipur Rani project (Wig et al. 1981) was one of the first systematic structured community intervention projects in India. The project was carried out in the Raipur Rani block of Ambala district in Haryana, north India, and covered a population of around 60,000 in about 100 villages. Neuro-psychiatric cases such as psychosis, epilepsy, mental retardation and depressive and anxiety neurosis were identified, and a limited list of needed drugs was drawn up for providing to the patients. At the primary health centre, a weekly psychiatric clinic was set up, which brought psychiatric care services closer to the community. It was seen that regular follow-up at the centre depended upon the accessibility and distance from patient's residence. Training of the health personnel was undertaken with the aim of building acceptability of services, easy access of care, expanding the workforce to deliver psychiatric treatment and maintain continuity of care. The services, especially that of follow-up care, were decentralised to the sub-centres, where brief assessment and provision of treatment was conducted by health workers under the overall supervision of psychiatrists. The project proved successful and paved way for other such projects.

Suman et al. (1980) studied 30 patients with schizophrenia attending a community clinic, exploring the problems encountered. Further interventions that were tried included regular home visits, family counselling, marital counselling, contact with social welfare agencies and providing an understanding about the illness. They observed multiple issues in these patients such as high level of expectation, excess emotional involvement, problems with long-term treatment, problems with marriage, rehabilitation issues and residual symptoms.

A project was initiated from National Institute of Mental Health and Neurosciences (NIMHANS) (Chandrashekar et al. 1981) catering to about 120 villages around the rural health centre of Sakalwara. The centre was manned by a psychiatrist, a psychiatric social worker and a psychiatric nurse. The strategies involved free prescription of drugs and rigorous attempts to keep the patient under follow-up. Severe and chronic psychotics showed a good response to treatment, and persuasive efforts were required to make patients accept long-term medications.

Apart from the Raipur Rani Project and Sakalwada Project, other community outreach and intervention programmes have been developed and introduced. The Bellary project was launched in Karnataka to cover an entire district (Murthy 1998), the success of which led to expansion of psychiatry through the National Mental Health Programme and the District Mental Health Programme to bring the services closer to the community.

In a set of studies by Pai and Kapur (1982, 1983), routine inpatient care was compared to home visits by nurses. The frequency of visits was determined by the severity of patient condition. It was seen that home visits by nurses was associated with better clinical outcomes. The nurse home care group had better social functioning of the patients and greatly reduced the burden on the families. This modality of intervention also was associated with lower costs. Chatterjee et al. (2003) in a community intervention study of patients with psychotic disorders concluded that an comprehensive intervention comprising psychotropic medication, psychoeducation, adherence management, psychosocial rehabilitation and support for employment was associated with greater reductions in disability. Thus, we see that community outreach has a positive impact on the outcome of patients.

3.4 Camps

The camp approach has been quite successful in providing mental health and de-addiction services to the community. In this modality, 'camps' are organised with the involvement of a host organisation involved in social welfare activities. Resources and infrastructure for the camp are mobilised from the community. Awareness is spread about of the conduct of the camp. During the camp, patients are evaluated by trained physicians and psychiatrists. Counselling is provided, and medications are supplied wherever possible. Aftercare and follow-up are provided, and referrals are made for serious cases. This kind of intervention helps those patients to seek help who otherwise do not approach structured health care systems.

The outcomes of these camps have been evaluated by many researchers. Purohit and Razdan (1988) conducted 14 camps for opioid-dependent patients in rural areas of Rajasthan. They found that many of the camp attendees never sought formal treatment and continued substance use. The outcome of patients treated at the camp was comparable to that of hospital-treated patients. Such an approach has been also found useful for the treatment of alcohol-dependent patients (Ranganathan 1994). It has been observed that the incidence of alcohol abuse decreases over time due to the community involvement consequent to the camps. In a study by Chavan et al. (2003), outcomes of camp inpatient detoxification were found to be comparable to hospital inpatient detoxification. Many other researchers have also concurred that camps have a positive impact in promoting abstinence (Chavan and Arun 1999; Raj et al. 2005).

3.5 Rehabilitation

Very few studies from India have focused upon the rehabilitation services of the patients with psychiatric disorders. Menon and Ramachandran (1976) in their study of patients with a diagnosis of chronic schizophrenia found that many patients could be gainfully employed in the occupational therapy section and then an industrial training centre. This suggested that when given adequate opportunities, patients can be reinstituted into productive vocations.

Nagaswami et al. (1985) assessed the rehabilitation needs of 59 patients with a diagnosis of schizophrenia using a structured questionnaire. The most important need endorsed was that for employment, stressing the requirement for rehabilitative job services. One-fourth of the men and about half of the women in this study expressed need for vocational training services. The authors had concluded that it would be meaningful to have a community-based approach to rehabilitation and provision of secure employment opportunities.

Chatterjee et al. (2009) in their cohort of patients with psychotic disorders found that intervention in the form of self-help groups, community networks and lay counsellors led to improved outcomes. It was seen that the majority of patients in the programme had been taking part in normative community activities such as attending marriages, participating in community festivals, visiting relatives in another village, attending *gram sabhas* and exercising electoral rights. A large proportion also secured employment in the National Rural Employment Guarantee (NREG) scheme consequent to the intervention. In another study, Chatterjee et al. (2003) found that the community-based rehabilitation programme fared better than usual outpatient-based services, especially in cases of non-compliant or poorly compliant patients.

Thus, studies from India suggest that psychosocial interventions would work in rehabilitation of patients with psychiatric disorders.

3.6 Interventions for Children

A psychosocial-based intervention has been described by Malhotra et al. (2002). The intervention had comprised of behavioural interventions in the form of communication enhancement and Treatment and Education of Autistic and related Communication handicapped CHildren approach (TEACCH), supportive interventions in the form of understanding and comforting the caregivers, and imparting educational information about autism and guidance about other facilities. The intervention was found to be helpful by the family members and could be better delivered in playroom setting in a comfortable environment. They found that the support, reassurance and empathy (understanding and comforting techniques) to be the most useful ingredients of this particular treatment package.

An inpatient-based family intervention has been developed by Narayanan et al. (1988) that focuses on the training of parents of children with mental retardation. The intervention included overlapping stages of detailed assessment and investigation, followed by priming the parents by giving information about mental retardation. Thereafter, individualised parent training was initiated, and targets were set for each child based on developmental level. The children were then discharged and followed up. Such an approach was found useful in demonstrating small gains with the help of training, thus improving the motivation of parents to train the child.

School-based programmes provide an excellent opportunity to target the youth who are at risk of developing substance use disorders. In a randomised controlled study, thirty schools in Delhi were randomly assigned to 3 conditions: school-based and family-based interventions, school-based intervention only, or control group (Reddy et al. 2002). A total of 4,776 seventh grade students were recruited. The school intervention included posters, booklets, classroom activities, debates and a signature campaign in relation to smoking. The family intervention involved home activities. The study showed that students receiving active intervention were significantly less likely than controls to have been offered, received or experimented with the use of tobacco. One of the programmes that involved 32 schools in two big cities of India (Chennai and Delhi) involved over 8,000 participants (Bate et al. 2009). The programme Mobilizing Youth for Tobacco-Related Initiatives in India (MYTRI) involved four components in the form of classroom sessions, school posters, parent postcards, and peer-led health activism. It was seen that conduct of the programme was associated with less likelihood of pupils receiving offers of using tobacco or using it themselves.

3.7 Disaster Situations

Psychosocial interventions focusing on mental health concerns of people affected by natural disasters have been studied. In the wake of the tsunami that affected the south eastern coast and Andaman and Nicobar Islands, psychosocial intervention had been carried out and the efforts documented (Vijaykumar et al. 2006). Immediately after the tsunami, the World Health Organization conducted an Orientation for Master Trainers who trained the relief workers serving the affected areas. In the wake of tsunami, the Schizophrenia Research Foundation (SCARF) conducted a rapid needs assessment in the areas surrounding Chennai. Requirement of psychological help was identified as one of the most prominent needs reported by 52 % of the participants. A short training course was provided to the staff of NGOs, self-help group members, volunteers and others native to the region focusing on understanding the reactions of the affected, providing counselling and referral of severe cases. A short film in Tamil about the tsunami was shown to dispel superstitious myths about it. The common reactions observed in the initial period after the tsunami were emotional outbursts, crying, lack of motivation, anxiety, depression, guilt and features of acute stress disorder. Active listening, emotional support, collective grieving, externalisation of interests (like recreation), guidance and practical help in housing helped in normal reintegration of most of the people. During the intermediate period post-traumatic stress disorder, depression, anxiety, drug and alcohol dependence and exacerbation of symptoms of previous mental illnesses were commonly encountered and were catered to using intensive counselling and medications. Another NGO—SNEHA—worked intensely in helping the tsunami affected, especially the youth. A temporary shelter was drawn up at one of the worst affected areas of Chennai, and support services to the individuals and families were provided. To bring back a semblance of normalcy at the locality, a cultural and sport activity was organised, with large participation, with the aim of encouraging creative expression and sublimation of grief and anxieties.

3.8 Others

Psychological interventions by lay health counsellors have been studied in patients with anxiety and depressive disorders presenting to the primary health care services (Patel et al. 2010). Clustered random sampling was utilised to allocate 24 public and private health centres into intervention (which included collaborative stepped-care case management and psychosocial interventions through lay health counsellor, supplemented by antidepressant drugs by the primary care physician and supervised by a mental health specialist) versus enhanced usual care groups. The lay counsellors from the community underwent 2-month training and delivered interventions in the form of psychoeducation and interpersonal therapy. Patients with ICD-10-confirmed common mental disorders in the intervention group were more likely to have recovered at 6 months than those in the control group. This suggested that lay counsellor-led collaborative care led to better outcomes in treatment at the primary care setting. Another integrated psychosocial treatment has been tested in patients with schizophrenia (Stanley and Shwetha 2006). The integrated intervention package included pharmacotherapy, psychosocial therapies and spiritual therapy. Significant reduction in patient symptoms as well as caregiver burden was found with intervention as was enhanced quality of life.

Patients with drug abuse problems often have difficulties in finding gainful employment and securing credit for setting up their personal businesses. To this effect, micro-credit-based rehabilitation has been studied in patients with opioid dependence being maintained on opioid substitution therapy (Yadav et al. 2010). In this project, 55 male patients were given small amounts of money to start their own enterprises. The micro-credit financing was successful in a proportion of patients and enabled social and occupational reintegration. Such micro-credit-based interventions have also been found to be useful in females with psychiatric illnesses that have a positive impact on the outcomes (Rao et al. 2011).

4 A Narrative View

Over the years, many experts and researchers have commented upon the need and implications of psychosocial interventions in India. Such views have been critical in developing services, shaping policies and stimulating research endeavours. They may not amount to evidence base in usual sense, but are true reflections of the ground realities and future promises.

Evaluating the family studies in the context of provision of care to patients with psychiatric illnesses, Murthy (2003) has made crucial recommendations. He suggests that families need to be supported by professionals to acquire skills of care and be supported emotionally; families should be supported financially by state at least partially due to economic disadvantage and hardships encountered, and partnerships of the professionals with the families should be developed for better care of the patients. The changing family lives in India has led to some issues including the growing urbanisation, breaking down of the traditional joint and extended families and their support, familial distress due to economic deprivation, social marginalisation, substance use, and chronic illnesses, and requirement of the elderly caregivers for the taking care of their psychiatrically disturbed wards.

Some authors suggest that NGOs can play a larger role in developing, testing and providing psychosocial-based interventions to the community (Murthy 2011; Thara and Patel 2003). These organisations can play an important part in suicide prevention services, school mental health programmes, education-based interventions, providing access to care, home visits and compliance enhancement, occupational rehabilitation and by many other means. Coordination between various NGOs can help to facilitate a dialogue, develop priorities, avoid duplication of efforts and to reorient services to meet deficits and gaps in services.

Rehabilitation services have been considered quite important in the patients with chronic mental health conditions. In one of the earlier reports, Gupta et al. (1968) found that many schizophrenic patients were being just kept in the hospital just for social reasons and the lack of rehabilitation services. They suggest that rehabilitation services need to be expanded and all mental hospitals should have at least one occupational therapist. Thus, rehabilitation work should be given an important consideration for patients to resume social roles.

Many authors have also expressed and emphasised the need to develop psychosocial interventions in different medical and psychiatric conditions (Chatterjee 2005; Chaturvedi 1994). This is usually based upon the demonstration of the magnitude of psychiatric problems in health-related conditions such as cancer. However, intervention studies have not kept up pace due to difficulties in conducting studies. Carefully planned psychosocial interventions can help answer questions about what kind of interventions may be helpful in such conditions.

5 Issues in Research for Psychosocial Interventions

Multiple issues need to be considered while evaluating psychosocial intervention research. The first and foremost involves the definition of the intervention. The psychosocial intervention being studied needs to be properly operationalised and the components distinguished. It should be clear in the programme content about what constitutes the intervention (e.g. psychoeducation sessions by lay workers) and what does not (e.g. cognitive behavioural therapy by psychiatrist). A manual may be developed to clearly define and document the workings of the intervention and how will it be delivered.

Another issue in such research involves what components of the intervention are actually of benefit. To answer such a question, a dismantling design is useful in which certain components of the intervention are delivered to specific groups and role of each part is evaluated. Another design that can answer such a question is one where each component is incrementally added and assessments are made at each level. Paying heed to such a question can help to retain the effective components in the programme and remove out the components that do not work.

The third issue involves obtaining a relevant and useful control. The control group provides a reference point for making comparisons while establishing efficacy. Randomisation is a well-accepted method of deriving control participants and tries to ensure equitable distributions of the confounders. Other methods of using controls include case–control design for retrospective data, intervention and non-intervention groups in cohort studies, and the wait list controls when using phased or delayed implementation of the intervention. A related issue involves what should be used as a control: whether no treatment, attention, wait list, another efficacious treatment should be used requires careful consideration. Getting a 'placebo' intervention may not be actually possible in a psychosocial intervention research situation. What constitutes a best control for a particular intervention is dependent upon many factors and should be considered carefully.

The fourth issue deals with blinding. Blinding of the participants is difficult if not impossible in studies involving psychosocial interventions. It has been seen that even therapist and intervention attention may lead to bias due to expectancy of effect. In such situations, it is prudent to use raters who are blinded to the group allocation and make efforts to minimise disclosure of information about group during the evaluation process.

Another issue that is quite relevant to psychosocial intervention research involves the ethical aspects. Whether and how consent is obtained, how confidentiality is maintained, whether effective treatment is withheld, and whether any harm due to the intervention is foreseeable are some of the queries that need to be adequately addressed by protocol of the research.

The sixth issue concerns establishing validity by independent replication of the findings by another group of researchers. Often, funded projects show good results in a particular place/institution till funding and resources are adequate. For the results to be generalisable, a replication of the results in another geographical setting by researchers unrelated to the ones who developed and professed an intervention is advised, but is infrequently attempted and established.

As in any research, the funding needs and constraints cannot be overlooked. For doing justice to the resources being utilised, the research should be able to answer clinically relevant questions and be translatable into practice.

The above-mentioned issues reflect upon the current research practices and make suggestions about considerations for future research endeavours. Probably in the future, more methodologically rigorous studies evaluating psychosocial interventions would be conducted. The present evidence base for psychosocial intervention research in India is fairly limited, and more work is desired and required. Pilot projects are useful means of testing whether an intervention is feasible to be carried out before launching on a larger scale to evaluate efficacy. Translating the initial findings of studies to a larger confirmatory study to clinical practice remains a challenge that needs to be answered.

6 Conclusion

Many psychosocial interventions have been utilised and evaluated in India for addressing mental health problems. These include a variety of individual as well as family-based interventions, conducted in the domains of psychoeducation, family involvement in treatment, rehabilitation services, school-based interventions, community outreach, camp-based approach and a combination of these. Further research interest would expand the evidence base of the psychosocial research in India and provide practical means of interventions for the benefit of the patients.

Acknowledgments The authors would like to acknowledge the commendable work done in psychosocial intervention area by individuals, organisations and institutions for patients with psychiatric disorders.

References

Avasthi, A. (2010). Preserve and strengthen family to promote mental health. *Indian Journal of Psychiatry, 52*, 113.

Bate, S. L., Stigler, M. H., Thompson, M. S., Arora, M., Perry, C. L., Reddy, K. S., et al. (2009). Psychosocial mediators of a school-based tobacco prevention program in India: Results from the first year of Project MYTRI. *Prevention Science : The Official Journal of The Society For Prevention Research, 10*, 116–128.

Chandrashekar, C. R., Isaac, M. K., Kapur, R. L., & Sarathy, R. P. (1981). Management of priority mental disorders in the community. *Indian Journal of Psychiatry, 23*, 174.

Chatterjee, P. (2005). Mental health care for India's tsunami survivors. *The Lancet, 365*, 833–834.

Chatterjee, S., Patel, V., Chatterjee, A., & Weiss, H. A. (2003). Evaluation of a community-based rehabilitation model for chronic schizophrenia in rural India. *The British Journal of Psychiatry, 182*, 57–62.

Chatterjee, S., Pillai, A., Jain, S., Cohen, A., & Patel, V. (2009). Outcomes of people with psychotic disorders in a community-based rehabilitation programme in rural India. *The British Journal of Psychiatry, 195*, 433–439.

Chaturvedi, S. K. (1994). Exploration of concerns and role of psychosocial intervention in palliative care—A study from India. *Annals of Academy Medicine, Singapore, 23*, 256.

Chavan, B. S., & Arun, P. (1999). Treatment of alcohol and drug abuse in camp setting. *The Indian Journal of Psychiatry, 41*, 140.

Chavan, B. S., Gupta, N., & Raj, L. (2003). Camp approach-an effective, alternate inpatient treatment setting for substance dependence: A report from India. *The German Journal of Psychiatry, 6*, 17–22.

Glass, T. (2000). Psychosocial Intervention. In L. F. Berkman & I. Kawachi (Eds.), *Social Epidemiology*. New York: Oxford University Press.

Gupta, P., Prabhu, M., & Prabhu, G. G. (1968). Rehabilitation of the chronic psychiatric patient. *Indian Journal of Psychiatry 10*, 157.

Gustad, J. W. (1953). The definition of counseling. In R. F. Berdie (Ed.), *Roles and relationships in counselling*. Minneapolis, US: University of Minnesota Press.

Hare, I. (2004). Defining social work for the 21st century the international federation of social workers' revised definition of social work. *International Social Work, 47*, 407–424.

Kohlmeyer, W. A., & Fernandes, X. (1963). Psychiatry in India: Family approach in the treatment of mental disorders. *American Journal of Psychiatry, 119*, 1033–1037.

Krishnamurthy, K., Venugopal, D., & Alimchandani, A. K. (2000). Mental hospitals in India. *Indian Journal of Psychiatry, 42*, 125.

Kulhara, P., Avasthi, A., & Sharma, A. (2000). Magico-religious beliefs in schizophrenia: A study from North India. *Psychopathology, 33*, 62–68.

Kulhara, P., Chakrabarti, S., Avasthi, A., Sharma, A., & Sharma, S. (2009). Psychoeducational intervention for caregivers of Indian patients with schizophrenia: A randomised—Controlled trial. *Acta Psychiatrica Scandinavica, 119*, 472–483.

Leff, J., Wig, N. N., Bedi, H., Menon, D. K., Kuipers, L., Korten, A., et al. (1990). Relatives' expressed emotion and the course of schizophrenia in Chandigarh. A two-year follow-up of a first-contact sample. *The British Journal of Psychiatry, 156*, 351–356.

Malhotra, S., Chakrabarti, S., & Nehra, A. (2002). Psychological intervention with parents of autistic children. *Indian Journal of Psychiatry, 44*, 108.

Manickam, L. S. S. (2010). Psychotherapy in India. *Indian Journal of Psychiatry, 52*, S366–S370.

Menon, S., & Ramachandran, V. (1976). Social and clinical factors in the outcome of schizophrenia. *Indian Journal of Psychiatry, 18*, 45.

Murthy, R. S. (1998). Rural psychiatry in developing countries. *Psychiatric Services, 49*, 967–969.

Murthy, R. S. (2003). Family interventions and empowerment as an approach to enhance mental health resources in developing countries. *World Psychiatry, 2*, 35.

Murthy, R. S. (2011). Mental health initiatives in India (1947–2010). *The National Medical Journal of India, 24*, 98.

Nagaswami, V., Valecha, V., Thara, R., Rajkumar, S., & Menon, M. S. (1985). Rehabilitation needs of schizophrenic patients—A preliminary report. *Indian Journal of Psychiatry, 27*, 213.

Narayanan, H., Embar, P., & Reddy, G. (1972). Review of treatment in family ward. *Indian Journal of Psychiatry, 14*, 123.

Narayanan, H. S., Girimaji, S. R., Gandhi, D. H., Raju, K. M., Rao, P. M., & Nardev, G. (1988). Brief in-patient family intervention in mental retardation. *Indian Journal of Psychiatry, 30*, 275.

Neki, J. S. (1975). Psychotherapy in India: Past, present, and future. *American Journal of Psychotherapy, 29*, 92–100.

Pai, S., & Kapur, R. L. (1982). Impact of treatment intervention on the relationship between dimensions of clinical psychopathology, social dysfunction and burden on the family of psychiatric patients. *Psychological Medicine, 12*, 651–658.

Pai, S., & Kapur, R. L. (1983). Evaluation of home care treatment for schizophrenic patients. *Acta Psychiatrica Scandinavica, 67*, 80–88.
Patel, V., Weiss, H. A., Chowdhary, N., Naik, S., Pednekar, S., Chatterjee, S., et al. (2010). Effectiveness of an intervention led by lay health counsellors for depressive and anxiety disorders in primary care in Goa, India (MANAS): A cluster randomised controlled trial. *The Lancet, 376*, 2086–2095.
Ponnuchamy, L., Mathew, B. K., Mathew, S., Udayakumar, G. S., Kalyanasundaram, S., & Ramprasad, D. (2005). Family support group in psychosocial rehabilitation. *Indian Journal of Psychiatry, 47*, 160.
Purohit, D. R., & Razdan, V. K. (1988). Evolution and appraisal of community camp-approach to opium detoxification in North India. *Indian Journal of Social Psychiatry, 4*, 15–21.
Raj, L., Chavan, B. S., & Bala, C. (2005). Community "de-addiction" camps: A follow-up study. *Indian Journal of Psychiatry, 47*, 44.
Ranganathan, S. (1994). The Manjakkudi experience: A camp approach towards treating alcoholics. *Addiction, 89*, 1071–1075.
Rao, K., Vanguri, P., & Premchander, S. (2011). Community-based mental health intervention for underprivileged women in rural India: An experiential report. *International Journal of Family Medicine, 2011*, 621426.
Reddy, K. S., Arora, M., Kohli, A., Prabhakaran, D., Perry, C. L., Nair, B., et al. (2002). Tobacco and alcohol use outcomes of a school-based intervention in New Delhi. *American Journal of Health Behaviour, 26*, 173–181.
Sethi, B. B. (1989). Family as a potent therapeutic force. *Indian Journal of Psychiatry, 31*, 22–30.
Shankar, R., & Menon, M. S. (1991). Interventions with families of people with schizophrenia: The issues facing a community-based rehabilitation center in India. *Psychosociological Rehabilitation Journal, 15*, 85.
Shihabuddeen, T. I., & Gopinath, P. S. (2005). Group meetings of caretakers of patients with schizophrenia and bipolar mood disorders. *Indian Journal of Psychiatry, 47*, 153.
Srinivasan, T. N., & Thara, R. (2001). Beliefs about causation of schizophrenia: Do Indian families believe in supernatural causes? *Social Psychiatry and Psychiatric Epidemiology, 36*, 134–140.
Stanley, S., & Shwetha, S. (2006). Integrated psychosocial intervention in schizophrenia: Implications for patients and caregivers. *The International Journal of Psychosocial Rehabilitation, 10*, 113–128.
Suman, C., Baldev, S., Murthy, R. S., & Wig, N. N. (1980). Helping the chronic schizophrenic and their families in the community- initial observations. *Indian Journal of Psychiatry, 22*, 97.
Thara, R., Padmavati, R., Lakshmi, A., & Karpagavalli, P. (2005). Family education in schizophrenia: A comparison of two approaches. *Indian Journal of Psychiatry, 47*, 218.
Thara, R., & Patel, V. (2003). *Meeting the mental health needs of developing countries: NGO innovations in India*. New Delhi: Sage Publications.
Varma, V. K. (1982). Present state of psychotherapy in India. *Indian Journal of Psychiatry, 24*, 209–226.
Verghese, A. (1988). Family participation in mental health care-the Vellore experiment. *Indian Journal of Psychiatry, 30*, 117.
Vijaykumar, L., Thara, R., John, S., & Chellappa, S. (2006). Psychosocial interventions after tsunami in Tamil Nadu, India. *International Review of Psychiatry, 18*, 225–231.
Wig, N. N., Murthy, R. S., & Harding, T. W. (1981). A model for rural psychiatric services—Raipur Rani experience. *Indian Journal of Psychiatry, 23*, 275.
Wolberg, L. R. (2005). *The technique of psychotherapy*. Lanham, Maryland US: Rowman & Littlefield Pub Inc.
Xia, J., Merinder, L. B., & Belgamwar, M. R. (2011). Psychoeducation for schizophrenia. The Cochrane database of systematic reviews CD002831.
Yadav, D., Dhawan, A., Balhara, Y. P. S., & Yadav, S. (2010). Occupational rehabilitation of opiate users on maintenance treatment in India: A microcredit-based approach. *Journal of Social Work Practice in the Addictions, 10*, 413–422.

Chapter 30
Rehabilitation Psychiatry

B.S. Chavan and S. Das

1 Introduction

Psychiatric rehabilitation or 'psychosocial rehabilitation', as it is now frequently termed, has been variously defined. The scope might include achieving social integration by reducing the impact of disability and handicapping conditions through various measures (WHO 1980), improving the capabilities and competence of a person suffering from mental illness through improvement in their environment (Anthony et al. 1984), helping a person to adjust to their deficits by using residual abilities (Benett 1978), or a therapeutic approach that encourages a mentally ill person to develop to his or her fullest capacity through learning and environmental support (Bachrach 1992).

In 1996, the World Health Organization (WHO) and the World Association for Psychosocial Rehabilitation (WAPR) jointly came out with a 'consensus statement' on psychosocial rehabilitation. This statement defines psychosocial rehabilitation as a strategy that facilitates the opportunity for individuals impaired or disabled by mental disorder to reach their optimal level of functioning in the community, by improving individuals' competencies and introducing environmental changes.

The essential elements of all rehabilitation programs are similar (Bachrach 1992):

(a) Enable a person with mental illness to develop to the fullest extent of their capacities despite the existence of mental illness.
(b) Rehabilitation has to happen in the context of the individual's environment.
(c) Rehabilitation is directed towards exploiting the individual's strength.
(d) Restoration of 'hope' for those with mental illness is a distinctive feature of rehabilitation.

B.S. Chavan, Professor and Head; S. Das, Assistant Professor

B.S. Chavan (✉) · S. Das
Department of Psychiatry, Government Medical College and Hospital, Chandigarh, India
e-mail: drchavanbs@gmail.com

S. Malhotra and S. Chakrabarti (eds.), *Developments in Psychiatry in India*,
DOI 10.1007/978-81-322-1674-2_30

(e) Optimism about vocational potential of people with mental illness.
(f) Reaching beyond work activities to cover other concerns of individuals.
(g) Active involvement of individuals and primary caregivers.
(h) Maintaining continued care.
(i) Establishing a strong relationship between patient and the caregiver.

People with psychiatric disabilities also have the same life aspirations and wishes as people without disabilities. They do desire to have their own houses, choice of education, career, social relationship, participation in community activities with equal rights and so on.

The overall philosophy of psychiatric rehabilitation in mental disorders comprises of two intervention strategies—*individual-centred* strategies and *ecological strategies.* Individual-centred strategies are aimed at developing patients' skills in interacting and handling the stressful environment, while ecological strategies are directed towards developing environmental resources to reduce potential stressors. Most of the persons with disability need a combination of both these approaches (Rossler 2006).

2 Steps in Psychiatric Rehabilitation

The starting point for an adequate understanding of rehabilitation is that it is concerned with the individual person in the context of his or her specific environment and is carried out under real-life conditions. Thus, rehabilitation practitioners have to take into consideration the realistic life circumstances that the affected person is likely to encounter in his or her day-to-day living (Bachrach 2000). The second step is helping the disabled person to identify their personal goals. This is not a process where the person simply lists his needs. Motivational interviews provide a better approach to identify the individual's personal costs and benefits associated with the needs (Corrigan et al. 2001). Assessing the individual's readiness for change is also required (Rogers et al. 2001; Liberman and Glick 2004). Subsequently, the focus of rehabilitation process is on the patient's strengths (Bachrach 2000). Irrespective of the degree of psychopathology in a given patient, the therapist must work with the 'well part of the ego' as 'there is always an intact portion of the ego to which treatment and rehabilitation efforts can be directed' (Lamb 1982). Often those with disabilities lack not only confidence, but also hope and so rehabilitation should also focus on restoring hope to such people. As Bachrach (2000) states, 'it is the kind of hope that comes with learning to accept the fact of one's illness and one's limitations and proceeding from there'.

Psychiatric rehabilitation cannot be imposed. The individual's right as a respected partner and endorsing his or her self-determination concerning all aspects of the treatment and rehabilitation process is important. The rehabilitation values are also incorporated in the concept of recovery (Farkas et al. 2005). Within the concept of the recovery, the therapeutic alliance plays a crucial role in engaging the patient in his or her own care-planning (Priebe et al. 2002). In addition to working with the patient, engaging the family in recovery planning is very crucial, more so in the Indian context where the family is closely involved in the recovery path. Research has also shown that social support is associated with recovery from chronic diseases, greater life satisfaction and enhanced ability to cope with life stressors (Rogers et al. 2004). Corrigan et al. (2005) have found that the most important factor facilitating recovery is the support of peers. Therefore, psychiatric rehabilitation is also an exercise in network building (Cutler 1985).

Finally, people with mental disorders and their caregivers prefer to see themselves as consumers of mental health services. This consumerism allows for due consideration of the affected persons' perspective and to seriously consider courses of action relevant for them (Kopelwicz and Liberman 1995). In this context, physicians should also acknowledge that disagreement about the illness between themselves and the patient is not always the result of the illness process (Bebbington 1995). Unlike the West, there is very little effort in our settings to engage the patient and his caregivers in the treatment planning, including rehabilitation. However, the consumerism movement and the rights-based approach have started making inroads in India and the families and patients, through self-help groups have started verbalising their needs and rights. In the experience of authors, the compliance and retention into care is better when the family was allowed to participate in treatment planning.

3 Role of Government in Rehabilitation and Recent Initiatives

3.1 Persons with Disability Act and Development of the Indian Disability Evaluation and Assessment Scale

The recognition of disability due to mental disorders came very late in India. Disability due to mental disorders was officially recognised for the first time when it was included as one of the disabilities in the 'Persons with Disability Act (PWD Act)' in 1995. Before this Act, care of the disabled as a whole was treated as a charity by the government and the civil society. They received whatever was left out after fulfilling the needs of so-called abled people, whose greed left very little for the persons with disability and the underprivileged. The PWD Act of the Ministry of Social Justice and Empowerment, Government of India, has been rated as the most powerful Act in the field of disability. It has restated that the persons with disability have similar rights and the government is duty bound to protect these rights. The most significant among these is the protection of employment. In addition to 3 % reservation in jobs (1 % each for physically, visually and hearing impaired), if a person acquires disability, including disability due to mental disorders, he or she cannot be removed from the job and will continue to get all the benefits including promotion and increment, at par with other employees. If a department does not have jobs where the person with disability can be engaged, he can be adjusted in other departments. The person with disability will retire at the due time. Before this Act, many patients suffering from major mental disorders used to hide their illness fearing loss of their jobs. The facilities and concessions under Persons with Disability Act such as income tax rebate up to rupees 75,000, concession in rail travel along with escort, free travel in the state roadways buses, free assistive devices, provision of passing on the family pension to persons with disability, and disability pension have helped many persons with disability. The Act also provide safeguards for protection of rights and any discrimination against a person with disability, such discrimination can be reported to the State Commissioner for Disability, who has been given judicial powers to summon a person and announce punishment, if found guilty.

For availing any benefit under the disability category, the disability certificate is a must which should indicate the type and degree of disability.

Initially, there was no tool to assess the degree of disability caused by mental disorders. Thus, the persons suffering from mental disorders were deprived of these benefits. This vacuum was filled after the development of the screening tool called the 'Indian Disability Evaluation and Assessment Scale' commonly referred to as the 'IDEAS'. The task for developing this tool was initiated by the Indian Psychiatric Society (IPS) and a tentative instrument formed was field-tested in eight centres all over the country with the Schizophrenia Research Foundation (SCARF) being the coordinating centre. The IDEAS was gazetted by the Government of India, Ministry of Social Justice and Empowerment, in February 2002 as the official instrument to measure psychiatric disability for the purpose of certification. Assessment with the IDEAS can be done by trained social workers, psychologists or occupational therapists, while the diagnosis and certification can be done by a psychiatrist only. This was thus a giant step towards rehabilitation of people with mental illness in India. The IDEAS gave importance to functional disability, rather than diagnosis alone. The disability score obtained after assessing personal care, communications, social interactions, work and duration of illness can be converted into percentage of disability.

The National Trust Act, 1999: The National Trust Act is also a landmark legal provision for the care and rehabilitation of persons with intellectual disability, autism, cerebral palsy and multiple disabilities. The Act has made it easier to appoint a guardian once the person has become major (more than 18 years as per our constitution). Instead of going to court, a local-level committee (LLC) at each district, consisting of the deputy commissioner, a person with disability and a parent representative of an NGO registered with the National Trust has been given semi-judicial powers to appoint a guardian. The LLC has powers to remove the guardian in case it is found that the guardian is neglecting the person with disability or not utilising the funds of this person properly. The guardian is supposed to file an annual return of all transactions to the satisfaction of the LLC. The parents of these children had a fear that their relatives and family members will grab the property and money after their death. After enactment of this Act, they are now satisfied that somebody is there to safeguard the interest of their wards, when they will be no more in this world. The National Trust Act has also created residential facilities for women, orphaned mentally challenged and 'below poverty line' families with a person suffering from any of the four disabilities in the name of SAMARTH. The emphasis of the National Trust Act is on family living, through empowerment of persons and their families through specific training programmes.

The Rehabilitation Council of India: Another landmark initiative by the government was the establishment of the Rehabilitation Council of India. The Parliament enacted the Rehabilitation Council of India (RCI) Act in 1992 to give powers to the Rehabilitation Council of India for regulating the training of rehabilitation professionals and maintenance of a central rehabilitation register for their registration and related matters. The vision of the body is 'to provide quality services to persons with disabilities, matching with the best in the World'. The RCI Act was amended in the Parliament in 2000 to make it more broad based. Thus, disability due to mental illness was included within the purview of RCI in 2000. Similar to the role of MCI in regulating the standard of medical education in the country, the RCI Act develops curriculum for various courses in the field of disability, inspects the institutions desirous of starting the course and supervises the examination standard.

4 Rights of Persons with Disabilities and the UNCRPD

The United Nations Convention on Rights of Persons with Disabilities (UNCRPD) was indeed a silver lining for the persons with disabilities, which clearly emphasised on the rights and privileges that this section of people should enjoy. The rights and privileges of people with various disabilities in general, and those with mental illness in particular, can be described aptly through an understanding of the UNCRPD. The UNCRPD was adopted by the United Nations General Assembly on 13 December, 2006 and was opened for signature on 30 March 2007. It came into force from 3 May, 2008. It is unique in the sense that it is both a development and human rights instrument. It is cross-disability and cross-sectoral and is also legally binding. India ratified the UNCRPD on 1 October, 2007. India was the 7th country in the world and one of the important countries to do so. The Convention sought to ensure equality and non-discrimination of the disabled people.

The following rights in the Convention have tried to bring those with disability at par with persons without disability:

1. Equality before the law without discrimination (Article 5)
2. Right to life, liberty and security of the person (Articles 10 & 14)
3. Equal recognition before the law and legal capacity (Article 12)
4. Freedom from torture (Article 15)
5. Freedom from exploitation, violence and abuse (Article 16)
6. Right to respect physical and mental integrity (Article 17)
7. Freedom of movement and nationality (Article 18)
8. Right to live in the community (Article 19)
9. Freedom of expression and opinion (Article 21)
10. Respect for privacy (Article 22)
11. Respect for home and the family (Article 23)
12. Right to education (Article 24)
13. Right to health (Article 25)
14. Right to work (Article 27)
15. Right to adequate standard of living (Article 28)
16. Right to participate in political and public life (Article 29)
17. Right to participation in cultural life (Article 30).

Thus, the Convention set out to promote, protect and ensure the full and equal enjoyment of all human rights and fundamental freedoms by all persons with disabilities, and to promote respect for their inherent dignity.

5 Facilities for Rehabilitation in Psychiatry

Half-way homes: A half-way home is a rehabilitation facility for individuals suffering from mental illness or substance use disorder who no longer require the complete facilities of a hospital, or other institutions, but who are not yet prepared to return to their communities. Half-way homes assist persons who have left highly structured institutions and are preparing to re-enter the society. These persons need to re-learn the societal norms, which they lost or failed to acquire due to mental illness. The intervention is targeted at improving social and interpersonal communication and to provide vocational training. In India, many half-way homes have come up, all established by NGOs. Some of the well-known ones are Richmond Fellowship India (Delhi and Bengaluru), Roshni (Guwahati), Paripurnata (Kolkata), Banyan (Chennai) and many others (Chavan et al. 2012a).

In Chandigarh, the Department of Psychiatry, Government Medical College, is running a half-way home for the chronic mentally ill patients. The patients are accepted on the recommendation of consultant psychiatrists. They are looked after by a trained and experienced medical social worker along with a caregiver. In fact, this half-way home is a joint venture of the department and a self-help group called 'Prayatan', which is formed by the family members of the patients. The facility is directly supervised by a faculty of the department. Transport facilities are also provided to the patients on nominal charges. Once the patient is admitted to this facility, a base-line assessment of dysfunction is done using the 'Dysfunction Anlysis Questionnaire'. The assessment is carried out again at the end of 3 months to find out the progress. During their stay in the half-way home, each patient is expected to participate in regular activities such as yoga, exercise, helping in the kitchen, nursery and gardening and envelope making. Vocational activities such as painting earthen lamps and making greeting cards are also undertaken for specific occasions such as Diwali and New Year. Additionally, there are daily activities, which include games, art competition, telling stories and singing songs. These daily activities are planned well ahead in the form of 'monthly activity'. Every day the patients are awarded 'token points' on the basis of their performance and participation. At the end of every month, the top three patients on the basis of their total points are awarded trophies, and their photographs and products are displayed in the home for next one month. Although, no formal assessment has been carried out to see the effectiveness of these facilities, the personal experience of the staff involved in the regular care of patients suggests that these facilities promote recovery and thus play an important role in rehabilitation.

Self-help groups (SHGs): Self-help groups (SHGs) are voluntary, small groups of persons facing similar problems, who come together for a special purpose. They are usually formed by caregivers who come together for mutual assistance for satisfying a common need, overcoming a common handicap or life disrupting problem. The initiators and members of such groups perceive that their needs are not addressed by existing government programmes and social institutions. Self-help groups emphasise face-to-face social interactions and the assumption of personal responsibility by their members. They often provide material assistance, as well as emotional support; they are frequently cause-oriented, and 'promulgate an ideology or values through which member may attain an enhanced sense of personal identity'. This definition, provided by Katz and Blender (1976), is possibly the most comprehensive definition of self-help groups (Chavan et al. 2012b).

The concept of SHGs originated in the West in the late nineteenth century. SHGs are involved in solving the practical problems and psychological sorrows of sufferers (Lock 1986) and are involved in curative, preventive, promotional, palliative and rehabilitative services (Nayar et al. 2004). SHGs are complementary to medical services and not substitutes to medical treatment (Moeller 1983). A characteristic of SHGs is that their members are service providers as well as receivers.

The effectiveness of SHGs is not easy to find out, and the evidence in their favour is, at best, equivocal. The members of the Alcoholic Anonymous (AA) have often claimed to have maintained abstinence for significant durations. Studies in India have also shown that among a cohort of 187 AA attendees at baseline, at one year, and at 5 years, the sobriety rate was 33.3 and 16.5 %, respectively (Kuruvilla et al. 2004; Kuruvilla and Jacob 2007). Systemic studies such as reviews and meta-analyses have also failed to give a clear picture. A literature review published in 2008 (Groh et al. 2008) argued for their effectiveness. Proponents of SHGs, however, reject attempts to make self-help 'evidence-based', stressing the need to understand health in a holistic way (Nayar et al. 2004). Moreover, evidence, which supports the positive role and good results achieved by self-help groups in the overall improvement of the mentally ill, does exist (Galanter 1988; Kennedy 1990; Kurtz 1988; Lieberman et al. 1979; Powell et al. 2000; Raiff 1984; Roberts et al. 1999). In Chandigarh, the Prayatan is a SHG of families of mentally ill persons, who got registered as a NGO, and are working closely under the guidance of the Department of Psychiatry, GMCH. This group has taken up few projects which are complimentary to the facilities provided by the department.

Day care centres and rehabilitation centres: These are meant for patients who can visit the centres and attend the available services regularly. The Schizophrenia Care and Research Foundation (SCARF) runs a day care centre at Chennai, which has about eighty regular patients. The 'Chetna' is a day care centre run by the Richmond Fellowship Society at Bengaluru and serves the needs of forty-five patients. The day care centres run by the Richmond Fellowship Society give admission to any person between 18 and 45 years of age with a diagnosis of schizophrenia, or any other major psychiatric disorder, or mild mental retardation. The facilities available include vocational training units for using computers, typing, printing, plastic moulding, tailoring and embroidery, arts and craft, yoga, vocational and instrumental music, dancing, painting, and vocabulary building. In addition to vocational training, the centre has therapeutic programmes such as structured daily activities and afternoon group activities, namely community meetings, group therapy, recreational activities such as going to movies, picnics, group games and horticultural activities. Regular individual and family therapy sessions and family support group meetings are also provided. The period of stay of members is generally up to 18 months. Therapeutic services are provided by a team of counsellors from the field of social work and psychology (Ponnachamy et al. 2005). At the 'Banyan', wandering mentally ill women on the streets are brought to the shelter and clinically assessed by a psychiatrist and put on medication. Various therapies are available such as individual counselling, music, art, yoga and vocational training (candle making, greeting cards, block printing on napkins, table linen, basket making, threading flowers and making bouquets, etc.). The inmates are entrusted with some housekeeping responsibilities and also take care of other residents. They are given an opportunity to attend meetings for a limited audience, to speak for their cause of inclusion. Recreation includes outings to the beach, movies, celebrating festivals and sports. As the inmate improves, her family address is elicited and traced. The family is educated about the illness, the woman's stay at the Banyan and the need for continuous medication. The duration of stay at the Banyan varies from less than 3 months to more than 3 years (Rao 2004).

6 Role of NGOs

Non-governmental organisations (NGOs) are institutions, recognised by governments as non-profit or welfare-oriented, which play a key role as advocates, service providers, activists and researchers on a range of issues pertaining to human and social development (Thara and Patel 2010). Currently, about 50–75 % of specialised mental health services are provided by the government sector and about 33–50 % by private sectors. Only 2–3 % of services are provided by NGOs (Desai et al. 2004; Arun et al. 2012). However, the facilities provided by NGO's might be much more in the field of rehabilitation. The mental health NGOs (MHNGOs) such as the SCARF have played an important role for patients with schizophrenia, providing facilities such as day care centres, residential centres, and even long-term care for some of the chronically ill. MHNGOs, such as the National Addiction Research Centre of Mumbai, also provide drug de-addiction services for the urban poor. In Chandigarh, 'Umeed' has been involved in rehabilitation of the mentally challenged persons for quite some time. In addition to these specific services provided to certain groups, the MHNGOs also provide domiciliary care, community-based programmes through community outreach clinics and suicide prevention services. Some of the MHNGOs have developed models of care and rehabilitation, which are replicable in diverse settings. The absence of trained staff to carry out psychosocial rehabilitation has led to the development of different modules of psychosocial rehabilitation in urban as well as rural settings by these MHNGOs. Activities carried out by these MHNNGOs towards rehabilitation include individual and group counselling, vocational rehabilitation and livelihood skills training, self-help groups, and recreation and leisure activities. Specific interventions for children and the elderly are also provided by these MHNGOs (Thara and Patel 2010).

7 Interventions for Specific Deficits in Mental Disorders

A person with mental illness, especially with severe mental illness, may have deficits in cognition, social skills as well as vocational skills. Often the deficit is in more than one area, severely affecting their quality of life. However, intervention strategies can be devised to help the individuals overcome these deficits.

(a) *Cognitive Skill Deficits*

Neurocognitive dysfunction has been postulated as a core deficit in many major mental illnesses. Individuals with schizophrenia present severe impairments in attention, executive functions, working memory and processing speed. Studies have suggested that patients with other psychotic disorders could also demonstrate a disruption of normal cognitive performance, but results have not always been consistent (Reichenberg 2010).

Two recent studies (Zanelli et al. 2010; Reichenberg et al. 2009) involving large epidemiological samples have compared neuropsychological functioning between psychotic patients with a diagnosis of schizophrenia, bipolar mania and depressive psychosis and have shown that differences in neuropsychological performance between schizophrenia and other psychotic disorders are quantitative and not qualitative. Cognitive deficits are present in all psychotic disorders, but are most severe and pervasive in schizophrenia, and least so in bipolar mania. Schizophrenia and mood disorders are characterised by deficits in various domains of cognition, e.g. learning memory, working memory, executive function, attention, verbal fluency and information processing. Cognitive disturbances are considered a major determinant of social outcome (Sumiyoshi 2012).

Assessment of Neurocognitive Deficits

(i) The NIMHANS, Neuropsychology Battery, (Rao et al. 2004) is based on Luria's method. It is the first neuropsychology battery developed in the country. It measures the domains such as speed (motor and mental), attention (focused attention, sustained attention, divided attention), executive functions (verbal fluency, category fluency, design fluency, working memory, planning, set shifting, response inhibition), comprehension, learning and memory (verbal and visual) and visuospatial construction. It comprises of 19 subtests.
(ii) The PGI battery of brain dysfunction or PGI-BBD (Pershad and Verma 1989) is used to assess cognitive dysfunctions in patients. Its subtests include the PGI Memory Scale, the Revised Bhatia's Short Battery of Performance Tests of Intelligence, the Verbal Adult Intelligence Scale, the Nahor Benson Test and the Bender Visual Motor Gestalt Test.

Cognitive enhancement therapy (CET) has been tried for overcoming deficits in social and cognitive domains among persons with chronic mental disorders. There are two main techniques in cognitive rehabilitation- remediation and compensatory approaches.

Cognitive remediation is designed to stimulate new learning, or re-learning of cognitive tasks, and thus, to improve domains of deficit. Early Cognitive Remediation (CR) programmes used paper and pencil tasks, but now most are computerised. Some remediation programmes use a mix of general educational software, but many train participants with specialised computer software designed to improve cognition. Often the software is adapted from computer exercises for remediation of age-related cognitive decline, brain injuries and patients with psychosis (Fisher et al. 2010; Hogarty and Flesher 1999). Many remediation programmes use a form of drill and practise training, which refers to the use of hundreds of trials of the same exercise to 'push' intrinsic learning systems, which are hypothesised to be intact in schizophrenia (Koch et al. 2007). However, as these are repetitive kind of exercises, the patients may get bored over time. So computer games with motivation and rewards, colours, noises, increasing scores, and encouraging words are used quite often. Several models of cognitive remediation are available. The features of the models of cognitive remediation vary from case to case. While some models emphasise drill practice of isolated cognitive skills (Delahunty et al. 1993), some are offered in conjunction with vocational training (McGurk et al. 2007).

The compensatory approach is designed to make improvements in the patient's functioning by avoiding areas of impairment and recruiting other intact cognitive domains, or by creating a supportive external environment (Kern et al. 2009). Compensatory approaches improve cognitive functioning by reducing errors in the learning process and also minimise impediments to activities of daily living. Errorless learning (EL) and cognitive adaptation training (CAT) are two compensatory approaches, which have demonstrated successful outcomes in patients with schizophrenia (Tomas et al. 2010).

The ultimate goal of all the programmes is the successful transfer of gains made in CR to improvements in functional outcome and quality of life. Multiple studies have shown improvements in measures of functional capacity or functional outcome after CR. In addition, improvements in global cognition as a result of CR have been demonstrated to mediate improvements in measures of functional outcome (Eack et al. 2010).

(b) *Social Skill Deficit*

Schizophrenia leads to substantial problems in cognition, affect and behaviour. Social deficits are prominent in this disorder (Bellack 1997) and generally take the form of social skill deficit (Bellack et al. 1990). Even in affective disorders, social skill deficits may be present and there is evidence to indicate that many people with depression exhibit deficits in social skills (Segrin 2000). Individuals with mental illness may have problems in expressing positive feelings, making requests, listening to others, expressing unpleasant feelings and so on. In order to restore harmony to these people, social skills training (SST) is very useful.

The term 'skills' refers to acquired behaviours, which are based on learning experiences (Kopelowicz et al. 2006). Social skills represent constituent behaviours, which when combined in appropriate sequences and used with others in appropriate ways, enable an individual to have success in daily living reflected by social competence (Bellack et al. 2004). Social competence can be defined as the ability to achieve legitimate personal goals through interacting with others in all situations: work, school, recreation, shopping, consumer services, medical and mental care and legal agencies (Knapczyk and Rodes 2001). Social skills training (SST) consists of behaviourally based instruction, modelling, corrective feedback, and contingent social reinforcement aimed to improve social competence, through the acquisition of social skills, self-care and independent living skills (Heinssen et al. 2000).

Social skills deficits may vary from person to person, so a thorough assessment of the social functioning is critical for SST to be effective. Information about the client should be gathered from a variety of methods. Interview with the client, indirect observation, direct observations that includes the Social Skills Checklist, role-play and the Maryland Assessment of Social Competence (MASC) can be used to find out the social functioning of an individual. Assessment is an ongoing process and continues till the end of treatment. Therapists can monitor homework and observe behaviour during sessions to gauge progress and evaluate the effectiveness of learned social skills.

The interventions may include simple advice in some cases, while in others, it requires elaborate combination of operant conditioning and social learning models. Steps involved in social skills training are as follows (Kaur and Rozatkar 2012):

1. Problem identification: Made in collaboration with patient by acknowledging 'barriers' and 'goals' of the patient.
2. Goal setting: Short-term, near-approximation goals that patient and therapist find feasible.
3. Behaviour rehearsal or role-play: Patient demonstrates the verbal, non-verbal and para-linguistic skills required for successful social interaction.
4. Corrective feedback: Required for behaviour exhibited in role-play.
5. Social Modelling: Demonstration by the therapist of desired interpersonal behaviour in a form that can be learnt by the observing patient.
6. Behaviour practice: Facilitate its use in real-life situations.
7. Positive social reinforcement: Contingent upon those behaviour skills, which showed improvement.
8. Homework assignment: To motivate the patient to implement the learned skill in real-life situations.
9. Positive reinforcement and problem solving: To address issues arising out of the patient's experiences due to the use of acquired skills.

Social skills training in psychiatric rehabilitation is now widely used. A proponent of social skills training, Robert Liberman has designed systematic and structured skills training since the mid 1970s (Rossler 2006). He and his colleagues developed skills training in the form of modules with different topics, which focused on medication management, symptom management, substance abuse management, basic conversational skills, interpersonal problem solving, friendship and intimacy, recreation and leisure, workplace fundamentals, community re-entry and family involvement. The modules are composed of skills areas, which are taught in exercises with demonstration videos, role-play and problem solving exercises and homework assignments (Liberman and Kopelowicz 2002; Rossler 2006).

Social skills training is now in use for more than three decades in developed nations. Its efficacy in diverse treatment settings, when by diverse practitioners such as psychiatrists, psychologists, mental health nurses and social workers, and covering a broad range of skills (illness management, smoking cessation, securing and retaining jobs), has shown gratifying results (Kopelowicz et al. 2006). SST has been found to be very effective, even in disorders such as schizophrenia. In recent times, Kurtz et al. (2008) conducted a meta-analysis of randomised, controlled trials of social skills training for schizophrenia. Outcome measures from 22 studies including 1,521 clients were categorised according to a proximal-distal continuum in relation to the presumed site of action of skills training interventions. Results showed content of mastery tests and performance-based measures of skills to be most proximal, community functioning, negative symptoms intermediate and general symptoms and relapse to be the most distal. Results revealed a large weighted mean effect size for content-mastery exams ($d = 1.20$), a moderate mean effect size for performance-based measures of social and daily living skills ($d = 0.52$), moderate mean effect sizes for community functioning ($d = 0.52$) and negative symptoms ($d = 0.40$), and small mean effect sizes for other symptoms ($d = 0.15$) and relapse ($d = 0.23$). These results support the efficacy of social skills training for improving psychosocial functioning in schizophrenia.

(c) *Vocational skill deficit*

The beneficial effects of work for mental health have been known for centuries (Harding et al. 1987; Rossler 2006). Work is considered therapeutic and essential for both the psychological survival and psychological well-being of people in contemporary societies (Chan et al. 1997; Perrone et al. 2000). Hence, vocational rehabilitation professionals have consistently advocated for work as a fundamental human right of people with disabilities (Rubin and Roessler 1995).

Vocational rehabilitation can be defined as, 'a dynamic process consisting of a series of actions and activities that follow a logical, sequential progression of services related to the total needs of a person with a disability. The process begins with the initial case finding or referral, and ends with the successful placement of the individual in employment. Many activities and developments occur concurrently and in overlapping time frames during this process' (Chan et al. 1997). Vocational rehabilitation is based on the idea that work not only improves socialisation, activity and productivity, but it also shows positive results in related areas such as self-esteem and quality of life. These in turn improve adherence to rehabilitation of even individuals with impaired insight. Work and employment helps an individual re-integrate into the society (McElroy 1987; Rossler 2006).

A person with chronic mental illness may have deficits in several areas, which may work in combination or independently, resulting in problems related to vocational activities and work. These may be in the form of physical deficits (mobility, balance and coordination), psychological deficits (such as lack of motivation, anxiety and apprehension regarding return to competitive employment), cognitive deficits (such as poor attention and poor problem solving capacity) and communication deficits and social skill deficits (such as ability to respect personal space of co-workers, spontaneously exchanging pleasantries and recognising position in the organisation). Hence, it is very important to do a detailed vocational assessment and evaluation of an individual before planning out the vocational strategies.

Vocational assessment is defined as the global appraisal of an individual's work or training background, general functional capacities, and social and behavioural characteristics. It usually includes an evaluation of medical factors, psychological makeup, educational background, social behaviours, attitudes, values, work skills and abilities (Chan et al. 1997). Vocational evaluation, on the other hand, is a *specific* process that involves the appraisal of a person's work-related characteristics, which are important for education and training to obtain and maintain employment. It includes a comprehensive review of specific work characteristics, including but not limited to occupational interests, specific job skills, worker traits, general intelligence, temperaments, physical capacities, strength, range of motion and other work-related functions and aptitudes (Chan et al. 1997).

Most vocational assessment takes a holistic approach. Following areas are usually assessed (Perry 2009):

1. History, education, employment and background.
2. Psychosocial strengths and development, including relevant psychological issues such as motivation, self-esteem, social and communication skills, and family situation.
3. Independent living skills such as self-care and grooming.
4. Literacy.
5. Knowledge of the world of work.
6. Abilities or aptitudes (assessing intelligence, dexterity, physical capacity and work tolerance).
7. Technical or job skills (by interviewing, using performance-based tests, and situational assessments).
8. Generic work behaviours (social and communication behaviours).
9. Job seeking skills (by interviewing, observation, and by result of job searching).
10. Job readiness (by looking at aspects such as realistic goals, management of money and understanding of the nature of job).

Vocational rehabilitation plan: The following strategies can be used for rehabilitation of patient suffering from mental illness.

(a) *Return to work*, i.e. re-employment by the same employer in the same job and work setting, with part-time hours until patient can build to full-time
(b) *Modified work,* i.e. re-employment by the same employer in the same job, but with changes or modifications to the work process or environment to accommodate the patient's physical or cognitive restrictions
(c) *Alternative work,* i.e. re-employment by the same employer in a similar or different position that is within the patient's limitations
(d) *Direct placement,* i.e. employment with a new employer in a new or pre-injury job that utilises remaining skills
(e) *On-the-job training,* i.e. employment with a new employer and new training to do a new job
(f) *Formal school or training,* i.e. vocational schooling or academic instruction for employment in a new position. Computer Preparation: Evaluation, Training, and Employment (COMPETE) is training for cognitively impaired young adults in information-age machines, such as computers and fax machines, which has resulted in the employment of a significant number of individuals (17 out of 27) who were unemployed before the training (Mann and Svorai 1994)
(g) *Self-employment,* i.e. establishing an independent, self-sustaining business
(h) *Transitional employment:* Here, a temporary work employment is provided to teach vocational skills which enables the person to move on to competitive employment
(i) Individual placement model (Robert Drake & Deborah Becker): Disabled persons are placed in competitive employment according to their choices as soon as possible and receive all support needed to maintain their position. The support provided is continued indefinitely (Rossler 2006).

Today, the most promising vocational rehabilitation programme is Supported Employment (SE) (Rossler 2006). In the past most studies evaluated short follow-up periods (12–18 months), and it was not known which individual would benefit from SE and who would not (Mueser et al. 1998). In recent times, it has been demonstrated that those who have found long-term employment through SE had improved cognition and quality of life and better symptom control (Bond 2004; Salyers et al. 2004).

Whatever be the model, there cannot be any doubt that vocational rehabilitation is required and is an important entity for those with mental illness.

8 Challenges and Future Directions

In India and other developing countries, opportunities for rehabilitation are limited either due to inadequate staff, infrastructure or training. Even where opportunities exist, occupational activities such as making of envelopes or baskets provide little initiative and may not change the quality of life (Deva 2006). Community-based rehabilitation under government agencies is virtually non-existent, leaving the field entirely to NGO run rehabilitation centres, which provide mainly shelter with very little emphasis on rehabilitation. These facilities are also quite expensive and unaffordable for the common people. Other than issues of infrastructure and manpower, various other factors are responsible for the poor focus on psychiatric rehabilitation. Mental illness in India has poor visibility due to a lack of cohesive patient and family groups to showcase the problems faced by this group of population. This could be attributed to stigma, poverty and poor awareness, and most of the caretakers' energies being expended on taking care of livelihood. The lack of visibility and lobbying for patients' rights lead to neglect in framing government rules and regulations, allocation of funds as well as providing other supportive programs such as vocational opportunities. For example, mental illness was the last group to be recognised as causing disability in the 'Persons with Disability Act', 1995. The aggressive marketing by the pharmaceutical industry is another reason for which the pharmacological interventions get precedence while caring for those with chronic mental illness. The industry offers pill for every deficit, and thus doctors are driven towards this pill. The research evidence brought forward by these companies is also often sponsored by them, thus doubting its genuineness. Most psychiatrists do not acquire all relevant skills needed in psychiatric rehabilitation during their training, which is predominantly hospital-based. Young psychiatrists are primarily trained in diagnostic procedures and prescription of medications, mostly to control symptoms, and not trained much in integrating pharmacological and psychosocial interventions (Liberman and Glick 2004; Rossler 2006). Thus, the whole training in psychiatry now requires an overhaul, so that there is enough trained manpower in the field of rehabilitation psychiatry. Exclusive centres and institutions are required to provide training to the professionals who are interested in rehabilitation. There is a need of developing newer and innovative strategies for training and rehabilitation of persons recovering from mental disorders. These approaches might vary from place to place depending upon the local need and resources. In Chandigarh, 'Umeed' has come up as an innovative and sustainable model for job placement of mentally challenged persons. This model was the best in the country in 2003 and received the national award. Currently, 60 mentally challenged persons are employed under Umeed. Similarly, the Department of Psychiatry, Government Medical College, Chandigarh, runs a half-way home in collaboration with 'Prayatan', a self-help group of family members of mentally ill persons for last 10 years. The patients who are discharged from the hospital after control of acute symptoms attend this half-way home. Through recreational, social and vocational skills training, patients are prepared to take up the work. Depending upon the interest and capabilities, some of the patients are engaged in production work carried out at the half-way home, and they are paid remuneration depending upon their production. Others are employed with Prayatan at its outlets at different places in Chandigarh. The profit from these outlets is paid as monthly wages. The wages are linked to profit rather than fixed salary.

However, the psychiatric rehabilitation or psychosocial rehabilitation has not made much progress in India. The government has to redesign and adopt policies enabling the disabled to re-integrate into the society. Keeping the UNCRPD in mind, a disabled friendly environment has to be created, which ensures equal rights and privileges for all. Reservation for the chronically mentally ill in jobs and availing of government facilities for self-employment is required. At present, only 3 % of the government jobs are reserved for the physically disabled in grade 'C' and grade 'D' posts. Sadly, there is no reservation for the people disabled due to mental illness. Likewise, though there is provision of 7.5 % reservation in dealerships or agencies provided by Oil Companies for physically handicapped or government personnel (other than defence personnel), disabled on duty or widows of government personnel (other than defence personnel who die in the course of duty), there is no reservation for persons with chronic mental illnesses.

Equal rights also means equal rights as citizen, including the right to vote, but again there is much confusion regarding the eligibility to cast vote by those with mental illness, especially when they are in remission. Again, the facilities for rehabilitation such as rehabilitation centres, half-way homes and day care centres should also be increased keeping in mind that at present in India there are over two crore persons with serious mental disorders and about 5 crore people with common mental disorders (Chandrashekar et al. 2009). These are but, a few instances where much is required to be done.

India has miles to go in the field of rehabilitation psychiatry, but we have surely taken our first step, and thus our journey begins.

References

Anthony, W. A., Cohen, M. R. & Cohen, B. F. (1984). Psychiatric rehabilitation. In J. A. Talbott (Ed.), *The chronic mental patient: Five years later* (pp. 137–157). New York: Grune & Stratton.

Arun, P., Patra, S. & Gupta, N. (2012). Voluntary sectors and NGOs. In B. S. Chavan et al. (Eds.), *Community Mental Health in India* (pp. 357–361). New Delhi: Jaypee Brothers Medical Publishers.

Bachrach, L. L. (1992). Psychosocial rehabilitation and psychiatry in the care of long-term patients. *American Journal of Psychiatry, 149*, 1455–1463.

Bachrach, L. L. (2000). Psychosocial rehabilitation and psychiatry in the treatment of schizophrenia-what are the boundaries? *Acta Psychiatrica Scandinavia, 102*(S407), S6–S10.

Bebbington, P. E. (1995). The content and context of compliance. *International Clinical Psychopharmacology, 9*(Suppl 5), 41–50.
Bellack, A. S., et al. (2004). *Social skills training for schizophrenia*. New York: Guilford Press.
Bellack, A. S. (1997) Social skills deficits and social skill training: New developments and trends. In H. D. Brenner & W. Boeker (Eds.), *Towards a comprehensive therapy for schizophrenia* (pp. 137–146). Goettingen (Germany): Hogrefe & Huber.
Bellack, A. S., et al. (1990). Analysis of social competence in schizophrenia. *The British Journal of Psychiatry, 156*, 809–818.
Bennet, D. H. (1978). Community psychiatry. *The British Journal of Psychiatry, 132*, 209–220.
Bond, G. R. (2004). Supported employment: Evidence for an evidence-based practice. *Psychiatric Rehabilitation Journal, 27*, 345–359.
Chan, F., et al. (1997). Vocational assessment and evaluation of people with disabilities. *Physical Medicine and Rehabilitation Clinics of North America, 8*(2), 311–325.
Chandrashekhar, et al. (2009). Innovations in psychiatry: Ambulatory services for mentally ill. *Indian Journal of Psychiatry, 51*(3), 169.
Chavan, B. S., et al. (Eds), (2012a). *Community mental health in India*. New Delhi: Jaypee Brothers Medical Publishers.
Chavan, B. S., Rozatkar, A. & Sidana, A. (2012b). Models of community mental health care. In B. S. Chavan et al. (Ed.), *Community Mental Health in India* (pp 269–280). New Delhi: Jaypee Brothers Medical Publishers.
Corrigan, P. W., et al. (2005). Some recovery processes in mutual-help groups for persons with mental illness; II: Qualitative analysis of participant interviews. *Community Mental Health Journal, 41*, 721–735.
Corrigan, P. W., Corrigan, P. W., & Corrigan, P. W. (2001). Motivational interviews as goal assessment for persons with psychiatric disability. *Community Mental Health Journal, 37*, 113–122.
Cutler, D. L.(1985). Clinical care update. The chronically mentally ill. *Community Mental Health Journal, 21*, 3–13.
Delahunty, A., Morice, R., & Frost, B. (1993). Specific cognitive flexibility rehabilitation in schizophrenia. *Psychological Medicine, 23*, 221–227.
Desai, N. G., Tiwari, S. C., & Nambi, S. (2004). Urban mental health services in India: How complete or incomplete? *Indian Journal of Psychiatry, 46*, 194–212.
Deva, P. (2006). Psychiatric rehabilitation and its present role in developing countries. *World Psychiatry, 5*, 164–165.
EACK, S. M., et al. (2010). Mechanisms of functional improvement in a 2-year trial of cognitive enhancement therapy for early schizophrenia. *Psychological Medicine, 22*, 1–9.
Farkas, M., Gagne, C., Anthony, W., et al. (2005). Implementing recovery oriented evidence based programs: Identifying the critical dimensions. *Community Mental Health Journal, 41*, 141–158.
Fisher, M., Holland, C., Subramaniam, K., & Vinogradov, S. (2010). Neuroplasticity-based cognitive training in schizophrenia: An interim report on the effects 6 months later. *Schizophrenia Bulletin, 36*, 869–879.
Galanter, M. (1988). Self-help groups as adjuncts to psychiatric treatment: A study of recovery, Inc. *American Journal of Psychiatry, 145*(10), 1248–1253.
GROH, D. R., Jason, L. A., & Keys, C. B. (2008). Social network variables in alcoholics anonymous: A literature review. *Clinical Psychology Review, 28*, 430–450.
Harding, C. M., et al. (1987). Work and mental illness. I. Toward an integration of the rehabilitation process. *The Journal of Nervous Mental Disease, 175*, 317–326.
Heinssen, R. K., Liberman, R. P., & Kopelowicz, A. (2000). Psychosocial skills training for schizophrenia: Lessons from the laboratory. *Schizophrenia Bulletin, 26*(1), 21–46.
Hogarty, G. E., & Flesher, S. (1999). Practice principles of cognitive enhancement therapy for schizophrenia. *Schizophrenia Bulletin, 25*, 693–708.
Kaur, P. & Rozatkar, A. (2012). Psychosocial rehabilitation in psychiatry. In B. S. Chavan et al. (Eds.), *Community Mental Health in India* (pp. 369–382). New Delhi: Jaypee Brothers Medical Publishers.
Kennedy, M. (1990). Psychiatric hospitalizations of GROWers. *Paper presented at the Second Biennial Conference on Community Research and Action*, East Lansing, Michigan.

Kern, R. S., et al. (2009). Psychosocial treatments to promote functional recovery in schizophrenia. *Schizophrenia Bulletin, 35*, 347–361.

Knapczyk, D., & Rodes, P. (2001). *Teaching social competence*. Champaign: Ill, Research Press.

Koch, K., Wagner, G., Nenadic, I., et al. (2007). Temporal modeling demonstrates preserved overlearning processes in schizophrenia: An fMRI study. *Neuroscience, 146*, 1474–1483.

Kopelowicz, A., & Liberman, R. P. (1995). Biobehavioral treatment and rehabilitation of schizophrenia. *Harvard Review of Psychiatry, 3*, 55–64.

Kopelowicz, A., Liberman, R. P. & Zarate, R. (2006). Recent advances in social skills training for schizophrenia. *Schizophrenia Bulletin, 32*(S), S12–S23.

Kurtz, L. F. (1988). Mutual aid for affective disorders: The manic depressive and depressive association. *American Journal of Orthopsychiatry, 58*(1), 152–155.

Kurtz, M., Mueser, M., & Kim, T. (2008). A meta-analysis of controlled research on social skills training for schizophrenia. *Journal of Consulting and Clinical Psychology, 76*(3), 491–504.

Kuruvilla, P. K., & Jacob, K. S. (2007). Five-year follow up for sobriety in a cohort of men who had attended and alcoholic anonymous program in India. *National Medical Journal of India, 5*, 234–236.

Kuruvilla, P. K., Vijaykumar, N., & Jacob, K. S. (2004). A cohort studies of male subjects attending an alcoholic anonymous program in India: One year follow-up for sobriety. *Journal of Studies on Alcohol, 65*, 546–549.

Lamb, H. R. (1982). *Treating the long-term mentally ill: Beyond deinstitutionalization*. San Francisco: Jossey-Bass.

Liberman, R. P., & Glick, I. D. (2004). Drug and psychosocial curricula for psychiatry residents for treatment of schizophrenia: Part I. *Psychiatric Services, 55*, 1217–1219. Washington, D. C.

Liberman, R. P., & Kopelowicz, A. (2002). Teaching persons with severe mental disabilities to be their own case managers. *Psychiatric Services, 53*, 1377–1379. Washington, D. C.

Lieberman, M. A., Solow, N., et al. (1979). The psychotherapeutic impact of women's consciousness-raising groups. *Archives of General Psychiatry, 36*, 161–168.

Lock, S. (1986). Self help groups: The fourth estate in medicine? *The British Medical Journal, 293*, 1596–1600.

Mann, W. C., & Svorai, S. B. (1994). COMPETE: A model for vocational educational, training, employment, and community for integration for persons with cognitive impairments. *American Journal of Occupational Therapy, 48*(5), 446–451.

Mcelroy, E. M. (1987). Sources of distress among families of the hospitalized mentally ill. *New Directions for Mental Health Services, 34*, 61–72.

Mcgurk, S. R., Mueser, K. T., et al. (2007). Cognitive training for supported employment: 2–3 year outcomes of a randomized controlled trial. *American Journal of Psychiatry, 164*, 437–441.

Ministry of law, justice and company affairs (legislative department), Government of India. (1996). *The Persons with Disabilities (Equal Opportunities, Protection of Rights and Full Participation) Act, 1995 (1 of 1996)*. New Delhi: GOI, Published In Part II, Section 1 of The Extraordinary Gazette of India.

Ministry of social justice and empowerment, Government of India. (2002). Indian Disability Evaluation and Assessment Scale, 2002. *Guidelines for evaluation and assessment of Mental illness and procedure for certification*. New Delhi: GOI, Published in the Gazette of India (Extraordinary), Part I, Section 1.

Moeller, M. L. (1983). Self help and the medical practitioner in Self Help and Health in Europe. In S. Hatch & I. Kickbusch (Eds.), *New approaches in health care* (pp. 68–76). Copenhagen: WHO Regional Office for Europe.

Mueser, K. T., et al. (1998). Models of community care for severe mental illness: A review of research on case management. *Schizophrenia Bulletin, 24*, 37–74.

Nayar, K. R., Kyobotungi, C. & Razum, O. (2004). Self help. What future role in healthcare for low and middle income countries? *International Journal for equality in health, 3*(1).

Perrone, K. M., et al. (2000). Assessing efficacy and importance of career counseling competencies. *Career Development Quarterly, 48*, 212–225.

Perry, D.(2009). The basics of vocational assessment. A tool for finding the right match between people with disabilities and occupation. Accessed on Jan 26, 2013 from www.ilo.org/public/english/region/asro/.../voc_assessment.pdf.

Pershad, D., & Verma, S. K. (1989). *Handbook of PGI battery of brain dysfunction*. Agra: National Psychological Corporation.

Ponnachamy, L., et al. (2005). Family support group in psychosocial rehabilitation. *Indian journal of Psychiatry, 47*, 160–163.

Powell, T. J., Hill, E. M., Warner, L., Yeaton, W., & Silk, K. R. (2000). Encouraging people with mood disorders to attend a self-help group. *Journal of Applied Social Psychology, 30*, 2270–2288.

Priebe, S., McCabe, R., Bullenkamp, J., et al. (2002). The impact of routine outcome measurement on treatment processes in community mental health care: approach and methods of the MECCA study. *Epidemiology and Psychiatric Sciences, 11*, 198–205.

Raiff, N. R. (1984). Some health related outcomes of self-help participation. In A. Gartner & F. Riessman (Eds.), *The self-help revolution*. New York, Human Sciences Press. (Chapter 14).

Rao, N. (2004). Rehabilitation of the wandering seriously mentally Ill (WSMI) women: The banyan experience. *Social Work in Health Care, 39*, 49–65.

RAO, S. I., et al. (2004). *NIMHANS neuropsychology battery manual-2004*. Bangalore: NIMHANS Publication.

Reichenberg, A., et al. (2009). Neuropsychological function and dysfunction in schizophrenia and psychotic affective disorders. *Schizophrenia Bulletin, 35*, 1022–1029.

Reichenberg, A. (2010). The assessment of neuropsychological functioning in schizophrenia. *Dialogues Clinical Neurosciences, 12*(3), 383–392.

Roberts, L. J., et al. (1999). Giving and receiving help: Interpersonal transactions in mutual-help meetings and psychosocial adjustment of members. *American Journal of Community Psychology, 27*, 841–868.

Rogers, E. S., et al. (2001). Assessing readiness for change among persons with severe mental illness. *Community Mental Health Journal, 37*, 97–112.

Rogers, E. S., Anthony, W., & Lyass, A. (2004). The nature and dimensions of social support among individuals with severe mental illnesses. *Community Mental Health Journal, 40*, 437–450.

Rossler, W. (2006). Psychiatric rehabilitation today: An overview. *World Psychiatry, 5–3*, 151–157.

Rubin, S. E., & Roessler, R. T. (1995). *Foundations of the vocational rehabilitation process* (4th ed.). Austin (TX): Pro-Ed.

Salyers, M. P., et al. (2004). A ten-year follow-up of a supported employment program. *Psychiatric Services, 55*, 302–308. Washington, DC.

Segrin, C. (2000). Social skills deficits associated with depression. *Clinical Psychology Review, 20*, 379–403.

Sumiyoshi, T. (2012). Essentials of neurocognitive assessment in clinical research. *Nihon Shinkei Seishin Yakurigaku Zasshi, 32*(3), 149–153. Article in Japanese.

Thara, R., & Patel, V. (2010). Role of non-governmental organizations in India. *Indian Journal of Psychiatry, 52*, 389–395.

Tomas, P., Fuentes, I., Roder, V., & Ruiz, J. C. (2010). Cognitive rehabilitation programs in schizophrenia: Current status and perspectives. *International Journal of Psychology and Psychological Thera, 10*, 191–204.

World Health Organization. (1980). *International classification of impairments, disabilities and handicap: A manual of classification related to the consequences of diseases*. Geneva: WHO.

Zanelli, J., Reichenberg, A., Morgan, K., et al. (2010). Specific and generalized neuropsychological deficits: A comparison of patients with various first-episode psychosis presentations. *American Journal of Psychiatry, 167*, 78–85.

Websites

www.uncrpdindia.org. Accessed on Jan 15, 2013.

http://www.rehabcouncil.nic.in. Accessed on Jan 19, 2013.

http://www.thenationaltrust.co.in. Accessed on Apr 8, 2013.

http://www.wapr2012.org/the-world-association-for-psychosocial-rehabilitation. Accessed on Apr 2, 2013.

Part X
Developments in Legal and Educational Aspects

Chapter 31
Challenges in Undergraduate Psychiatric Training in India

R. Gupta and H. Khurana

> *The principle fault of the present-day medical curriculum is that it is mainly cadaver centred, lab oriented and organ minded. The whole man never finds a place in the medical curriculum. Our whole medical system is oriented towards living long and not living well*
>
> Neki et al. (1965).

1 Introduction

On examining the current medical curriculum including psychiatry at undergraduate level, the above statement of 1965 seems to hold true even today. Undergraduate medical training in India suffers from a multitude of problems. It is ineffective and lacks practical and scientific application. It needs modifications keeping in view the ever-increasing load of mental health problems. Moreover, it has no parity with the medical education in the developed countries. In India, undergraduate psychiatry teaching needs to be upgraded, as at present, it is appended to medicine without proper emphasis.

R. Gupta, Senior Professor and Head; H. Khurana, Professor

R. Gupta (✉) · H. Khurana
Department of Psychiatry, Pt. B.D. Sharma PGIMS, Rohtak 124001, Haryana, India
e-mail: rajivguptain2003@yahoo.co.in

R. Gupta · H. Khurana
Pt. B.D Sharma University of Health Sciences, Rohtak, Haryana, India

S. Malhotra and S. Chakrabarti (eds.), *Developments in Psychiatry in India*,
DOI 10.1007/978-81-322-1674-2_31

2 Magnitude of Mental Health Problems

The magnitude of people suffering from mental disorders in the country is alarming. At any given point of time, 20 % of adult population is likely to be suffering from mental illness (Math and Srinivasaraju 2010). The Government of India's National Commission on Macroeconomics and Health Report (2005) highlighted that, even on ignoring minor mental illnesses, rough estimates suggest that nearly 70 million people in the country are seriously mentally ill. This population is more than the population of many European countries. Further, these disorders contribute much more than the physical illnesses such as tuberculosis, HIV, cancers and chronic obstructive lung diseases to the disability-adjusted life years (DALYs) (Thiruvanakasru and Thiruvanakasru 2010). The morbidity and mortality statistics are certainly important in planning the health care services, but in the case of chronic diseases that affect the productivity and growth of a nation, DALYs has advantages over mortality statistics.

3 Manpower for Health Care

India has around 355 medical colleges with an annual intake of 44,250 MBBS students per year (MCI 2013). The potential of our medical graduates and postgraduates can be realised from the fact that nearly one-third of them migrate to other countries, including the United States and the United Kingdom for higher education or employment every year (Supe and Burdick 2006). As our undergraduate course is not recognised in most of the European countries, health professionals of Indian origin face a lot of hardship in getting acceptance in these countries, but once accepted, their contribution in health care programmes of other countries is openly acknowledged (Chaudhry 2010; Ghambheera and Williams 2010; Kalra and Bhugra 2010; Srivastava and Natrajan 2010).

Compared to the resources for undergraduate training, we have only 142 medical colleges providing facilities for postgraduate courses in psychiatry and 49 colleges have facilities for training for Diploma in Psychological Medicine (DPM). Surprisingly, training facilities in psychiatry are available only to about 0.4 % of graduates passing out every year (MCI 2013) in the country that supports 16 % of the world's population. The number of psychiatrists available is much less than required. The survey of national mental health resources based on the 2001 census suggests a gross deficit of mental health professionals in the country. Taking the ideal requirement as 1 psychiatrist for one lakh population, there is a shortage of psychiatrists in almost all the states, ranging from 50 to 90 %. Only few states such as Chandigarh, Delhi, Goa and Pondicherry are exceptions and have a surplus of psychiatrists (Thiruvanakasru and Thiruvanakasru 2010).

The ideal requirement for psychiatrists one per lakh population recommended by the Health Survey Report (2002) as cited by Thiruvanakasru and Thiruvanakasru (2010) is calculated arbitrarily. This requirement is much less than what is projected by the Western countries. Even on accepting that, we have not been able to catch up with the targets suggested at that time, and the situation is likely to deteriorate. The District Mental Health Program (DMHP) was launched in 1983 with the hope of providing mental health care at the primary care level. But, its implementation has been quite slow due to administrative, financial and time resources and manpower reasons. It is currently only being implemented in 127 of 625 districts (Murthy 2011).

Another approach to improve mental health care resources could be to strengthen our undergraduate medical curriculum in psychiatry so that we may reach the unreached (Jugal et al. 2007). The medical graduate and a primary care physician of the present day have a negative attitude towards psychiatry. Even psychiatric consultation is not utilised by physicians. Physicians could help their patients better or seek psychiatric consultation, if they had been properly exposed to psychiatry during their undergraduate training (Chadda and Some 1996).

This scenario of training the doctors in mental health skills in India opens up a pile of questions about the mental health care delivery in the country. We have a handful of psychiatrists in the country. The Directory of the Indian Psychiatric Society (IPS), 2012, lists 3,947 psychiatrists in its membership till 2011(IPS 2012). This is about 25 % of the required strength of psychiatrists in the country. Our postgraduate training programme would take at least 50 years to make up the numbers required for the present. On the other hand, training undergraduates adequately seems to provide a viable solution within five years. Therefore, the focus must be on the mental health training at undergraduate level. The advantage of teaching psychiatry at the undergraduate level would provide adequate manpower to manage the burden of mental illness in a cost-effective manner. It would also improve the attitude of physicians and community towards mental health.

4 The Challenge of Undergraduate Training

Long ago in 1975, the World Health Organization (WHO) had recommended that mental health objectives in each country should be defined by taking into account the nature, extent and consequences of the mental disorders, the resources available and time constraints (Wig et al. 1981). However, it seems that while planning our mental health care policy, we somehow forgot about the resources and time limits. For a long time, it has been realised that our mental health training at the undergraduate level has been unsatisfactory for a variety of reasons. Some of these reasons, which have been highlighted, include insufficient teaching hours, inadequate teaching faculty, ambiguity and controversies surrounding many psychiatric concepts, lack of interest and sensitivity of the students and non-psychiatric faculty towards psychiatry and mentally ill, stigmatisation, no separate examination for the subject and inadequate training during internship (Bhaskaran 1990). On flipping the pages from the archives of the Indian Journal of Psychiatry, it is evident that inadequacy of teaching of psychiatry has frequently been emphasised by many medical educationists and psychiatrists (Kallivayalil 2012; Reddy 2007; Thirunavukarasu 2007). Integrating psychiatric training with that of community medicine, which at present is a full subject in the

Table 1 The challenges of undergraduate teaching in Psychiatry

1. Shortage of mental health trainers
2. Inadequate orientation to the needs of undergraduate among trainers
3. Negative attitude towards psychiatry in community, among physicians and students
4. Improper cultural orientation towards psychiatry
5. Inadequate exposure to social sciences in the early MBBS years
6. Inadequate emphasis on psychiatry as a full subject
7. Lack of political and administrative motivation towards psychiatry

MBBS curriculum, seems to be viable solution to make up for the deficiency in the mental health training. But, training in mental health needs to be allotted sufficient time (Sood and Sharan 2011, 2012). However, the efforts done to improve upon these deficiencies had been lacking. We must have the answers to the reasons for our failure to overcome these problems, before we embark upon any new strategy (Table 1).

5 Undergraduate Psychiatry Is Not a Mini Postgraduate Training

The psychiatric trainers in our country have undergone training, which is not in keeping with the aims and objectives of undergraduate curriculum. Due to the shortage of mental health professionals in the country, the psychiatric trainer in most of the medical colleges today is a young postgraduate, who has undergone training based on Western models. He or she has had practically no exposure to psychiatry at undergraduate level. During postgraduate training, the trainee has extensively dealt with the diagnostic and therapeutic controversies of major psychiatric syndromes. He or she has had extensive clinical exposure in the hospital, but has rarely gone to the community to know whether the mental health needs there. In other words, the psychiatric teacher of today has been trained as a specialist clinician and researcher, rather than a health care provider at community level, which is the aim of undergraduate medical training. On the other hand, a teacher for psychiatry for undergraduates needs to be sensitive about the needs of the students and the expectations of the community. Due to inappropriate training at postgraduate level, undergraduate teaching gets reduced to a stereotypic ritual of telling them about how to fit a patient in the category of schizophrenia or bipolar disorders, instead of focusing upon the common mental disorders seen in the medical outpatient clinics. MBBS students who are new to psychiatry find the postgraduate trainers talk full of ambiguities, technicalities and dry jargon. This kind of exposure strengthens the culturally prevalent stereotyped image about the psychiatry and psychiatrist. Undergraduate students never seem to get taught about what the community needs from a mental health care provider. However, postgraduate students can be an asset for undergraduate psychiatric training for two major reasons; firstly, they are mostly engaged in clinical work; therefore, they can give the "actual feel" of patient with psychiatric problems; secondly, they make up for the shortage of trainers in psychiatry, which is likely to persist for many years to come (Polan and Riba 2010). Therefore, the postgraduate trainer too needs to train well according to the needs of the community. Due to the gross discrepancy between our community mental health needs and the Westernised training at postgraduate level, psychiatrists prefer to go abroad whenever there is an opportunity and prefer never to come back, despite the adverse mental health situations and attitude of the country (Patel 2003; Mellor 2003; Thirunavukarasu 2007). Those who get trained in psychiatry abroad would naturally feel less interested in coming back to India (Patel 2003).

As teachers in psychiatry, we have observed over years that many of aspirants choose psychiatry for postgraduate training not as a choice but as compulsion. The moment they see a chance, the choice of discipline is quickly changed. All these facts, though not very well researched, are common knowledge. During the postgraduate career in psychiatry, due to many constraints including manpower, the doctor is primarily trained as a "psychiatric drug prescriber" and a "psychiatric philosopher", rather than an undergraduate teacher. To impart a community-need-oriented training at undergraduate level, we need to reorient our postgraduate training curriculum too. We need to make it more Indian with a focus on community mental health needs.

6 Providing Need-based Training

There is so much of cultural influence on understanding and practice of psychiatry that it cannot be refuted by any argument (Avasthi 2011). The students both at the postgraduate and undergraduate level read either Western or Westernised textbooks on psychiatry, which are devoid of any description of Indian culture. We have a strong need of mental health literacy in India, and this need is qualitatively different from the Western needs due to the sociocultural influences. We need to follow a different Indian approach to the treatment of psychiatric, especially neurotic disorders. The Western psychotherapeutic approach to such disorders may not be equally suitable to our patients due to cultural inappropriateness and inadequate mental health resources. Indian patients are not aware of their rights as in the West. Consequently, doctors in India have more accountability towards the health of their patients. Most of the patients instead of being an equal partner in the treatment process prefer to leave the decision on the doctor and follow his or her advice. Under such circumstances, the doctor–patient relationship is much more important than anywhere else in the world. The undergraduate curriculum of psychiatry, adopted by the MCI, the discipline that should emphasise this aspect of treatment the most, does not lay any emphasis on it. Going further, most of our patients enjoy good family support. Dr. Vidya Sagar recognised this fact and involved the family members along with the patient in mental hospitals. Unfortunately, none of these aspects are adequately addressed in the present-day academic curriculum for undergraduates (Undergraduate taskforce-IPS-2010).

Even when we know what we need to train about, how we need to train our undergraduates has been a matter of concern to all of us for a long time (Sharma 1984).

7 Changing Attitudes: Stigma a Silent Inhibitor

Before joining medical school, the undergraduate student carries the cultural stereotype image of psychiatric patients with him or her. When suddenly exposed to the patient with psychiatric problems with inadequate preparation, this often evokes a feeling of fear and hate in the student. During the two-week posting in the psychiatric ward, each student is exposed to two or three patients. The history and mental status examination recorded by them clearly reflect their anxiety and disinterest in the patient. Many students find it very easy to skip the posting as they need only 50 % attendance in psychiatric theory and clinics. When they leave the posting, they carry the same negative attitude with them, which they had brought (Chawla et al. 2012; Lingeswaran 2010). Even at the end of two-week posting in psychiatry, students are still not able to empathise with the patient. They are not aware of aetiological factors for mental illness and believe supernatural factors responsible for the mental disorder. Modified ECT remains an undesirable treatment option to them. Majority of the students even after their posting are not very keen on choosing psychiatry as career (Chawla et al. 2012). The earlier studies too highlighted that fact that only a few final year students wish to take up psychiatry as their career, as they too find it less rewarding (Alexander and Kumaraswamy 1993; Tharayan et al. 2001). Perhaps the current medical curriculum is not designed to dispel the myths and stereotypes a medical student carries as a part of societal beliefs. Even today, people with minor emotional and psychological problems approach the general physician at first level. With such negative attitudes even if the student prefers to become a general physician, the impact on the community about patients with psychiatric problems would still be the adverse. The studies quoted above all reflect a need to modify the psychiatry training curriculum at MBBS level.

8 Inadequate Duration for Training

The MCI has neglected psychiatric training at the undergraduate level (MCI 1997; Sethi 1978). The council recommends 20 h of didactic lectures and two-week posting in the psychiatry ward during MBBS course. The duration is much less in comparison with our national needs (Jacob 1998; Kattimani 2010; Yerramilli and Murty 2012; Chawla et al. 2012; Rajagopalan and Kuruvilla 1994). The time allotted for teaching is just about 1.4 % of the total training time during the four-and-a-half-year MBBS course (Thirunavukarasu and Thirunavukarasu 2010). In the United Kingdom, which has a population comparable to any single state of India, the General Medical Council recommends training for 80 h in behavioural sciences and a 36-week clinical posting. In Denmark, the psychiatry curriculum has much superior status compared to paediatrics and gynaecology. The current training is not sufficient as the medical graduates are unable to diagnose common psychiatric problems in the emergency room (Balhara et al. 2010).

9 Psychiatry Is Not a Main Subject in the Undergraduate Curriculum

For decades, the IPS is fighting for psychiatry to be accorded the status of a full subject. However, such efforts have not yielded the desired results. The biggest problem at present seems to be creating some space for psychiatry in the already overburdened undergraduate curriculum. It must be realised that a positive attitude towards a particular discipline and its growth is not feasible till it is allowed to be an essential part of the curriculum. Certain specialities such as paediatrics and orthopaedics are good examples of this approach. The clinical posting and number of theory lectures prescribed in these subjects far exceed what has been prescribed for psychiatry. Not just that attending classes in these subjects is compulsory, but the students at undergraduate level are also examined in these subjects in their final examination by the concerned specialists. Both these compulsions make the undergraduate student "serious" towards the speciality. Certainly, creating space for any speciality in the undergraduate curriculum is an uphill task, when the demands of already existing subjects are also increasing due to the rapid advancements in the field. In the UK, it was felt that the undergraduate curriculum is loaded with unnecessary factual details, which a student simply needed to reproduce as such without any advantage in the training. Omitting these details reduced the academic burden by about 35 % of the training time (GMC 1993). Similarly, there is an urgent need to revise our training programme so as to make it suitable for the needs of the community, to make it less burdensome for the students and get sufficient time slots for the subjects such as psychiatry. The MCI seems to have overlooked the state of the country's mental health problems, while responding to the call from the IPS for making psychiatry a complete subject at the MBBS level. The MCI, in its letter dated 20 August 2011, as stated by Kallivaylil (2012) gave psychiatry a respectable status in the MBBS curriculum, but denied the status of full examination subject due to the overburdened curriculum. This step is, thus, less likely to bear the desired results as we know that students take a subject seriously only if they have to take up an examination in the subject. The current MBBS curriculum is considered as one of the most overloaded of all academic curricula. Mental health needs special attention in the undergraduate curriculum (Das et al. 2002) and should be given the need-based priority it deserves. It needs to be revised according to the recommendations of the Taskforce on Undergraduate Training of the IPS and the World Psychiatric Association to meet the national needs and international standards (Murthy and Khandelwal 2007).

10 Political and Administrative Motivation

India is a large developing country. It has multiple demands and needs for adequate community and economic development. For that reason, priorities for development keep on changing from time to time. It has been realised that only those issues for which our leaders are sensitised get a place in policies and become a priority for development. The IPS has made seminal efforts to make the administrators and policymakers aware of the mental health needs of the country. However, political still seems to be lacking. Policymakers either have a negative attitude towards mental health needs or seem to be unaware of mental health problems. It is possible that this is the reason why whenever mental health issues of the country are a matter of concern, policymakers find it very easy to circumvent this priority (Mellor 2003).

11 Our Effort to Improve Undergraduate Psychiatry

As per a national report, 856,065 MBBS doctors who are registered were with the Indian medical register till 31 July 2011 (PTI 2011). India ranks 67th among the developing countries, with the doctor–population ratio in the country estimated to be around 1:2,000 (PBI 2013). But, this number is quite significant keeping in view that many graduates opt for training or working abroad despite facing hardships. On the other hand, we have only 23 % of the required number of psychiatrists in the country (TNN 2011). We must bear in mind that the health care system in India is still based on the quality of primary care. It is, therefore, the quality of training at the undergraduate level, which influences the health care outcome. Thus, we need to strengthen mental health training at the undergraduate level in order to meet the current mental health needs of our country. In 1946, the Bhore Committee recommended setting up of separate departments of psychiatry in the existing general hospital for specialist training within the teaching institution itself, instead of sending the students elsewhere for training (Bhore 1946). This suggestion led to opening up of many general hospital psychiatry units and psychiatry departments within the medical colleges. Consequently, we now have 149 medical colleges offering postgraduate training in psychiatry in comparison with almost none in the 1950s. Since then, the efforts to improve undergraduate training in psychiatry have been continuing. The Committee also stressed that the aim of undergraduate training in psychiatry should be to enable the medical student think, observe and take decisions by themselves. Training the medical graduates in social aspects was also recommended so that the undergraduate student became aware of mental health needs of not just patients with mentally illness, but also of the emotional problems of patients with medical problems. The social aspect of training could never be properly imparted due to the lack of sufficient trainers. Consequently, undergraduate students continue to have negative attitudes towards the mentally ill patients and psychiatry. The first seminar on teaching psychiatry to undergraduates was held at the Central Institute of Psychiatry (CIP), Ranchi, in 1965. A task force for training in psychiatry at undergraduate level was also constituted. In the first meeting of the IPS Subcommittee on Undergraduate Psychiatric Education (1965), it was pointed out the "if all five year plans are geared to make up for the deficiency of psychiatrists in the country, it would take 100 years to fill the gap". Undergraduate students were also found apathetic to psychiatry. The reasons for such apathy that could be identified are as follows:

1. They had poor background of the basic subjects such as psychology and sociology
2. Inadequate use of the teaching methods
3. Non-integration of psychiatry in the mainstream teaching
4. Lack of regulations for compulsory attendance in psychiatry
5. Lack of post-MBBS house surgeon posts in psychiatry departments.

Due to all these factors, medical graduates considered psychiatry as the odd man out in the whole academic curriculum. To overcome these deficiencies, the following reforms were proposed by the task force (Neki et al. 1965):

1. Introduction of basic behavioural sciences in the preclinical years
2. Modular teaching methods involving use of multiple teaching technology, reality and practice based instead of didactic teaching
3. Introduction to psychopathology and history taking in the early clinical years with exclusive psychiatric teaching to make the student identify and manage common psychiatric syndromes and emergencies. One month of such training was felt to be the bare minimum in order to give the medical student a "feeling" of psychiatric disorders
4. Collaborative teaching: teaching psychiatry to the undergraduate students in community settings or in the liaison clinics with other specialties
5. Accommodating the psychiatric curriculum in the main curriculum. The committee proposed to include psychiatry as one of the main subjects, with "bare minimum" requirements, keeping in view the already overcrowded medical curriculum
6. At the end of the course, an examination was also considered necessary
7. The expert committee also proposed the staff requirements, minimum infrastructural requirements for the "minimum curriculum".

In the mid-1970s, the Srivastava Committee, a group of educators commissioned by the Indian government, advocated reorientation of medical education in accordance with national needs and priorities. They recommended the formation of a medical education committee to implement reforms. A National Workshop on Undergraduate Training in Mental Health was held at Jawaharlal Institute of Postgraduate Medical Education and Research, Pondicherry (JIPMER), in 1983. A National Workshop on Social and Behavioural Sciences in Mental Health was held at the All India Institute of Medical Sciences, New Delhi (AIIMS), in 1994. It was observed that the one of the main reasons for the undergraduate not being keen on studying psychiatry was lack of orientation towards behavioural sciences. A workshop and teachers' training programme on undergraduate training in psychiatry was held in the National Institute of Mental Health and Neurosciences, Bengaluru (NIMHANS), in 1989, for teachers from 10 medical colleges, which identified the necessary steps to improve undergraduate training and teaching. One of the important recommendations of this workshop to the MCI was giving psychiatry the status of a full-fledged subject at the MBBS level. We still need to persist in our efforts for this status for psychiatry.

In 1986, the Bajaj Committee and, in 1993, Katker and Adkoli advocated to updating the course content, introducing revisions in student assessment and innovative teaching methodology. To implement these changes, they suggested faculty development, establishing medical education units and making educational funding more transparent. These recommendations were reiterated in 2004 by the Majumdar Committee in a government-commissioned report, in which the need for political commitment and leadership to achieve relevant, evidence-based medical education was emphasised. Efforts were continuously put in. But these could not bring any noteworthy change in the medical curriculum, especially in psychiatry (Reddy 2007; Thirunavukarasu 2007). This undergraduate psychiatry task force is continuing to review undergraduate training and submitted its latest recommendations under the leadership of Prof. Jiloha and Prof. Parkar in 2010 to the MCI (Jiloha and Parkar 2010; Manohari 2013). They stated that a medical student on graduation should be able to deliver mental health services at primary care level as was proposed by Trivedi (1998). The following were listed as the main objectives for undergraduate teaching:

1. Ability to identify signs and symptoms of common psychiatric illnesses
2. Ability to identify developmental delays, including cognitive delays
3. Ability to understand the nature and development of normal human behaviour
4. Ability to appreciate the interplay between psychological and physical factors in medical presentations
5. Awareness of common psychopharmacological interventions in clinical practice of psychiatry
6. Ability to apply basic counselling skills and be comfortable while discussing common psychiatric issues with patients or their relatives
7. Awareness of statutory and educational provisions with regard to psychiatric illnesses and disability
8. Ability to develop a helpful and humane attitude towards psychological, psychiatric and behavioural difficulties
9. Ability to deliver mental health services at the primary care level.

As cited by Kallivayalil (2012), responding to these recommendations, the MCI, in a letter dated 20 August 2011 addressed to the Ministry of Health and Family Welfare, Government of India, stated that the following have been incorporated into the curriculum for psychiatry, for the undergraduate MBBS course:

1. The teaching hours in psychiatry were to be increased from 20 to 40 h
2. The clinical posting in psychiatry was to be increased from 2 to 4 weeks
3. Marks for questions in psychiatry in the theory paper for medicine were to be doubled to 20, and it was agreed that the questions for psychiatry would be made mandatory
4. Internal assessment in psychiatry was to be made mandatory for the final examination
5. Psychiatry posting in internship was to be made mandatory, instead of it being an elective posting
6. The subject was to be taught in an integrated manner, especially with community medicine.

Of these recommendations to the Ministry of Health, there are still many yet to be implemented. There is still a 20-h teaching course in psychiatry, and questions on psychiatry have not been made mandatory in the final examination. Internal assessment in psychiatry too has not been uniformly adopted by the all medical colleges. Integration with the other subjects is also pending.

The IPS is continuing in its efforts to get psychiatry the status of complete undergraduate subject and has represented to the MCI and the Ministry of Health regarding this. On 25 November 2011, the Ministry of Health seemed to be convinced with the evidence provided by IPS on granting psychiatry the status of full subject with separate exam. The decision, however, is still pending for implementation (Kallivayalil 2012). Clearly, our record on psychiatric teaching at the undergraduate level has been dismal. Despite several good recommendations of many Indian and international bodies, we still need to improve our teaching psychiatry for medical students. Teaching psychiatry in an effective, need-based manner is the immediate requirement. We do hope that through repeated

Table 2 Steps to improve Skills, Aptitude and Training in Psychiatry (adapted from Kallivayalil 2012)

Changing negative attitudes of clinicians towards psychiatry by working with them
Convincing policymakers about the burden of psychiatric disorders
To convince students that they need psychiatry for their professional and personal development, by incorporating behavioural sciences class in the preclinical curriculum
Making psychiatric teaching needs based by giving more importance to anxiety disorders, depressive disorders, substance use disorders, medically unexplained somatic symptoms, psychosomatic symptoms and suicidal behaviour than schizophrenia or mania
Emphasise more on consultation liaison psychiatry and general hospital psychiatry than on specialised psychiatry
Make clinical postings interesting by incorporating new teaching methods such as demonstrating a video recording of interviewing a patient and asking students to evaluate the skill of interviewer
Encourage humanities in medicine, such as arts and literature to orient students to social sciences and its application to the medical sciences
Soft skills such as communication skills, stress management and study techniques, which may help personal development may be included in training
Uniformity in training and examination schedule and module throughout the country based on some national guidelines for syllabus, class room teaching hours and practical training
An objective method of examination that should include multiple choice questions for evaluating psychiatric knowledge, objective structured clinical examination and objective structured long examination review in place of personal idiosyncratic methods of assessment in clinical skills and knowledge
Integrating psychiatric teaching with other clinical subjects such as general medicine (to demonstrate a case of anxiety, depression or somatoform disorder) and specialties such as dermatology (obsessive–compulsive disorder, trichotillomania, delusional parasitosis), cardiology (panic disorder or depression), gastroenterology (irritable bowel syndrome, peptic ulcers), surgery (delirium, head injury), neurology (dissociative disorder) and paediatrics (attention deficit hyperkinetic disorder, mental retardation) would decrease academic load and make teaching interesting

regulations, the MCI would be able to do something to make psychiatric teaching effective. Making psychiatry a full subject with a separate examination at the MBBS level conducted by the psychiatric faculty is the only way to make the undergraduate student appreciate the importance of the subject and help him or her to understand psychiatry better. At present, we need to be prepared with a proposal of 100 h of psychiatry teaching and examination scheme for the undergraduates. Kallivayalil (2012) had proposed an action plan to improve psychiatric training, which is depicted in Table 2.

12 World Perspective on Undergraduate Psychiatry

The shortage of psychiatrists is not an Indian phenomenon, but it is globally prevalent depending upon the mental health needs of different countries (Bhugra 2009). Different countries differ in their emphasis upon psychiatric teaching during the undergraduate years. Denmark has put in the best effort making psychiatry a full subject at the undergraduate level. Teaching of psychiatry at the undergraduate level was well established in Denmark by 1912, and psychiatry acquired the status of a major clinical subject in the 1950s, rising to third place after surgery and medicine with approximately 240 h of teaching in psychiatry. In the USA, during the first 2 years, there are about 60 h of teaching in various psychosocial areas. In the third year, 30 h are devoted to practical teaching of psychiatry. In the fourth year, there is a full-time posting of 8 weeks of psychiatric clerkship. Sri Lanka and Nepal give prominence to psychiatry, and medical students need to pass an examination in psychiatry to qualify for medical degree (Kallivayalil 2012). But, in most countries, the status of psychiatry at the undergraduate level is in a developing phase.

There has been a global initiative on improving the undergraduate medical education. The undergraduate curriculum has been recognised to be over-burdened since the middle of the nineteenth century. The recommendations of the General Medical Council of the UK in 1957 and 1967 were felt to be such that it needed the student to produce more factual data and restricted him or her from developing independent thinking. It was felt that about 35 % of the load due to factual data could be reduced from the medical curriculum. Along with this, a strong emphasis on public health aspects, i.e. preventive and promotional aspects, instead of learning more about diseases and their diagnosis and treatment was required. It was also stressed that the curriculum should incorporate the latest advances in the field of medicine and surgery and should encourage self-learning by the student, instead of memorising facts. Emphasis was also laid on changing epidemiological trends, disability and distress, family experiences in the wake of a disease, and the ability to recognise "non-organic" aspects of disease, so as to make the curriculum oriented towards human disease, instead of conventional orthodox views of illnesses. Besides making the curriculum less heavy, emphasis was also placed on making it oriented to self-learning. A sound examination with the ability to test the students' skills as per the aims of the undergraduate training and test his or her ability to practice independently was also recommended. In order to meet these requirements, a core curriculum based upon modular learning was proposed. The basic structure of psychiatric module was as follows:

1. The prevalence, presentation, aetiology and basic management of "core" psychiatric conditions were made mandatory. "Core" conditions included the following: affective disorders, substance dependence, anxiety, panic and phobias, post-traumatic stress disorder, normal and abnormal grief and adjustment reactions, psychological problems complicating physical illnesses, acute confusional states, dementias, obsessive–compulsive disorder, conduct and emotional disorders of childhood and adolescence, and schizophrenia. Additionally, conditions such as somatic manifestations of psychological distress, eating disorders, psychosexual disorders, disorders of personality, developmental disorders and attention deficit disorders were also included
2. The conditions, under which patients may be detained and treated against their will, were to be taught
3. Common physical treatments in psychiatry, their indications, mechanisms of action and unwanted effects were included
4. The principles of psychotherapy were to be taught
5. The range of services and role of professionals in the community and the hospital in care of the mentally ill were to be taught
6. Common psychiatric conditions among people with learning disability and the range of services available for them were included
7. The ability to communicate effectively with the mentally ill, take a history and carry out a mental state examination was to be taught
8. The ability to produce a formulation commenting on differential diagnosis, aetiology, management and prognosis was to be taught
9. Assessing family relationships and their impact on family members was to be taught
10. Assessing the need for physical investigations and further psychometric assessment was to be taught
11. Assessing a patient's potential risk to others was to be taught
12. Assessing a patient's risk of suicide was to be taught
13. Facilitating referral to more specialist health services was to be taught
14. Demonstrating empathy, an understanding of the emotional problems of patients and of the psychological dimension of illness, was to be taught
15. Demonstrating a commitment to maximising social integration of patients with mental health problems and a sensitivity to patient concerns about stigma was to be taught
16. Appreciation of the importance of multi-disciplinary working in the field of mental health services was to be taught.

The GMC did not make the curriculum specifically assessment based, but issued only the guidelines for the individual schools to make their own assessment plan to include the different aspects of knowledge, skill and attitude.

Table 3 Essentials of psychiatry training for undergraduates (WPA Recommendations, 2002)

1. Clarifying what does a non-psychiatrist physician need to know about recognising and treating psychiatric problems and when to obtain a psychiatric consultation or make a referral
2. Develop six core competencies: patient care, medical knowledge, practice-based learning and improvement, interpersonal and communication skills, professionalism and systems-based practice
3. Faculty supervision of the medical students' clinical work is central to all medical education, for integration of knowledge, clinical skills and attitudes to occur
4. The evaluation of the learned skill should be done in a phased manner depending upon what is the focus of learning at a particular stage
5. A permanent education committee, either for students chaired by the director, including representatives from faculty responsible for major didactic and curricular components should evaluate and monitor the curriculum
6. Of equal to the importance of training is the attention to cultural and political influences on education. This requires acknowledging both the cultural context in which training is taking place and the anticipated practice locations of trainees
7. Health care financing must be taken into consideration for planning the curriculum, as inadequate number of psychiatrists and lack of finances make certain aspects of care, such as psychotherapeutic interviews an uncommon or non-existent part of clinical practice. However, appropriate financing for patient care and training is advocated
8. The use of technology and computer-based instruction may be preferred. Studies have found that lecture-based instructions and learning are cost effective, but computer-based instructions are far more time effective

The World Psychiatric Association collaborated with the World Federation on Medical Education and recommended that psychiatry be an independent subject at the undergraduate level (WPA 2002). The structure of undergraduate training in psychiatry was developed with the task force's appreciation of the tremendous diversity in psychiatric education across the globe. These recommendations of the task force were based on the observations that there was a massive burden of mental health problem around the globe. The need for treating mental disorders was obviously a pressing one in both developed and developing countries. Due to the global shortage of psychiatrists, it was, therefore, evident that all physicians must know how to detect and manage psychiatric disorders and when to refer patients to a specialist. The recommendations of the WPA for improving mental health teaching for undergraduates are included in Table 3.

In the United States, the Accreditation Council on General Medical Education (ACGME) has outlined six core competencies: patient care, medical knowledge, practice-based learning and improvement, interpersonal and communication skills, professionalism and systems-based practice (ACGME 2012). This is in addition to the extensive specialty-specific competencies. Focusing on specialists, the European Union of Medical Specialties (UEMS) outlines the psychiatrist's main roles as expert or clinical decision-maker, communicator, collaborator, manager, health advocate, scholar and professional. The required competencies, according to these organisations, are based on an educational framework, within which practical decisions are made, that allows a consistent approach to the formulation and monitoring of the curriculum's performance (WFME/AMSE 2007).

Keeping in view the above recommendations, our psychiatry curriculum for the undergraduates needs a thorough overhauling. The recommendations by the international bodies are based on the local and largely the global variations in the mental health needs of different regions. Hence, these guidelines can be followed to tailor the curriculum to suit the requirements of the country.

13 Future Directions

The proposed action plan for undergraduate training in psychiatry is presented in Table 2. There is an urgent need to include psychiatry in the main MBBS curriculum. It has been recognised for long that the stigma of psychiatric disorders cannot be removed, and adequate care of patients with such disorders cannot be ensured unless the primary care doctor is aware of the needs of patients with psychiatric disorders. If psychiatry can be included in the main curriculum, it would be much cost effective than the DMHP and training at the postgraduate level. Postgraduate training is needed in order to develop trainers in psychiatry and patient friendly treatment options in the field of mental health. The ultimate aim of the undergraduate training should be to provide comprehensive care to the psychiatric patient according to the international standards and not just the treatment of common mental disorders. The international guidelines for the undergraduate training must be followed in the time to come.

We have the following suggestions for all medical educationists to reform the medical curriculum for the complete health care of the person and his or her mind.

1. Psychiatric teaching needs to be vertically integrated with the whole medical curriculum. In the preclinical years, relevant portions of psychology, sociology and anthropology should be focussed upon, so that the student gets primed to understand the human behaviour and its determinants. This teaching would also help him in understanding biopsychosocial models of the disease and its treatment
2. The student must develop adequate skills in assessment of psychiatric disorders. Assessment should be primarily communication based, which is possible through development of good language skills, understanding of the patient's culture and empathic understanding and establishment of rapport. Psychiatry emphasises these skills a lot. Broadly speaking, these skills are not just required for psychiatry, but are important in all healthy human interactions. So later on, even if a medical graduate does not choose psychiatry as specialty for further training, these skills would be helpful in developing a good doctor–patient relationship
3. During clinical years, psychiatry should be taught taking cultural aspects into consideration. Medical undergraduate should be informed about the influence of culture on the mental disorders. The popular cultural beliefs, myths and practices should be a major focus of teaching psychiatry to them. A specific mention about the Indian contribution of psychiatry at the international level must be a

focus, so that the students should "feel" psychiatry getting "Indianised", and not just a Western speciality. Indian methods of treating neurotic patients would also be helpful in de-stigmatising psychiatry for the young minds

4. Drug treatment should focus on only few essential drugs for the treatment of psychiatric disorders, rather than loading them with complete textbook information on psychopharmacology
5. Wherever possible an integrated "psychosomatic" approach towards the management of physical and psychiatric disorders should be followed, i.e. while discussing the medical disorder, psychological and emotional aspects should also be touched upon. This approach would help in better understanding about clinical features and management of physical disorders. This approach would also help in accommodating psychiatry in an effective manner in the already overloaded MBBS curriculum. We must make adequate room to accommodate the advancements in the other medical fields also. This approach may be difficult but once applied its benefits outweighs the difficulties (Doraiswamy and Radhakrishnan 2013; Jacob (1998))
6. During clinical years, the focus should be on the understanding and management of common psychiatric disorders such as anxiety, somatoform and dissociative disorders, rather than the stereotyped descriptions of schizophrenia and bipolar disorder. The understanding and medical management of the widely prevalent substance use disorders should be taught
7. Psychiatry should be made a full subject at the MBBS level, with an examination at the end of the training, so that the whole training is taken seriously. At present, psychiatric curriculum for BSc. Nursing is much better theoretically and practically, compared to the MBBS curriculum
8. Classroom blackboard-lecture-based teaching has become outdated with the recent advancements in mass communication technology. The students generally do not prefer the old-fashioned techniques. The best possible use of audio-visual aids should be made. Instead of monotonous lectures, teaching should be didactic and interactive to gain attention of the students for the most of the time during teaching hours.

References

ACGME. (2012) Data Resource Book Academic Year 2011-2012, Accreditation Council of Graduate Medical Education, Chicago http://www.acgme.org/acgmeweb/Portals/0/PFAssets/PublicationsBooks/2011-2012_ACGME_DATABOOK_DOCUMENT_Final.pdf. Accessed 21 Apr 2013.

Alexander, P. J., & Kumaraswamy, (1993). Senior medical students attitude towards psychiatry: Relationship with career interest. *Indian Journal of Psychiatry, 35*(3), 221–224.

Avasthi, A. (2011). DLN Murthy oration: Indianizing psychiatry—Is there a case enough? *Indian Journal of Psychiatry, 53*, 111–120.

Balhara, Y. P. S., Sagar, R., & Chawla, J. M. (2010). Undergraduate psychiatric training: Insights from emergency room. *Delhi Psychiatric Journal, 13*(2), 287–290.

Bhaskaran, K. (1990). Undergraduate training in psychiatry and behavioural sciences—The need to train the trainers. *Indian Journal of Psychiatry, 32*(1), 1–3.

Bhore ,J. (1946). *Health survey and development committee*. Government of India New Delhi.

Bhugra, D. (2009) Fears of mental health crisis prompted by shortage of specialist doctors. www.mailonline.com. dated 21 June 2011. Accessed 24 Apr 2013.

Chadda, R. K., & Some, S. (1996). Psychiatric aspects of clinical practice in general hospitals: A survey of non-psychiatric clinicians. *Indian Journal of Psychiatry, 38*, 86–93.

Chaudhry, H. R. (2010). Indian psychiatry and research in Pakistan. *Indian Journal of Psychiatry, 52*, 72–75.

Chawla, J. M., Balhara, Y. P., & Sagar, R. S. (2012). Under graduate medical students attitude towards Psychiatry. *Indian Journal of Psychiatry, 54*, 37–40.

Das, M., Gupta, N., & Dutta, K. (2002). Psychiatric training in India. *The Psychiatrist, 26*, 70–72. doi:10.1192/pb.26.2.70.

Doraiswamy, R., & Radhakrishnan, S. (2013). Effectiveness of integrated teaching over traditional teaching among first year MBBS students. *Medical Journal of DY Patil University, 6*(2), 139–141.

Ghambheera, H. C., & Williams, S. (2010). Shared Challenges in Psychiatric research in India and Sri Lanka. In T. S. S. Rao (Ed.), *Indian research in Psychiatry* (pp. 159–164). Mysore: Indian Psychiatric Society.

GMC. (1993). *Tomorrow's doctors: Recommendations on undergraduate medical education*. London: General Medical Council.

IPS. (2012) Indian Psychiatric Society-Membership Directory-2012, Indian Psychiaric Society Headquarters, Gurgaon.

Jacob, K. S. (1998). Psychiatric education for medical students. *National Medicine Journal of India, 11*(6), 287–289.

Jiloha, R. C., & Parkar, S. (Ed.), (2010). Recommendation for under-graduate (MBBS) syllabus in psychiatry. Psychiatry education committee-2010. Indian Psychiatric Society. Available from: http://www.ips-online.org. Accessed 4 Dec 2012.

Jugal, K., Mukharjee, R., Prashar, M., Jiloha, R. C., & Ingle, G. K. (2007). Short communication-beliefs and attitude towards mental health among the medical professional in Delhi. *Indian Journal of Community Medicine, 32*(7), 198–200.

Kallivayalil, R. A. (2012). The importance of psychiatry in undergraduate medical education in India. *Indian Journal of Psychiatry, 54*(3), 208–216.

Kalra, G., & Bhugra, D. (2010). Mutual learning and research Messages. In T. S. S. Rao (Ed.), *Indian research in Psychiatry* (pp. 114–130). Mysore: Indian Psychiatric Society.

Kattimani, S. (2010). Undergraduate clinical posting in psychiatry: Are we paying enough attention? *Indian Journal of Psychiatry, 52*(2), 194.

Lingeswaran, A. (2010). Psychiatric curriculum and its Impact on the attitude of indian undergraduate medical students and interns. *Indian Journal Psychology Medicine, 32*, 119–127.

Manohari, S. M., Johnson, P. R., & Galgali, R. B. (2013). How to teach psychiatry to medical undergraduates in India?: A model. *Indian Journal of Psychology and Medicine, 35*(1), 23–28.

Math, S. B., & Srinivasaraju, R. (2010). Indian psychiatric epidemiologic studies, learning from the past. In T. S. S. Rao (Ed.), *Indian research in Psychiatry* (pp. 194–212). Mysore: Indian Psychiatric Society.

MCI (1997). www.mciindia.org/rulesandregulations/Thegraduatemedicaleducationrules1997.aspx. Accessed 22 April 2013.

MCI. (2013). http://www.mciindia.org/InformationDesk/MedicalCollegeHospitals/List of colleges. Accessed 20 April 2013.

Mellor, D. (2003). Commentary: Recruitment is ethical. *BMJ, 327*, 928.

Murthy, R. S. (2011). Mental health initiatives in India (1947–2010). *The National Medical Journal of India, 24*(2), 98–106.

Murthy, R. S., & Khandelwal, S. (2007). Undergraduate training in psychiatry: World perspective. *Indian Journal of Psychiatry, 49*, 169–174.

Neki, J. S., Masani, K. R., Dube, K. C., et al. (1965). Reports of the subcommittee on undergraduate teaching in psychiatry. *Indian Journal of Psychiatry, 7*, 63–74.

Patel, V. (2003). Recruiting doctors from poor countries: The great brain robbery? *BMJ, 327*(7420), 926–928.

PIB. (2013). *Doctor patient ratio in the country-Release ID :77859)*. Delhi: Press Information Beurau.

Polan, H. J., & Riba, M. (2010). Psychiatry's reliance on residents as teachers. *Academic Psychiatry, 34*(4), 245–247.

PTI (2011). Doctor-population ratio at 1:2000 in India. www.Zeenews.com Nov 29, 2011. Accessed 20 April 2013.

Rajagopalan, M., & Kuruvilla, K. (1994). Medical students's attitude towards psychiatry: Effect of two weeks training. *Indian Journal of Psychiatry, 36*, 177–182.

Reddy, I. R. (2007). Undergraduate psychiatry education: Present scenario in India. *Indian Journal of Psychiatry, 49*, 157–158.

Sethi, B. B. (1978). Undergraduate psychiatry. *Indian Journal of Psychiatry, 20*, 97.

Sharma, S. D. (1984). General hospital psychiatry and undergraduate medical education. *Indian Journal of Psychiatry, 26*(3), 259–263.

Sood, M., & Sharan, P. (2011). A pragmatic approach to integrating mental health in undergraduate training: The AIIMS experience and work progress. *National Medicine Journal of India, 24*, 108–110.

Sood, M., & Sharan, P. (2012). Letters to editor: Undergraduate training in psychiatry at AIIMS: Integration with community medicine. *Indian Journal of Psychiatry, 54*(1), 93–94.

Srivastava, A., & Natrajan, D. (2010). Psychiatrists and neuroscientists of Indian origin in Canada. In T. S. S. Rao (Ed.), *Indian research in Psychiatry* (pp. 131–138). Mysore: Indian Psychiatric Society.

Supe, A., & Burdick, W. P. (2006). Challenges and issues in medical education in India. *Academic Medicine, 81*(12), 1076–1080.

Tharyan, P., John, T., Tharyan, A., & Barganza, D. (2001). Attitude of "tomorrows Doctors" towards psychiatry and mentally illness. *National Medicine Journal of India, 14*(6), 355–359.

Thirunavukarasu, M. (2007). Psychiatry in UG curriculum of medicine: Need of the hour. *Indian Journal of Psychiatry, 49*, 159–160.

Thiruvanakasru, M., & Thiruvanakasru, P. (2010). Training and national deficit of psychiatrist in India. In T. S. S. Rao (Ed.), *Indian Research in Psychiatry* (pp. 165–179). Mysore: Indian Psychiatric Society.

TNN. (2011, December 22). Mental healthcare in dire straits. The Times of India.

Trivedi, J. K. (1998). Importance of undergraduate psychiatric training. *Indian Journal of Psychiatry, 40*, 101–102.

WFME/AMSE International Task Force. (2007). WFME Global standards for quality improvement in medical education: European specifications for basic and postgraduate medical education and continuing professional development. WFME Office University of Copenhagen, Denmark.

Wig, N., Murthy, R. S., & Harding, T. W. (1981). A model for rural health services: Raipur Rani experience. *Indian Journal of Psychiatry, 23*(4), 275–290.

WPA. (2002). World psychiatric association institutional program on the core training curriculum for psychiatry. World Psychiatry Association, Yokohama.

Yerramilli, S. S. R. R., & Murty, Y. V. S. S. (2012). VIEW POINT: Psychiatric education in India: need for reforms, Andhra Pradesh. *Journal of Psychology and Medicine, 13*(1), 17–22.

Chapter 32
The Mental Health Act of India

R.C. Jiloha

1 Introduction

Science has progressed immensely in the realm of curing and treating various diseases and disorders. The legal framework pertaining to diseases and disorders is also being strengthened with time. However, the same has not been the case of persons suffering from mental illnesses. Being a vulnerable section of the society, persons with such illnesses have been recurring victims of cruelty, ridicule, abuse and neglect of their legitimate rights. Mental disorders account for 13 % of the global burden of diseases (Kamra and Tiwari 2012).

Only 59 % people worldwide live in a country, where there is dedicated mental health legislation.[1] In India, we have over 10 crore people suffering from a mental illness, there are just 43 mental hospitals and about 4,000 psychiatrists.[2]

Mental health services in the Indian subcontinent began with the establishment of mental hospitals. The need and demand of mental hospitals during the early British rule were influenced by the ideas and concepts as prevalent in England during that period (Sharma 1987). The idea behind incorporating any measure with respect to mental illness was to isolate the affected patients, preferably in an institution, and keep them away from the mainstream society as much as possible.

R.C. Jiloha, Director, Professor and Head

---

[1] http://whqlibdoc.who.int/publications/2011/9799241564359_eng.pdf, visited on Jan 24, 2013.

[2] http://week.manoramaonline.com/Cgibin/MMOnline.dll/portal/ep/theWeekContent.do?contentId=11632435&programId=1073755753, visited on Jan 23, 2013.

R.C. Jiloha (✉)
Department of Psychiatry, Maulana Azad Medical College and G.B. Pant Hospital,
New Delhi, India
e-mail: rcjiloha@hotmail.com

S. Malhotra and S. Chakrabarti (eds.), *Developments in Psychiatry in India*,
DOI 10.1007/978-81-322-1674-2_32

Primarily, these hospitals or asylums were constructed away from the cities with high enclosures. The rules and the laws with respect to the admission care and discharge of the mentally ill have their origin in the English Acts such as Act for Regulating Private Mad Houses, 1774 and Country Asylums Act, 1808 (Kathleen 1972). In the middle of the nineteenth century, Lord Ashley introduced three amended acts, the Lunacy Regulation Act, 1853, the Lunatic Care and Treatment Amendment Act, 1853 and the Lunatic Asylums Act, 1853 (Sharma 1987).

After the British Crown took over the reins of India from the East India Company, it enacted the first Indian Lunacy Act (No 36) of 1858 providing guidelines for establishment of lunatic asylums and to regulate procedure for admission of the mentally ill. This Act was later modified in 1883, with more elaborate instructions for admission and care of the mentally ill. The sole purpose of establishing lunatic asylums was to segregate mentally ill who were considered as troublesome and dangerous to the society. It is obvious that the asylums constructed at that time were simply places for detention.

Due to deplorable condition of mentally ill in lunatic asylums and growing public concern, the government contemplated having a central supervision of these asylums in 1906 and Indian Lunacy Act 1912 (No 4) came with a racial bias. Separate institutions were established for European and Indian patients. In 1920, nomenclature was changed and the name Mental Hospital was substituted for lunatic asylum . Administrative control of these institutions was passed on to the civil surgeon of the district from the prison authorities (Kathleen 1972).

The Lunacy Regulation Act, 1853, the Lunatic Asylums Amendment Act, 1853, the Indian Lunacy Act, 1858 and the Indian Lunacy Act, 1912 were some of the archaic legislations that dealt with mental illness where persons suffering from such an illness were referred to as lunatics or idiots, were provided only custodial care, thereby ignoring the overarching principles of equality and dignity of individuals, as well as the International Instruments such as the Universal Declaration of Human Rights, which inter alia provides that all human beings are born free and equal in dignity and rights.[3]

The developments during the first half of the twentieth century brought newer insights into the understanding of mental disorders as medical illness requiring humane and sympathetic treatment. Introduction of general hospital psychiatric units (GHPUs) and electroconvulsive therapy (ECT) in the fourth decade of twentieth century and anti-psychotics and anti-depressants in the 1950s and 1960s revolutionised the concept of treating mental disorders. The mentally ill no longer remained subjects of amusement, ridicule, neglect or affliction by supernatural powers, and they came in the domain of treatable medical conditions (Wig 1978).

The Indian Lunacy Act of 1912 fell short and could not keep pace with the fast-developing field of psychiatry. It soon outlived its utility as it was no longer relevant to the needs of the society and the mentally ill. The Bhore Committee Report (Sharma 1987) pointed out that the existing mental hospitals were quite

---

[3] http://www.firstpost.com/living/suicide-nation-can-the-mental-health-bill-change-anything-in-india-503557.html, visited on Jan 24, 2013.

out of date and were designed for detention and custodial care without regard for curative treatment. In 1949, the Indian Psychiatric Society drafted 'Indian Mental Health Act Bill' (Varma 1953). The Bill was introduced in the parliament several times, but due to political reasons, it took many years to be enacted. After 40 years of independence, in 1987, came the Act, arousing expectations, raising hopes, making promises and generally heralding a new, a better and a more decent life for the mentally ill living a stigmatising existence. The Indian Mental Health Act (Act 14), 1987 replaced the Indian Lunacy Act, 1912 and the Jammu and Kashmir Lunacy Act, 1977.

Following are the objectives of the Act:

1. The attitude of the society has changed, no stigma should be attached with mental illness and the mentally ill persons should be treated like any other patient.
2. With the rapid advancement in medical sciences and mental health, the Indian Lunacy Act, 1912 has become outmoded, and it is necessary to have fresh legislation with provisions of treatment.
3. It is considered necessary:
   (a) To regulate admissions and to protect the rights of the inpatients.
   (b) To protect the society from patients who become a danger and a nuisance.
   (c) To protect citizens from being detained without sufficient cause.
   (d) To regulate responsibility for maintenance.
   (e) To provide facilities for establishing guardianship or custody of mentally ill who are unable to look after themselves.
   (f) To establish Central and State Authorities for Mental Health.
   (g) To regulate the powers of the government in relation to mental health.
   (h) To provide legal aid to mentally ill at state expense in certain cases.

The general expectation was that the legislation would usher in a new era of proper care and dignified life for the psychiatric patients.

2 The Mental Health Act, 1987

The Act that is spread over 10 chapters and 98 clauses extends to whole of India and came into force on 1 April 1993. The Act represents a departure from the earlier Act by bringing the latest concepts and knowledge in the field of mental health. Following are the important features of the Act:

1. **Nomenclature:** The Indian Lunacy Act used terms, which were derogatory at the time and context. They undermined the human dignity of the mentally ill and were replaced by acceptable terms. Mental hospitals are known in the Act by the terms psychiatric hospitals or psychiatric nursing homes. The patients are not to be called as lunatics, meaning thereby idiots or persons with unsound mind. In the new Act, they are known as psychiatric patients who are in need of treatment. An important departure from the earlier Act is that the mentally challenged

(retarded) have been excluded from the ambit of this Act, which has evoked a mixed response from the professionals. Change in nomenclature brings psychiatry at par with other medical disciplines and de-stigmatises mental illness.

2. **Supervision of psychiatric hospitals:** The Chapter II of the Act deals with the creation of Mental Health Authorities both at centre and state levels, as watchdog bodies to assure quality of services. This brings mental health services under the ambit of the Mental Health Authority, making the services accountable and responsible for the care of mentally ill. However, licensing of psychiatric nursing homes is perceived to be a different yardstick for those who wish to establish a private hospital or a nursing home (Antony 2000).
3. **Admission procedures:** While retaining the earlier modes of admission, i.e. voluntary and under reception order, a new category of admission procedure has been introduced under Section 19 (Chapter IV), which does not involve judiciary to admit an uncooperative or unwilling patient for a period of 90 days with the support of two medical certificates. This provision is helpful in emergency situations where the patient requires immediate medical intervention, but is unable to give his consent. Experiences reveal that many professionals make use of this mode of admission as an easier option for admitting a patient who is unable to give consent. The procedure for admitting a voluntary patient is also simplified. Approval of members of Board of Visitors is not required for admitting a voluntary patient according to the Mental Health Act, 1987.
4. **Functioning of the Board of Visitors:** Chapter V deals with inspection, discharge, leave of absence and removal of mentally ill. The Act insists on inclusion of psychiatrists and social workers as members of the board giving clear directions with respect to its working. Subsequently, members from judiciary were also added to the team. Patients' records considered to be confidential by the medical officer incharge may not be accessible to the members of the board. To ensure regularity in members, visits to the hospital, the Act provides that a member absenting himself for three consecutive months forfeits his membership.
5. **Judicial safeguards for patients' rights:** Chapter VI deals with judicial inquisition regarding alleged mentally ill persons possessing property, custody of his person and management of his property. It incorporates some newer provisions, which are consistent with other civil laws and procedures governing management of such property by managers. The Mental Health Act, 1987 provides safeguards for the patients, and there is greater penalty for misuse of property by managers. Liability to meet cost of maintenance of mentally ill by government in certain cases is elaborately described. There is also a provision by which persons legally bound to maintain mentally ill persons are not absolved from such a liability.
6. **Humanitarian provisions:** Chapter VIII (Section 81) of the Act contains a progressive and explicit provision on 'protection of human rights' of the mentally ill persons. No mentally ill person during treatment is to be subjected to any indignity. No research, unless of direct benefit in diagnosis and treatment of the patient can be conducted. Letters or other communications of the patient cannot be intercepted, detained or destroyed.

7. **Penalty for detaining a patient in psychiatric hospital or nursing home other than the licensed ones:** The Act provides for the punishment for detention of a patient in a hospital or nursing home other than the licensed ones.

The Act defines a mentally ill person to be a person who is in need of treatment by reason of any mental disorder. However, mental disorder as such is not defined (Trivedi 1989). The definition of mental illness excludes mental retardation, without providing alternative options for the care of the mentally retarded. As a result, persons with severe and profound mental retardation who need comprehensive care from mental health experts are deprived of these services. While defining the psychiatric hospital or psychiatric nursing home, the Act includes these institutions established and maintained by government or another person and excludes general hospitals or nursing homes established and maintained by the government, but not those established and maintained by any other person. It means that the private general hospitals or nursing homes admitting psychiatric patients are treated like psychiatric hospitals or nursing homes meaning thereby, they have to follow the rules as laid down for psychiatric hospitals or nursing homes. This discriminatory approach has led to resentment among the psychiatrists, and it is observed during these 20 years that many psychiatrists do not admit their patient in privately run general hospitals for want of a license (Antony 2000).

The provision of admitting patients under special circumstances (Section 19) is indeed a welcome option for admitting unwilling patients without involving the judiciary (Sharma 1987). However, for some professionals, the experience of admitting patients under special circumstances has not been encouraging, because friends or relatives on whose behalf the patient was admitted fail to turn up to take the patient back after discharge (Dutta 1995).

Section 23 of the Act empowers the police officer to take in his custody the wandering patient incapable of looking after himself, one who is dangerous to himself or to others, or the one who is cruelly treated in the household, within his jurisdiction and produce him before the magistrate within 24 h for reception orders.

However, a large number of mentally ill persons be wandering in public places in conditions of total neglect and squalor can still be seen. Police officials are very much aware of this fact. When we have such a large number of neglected patients in the public places, in all probability, we have a much larger number who are neglected, denied elementary creature comfort, cruelly treated in their home, and are allowed to perish. This shows that provision in the Act has failed to achieve the objective. Police officials need to be sensitised about their duty towards mentally ill (Trivedi 2002).

The lawmakers, with a lot of empathic consideration about human rights and human dignity issues of patients with psychiatric disorders, have introduced the provision of magistrate enabling to 'consider applications for reception order in camera …' [Section 22(7)]. The active role played by the Human Rights Commission and certain NGOs has brought tremendous improvement in the living conditions of most of the psychiatric hospitals in the country.

No doubt, the Act provides punishment for detention of a patient in a hospital or nursing home in contravention of the rules laid down. It is true that the Act is stringent with erring hospitals and nursing homes, but it does not address the prevailing socially sanctioned customs permitting detention and treatment of mentally ill in an unscientific manner. The Act fails to achieve its objective of reducing stigma attached to mental illness. If the law does not address the social issues responsible for maltreatment of patients with psychiatric disorders, the prevailing attitude towards the mentally ill will continue to exist.

The directive of the Supreme Court for implementation of the Mental Health Act in its present form has brought about many controversies due to lack of proper understanding of the Act on the part of the government and the absence of organised Mental Health Authorities in some states. The Act gives more of a legal flavour and shows very little consideration for clinical and medical aspect of mental illness (Kamra and Tiwari 2012). Though it incorporates provisions relating to treatment and care, it retains the concept of custodial care and segregation of the patients from the community (Sharma 1987). In some states, even for running a psychiatry outpatient clinic, the government insists that a license has to be procured (Trivedi 1989). No doubt, the Mental Health Act, 1987 is a positive step towards ameliorating the conditions of persons with mental illnesses in the country, and it has brought a lot of positive changes from the erstwhile draconian legislations, yet it has left a lot to be desired, particularly with respect to the fast-changing knowledge and attitudes in relation to mental illness (Kamra and Tiwari 2012).

The Persons with Disabilities Act (1995)[4] includes mental illness as a disability; however, it does not clearly define what mental illness actually amounts to. India is a signatory to the Convention on Rights of Persons with Disabilities, 2006 and has ratified the said instrument in October 2007. The convention inter alia provides that every person with disabilities has a right to respect for his or her physical and mental integrity on an equal basis with others (Article 17).[5]

The states who are parties to the Convention must recognise the equal right of all persons with disabilities to live in the community, with choices equal to others, and shall take effective and appropriate measures to facilitate full enjoyment by persons with disabilities of their rights and their full inclusion and participation in the community (Article 19). Such states shall protect the privacy of personal health and rehabilitation information of persons with disabilities on an equal basis with others (Article 22). These states must recognise that persons with disabilities have the right to the enjoyment of the highest attainable standard of health without discrimination on the basis of disability (Article 25).

The National Health Policy, 2002[6] has also dealt with mental health, recognising that mental disorders have serious bearing on the quality of life of the person

[4] The Persons with Disabilities (Equal opportunities, Protection of Rights and Full Participation) Act, 1995 (1 of 1996) Published in part II, Section I of the extraordinary gazette of India. Ministry of Law, Justice and Company affairs. (Legislative Department), New Delhi.

[5] Convention on the Rights of Persons with Disabilities, Dec 13, 2006, A/RES/61/106, Annex I, Accessed on Jan 29, 2013, from http://www.unhcr.org/refworld/docid/4680cd212.html.

[6] The Ministry of Health and Family Welfare, Government of India, New Delhi. http://www.mohfw.nic.in/NRHM/Documents/National_Health_policy_2002.pdf.

affected by it. The plan had envisaged a network of decentralised mental health services.

The World Health Organization in a document[7] lists the 10 basic principles of mental health care law, which are as follows:

1. Promotion of mental health and prevention of mental disorders.
2. Access to basic mental health care.
3. Mental health assessments in accordance with internationally accepted principles.
4. Provision of health care which is the least restrictive.
5. Self determination, i.e. consent is necessary before any type of action can be taken with respect to that individual.
6. In case of difficulty in exercising consent or understanding the implications of the decision, the person may seek assistance with regard to the same from a known third person of his or her choice.
7. Availability of a review procedure in case of decisions made by officials or surrogate decision makers.
8. Automatic review system in certain cases.
9. Decision makers to be qualified individuals.
10. Respect for rule of law.

Mental health care has found mention in the approach paper for the 12th Five Year Plan. It has been provided that there must be a focus on the special requirements of different groups, e.g. integrated health care and other needs specific to the elderly, adolescents, health support services (and counselling) for victims of sexual or substance abuse and those infected with HIV/AIDS. Mental health services, including psycho-social care and counselling, should be prioritised, in settings of transition due to migration, areas of conflict and disturbances.[8]

In view of the fast-occurring changes, the experience with Mental Health Act, 1987, has been far from satisfying. In order to devise a strong mechanism to address the concern of persons suffering with mental illness and to ensure compliance with international instruments, the Draft Bill on Mental Health Care[9] (Draft Mental Health Care Bill 2012[10]; Chatur 2012) has been prepared by the Ministry of Health and Family Welfare.

---

[7] Prevention and Promotion in Mental Health, World Health Organization. http://www.who.int/mental_health/media/en/75.pdf, visited on Jan 24, 2013.

[8] Issues for the Approach to the Twelfth Five Year Plan. http://planningcommission.nic.in/plans/planrel/12appdrft/appraoch_12plan.pdf.

[9] http://judis.nic.in/temp/334200131242002p.txt, visited on Jan 24, 2013.

[10] Draft Mental Health Care Bill 2012, http://clpr.org.in/the-mental-health-care-bill-2012-an-overview/, visited on 24.1.2013.

3 Draft Mental Health Care Bill (2012)

The Bill seeks to protect, promote and fulfil the rights of persons with mental illness and to provide treatment, care and rehabilitation to improve the capacity of the person to develop his or her full potential and to facilitate his or her integration into community life. The Mental Health Care Bill attempts to remedy the inaccuracies and ambiguities in definitions with respect to mental health.

Section 2(j) defines the term 'least restrictive alternative'. This definition assumes importance as the Bill seems to comply with the basic requirements laid down by the WHO with respect to mental health legislation. Least restrictive alternative, option or environment means offering an option for treatment that meets with a person's treatment needs and imposes the least restriction on person's rights.

Section 2(r) defines 'mental illness' as 'disorder of mood, thought, perception, orientation and/or memory, which causes significant distress to a person or impairs a person's behaviour, judgment and ability to recognise reality, or impairs the person's ability to meet the demands of normal life, and includes mental conditions associated with the abuse of alcohol and drugs, but excludes mental retardation'. The Bill also lists the factors upon which mental illness shall be determined in accordance with Section 3.

The definition of 'mental illness' is a major improvement from the earlier Act which did not provide any guidance as to what would constitute mental illness except for stating that a person who was mentally ill was anyone needing treatment and who did not come under the definition of mental retardation, while the 2012 Bill seeks to understand mental illness from a social model, giving a broad and inclusive definition as to what may constitute mental illness. Section 20 of the Bill seeks to ensure that all persons with mental illness shall have a right to live with dignity and be protected from cruel and inhuman treatment.

Unlike the Mental Health Act, 1987, Section 25 of the Bill provides that patients will have the right to access complete information about their treatment, including all medical records. Such information shall only be withheld in exceptional circumstances where there is likelihood of harm to the patients or other persons. The Bill imposes a duty under Section 23 upon health professionals treating the patients to keep information relating to their mental health strictly confidential.

Mental health services are sought to be integrated into general health-care services at all levels of health care including primary, secondary and tertiary care level of health services and in all health programs run by the Government as provided under Section 18(5). The Insurance Regulatory Development Authority (IRDA) (1999) under the IRDA Act 1999 shall endeavour to ensure that insurance shall be provided for treatment of mental illness at par with that of physical illness as given under Section 21(2).

The Bill provides that any person with mental illness and his or her 'nominated representative' has the right to complain regarding deficiencies in provision of care or services, in the mental health establishment to the medical officer or psychiatrist incharge of the establishment, and if not satisfied with the response to the State Mental Health Authority and if not satisfied with the response to the State Panel of the Mental Health Review Commission.

The Bill seeks to create various new bodies and completely overhaul the existing mental health-care system in the country. It provides for the establishment of the Central and State Mental Health Authorities, which would be responsible for the registration and oversight of mental health establishments by laying down minimum standards and a monitoring mechanism to ensure statutory compliance. The Bill also sets up the Mental Health Review Commission (MHRC) and state-wise Mental Health Review Boards (MHRB).

The MHRC and MHRB are to be equipped with several administrative and adjudicatory functions and will form the first level of interaction of any person with mental illness or his or her representative with the mental health-care system for violation of any of his or her rights. With the introduction of these new bodies, for the first time, a person with mental illness can directly approach a forum for protection of his or her rights.

The Draft Bill lists the following treatments that are prohibited from being performed on persons with mental illness under Section 104:

1. The present Draft Bill seeks to prohibit the use of ECT treatment completely in case of minors. However, after consultation with doctors, administrators and state government officials, it was decided that such therapy could be allowed under anaesthesia and with the consent of the guardian and prior permission of the concerned board since in certain extreme cases involving minors it does prove to be a life saving exercise.
2. Prohibiting the sterilisation of any person with mental illness.
3. The Apex court took suo moto cognizance of the Erwadi episode (Venkatesan 2002) and ordered [W.P (C) 334 of 2001] (see Footnote 7) a ban upon chaining of patients suffering with mental illness. The present Bill seeks to prohibit the chaining of patients in any manner.
4. Restrictions on the use of psychosurgery as a treatment has also been incorporated (Section 105) for persons with mental illness, and such a procedure shall only be undertaken when there has been an informed consent of the person upon whom the surgery is to be performed and when an approval from the State Mental Health Authority has been taken to perform the surgery.

According to a recent report, WHO (Patel et al. 2013) estimates that about 170,000 deaths by suicides occur every year in India. The maximum suicide rate is in the age bracket of 15–29 years. The Bill seeks to decriminalise attempt to suicide due to mental illness under Section 124. Any person who attempts to commit suicide shall be presumed to have mental illness, and no investigation or prosecution shall be carried out. The government shall be duty-bound to take care of such a person and ensure his proper treatment and rehabilitation to reduce the risk of suicide attempts in future.

A provision under Section 114 has also been incorporated whereby a proof of a person's past or present admission or treatment in a mental health establishment for mental illness shall not be a ground for divorce.

Section 116 and Section 117 of the Act prescribe that mental health establishments which have not been registered shall also be dealt with severely. A fine of 50,000 rupees shall be imposed for the first offence. A fine of 2 lakh rupees and thereafter a fine of 5 lakh rupees shall be imposed for subsequent offences. Persons knowingly serving in such unregistered mental health establishments shall also be liable to pay a fine of 25,000 rupees.

Contravention of any provision entails punishment by the State Panel of Mental Health Review Commission with imprisonment for a term up to 6 months and fine of 10,000 rupees. In case of a subsequent offence, the imprisonment shall be for 2 years and a minimum fine of 50,000 rupees, which may extend to 5 lakh rupees. Under Section 91(4), where a mental health establishment does not comply with the orders of the Commission or the board, or wilfully neglects such order or direction, the Commission or the Board may impose a penalty of 5 lakh rupees, or can also order the central or state authority to cancel the registration of such establishment.

Chapter XII of the Bill deals with 'Admission, Treatment and Discharge'. The Bill provides that as far as possible all admissions to the mental health establishments should be independent admissions, i.e. where a person suffering from mental illness has the capacity to take decisions regarding his or her illness without depending on anyone. But, it is imperative to understand that in certain cases, supported admissions become a necessity.

The Bill covers the circumstances of discharging independent patients; however, clarity is still lacking on the fate of patients who are unable to fathom the consequences of their judgment. The Bill also restricts the duration to 72 h under Section 103, for which emergency treatment in exceptional circumstances may be carried out.

Even though the previous legislations on mental illness incorporated provisions for ameliorating the conditions of persons with mental illness, there was no provision or step considered necessary to reduce social stigma attached to such an illness. Unless this issue is addressed no matter how strong legislation may be drafted, the predicament of such persons shall never cease.

In 2009, the Delhi High court had ordered the creation of wards for women with mental illness, when a former model was found begging on the streets of Delhi.[11] The present Bill mandates the government to take measures so that the provisions of the Bill are publicised and communicated to the general public. In order to reduce social stigma associated with mental illness, programmes shall also be devised and implemented.

Despite the attempts in the Bill to ameliorate the conditions of the mentally ill people, the Bill has been criticised severely, by disabled rights activists as an 'apartheid' against mentally ill people, making it easier to forcibly confine a person into a mental asylum. Some call it 'anti-patient' and some label it a 'pro-doctor' Bill (Kamra and Tiwari 2012).

Thus, even before the draft has been tabled in the parliament, there have been protests from all corners as to certain provisions of the Bill, claiming that the Bill

[11] Special-units-for-mentally-ill-women-in-Delhi. http://www.igovernment.in/site/.

still allows the practice of involuntary admissions. However, it must be seen in the context that sometimes there are circumstances when the patient is unable to take a decision on his or her own treatment, and due to the nature of his illness, it becomes imminent that special care be taken.

The Bill addresses even this issue by limiting such forced admissions to 30 days (Section 98). There is appreciation of patient autonomy as a 'medico-ethical' principle and in the absence or reduction of this decision-making capacity, the second principle of 'beneficence' supersedes it. The question of surrogate decision-making arises in this context across all medical fields, psychiatry included.

It is also deprecated, implying that it is argued that under the Bill, mental health-care professionals such as psychiatrists have been given power to decide whether a person needs to be put in a mental asylum or not. Under the Mental Health Act, 1987, such a power was with the Magistrate. Any mentally ill person admitted to a mental health establishment, or his or her relative or friend, may apply to the Magistrate for discharge of such person.

Under the Bill as mentioned, the Magistrate is removed from the picture completely and is replaced by mandatory reviews of all such cases by mental health panels, which comprise judges, and also administrators and persons with mental illness and their caregivers. This has been called as taking away the voluntary admission aspect. But it should be noticed that, in a way this whole new regime is an improvement over the unbridled power to the Magistrate in the mental health system, which has now been reduced to only a few specific cases.

Also, it is argued by many groups that, even though there is a provision for an advance directive in the bill, which provides for a person to detail in advance as to what treatment he prefers in case of mental illness in future, the provision is watered down by giving the caregivers, relatives and NGOs the right to seek cancellation of such directives by appealing before the Mental Health Review Commission. It is also said that in a way, if the electroconvulsive treatment for children and without anaesthesia is barred, it would be much against scientific and logical thinking. Such things are best left to the experts. So is the restriction of the period of treatment, which should again be a professional case-by-case decision.

Moreover, the lenient rules regarding establishment of mental health establishments or institutions with a general form and provisional registration within 10 days is totally underestimating the importance of expertise needed in the treatment and care of mentally ill people. India has ratified the United Nations Convention on Rights on Persons with Disability in 2007, which advocates community health care, rather than the rapid mushrooming of such institutions, without any deterrents for those who run such institutions illegally. There is an argument for more community health-care provision, than more psychiatric facilities.

India needs to look at the experience of countries that have moved away from asylum-based treatments and embraced community integrated psychiatry as the treatment model, which has also been stressed by the Rights of Persons with Disabilities Bill 2012 recently unveiled by the Ministry of Social Justice and Empowerment (MSJE), which guarantees the 'legal capacity' and the 'right to choice' of all persons with disabilities, including those with psychosocial disabilities.

It is an undisputed fact that this Bill has addressed many problems faced by the persons with mental illness. It has definitely encouraged people to have a healthy discussion and debate on the protection and promotion of rights of the persons suffering from mental illness. The very fact that the Bill recognises that The Mental Health Act, 1987, has not been able to adequately protect the rights of persons with mental illness and promote access to mental health care in the country is a welcome step.

The proposed Mental Health Act, in its final form, should ensure proper care for the mentally ill, who are at the risk of harming either themselves or others. Provisions in the Act to make amendments based on feedback from stakeholders will go a long way in reducing concerns, which may arise out of local variations of needs and societal mores.[12]

Thus, persons with mental illness should be treated like other persons with health problems, and the environment around them should be made conducive to facilitate recovery, rehabilitation and full participation in society. The Bill brings about a rights-based protection of mentally ill persons, for the first time and definitely gives a humane perspective to the issue.

References

Antony, J. T. A. (2000). Decade with the mental health act 1987. *Indian Journal of Psychiatry, 42*(4), 347–355.

Chatur, D. (Nov 5, 2012). Available at http://clpr.org.in/ visited on Jan 24, 2013.

Dutta, A. B. (1995). Medico-legal problems of psychiatrists in private practice. *Journal of Clinical Psychiatry, 1*(1), 7–14.

Insurance Regulatory Development Authority Act, 1999 http://en.wikipedia.org/wiki/Insurance_Regulatory_and_Development_Authority visited on Jan 24, 2013.

Kamra, A. & Tiwari, G. (2012). Mental Health Care Bill 2012 The Lex-Warrier, *Online Law Journal* ISSN 2319-8338, Nov 6, 2012.

Kathleen, J. (1972). *A history of mental health services*. London: Routledge and Kegan Paul.

Patel, V., Ramasundarahettige, C., Vijayakumar, L., Thakur, J. S., Gajalakshmi V., Gururaj, G., Suicide mortality in India: A nationally representative survey. In W. Suraweera, & P. Jhathe (Eds.), *Million death study collaborators*. http://press.thelancet.com/indiasuicide.pdf, visited on Jan 24, 2013.

Sharma, S. (1990). Indian Mental Health Act 1987: A critical assessment. In: *Mental Hospitals in India*. New Delhi: DGHS Publication.

Trivedi, J. K. (1989). Ethics in psychiatry. In A. K. Agarwal, J. K. Trivedi, P. K. Sinha, & M. Katiyar (Eds.), *The Mental Health Act 1987* (pp. 158–160). Lucknow: LPH.

Trivedi, J. K. (2002). The Mental health legislation an ongoing debate. *Indian Journal of Psychiatry, 44*(2), 95.

Varma, L. P. (1953). History of psychiatry in India and Pakistan. *Indian Journal of Psychiatry, 4*(1–2), 26–53.

Venkatesan, J. (2002, April 18). Prevent recurrence of Erwadi-type incidents: SC. *The Hindu Online edition of India's National Newspaper*.

Wig, N. N. (1978). General hospital psychiatric units: Right time for evaluation. *Indian Journal of Psychiatry, 20*, 1–3.

[12] http://www.thehindu.com/opinion/op-ed/dr-jayakumar-menon-responds/article4055360.ece.

Erratum to: Psychiatric Nosology, Its Philosophy and Science

P.K. Singh

Erratum to: Chapter 5 in: S. Malhotra and S. Chakrabarti (eds.), *Developments in Psychiatry in India*, DOI 10.1007/978-81-322-1674-2_5

On page 67, the designation of the author P.K. Singh is incorrectly mentioned. His correct designation is as below:

P.K. Singh, Professor and Head

The online version of the original chapter can be found under
DOI 10.1007/978-81-322-1674-2_5

P.K. Singh (✉)
Department of Psychiatry, Patna Medical College, Patna, India
e-mail: pkspostline@yahoo.com

S. Malhotra and S. Chakrabarti (eds.), *Developments in Psychiatry in India*,
DOI 10.1007/978-81-322-1674-2_33

Reminiscences

Savita Malhotra:

The Golden Jubilee of the department is an opportunity to reflect and reminiscence about one's life and journey in the department. I joined the department in 1974, as a house physician (when I was just 23 yrs of age) and never left it till today, which makes it 40 yrs so far, the longest anyone has ever spent.

A life time and the best time of my life have been given to the department. So great was the work environment and work culture that I had tremendous admiration for the place. Prof. NN Wig and Prof. VK Varma were my teachers and mentors who taught not only the basics of psychiatry but also the highest ethical and moral values associated with the discipline and practice of psychiatry. The department then was small with only eight Junior Residents, two Senior Residents and four faculty members. Interaction was close and personal. From housejob to residency, then joining the faculty in 1979, and career progression thereafter was smooth sailing. Being a junior faculty member working with Dr Wig and Dr Varma was the greatest joy and honour.

Professionalism, pride in specialty, attention to detail, pursuit of perfection were some of the most valuable learnings. I could never imagine that this journey would be so intense, productive, and fulfilling. Each day for me, had a new lesson of life; was better and more exciting than the previous one.

I am thankful to the almighty and humbled to have reached the position of head of the same department that was headed by Prof. NN Wig, occupying the same office as he did. I always used to hold the magnificent facade of the Kairon Block of PGI in awe, and having an office in Kairon Block as Dean of PGI has been the crowning touch in my life.

I have had great friends and companions, and excellent juniors and students, who kept me young, contributed to my life, shared my joys and sorrows, and enriched my experience. Looking back, I have the greatest sense of satisfaction for being able to serve the department and the profession with my best possible ability.

S. Malhotra and S. Chakrabarti (eds.), *Developments in Psychiatry in India*,
DOI 10.1007/978-81-322-1674-2

A. Avasthi: A Journey Well Wrought

Since the time of my joining as a Senior Resident at Postgraduate Institute of Medical Education and Research (PGIMER), Chandigarh, I observed that trainees and clinicians have been hesitant in exploring marital and psychosexual history. Hence, I decided about learning and imparting training about marital and psychosexual problems in a structured manner to the residents, so that they do not overlook the patient's complaints and delve deeper when situation requires. I started working with patients presenting with psychosexual and marital relationship problems since 1982 with the active encouragement and guidance of Prof. V.K. Varma. This work was discontinued after I left PGIMER to work abroad for a while. After joining as a faculty member in PGIMER in 1987, a formal Marital and Psychosexual Clinic (MPC) was started for dealing with cases where marital and psychosexual issues were of prime concern. The MPC was a weekly clinic, in which junior residents worked up patients and discussed with consultants. By that time, little amount of research on psychosexual matters had been undertaken in the country. The MPC gave an opportunity for structured research in psychosexual disorders and many studies were initiated. Liaison was also established with other departments like urology and endocrinology. At the time MPC was established, pharmacological agents for treatment of sexual disorders were virtually negligible. Things changed with advent of sildenafil for potency disorders, though it was realised that many patients could not be helped by medications alone and psychotherapeutic interventions had a definite role. The MPC provides guidance for providing psychotherapy for marital and psychosexual disorders. The training imparted through the MPC hopefully has helped a generation of psychiatrists in the past and would surely be of use for a generation to come. With augmentation of resources, MPC should run daily with the primary responsibility of care shifting to senior residents with greater commitment of consultants in charge. Supervised training of junior residents can then focus upon sharpening their skills in psychosexual therapies, marital and family therapies, and group therapies.

D. Basu: My Department and I—A Psychodynamic Formulation

I have been in the Department since 1987 till date—26 years: exactly half my age. Of these 26 years, other than 3 years abroad, the remaining 23 years of my existence has been in the Department—starting as a callous but rebellious Junior Resident (suspected to be a 'latent schizophrenic' by the then Acting Head of the Department), through by-my-standard hard-working years of Senior Residency and then through various stages of Faculty positions till I gloriously reached the "level of my incompetence" as Professor, faithfully demonstrating Peter Principle all along the way.

Practically a piece of departmental furniture now (like the easy chair meant for the Consultant in the Rounds Room, which I have been seeing for all these years and which, it is rumored, hails from the times of Le Corbusier), I have virtually internalized the Department; or should I say, the Department has internalized me. It is said that the post-Eliot modern poets (or post-Tagore, in Bengal) all tried to vehemently defy their powerful predecessor in a conscious but vain attempt to get out of their towering influence in order to find their own style and identity in poetry. I have tried in my younger years, in vain, to defy, vilify, antagonize, rebel against and even ignore my department, to come out of my Oedipus Complex; waging a hopeless battle against the towering father figure of my Department. After suffering my quota of castration anxiety, I finally grew out of it exactly as old Freud would have predicted—by starting to assimilate the values of my Department, by identifying myself with its ethos and its culture, its beauty and its power, its dominance and its love, ...by becoming proud of it, by gradually developing the internalized departmental superego structure in my struggling psyche.......by becoming my Department.

P.B. Behere

The Post-Graduate Institute of Medical Education and Research (PGIMER) is one of the institutions of national importance for postgraduate medical education and research. The present author spent 1976–1979 and worked with stalwarts of Indian psychiatry. The author got an opportunity to work in various projects like '*Strategies for Extension of Mental Health services,*' '*Determinants of Outcome of Severe Mental Disorders,*' '*Standardized Assessment of Depressive Disorders,*' and many more. This Department has been a leaderin many important areas of psychiatry and one of them was in community psychiatric research. This author has been privileged to be part of the community psychiatry research team at PGIMER that published many articles in this area. The author has also won many prestigious awards like the Marfatia award in 1981, the WHO fellowship in community Psychiatry in 1986, and the Dr. B.C. Roy National Award in psychosocial relief in 2006. In PGIMER, the author got interested in community psychiatry and decided to work in rural areas for the uplift of mental health services to rural masses. He is since then working for the rural community and dealing with farmers' suicides in Vidarbha in Wardha, Maharashtra.

R.K. Chadda

I am currently Professor of Psychiatry, at the All India Institute of Medical Sciences, New Delhi. I finished my MD in psychiatry from Post Graduate Institute of Medical Sciences and Research, Chandigarh (PGIMER) in June 1985 and later worked as senior resident till January 1987. I was in the Department from January

1983 to 1987. I have served as faculty in a number of prestigious institutions of the country, from 1988 to 1995 at the University College of Medical Sciences, Delhi, and from 1995 to 2004 at the Institute of Human Behaviour & Allied Sciences, Delhi. I have also served as a visiting faculty in March–April 1997 at the BP Koirala Institute of Health Sciences, Dharan, Nepal. I have also worked as a consultant psychiatrist in National Health Service of UK from April 2004 to July 2005 under International Fellowship Scheme.

I am currently the President of the Indian Association for Social Psychiatry. I have been a past President, Indian Psychiatric Society, North Zone. I am a Distinguished International Fellow of the American Psychiatric Association, a Fellow of the Royal College of Psychiatrists of UK and the National Academy of Medical Sciences (India).

I have about 160 publications to my credit, including 4 books. I have worked in areas of somatisation, caregiver burden in severe mental disorders, *Dhat* syndrome, help-seeking behaviour and psychiatric rehabilitation. I have been has been a recipient of 9 national awards in psychiatry including Indian Council of Medical Research's Tilak Venkoba Rao Award and the National Academy of Medical Sciences' Dr. Vimla Virmani Award.

I have very fond memories of the department of psychiatry at PGIMER, especially the 8 A.M. teaching programme, psychotherapy and psychodynamics classes by Professor Vijoy Varma, learning of presentation skills, annual picnics, the weekly movies at the Bhargava Auditorium, and visits to the faculty's homes on occasions of Holi. It was a really a wonderful phase of my life.

S.K. Chaturvedi : Training at PGI

I completed my MD in Psychiatry at PGI from June 1979 to 1981, and later worked as a Research Officer and Senior Resident for a few months, before taking up a faculty position at the National Institute of Mental Health & Neurosciences, Bangalore. It was during the post MD period that I worked as a Research Officer in the ICMR pain project, which became an area of work and interest till the present time.

The period of my training at PGI had some exciting developments. Professor Wig left PGI and joined AIIMS mid way of my post-graduation. It was also the short period during which we did not do any formal thesis or dissertation; rather, we were expected to do a small study to learn research methods. I did my research work on 'Parental attitudes towards mental retardation'—a home based study, going all over Chandigarh in the Institute and department autos and jeep. I also got to do an exciting study completed in just a week, on renal transplant recipients and donors, who had assembled in PGI for a sports meet. This formed the research work of Dr. VLN Pant (now known as Dr. Voruganti). Same way, I was involved in Dr. Deepak Kelkar's research work on Psychiatric emergencies in the Casualty and emergency department of PGI.

On leaving PGI, I continued my association with the ICMR Project on chronic pain and cancer pain till about 1985. In 1986, I got an opportunity to present the renal transplant work at a Psychonephrology conference in New York and got a chance to visit to Memorial Sloan Kettering Cancer Centre, New York to work with Dr. Jimmie Holland. I had already started working and writing on cancer pain, since 1985, when I was a founder member and first vice president of the Indian Society for Study of Pain.

The major thrust on my work and interest on psycho oncology grew from 1988 to 1990, when I was awarded the Commonwealth Medical Fellowship at Christie Hospital Manchester, UK, with Dr. Peter Maguire. I did small studies on use of antidepressants in cancer patients and Somatization in cancer. I trained in Communication skills training. This also started a series of studies on quality of life, starting with QOL studies in cancer. The next decade saw close work with cancer centers and Institutes, on many areas including detection of psychiatric morbidity, quality of life (QOL) and subjective well being, head & neck cancers, awareness of diagnosis and on palliative care. Workshops on communication skills were held at regular intervals, as were other workshops on psycho oncology, grief, counseling and staff stress, with the help of international authority like Dr. Peter Maguire. Since 1996 there is an active collaboration and association with Palliative care centres and Hospice, Karunashraya, at Bangalore.

B.S. Chavan

I joined the Department of Psychiatry at the Postgraduate Institute of Medical Education and Research (PGIMER) in January, 1985 as junior resident, along with three other residents. Under the leadership of Prof. V.K. Varma as Head of the Department and Dr. P. Kulhara, Dr. Savita Malhotra, Dr. S.K. Varma, Dr. Dwarka Pershad and Dr. Ajit Avasthi, the learning in psychiatry started with a positive note. The atmosphere in the department was very strict, but stimulating for learning. In addition to psychiatry learning, there were many other things which attracted all of us. The department at that time enjoyed a prestigious position in the country. We saw our faculty enjoying excellent reputation and recognition in the field of psychiatry. This made us feel proud. Although the atmosphere in the department was quite strict and tough, the smile on the faces of our seniors made us feel relaxed and hopeful. They became our guides and taught us not only psychiatry but also the working style and personal preferences and mannerism of each faculty. Since they were the first one to cross the tight boundary created by some of the faculty, we started becoming closer to them. Gradually we were taught the culture in the department, which included how to behave in the coffee room, during the rounds, how to present a case and how to enter in the office room of each faculty. Prof. Varma was an excellent teacher and human being. We enjoyed his psychotherapy classes. In fact, he also enjoyed teaching us. I still remember long discussions on small points. On occasions we took advantage of his cooperative nature and drew his attention to irrelevant topics and made the excuse that we did not understand anything, and whatever was being taught has no basis. However, we never saw annoyance on his face. These are the qualities of a good teacher- be firm and strict where it is must, but don't get biased and preoccupied and allow the students to clarify their doubts. Prof. P.K. Kulhara was another loveable teacher. He was very friendly with the residents and it was easy to interact with him. I still remember all the residents walking with him to have a cup of coffee after the rounds in the small cafeteria. He was very helpful and gave a lot of breathing space to the residents. Dr. Kulhara was full of knowledge and his interest in research motivated us to initiate at least thinking about it at that time. Dr. Savita Malhotra, the present Head of the Department was projected as a very tough teacher by our seniors and it made us scared to face her. As time went on, we found her strict and target oriented and it was impossible to escape the assigned work. I personally think, some degree of strictness is required for the students in the beginning of their career. Dr. Ajit Avasthi had joined the department just few months before our final exams. He did try to contribute to our training, but there was passive resistance from us. By that time, we had started feeling that our training and learning has already occurred and we were not prepared to learn new things. But, Dr. Avasthi could do it despite resistance. Now, I realize that we were wrong in our thinking, as the learning is never complete and definitely not when we were still students. I feel the department which has more variety will be more visible and will be remembered for long and the Department of Psychiatry, PGIMER left permanent impression on our mind and heart which will never be erased. The rich culture of the department, in addition to training, including the annual picnic, annual dinner, the celebration of festivals and other functions in the ward with patients and their relatives, were all great occasions to bind us to the department. Many of these events have been used by many of us to lay the foundation of new department and I personally found it easier to develop a cohesive department. The legacy of the department has spread to many parts of the country and even to many parts of the world.

I joined AIIMS as faculty in May, 1988 and continued working there till March 1996. We were seven faculty members who joined together at various positions in the National De-addiction Centre. Since the centre was a new service to be set up, there was not much work in the beginning and thus we had time to know each other and to get settled at the new place. Gradually, we started planning to add new services to the existing facilities, but faced lot of resistance from the residents and the Head of the Department, Prof. D. Mohan (who is no more now). Most of us were expected to work for the agenda driven by the head, with very little scope of innovation and variety. Such a culture led many of the faculty to start searching for alternatives and most of us did it at appropriate times. I feel that the head has very important role to make a department, but also to damage it. The damage is faster and I saw it happening. However, my stay of 8 years at AIIMS from 1988 to 1996 was still productive and shaped my further growth and direction. I, along with my other colleagues, learnt to set—up the new service. In addition to clinical services, we were involved into networking with government and NGO, development of health education material, and training. Lack of patients in the centres compelled us to look for them in the community and that was the beginning of my interest in community psychiatry. Later, I got an opportunity for WHO Fellowship in Community Psychiatry in Australia. This was the beginning of my journey of community mental health, which is still continuing.

After joining the department of psychiatry at Government Medical College in 1996 as professor and head, as I was in the process of setting—up the clinical facilities in the department along with Dr. Priti Arun, I got an opportunity to take care of a government institute for mentally challenged children (the GIMRC), which was with education department earlier, but the education department had declined to run it due to lack of expertise. This opportunity allowed me to convert my ideas of rehabilitation into reality. I started new vocational courses for these children and initiated newer and innovative models of rehabilitation. The best of these is the 'UMEED' model in the field of job placement and it was declared as the best in the country in 2003 in the category of placement of mentally challenged children and I was given a presidential award for this work, by then President of India, Dr. A.P.J. Abdul Kalam. Since then, 'Umeed' has grown much bigger and has successfully employed 60 mentally challenged children at various outlets at important tourist places in Chandigarh. The 'Umeed' model of rehabilitation is self sustaining, replicable and rights based. In addition to earning a livelihood, there is inherent mechanism of social and personal growth. The skills learnt by these children before placement were just enough to seek employment, but the social and management skills required for the business are taught while working (on the job training). The expansion and addition of new services at GIMRC attracted many new families of children with special needs (CWSN) and gradually the space became inadequate. I was able to convince the Chandigarh Administration to allocate bigger space. Gen (Retd.) JFR Rodriques, who was then the Administrator of Chandigarh and his wife Jean Rodriques had special sensitivity towards disability, and I was able to capitalise on this. The Chandigarh Administrator allotted 10 acres of land for setting-up Regional institute for mentally challenged Children (RIMH), which is being developed into state of art facility. RIMH is providing medical care, special education, vocational training, training courses in disability (approved by the Rehabilitation Council of India), school readiness programme, disability assessment and certification and community outreach activities for CWSN. RIMH caters to four disabilities- mental retardation, cerebral palsy, autism and multiple disabilities and currently it has approximately 400 children on its roll, this is in addition to daily intervention through intervention at OPD level.

My experience of setting up RIMH has been quite rewarding. I could contribute to field of disability and rehabilitation. This was my voluntary decision to take over the functioning of the GIMRC (now called the RIMH), but decision of mine has been instrumental in shaping my future work. Although, there were many challenges to begin, but I was successful in overcoming them. The biggest inspiration to continue my journey was the little children, whose innocent smiles made me happy and satisfied. Their parents who followed me blindly continued to provide more energy as small improvement in the child made them happy, and this happiness was shared with me.

The success of setting-up rehabilitation services for mentally challenged also encouraged me to start new services for mentally ill also. Some of these services include half way home, promotion of self help group of caregivers, promoting non government organizations (NGO's) in the field of mental health, and day care services for persons with chronic mental disorders.

K. Deka

It is indeed a great pleasure for me to be a part of the golden jubilee celebration of my Alma mater. I have been associated with PGI (Post Graduate Institute of Medical Education and Research) since 1991 when I joined into postgraduate course in psychiatry. Further I have done senior residency for almost a year. At present I am working at Assam medical college, Dibrugarh as Professor of Psychiatry. Moments and memories of PGI are still fresh and alive. Flashbacks of seminar room, case conferences, discussions, experiences at the Child Guidance Clinic, the Psychosexual Clinic, of psychotherapy sessions, the Drug De-addiction and Treatment Centre and others still give me goosebumps. I have experienced the fragrance of excellent faculty and exuberant researchers, which the department is filled with. I am fortunate to have trained under such dedicated and wonderful teachers. To be named in the author's list of the commemorative book to be published on the occasion of golden jubilee celebration will genuinely remain as an achievement.

S.C. Girimaji: A Personal Note on my Experiences at PGI

When I went to report to dept after selection in 1980, it was vacation time and Dr. Srinivasa Murthy was the in-charge head. To our amazement and pleasure we discovered that he and my mother came from same place—Kollegal—a small town in Karnataka. This started a long association that continued in NIMHANS and I drew upon his dynamism and commitment.

The holistic, bio-psychosocial approach taught and practiced at the Department provided me a solid foundation and has had an enduring effect on my professional development. The rich academic zeitgeist and encouragement for independence of thinking were great influences on shaping my career. Chance to interact with colleagues from other Departments especially in the psychosomatic case conferences and referral postings were great learning experiences in how to effectively communicate and work along with our medical colleagues.

The nuances of child psychiatry that I learnt from Dr. Savita Malhotra helped me a lot when I moved to child psychiatry unit at NIMHANS. The scholarly and insightful lectures on psychotherapy and supervisory session by Dr. V.K. Varma kindled my interest in psychotherapy, which continues even today. The bonhomie that existed between my peers, senior residents and staff and trainees from sister disciplines made life quite enjoyable and full of vivid memories.

R.C. Jiloha

The author of the chapter, The Mental Health Act of India, has been a student of PGIMER Chandigarh. He entered the department of Psychiatry at PGIMER Chandigarh as a post-graduate student on 1st January 1979. After completing his MD he worked in the department as a senior resident and research officer on a WHO research project on 'Outcome of Acute Psychosis'. He left PGI on 18th March 1983. His training in psychiatry and exposure to research methodology and clinical and academic areas shaped his future career to be a successful clinician, teacher and researcher.

Immediately after leaving PGI, he joined the faculty at Maulana Azad Medical College & GB Pant Hospital, New Delhi, a premier medical institution known for its best clinical care and highest academic standards. He rose to be professor of Psychiatry in 1991 and head of the department in the year 2001. Currently he is heading the department in the capacity of Director Professor. During this period he has published around 140 research papers, received several academic awards, produced around 50 post-graduates in psychiatry and has conducted several national and international research projects.

Dr. Jiloha is closely associated with the working of Mental Health Act 1987. As a member of Board of Visitors to Institute of Human Behaviour and Allied Sciences he has closely seen the implementation of the Act and the difficulties faced thereof. As a member of the Mental Health Authority of Delhi state, he has been closely linked to licensing of psychiatric nursing homes of Delhi under the Mental Health Act. These experiences have taught about the limitations and the good points of the Act. As a member of the Draft Committee of the Mental Health Care Bill, he has contributed his inputs and has closely seen its drafting.

P. Kulhara

My association with the Department began in 1969 with my interactions with Prof. Wig, my teacher and mentor and departed from the Department end October 2011. It is not easy to condense all these years, full of sweet memories, in few lines. The time spent with teachers (Profs. Wig and Varma), which honed my skills and built my capacity, will always remain the most fond and cherished memories of life. The mentorship of Prof. Wig and the involved discussions with Prof. Varma still remain with me; the Coffee Room, and its tidbits, is still etched on my mind. Rejoining the Department after 12 years sojourn in the UK and then continuing till superannuation has its exciting, dull, frustrating and happy moments, so full that these defy penning down in few lines. The love, affection, respect and admiration that I got from colleagues and students has made my life so rich that without any hesitations I would opt for the same time and life again!

R. Nehra: My Experience

The importance of clinical psychology in psychiatric practice cannot be overemphasised. The role of clinical psychologist remains a crucial one in competent clinical practice, through the use of structured psychological assessments and psychodiagnostics. A lot of subtle and latently manifest findings may be gleaned from a patient or client, by a trained clinical psychologist. Thus, a clinical psychology is an extremely important field which complements and supplements the care of patients with psychiatric disorders who seek help.

I joined the Division of Clinical Psychology of the Department of Psychiatry in PGIMER, Chandigarh, in 1983. It had come under my observation that difficulties were experienced in utilising psychological instruments in the Indian scenario. Firstly, few instruments were available which were validated for the Indian setting, as many of the scales originating from the West were not culturally relevant. Secondly, the average patient in the department was not always psychologically sophisticated. Hence, I developed a keen interest in developing and adapting scales and instruments, which could be utilised in the clinical practice in India.

Over the years, many tests were developed by me and my colleagues at PGIMER. Few of these tests include Social Support Questionnaire, Sexual Knowledge and Attitudes Questionnaire, Scale for Knowledge and Attitudes towards Condom Use, Coping Checklist, EAT 26, Body Shape Questionnaire, and the PRIME MD Patient Health Questionnaire (PHQ). These scales were validated in our clinical and community populations. Many of these tests have been utilised in research originating around the country.

My role as a clinical psychologist at PGIMER, Chandigarh has been a satisfying and stimulating one. However, the journey of extending help to the patients is still unfinished. There is a need for greater endeavour for developing psychological instruments with wide applicability and ease of administration that gains widespread utilisation. The present clinical practice can also be enriched by further utilisation of the psychological and psychometric tests that have been developed till now.

S.K. Padhy

The department has a dynamic learning environment for professional and personal growth, brings information, makes the individual realise what is adaptive stress with real "guru-chella" relationship.

B. Pradhan

The Postgraduate Institute of Medical Education and Research (PGIMER) is one of the pioneering educational institutions of Asia for postgraduate medical education and research. To this present author (M.D. in Psychiatry from PGIMER in 2004) who had the good fortune of working with and being mentored by some of the prominent leaders in Indian psychiatry, PGIMER has been a temple of learning. The Department of Psychiatry at the PGIMER was one of the first major academic departments of psychiatry in a general hospital psychiatry unit (GHPU) setting. This Department has been a leader not only in many crucial aspects of psychiatry including community psychiatry, schizophrenia, mood disorders and psychometric research, but also in some of the major and pioneering research in child psychiatry. This author has been privileged to be part of the child psychiatry research team at PGIMER that published the first Indian study on incidence of childhood psychiatric disorders.

V.K. Sharma: Memories of PGIMER

PGIMER gave a complete package of professional and personal learning for me. Who can forget the trail of outstanding fragrance at 7.45 A.M. in the corridors; coffee breaks at 11 A.M. with everyone; book clubs on Sunday mornings and long rides to Raipur Rani in an imported (Renault) car?

In my time the department was full of psychiatry giants, with Prof. Wig as the departmental father figure, Prof. V.K. Varma, Dr. R.S. Murthy, Dr. Raja Ghosh and Dr. Savita Malhotra (then Gupta) supported by Dr. Verma and Dwarka Prasadji and with Prof. Morris Carstairs as a special appearance.

English being a third language at school, I struggled with my English at PGI. One morning, when I presented a case to Dr. Varma, he quietly commented "*Istarah to kam chalega nahiji; tum ko English keliye kuch karna padega*" ("This won't work. You have to something to improve your English."). I thought that was the end of PGI for me! Any way Dr. Varma went to USA soon after for a period of three months that gave me a huge relief. On his return, I was very nervous to present cases to him, but had no choice. One day after my presentation he commented—(I was shivering inside)—"*Aap ko kya ho gayaji- English itnee improve kaise kar lee?*" ("How did you improve your English so quickly?"), and you know what, I later emigrated to England!

S.K. Verma

It is not possible to live for 50 years in a place without falling in love with it—with all that are associated with it. It still seems to say:

"Grow old with me,
The best is yet to be".

I had spent less than 50 years with my late wife and know what it means to me, even now—Although I also know that—change is the law of nature.

"The old order changeth, yielding place to New. Lest one good order should corrupt the world." People come and go. The staff and students come and go, leaving old memories and unfinished works to be completed by another generation. This is how progress is made and civilization, culture and their products grow. Change is always for better—and growth takes time. Speed of growth varies with time, place and persons. It can never remain static. While taking credit for the growth, one also has to accept the responsibility for the slowness and other related drawbacks. Everything cannot be achieved at once, but one has to oil the machinery and keep it ready to achieve more in future by better persons, with greater resources at their command. We can only hope and pray for the same.

It was indeed a privilege to have joined the Department of Psychiatry under the able guidance and leaderships of Professor N.N. Wig, so soon after getting the degree of Clinical Psychology and during the early stages of the Department itself. Both the things provided the necessary scope of developing professionally and personally. I was lucky enough to get this opportunity which proved to be a cornerstone in my professional life. I also did my Ph.D. work under his guidance in the department.

I have always believed that—
Work is worship, therefore—
The place of work is a place of worship,
Where I can enter only as a devotee—
In order to grow professionally and personally.

This faith got further strengthened with time in this ideal and beautiful environment. Even after 14 years of my retirement in 1998 from my active professional life in this beautiful place, it only reminds of what the poet Keats wrote many years ago:

"A thing of beauty is joy forever.
Its loveliness increases,
It will never pass into nothingness…"

I worked in this department for well over 30 years before my retirement, but I still love to visit this great Department—as and when I can and love to see the staff and students working there. But I hate to even think of my presence there distracting their attention—even for a moment from their work. This rather ambivalent attitude (of love—hate relationship) still prevails—and prevents me from visiting the Department as frequently as I would have wished.

We all live in this world of sweet dreams, trying our best to convert those dreams into reality. But the cruel fact remains that all dreams however sweet they might be for us, are product of our own imagination and can never be fully realized in one lifetime, which by nature is a very short period. Besides, what a sweet dream may be for one person may not be the same for another person—who lives now, replacing us in time and place. Perception of "burning issues" of things change with person, place and time. Also, the new generation of workers are entitled to have their own sweet dreams, which they want to realize in their own lifetime. Dreams differ, priorities differ, especially when there is limited time and resources to fulfill all our aspirations—past and present. I remember reading somewhere that "You must be mad working here, but if you are, it helps."

There is quite some truth in this blunt statement of facts—however unpleasant it might be for some of us, who love our dreams and are always making some attempts to realize them. Personally I would still prefer to be called "mad" rather than be called "unfaithful" to my dreams. Others are entitled to have their own preferences and priorities.

Another thing this beautiful place of worship provides us is the opportunity to grow, by learning even while you are teaching. I have done both, working at this place in both capacities and seeing for myself how both the things (teaching and learning) go side by side—provided one keeps ones eyes, ears and mind open to receive it. In a sense, it is often difficult to keep them separate. Gaps in our limited knowledge are automatically filled up by what the Gestalt school describes as closure principle and what others also call as insight or, Aha experience. For some, it can come as a shocking experience when suddenly it breaks the barriers in time, place and meaningfully joins different parts into a whole experience—generating something new/original at times—from old and frequently seen experiences. This is an ongoing process and capable of being continued throughout our life, no matter where one might be at the moment. Time and opportunities never wait for anybody. We have to grab it by the neck whenever opportunity comes, or, live to regret it forever. We can be wiser if we grab it in time and live wisely thereafter. Newer learning help also, by creating newer opportunities and finding new uses for old learned experiences and tools. Surprisingly for some, as our knowledge goes on increasing, we also became more aware of our shortcomings—so far being ignored and/or denied. Our resolve to know more and to achieve more gets further strengthened this way. Instead of complaining that the glass is half-empty, we learn to see it as half–full, with need to fill is further to make it full. Our own students—by asking specific, pointed, critical and important questions—draw our attention to some areas ignored so far and thereby help us in looking for their answers. So, we all learn while we teach. We tend to look at old things with newer attention, thereby strengthening our need-achievement and need-knowledge. Working together in the Department, we develop a new sense of belonging—we belong to the Department and the Department also belongs to us. Social get-togethers within the Department, add to this sense of belonging and here one can see the social contribution of Mrs. Wig also, who almost always participated in all such functions along with Prof. Wig, interacting with staff, students and their families also. Increasing cohesiveness contributes indirectly to group morale. It reminds one to share each other's experiences, achievements and efforts. The effect can be seen in sharing in each other's researches also. In these functions, we tend to know more about each other's extra-curricular activities and welcoming new comers to the Department. Sharing each other's happiness, which include awards, marriages, parenthood, promotions etc all add to the feeling of oneness in the Department. Timely publications of decades of progress includes achievements of the Department, bringing it the notice of all participants and gives further directions, that all can take to grow individually and socially. Direction for newer objectives like extension of services like rural community work, school counselling, drug addiction, etc. also find its place. The Department also encourages us to participate more and more in National Conferences of Psychiatry in India and abroad. We are encouraged to participate, to learn what other researchers are doing everywhere and to show others what we ourselves are doing. Looking at the work and contributions of the whole Department, we often get a feeling of our own 'dwarfness'—yet it adds to our sense of pride that however small and tiny we might be, still we remain part of this great department. It gives us additional strength to contribute more and more to make it all the more strong and rich, while contributing to the mental health of the community and the nation. We can only hope and pray for more success in future years.

CPSIA information can be obtained at www.ICGtesting.com
Printed in the USA
LVOW01*0004040815

448621LV00010B/427/P

9 788132 216735